CW00523664

1 MONTH OF
FREE
READING

at

www.ForgottenBooks.com

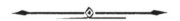

By purchasing this book you are eligible for one month membership to ForgottenBooks.com, giving you unlimited access to our entire collection of over 1,000,000 titles via our web site and mobile apps.

To claim your free month visit:

www.forgottenbooks.com/free793784

* Offer is valid for 45 days from date of purchase. Terms and conditions apply.

ISBN 978-0-483-11231-5
PIBN 10793784

This book is a reproduction of an important historical work. Forgotten Books uses
state-of-the-art technology to digitally reconstruct the work, preserving the original format
whilst repairing imperfections present in the aged copy. In rare cases, an imperfection in
the original, such as a blemish or missing page, may be replicated in our edition. We do,
however, repair the vast majority of imperfections successfully; any imperfections that
remain are intentionally left to preserve the state of such historical works.

Forgotten Books is a registered trademark of FB &c Ltd.
Copyright © 2018 FB &c Ltd.
FB &c Ltd, Dalton House, 60 Windsor Avenue, London, SW19 2RR.
Company number 08720141. Registered in England and Wales.

For support please visit www.forgottenbooks.com

THE

ANNALS OF HYGIENE.

THE OFFICIAL ORGAN OF

THE STATE BOARD OF HEALTH

OF PENNSYLVANIA.

EDITED BY

JOSEPH F. EDWARDS, A. M., M. D.

A. L. HUMMEL, M. D., Managing Editor.

VOLUME V.

JANUARY TO DECEMBER, 1890.

PHILADELPHIA, PA.:
THE HYGIENIC PUBLISHING COMPANY,
224 South 16th Street.

CONTENTS VOL. V.

14780

THE
ANNALS
OF
HUGIENE

✳

VOLUME V.

Philadelphia, January 1, 1890

NUMBER I.

COMMUNICATIONS

PORK.*

BY D. H. BECKWITH, M. D.,
of Cleveland, Ohio,
President of the Ohio State Board of Health.

LADIES AND GENTLEMEN:

We are deeply grateful to the good people of your beautiful city for the opportunity which their kindly interest in the proceedings of our Association affords us of contributing, in an humble way, a moiety to the great movement of reform now in progress throughout the civilized world. Other reformations the world has seen and benefited by—but they have been characterized by the bonds of tribal union ; the impulses of honor ; the dread of infamy ; or the sanctions of religion, while the present world-wide movement knows no selfish end, but seeks simply to ameliorate the condition of the whole human race through self-forgetfulness in the family and social relations ; purity and honor in public life ; true worth in manhood and womanhood ; and noble, untiring, self-sacrificing effort in the whole sphere of public action.

Seven years ago the Ohio State Sanitary Association was organized in Columbus, and began its labors in this new field. To-day it points with pardonable pride to a State Board of Health, and nearly two hundred local boards in various parts of the great State of Ohio. It has enlisted the active support of the very best element in society. It has drawn a devoted following from pulpit and bar, from counting-room and workshop, from the busy marts of trade and the quiet walks of private life. With no sectarian leanings—no hope or promise of personal gain, or partisan reward, it has but one aim—that of preserving health and prolonging life. Its deliberations have been published and scattered broadcast throughout the land. The seed thus sown has been nurtured into activity, and everywhere are seen the evidences of a bountiful harvest rich in blessings for neglected humanity. We may not see the full fruition in our time, but we may continue the part of the trustful husbandman, in the spirit of the great painter Reubens, who, when asked why he devoted so much time to a single picture, replied, " I paint for posterity." We do not know that harvest will follow the seed-time, but the trust which God has planted within us is so strong

*The Presidential Address before the Ohio State Sanitary Association, November 21, 1889.

that it answers the purpose of foreknowledge, and gives us a basis for the plans necessary to the full consummation of our work. But I must not forget that the main purpose of my address is to present a paper. The subject is a very commonplace one. It relates to the use of that small-sized pachyderm, zoologically known as *sus scrofa*, as an article of food. This four-footed, omniverous, cartilagenous-trunked, and sub-cutaneous-fat-secreting animal, is vulgarly called

THE HOG.

The hog differs widely in its general appearance—ranging from the attenuated razor-backed, forest-roaming denizen of the South, with features sharp enough to drink buttermilk from a jug ; to the plump, rosy-skinned, sumptuously faring domestic pet of the North, with a double chin and laughing face of the contented epicure. The hog discovered America shortly after Columbus—in fact he accompanied the latter on his second voyage in 1493, and landed in Hayti. He made his way subsequently into Florida with De Soto, about the year 1538. These hogs, however, differed widely from the hog of to-day. They were coarse, large boned, and deficient in fattening qualities. The first importation of a finer stock was made by General Washington,—rather General Washington was the recipient of a present from the Duke of Bedford of a trio of improved breed to which Washington gave the name of Bedfords, as a grateful acknowledgment of the Duke's kindness.

The finer breeds for which the United States is to-day noted include the Chester Whites, the Poland Chinas, the White Suffolks, the Isles of Jerseys, the Red Cheshires, the Victorias, and the Berkshires. All of these owe their finer qualities to a common parent stock of China and Neapolitan strains. ·

The hog being an omniverous animal, owes its highest development to a very generous diet. During its early and rapid growth, its food should contain a large percentage of the phosphates and nitrogenous compounds, or bone and muscle producing elements, and a small percentage of the carbonates, or fat-producing compound. Indian corn is rich in the latter, and is used almost exclusively in preparing the hog for the market.

Clean, wholesome diet brings pork to its highest perfection, when used as an article of food ; but the most careful diet, and thorough breeding, has .failed to eliminate certain disorders which are a constant menace to good health to consumers of pork ; of these disorders we will mention two—scrofula and trichinosis.

From remotest antiquity the unclean habits of the hog have challenged man's aversion and disgust. The Egyptians, the Ethiopians, the Libians, the Comani, the Scythians, the Galatians, the Zabbi, the Hindoos, and the Phœnicians abominated and detested the dirty, mire-loving swine. "Mohammed denounced its use as food, and the Bedouins consider it the only object whose touch is pollution. The Egyptian priests inveighed against it, declaring that it engenders" many superfluous humors. The Talmud, or general code of Jewish laws, states that " ten measures of pestilential sickness were spread over the earth and nine of them fell to the share of pigs." Plutarch and Tacitus speak of the detestation in which the hog was held by the people of their time on account of the " leprous emanation appearing upon his belly." Herodotus, and a host of more recent chroniclers, unite in ascribing various disorders to the use of pork as food. What the hog was 2000 years ago he is to-day. No animal has such filthy habits. No place exists so foul and loathsome that will exclude him. Animal carcasses, undergoing decomposition and filling the air with pestilential odors, are sought after by him with epicurean gusto. He will leave a repast of nuts in the southern woods to dispute with the buzzard the possession of the putrid remains of a defunct mule. He is the scavenger of the shambles. He is voted the freedom of our village streets, to act as a sanitarian in removing the filth and garbage therefrom.

These filthy habits are natural, not acquired, and no amount of careful breeding will ever modify them. Is it then surprising that among all nations and in all ages the flesh of the hog has been supposed to "engender many superfluous disorders?" The derivation of the terms "scrofula" and "choiras," applied to a disease alarmingly frequent, the former from the Latin scrofa, meaning a "breeding sow," the latter from the Greek "Xoipos," meaning "a hog," indicate that the ancients had good reasons for excluding the flesh of the hog from their dietary regimen.

Examination of the lungs, liver and spleen of hogs killed in slaughter-houses as well as of those raised and fattened by farmers for their own consumption, have often revealed the presence of tubercles, although no outward symptoms of disease were apparent. These tubercles may be easily communicated to man through the alimentary canal, appearing as the modern "bacillus tuberculosis," and producing consumption and scrofulosis. In all cases their presence invites disease, and nearly ten per cent. of the mortality of Ohio is directly traceable to scrofulous disorders. During the war of the Rebellion the records of five years and two months show 5,286 deaths from consumption, while 20,403 soldiers were discharged suffering with tuberculosis, and many others who died from other diseases were found on post-mortem examination to have tubercles. The death rate from scrofulous diseases in the armies of the world is appalling. It is true that their soldiers are exposed to sudden climatic changes, long and exhaustive marches, broken rest and irregular dietary habits, but when recruited they are the finest specimens of manhood that their countries afford, well adapted to the vicissitudes of war; yet statisticians tell us that twenty-seven per cent. 'of the death-rate among the Prussians, twenty-five per cent. among the Austrians, twenty-four per cent. among the French, thirty per cent. among the Hanovarians and Belgians, and twenty-three per cent. among the enlightened Britons, are directly charged to scrofulous affections. One of the chief articles of food for soldiers in the field is *pork*, in one shape or another, *contract pork*, hastily inspected, half cured, and imperfectly cooked, if cooked at all; and to its use as food rather than to the hardships of a campaign may be attributed this frightful mortality. Virchow, the celebrated scientist, holds to the doctrine that scrofulous constitutions imply liability to consumption, and that whenever tubercles are found in man, or any other animal, it is indicative of a scrofulous diathesis. The dietary laws of the Levitical code, given by Moses to the Hebrew people, are invested with so much religious solemnity and binding moral power that we are almost persuaded that they were more intimately allied to Hebrew theology than to Hebrew sanitation. But it must be remembered that the practical ends of life in that day were gained largely through spiritual means; and accepting the testamentary evidence of cotemporaneous writers, we must be convinced that Moses sought quite as much the temporal as the spiritual welfare of his followers in the prohibitory enactment respecting the use of pork as food. For if we go back to the early sources of Hebrew knowledge, we learn that man abstained from all animal food, and subsisted upon vegetable food alone. Wherefore we reason that if by degeneration man had made animal food a necessity, then the prohibitory clauses of the code against the use of certain kinds of animal food were given as a means of promoting the physical welfare of the people.

The teachings of the Parsees, the Hindoos, and the Pythagoreans were against all flesh as food—their practice in favor of certain kinds. The flesh of the hog has always been the exception from the remotest antiquity, and to-day the antipathy against its use is more marked than ever before—among scientific men and believers in the infallibility of modern means of research—on account of the discovery in the flesh of apparently healthy hogs, of a small thread-like parasite, to which has been given the name of

Trichina Spiralis.

The discovery of this little animal is comparatively new, although his ancestry is quite as old as that of the hog. To Sir James Paget, of London, belongs the honor of the discovery. Other anatomists, chemists and physiologists have failed to detect its presence, owing, perhaps, to its minute size. Taken, with the pork it infests, into the stomach of man, it produces symptoms of the most painful character, causing death in the most robust person in a few weeks. Previous to the discovery of Trichina the symptoms attending its depredations were ascribed to some new disease analogous to typhoid, etc.

Trichina may sometimes be detected by the naked eye, and appears as small round, or nearly round, specks. The best method for examination, however, is to place a small thin slice of the diseased pork under a microscope of from 50 to 100 diameters. If the pork be first saturated with a solution of liquid potassa one part and distilled water eight parts, which can be accomplished by ten or fifteen minutes' immersion ; the muscles will become clear, when the Trichina can be more readily observed. A few drops of sulphuric ether applied to the pork will also assist in bringing the parasites to view, if the sample under consideration be lean. In a full state of maturity the *trichina spiralis* measures about $\frac{1}{20}$ of an inch longitudinally, and $\frac{1}{100}$ of an inch transversely. The eggs measure only the $\frac{1}{1270}$th of an inch in their long diameter. Their power of multiplication is marvelous. Their mode of reproduction is viviparous, and many of the females contain from 200 to 500 ova. If any one of my audience should partake of an ordinary dinner of pork, well supplied with live trichina, he would, in a short time, become infested with half a million of these interesting creatures, a delightful thought for pork-eaters—especially those who have a penchant for underdone or raw hams. Prof. Dalton, the physiologist, says that 2,000,000 trichina have been estimated in the muscles of a man who died of the disorder. Dr. Voss, of New York, removed a small portion of a muscle from a living subject, and detected enough in it to warrant an estimation of over 7,000 to the cubic inch.

Dr. Wilson cites a case that proved fatal, wherein 104 trichina were counted in a piece of muscle measuring $\frac{1}{12}$ of an inch square, and $\frac{1}{12}$ of an inch thick, or 180,000 to the cubic inch. About 60 per cent. of the constituent element of the human body consists of muscles. In an individual weighing 150 pounds, there are, therefore, about $1\frac{4}{10}$ cubic feet, or $2,419\frac{2}{10}$ cubic inches, which multiplied by 180,000, as estimated by Dr. Wilson, will give 435,456,000 of these interesting creatures in his carcass.

"In a small country town in Prussia, near the Hartz Mountains, numbering from 5,000 to 6,000 inhabitants, 103 persons sat down to an apparently excellent dinner, most of them in the prime of life. Within a month more than 20 persons had died, and more than 80 persons more were then suffering from the fearful malady ; while those who were apparently unscathed were in hourly fear of an outbreak of the encapsulated flesh-worm. The dinner had been ordered at a hotel, and it had been arranged that the introduction of the third course, should consist of ' Rostewürst.' The sausage-meat was, therefore, ordered at the butcher's the necessary number of days before, and in order to allow of its being thoroughly smoked, the butcher, on his part, went to a neighboring proprietor of pigs, and bought one of the two pigs from the steward of the pig farm. The steward, unfortunately, sold a pig which his master intended should not be sold, because it was not considered to be in good condition. Nevertheless, for this time at least, the butcher got the ' wrong sow by the ear.' The ill-conditioned pig was the one that was killed and worked up into sausages. These were duly smoked and delivered at the hotel, and after being toasted before the fire they were served to the guests at the dinner-table. One day, after the dinner, the persons who partook of the sausages were prostrated and an epidemic of typhoid fever was anticipated by the physicians, or some poison must be at the bottom of the outbreak ; but when the muscles of the calves of the legs became affected in some of the sufferers, trichina were immediately anticipated ; on removing a small piece of the muscle it was found to be swarming with the little parasites. The catastrophe awakened sympathy and fear throughout the whole of Germany. Leading physicians were consulted and many visited the sufferers—none could give relief or cure. Case after case died, a slow and lingering death."

A few years ago the Chicago Academy of Sciences appointed a committee to examine hogs in the different packing houses in the city, to ascertain if trichina pork was in the market. Portions of muscles were examined from 1,394 hogs, and trichina were found in the muscles of twenty-eight hogs, from which the examiners concluded that one hog in fifty in the Chicago market had trichina to a greater or less degree. For the past eight years in Cleveland about twenty-five cases have been reported to the Health Office, which have been verified by finding *trichina spiralis* in the meat from which the persons afflicted had eaten portions.

Some of the cases were dangerously sick, and their sickness long continued, from five, eight, to ten weeks ; none died. Undoubtedly the above number were a very small portion of cases that have actually existed in Cleveland, as only a few physicians would report the cases to the Board of Health. The American people are well aware that by *thoroughly cooking pork* the trichina will come to an untimely end, and hasty meals and careless cooks should therefore be avoided when pork is used as food. A temperature of 170° Fh. will destroy trichina. In cooking hams to be sliced as cold meat there is great danger that the interior will not reach a temperature of over 130° Fh., and the encapsulated trichina will not be destroyed until a much higher temperature is reached. Smoking and salting meats have no perceptible effect, and trichina are found in meat that has undergone long and thorough curing in this manner.

This fact should be strongly impressed upon the public as one of vital importance, as pork enters so largely into the diet of the American people, especially among the laboring classes. Too much care cannot be taken on this point--*thorough cooking* of pork whenever it is prepared for table use.

It is a question if the civilized world would not be healthier and life extended, provided the old Levitical Law was still in force, and the eating of pork strictly forbidden, for the Jews as a people are to-day less subject to scrofulous diseases than the pork-eating community.

To my mind the Divine decree given to them by Moses, to abstain from the use of pork, was to improve the race to which he belonged: to prolong their lives and prevent diseases which he believed the eating of pork would engender.

I desire, in closing, to compare the sanitation of a few centuries ago with that of the present time. About six hundred years ago the Old World was visited by the most dire scourge that ever devastated fair mother earth. For a quarter of a century people stood silent with fear or raved with terror; families deserted their hearthstones, parents forsook their children, and children their parents, merchants fled the cities, leaving behind their goods and gold; prayers and incantations were mingled with curses; bishops and priests barred the doors of their churches and the gates of their monasteries; cemeteries were filled with the dead; pits were dug, and thousands were thrown into them, unshrouded and unmourned. The unburied dead clogged the streets and by-ways, and, festering under the scorching rays of the sun, gave wings to the terrible scourge. Over 13,000,000 died of the plague in China alone, Syria and Tartary were literally covered with the dead. In Carminia and Cesarea no one remained to bury the dead. India was nearly depopulated; Italy lost over one-half her population; Germany 200,000; England counted one dead for every one living. To die was far preferable to wander among the dead and dying. No tongue can tell, no pen describe, the misery of that period. Physicians and philosophers prostrated themselves before the god of superstition, and forgot their calling. The Royal College of Surgeons at Paris,—the boasted city of learning at that time,—ranked as the first in the world, and to its learned professors the whole of suffering humanity looked for aid in checking the devastation of the plague. The French Government called a medical council together, consisting of the professors of the Royal College and other noted medical men of Paris. This council was instructed to ascertain what means there were, if any, to arrest the progress of the scourge. After many learned dissertations and prudential discussions, the council issued a bulletin, which, I believe, has no equal, and I am informed is still preserved in the government archives of Paris. It reads as follows :

Causes. "Constellations which combatted the rays of the sun, had struggled with the waters of the great sea and originated vapors, that the sun and fire had attracted a great portion of the sea to themselves and the waters were corrupted and the fish died and the vapor overspread the earth like a fog, and the like would continue so long as the sun remaineth in the sign *Leo*."

Prevention. "Constellations striving with the aid of Nature, by virtue of their divine might to protect and heal the human race, burning of vine-wood and green laurel, also that the fat man should not sit in the sun, nor rain water be used in cooking."

It seems almost incredible that science, as it embodied itself in the thought and investigation of so learned a body, should have overlooked so completely, if not the first cause of the plague, at least the reason that it became so fatal all over Europe from natural causes.

Absurd as these conclusions of the French savants may appear to us, their ingeniousness and profundity challenge our highest admiration and serve as an example of the superiority of the good common-sense of to-day to the great learning of that time, dissociated from those qualities and powers which can make it useful in the solution of the vexed questions which arise in practical every-day life. We have outgrown the narrow, proscribed limits of that age. We have shaken off the shackles of blind, unreasoning routine, of devotion to professional arrogance and time-honored customs and launched forth into intelligent and rational experiment.

The investigations of to-day are conducted in such a thorough and scientific manner by Boards of Health, that epidemics do not jeopardize the safety of any community. To ascertain the cause of disease, the microscopist and the chemist bring their united forces into play.

Drinking water is analyzed, the sewerage, ventilation, etc., of our homes is examined, and thus they point out, not only to the intelligent, but to all classes of society, the natural causes that produce epidemics, and their envenomed sting is withdrawn before their fury is aroused.

The good work that has been done for public health by this organization for the past seven years is well known to you all, and the labor before us sanitarians is still great ; what there is to accomplish in Ohio is vast and important. Among the co-workers are the best thought and intellect; and whether we continue as a seperate organization, or allow the State Board to carry on the work, it matters not to us providing the seed that we have planted be properly cared for until the harvest has come. Members are here to-day who have never failed to attend our annual meetings. They come without any pecuniary reward, and the only compensation they will ever receive is, that their work has not been in vain ; that, by their advice and instruction, human lives have been prolonged, and society has received the benefit of their efforts in sanitary work.

> " For Heaven's gate may be closed to him that comes alone,—
> Save thou a life, and thou shalt save thine own."

I thank the members of the Ohio State Sanitary Association for selecting me as their presiding officer. My tenets are so at variance with most of theirs that I never anticipated the honor that their suffrage conferred upon me at our last session, and for their trust and confidence I again thank them many, many times.

The Disinfection of Books.

The Boston Health Board has ordered that the public library ticket, held by any person in whose family a case of contagious disease has occurred, be stamped so as to show the presence of such disease. All books returned with a card so stamped are to be disinfected, and no other books can be taken out on this card until an official notification is received that the danger of contagion no longer exists.

The Proper Food for Man.*

BY J. D. BUCK, M.D.,
of Cincinnati, Ohio.

Foods are those substances which when introduced into the body are capable of renewing and maintaining its structure and vitality. Aside from the direct renewal of tissue and vitality there are certain substances that have a more direct relation to the heat of the body. These are classed with foods though alone they are incapable of renewing the tissues. The normal temperature of the body bears always a direct ratio to its vitality, and these heat-producers, like the fats and oils, are more or less incorporated with albuminates in the production of tissues. There is again another class of substances—the product of fermentation and distillation—classed as stimulants, heat-producers and yet not, strictly speaking, nutritious. Just as the fats are capable of being rapidly oxydized and so to increase the heat of the body, so malt and alcoholic liquors act as a stimulant to the vitality of the organism so that a larger amount of energy may be expended within a given time, but to be followed by proportionate after exhaustion. To the substances already named must also be added water and air as promoting both nutrition and vitality.

Medicines and foods may be contrasted in this wise. Medicines are directly related to the forces of life and indirectly to the tissues; while foods are directly related to tissues and indirectly to vitality.

The present is, however, not the place or time for an elementary treatise on foods, stimulants or medicines. These subjects have been carefully investigated and the results are easy of access. The point to which I desire to draw attention is the two great classes of foods derived in the one case from the vegetable kingdom, and in the other from the animal world, or vegetable and animal foods. Of these two classes the vegetable foods are inclusive and animal foods exclusive. So far as the chemistry of nutrition is concerned every element really necessary for the maintenance of animal or human life is to be derived from the fruits and vegetables, while strictly animal substances, both in theory and in fact, can furnish but a part of the necessary and healthy nutriment of man. In other words, animal substances furnish nothing necessary for man that cannot be found in fruits and vegetables.

It is not my purpose to recite statistics or the result of experiment in support of this statement, though these are by no means wanting. There have been not only whole communities, but whole nations, who have entirely excluded animal foods from their bill of fare, and statistics show that such peoples have been remarkably free from both disease and crime. Aside from mere chemism and the equivalents of energy, there is a more subtle quality involved, and it is this quality that I regard as of prime importance. It is an old saying that "man grows like what he feeds on," and if we take into account the quality as well as the quantity of energy to be derived from foods, the discussion narrows down to our aims and ideals." If our aim is to breed a warlike race, who shall cut throats without compunction and be enthusiastic subjects of tyrannical aggression, we should feed them largely on beef and rum. We have here the concentration of energy of the grossest form; but the vitality of animals is inseparable from the disease of animals. A short, wild, brutal life is the inevitable result of such feeding. While it is true that meat-eaters and rum-drinkers have

* Read before The Ohio State Sanitary Association.

sometimes reached a ripe old age, it is not true that the quality of the life forces of these have exhibited the higher human attributes in any large degree. On the other hand, it is true that a great majority of those persons who have been noted for longevity have been exceedingly temperate and abstemious, if not exclusive vegetarians. It is well known that animals like the beef, the sheep, and the hog, are subject to many diseases that affect human beings. Catarrhal diseases of the intestinal tract and air-passages, diseases of the liver and kidneys, are very common in all these food-animals. Nor is the presence of these diseases to be detected from examination of the carcass after the diseased organs have been removed. Beyond these undetected taints of animal foods, there are others known to food-inspectors of so gross and palpable a nature as to be easily seen, and where hucksters are so often detected in exposing for sale meats palpably diseased, it may readily be inferred that no conscientious scruples will induce them to destroy foods that present no visible taint, even when known to be present.

With fruits and vegetables the case is very different. Freshness and soundness can easily be determined by anyone, and were such not the case the poisonous effects arising here are in no way comparable to those arising from the diseased animal carcass. We are indebted to the hog and the sheep for trichina and tape-worm, though these are doubtless among our lesser obligations. If the superiority of man over the animals is manifest in the shambles and the reeking *abattoir*, our dumb brothers manage to balance the account by transmitting to us all their diseases.

I hold that meat-eating is an acquired appetite—unnatural and unnecessary—not justified by any known law of physiology, and that it is the cause of many diseases. If mere brawn, strength of muscle and endurance are the only things desired, the horse and the ox certainly get these from grass and grain ; but if we are not satisfied in developing these but must develop the tiger and the goat, we can become both blood-thirsty and salacious at once by living largely on animal foods.

Every physician is aware that the average citizen is not remarkably abstemious or temperate ; he eats far more than either health or comfort require, and many diseases are directly traceable to over-feeding. It is just this tendency to over-feeding that meat-eating stimulates. The vegetarian seldom suffers from hunger, and yet eats with relish at the allotted time. There are probably more diseases due to over-feeding than to strong drink, and yet this form of intemperance is but slightly condemned.

The diet of the sick offers no exception to the foregoing suggestions. The idea that the sick or those debilitated by disease must be fed on animal broths, beef tea, and the like, is a relic of barbarism. Fats and phosphates are generally the elements needed in such cases, and animal substances are rendered necessary only on account of previous habits and long generations of acquired and unnatural appetites. The white of an egg in a glass of milk contains far more real nourishment than an equal quantity of beef tea.

I am perfectly well aware that in expressing these views I am in a minority of the medical profession. So long as the venders of liquid filth, with every characteristic of carrion, can amass fortunes by the aid and "indorsement" of the medical fraternity , the minority to which I belong will be designated as cranks and croakers. The facts of nature, however, always disregard majorities, and the lessons of human experience are the only real tests of theories.

The promotion of health and the prevention of disease is beginning to be regarded as superior to all attempts at the cure of disease, and Boards of Health are emphasizing this higher aim and larger beneficence.

The time is not far distant when the question I have herein raised will be recognized as most vital in the prevention of disease, in the promotion of long and happy lives, and in the elevation of the mental and moral status of mankind. Then majorities will change sides, and it will be seen that the commandment "*Thou Shalt not Kill*" is without regard to the degree or quality of life. There will be no longer a "blood offering" to human appetite, and the "ruddy hue of health" will be no longer derived from the shedding of blood, but from the pure air and the sunlight where the fruits of the orchard and the flowers of the field get their beauty and bloom.

Will General Sanitation Ever Become Popular?*

BY JOHN McCURDY, M. D.,
of Youngstown, Ohio.

What we mean is, will those laws that secure good health, long life, and a vigorous physical and mental condition be cheerfully learned and practiced?

In other words, will that branch of medicine known as preventive medicine, which can be learned and practiced by all laymen, be acquired and utilized?

It would seem natural to answer this in the affirmative when we call attention to the deadly epidemic known as the plague that visited Russia, Germany, Italy, England, and all nations in Europe, taking its hundreds of millions of victims in the aggregate; Hecker telling us that this disease alone swept from the earth 25,000,000 of people from the years 1347 to 1351. London alone having lost by it 100,000 a month, Venice the same, Paris 50,000, Avignon 60,000 in the same time, and it is believed that in England not one-tenth of her population escaped from this cause.

By the observance of the simplest sanitary injunctions this plague was barred from entering one nation after another, until the doors of all are now closed against it, and it has perished as a pestilence and a terror from the face of all civilized nations, and is not known to any of them even by name.

We can point to the visitations of cholera in France, Russia, Germany and England, and show that in the years 1831–32 the number of victims went up into the millions; but when this same disease visited these same countries, in 1873, so well was it understood, that its fangs were extracted just as civilization advanced.

In England it did not even attain the importance of an endemic.

We can turn to our own country and look at the condition of things in 1831–32, and note the incalculable ruin it wrought to life and industries; but pointing again to the same disease when it visited us in the years 1834–66, we see that its march was like that of a lion, paralyzed, with fangs extracted, all along the eastern part of our country, for the laws of preventive medicine were respected. The filthy South and West alone suffered severely.

---

* Read before the Ohio State Sanitary Association.

The typical filthy city of America is New Orleans.

Cholera visited it and the Mississippi River in the years 1832-34-48-66, gathering, as usual, a large number of victims, while the good sanitary condition of the East secured for her complete safety. Yellow fever has appeared in our country and the West Indies 180 times. It is safe to say that the South never escaped, and this disease continued to harvest its victims in it without opposition until the year 1863, when both General Butler and it started for New Orleans.

The General reached there first, bringing with him all the elements, both of yellow fever and cholera, in the large bodies of men with the indispensable host of camp-followers, who are entirely irresponsible in their habits of life ; and added to these the vast numbers found in the city, depressed in body and mind by poor and scanty food and fright : people who were too ignorant, too poor, and too helpless to get away from it, and added to this the vast number of animals indispensable in the movement of large bodies ; and to complete the above unfavorable conditions, the reeking filth and loathsome condition of this city with the germs of these diseases that had never left this old camping ground. What was there now wanting to generate a cyclone of death equal to that which ever visited any country ?

While that city was held in the grip of General Butler, he, in turn, yielded ready obedience to his sanitary engineers, sanitary inspectors and medical officers, aiding them with just such an intelligent, earnest and ample force as they needed to carry out in a prompt and effective manner all plans for the securing of cleanliness.

So marked was the immunity from disease that not only were the eyes of all people cast upon it, but to this day it has been spared from both epidemics. How largely this single factor entered into the solution of the greatest governmental question of all time can be realized by all who have witnessed an epidemic in a crowded city.

The problem of self-government is watched by all intelligent, liberty-loving people upon the globe, and their eyes are all upon us, as we are the only example of a powerful people governing themselves voluntarily.

Suppose yellow fever and cholera had attacked our armies as pestilential diseases did large bodies of men of old. Where would have been the republic we to-day enjoy ?

We can point to Memphis in 1879, with its yellow fever scourge.

There is not a city in our country we cannot point to for proof of the profit and vital importance of observing the laws of preventive medicine.

I shall cite a few extracts from the pen of that classical lay writer, Charles Dudley Warner, who in writing of our great West, as he saw it, says of the city of Memphis : " The student of social science will find in the history of Memphis a striking illustration of the relation of sanitary and business conditions to order and morality. In 1878 the yellow fever came as an epidemic, and so increased in '79 as to nearly depopulate the city ; its population was reduced from 40,000 to about 14,000, two-thirds negroes. Its commerce was absolutely cut off ; its manufactures were suspended ; it was bankrupt. The turning point in its career was the adoption of a system of drainage and sewerage which immediately transformed it into a fairly healthful city. The inhabitants were relieved from the apprehension of the return of a yellow fever epidemic.

"Population and business returned with this sense of security and it can now truthfully claim between 75,000 and 80,000." In practical sanitary reform, England first started, and is still in the lead, and she has no city which has profited more by it than her great manufacturing city, Manchester, with her more than half million people. Her sanitary records show that for all expenses of every kind, $435,000 were paid out in one year and for this, the actual saving of life was 2,301, about 1,000 of them between 20 and 70—or a gain of $1,000,000, at the rate of $1,000 per person; add to this the saving for funeral expenses, about $75,000, and a gain of $250,000, that would have been spent in the treatment of 103,000 citizens preserved from sickness, and another $250,000 for the wages they must have earned; and then, at a very moderate computation, we have a gain of more than $1,500,000, to be set against the expenditure of $435,000—not including the bodily suffering of the sick, and the mental distress of the friends.

Professor Pettenkofer, of Munich, Germany, has made careful estimates of the German cities with about the same showing. New York, in our country, is the great sewer into which is poured, more than any single city, the scum and slush of Europe and the West Indies, in addition to her own; and although, invaded by every form of pestilence, nearly every day in the year, her health department has demonstrated again and again its ability to starve or stamp it out, till now every family and individual feels that nothing can molest or make them afraid; although before her health department was organized, one case would put "a thousand, and two, ten thousand to flight."

It would seem, from what has been said, that the people would cheerfully respond and be eager to enforce sanitation, but exactly the opposite is true.

That city does not exist upon the globe to-day with a sense of cleanliness strong enough to keep herself clean voluntarily. The determination and deadly resistance between the health department and the great bulk of the people, corporations and many manufacturers is as deep and desperate as that displayed at the Battle of Gettysburg. People will not keep clean. The natural bent of human nature is to filth and poverty, and the virtue of personal and property cleanliness, like all others, is secured by hard and persistent effort; by driving up hill the vice, ignorance, laziness and poverty that stand in the way. The refined, the educated, the self-respecting and the enterprising only are the friends of cleanliness. The advocates of protective medicine show facts clear and strong as the sunlight in the protective powers of vaccination, but it avails not. In Paris, where vaccination is lax, there there are yearly 10 deaths to each 100,000 inhabitants; and in Zurich, where the mortality was 8 in 100,000, the vaccination ordinance was repealed, and at once the deaths rose to 85 per 100,000. Then, look across to Germany, where it is enforced by law, and in the face of all those elements so productive of contagious diseases—as large standing armies and immense numbers of poor—there is not $\frac{1}{2}$ of one to the 100,000; and in London, where the law is rigidly enforced, there is only $\frac{6}{10}$ of one to 100,000, and this, too, in the face of poverty, squalor, vice, ignorance and filth. Yet in all the latter countries the enemies of vaccination are so numerous, fierce and persistent, that they are organized and expend large sums of money trying to defy the law and have it obliterated. We point them to Germany, England and France and the United States, and show them the lives lost, and the fabulous sums of money filth costs in disease, and still every city and town presents an army of determined opposition to preventive measures. We hold the figures up before their eyes, and show them that on the beggarly basis of valuing a life at $750, we lose $500,000,000 a year; that we lose more than 250,000 citizens from strictly preventable diseases, and that with scarcely an exception, in every town, each inhabitant would be taxed at least $8 per head for its filth and sanitary neglect.

Yet in what community has not the election of officers been fought on the sanitary issue—and where is the place where people, not only of ignorance and narrowness, but even the so-called cultured, do not keep in open rebellion on all preventive measures?

We can point to our opponents, and show them that in a city like Boston the mortality from preventable diseases was 34 per cent. of the whole, and then by but moderate cleanliness it was reduced to 18 per cent., and kept at that as long as wished. Yet the people of Philadelphia not only insist on being dirty, and drinking water that has been shown to be directly destructive to human life, but they will break open the pumps and hydrants, and defiantly drink said water, and discharge the officials who dare oppose them; and this sort of mob is headed by a person no less than the so-called honorable Mayor .

We can point to Plymouth and Bellaire, towns in vast numbers, and trace for our opponents the course and cause of typhoid fever and diphtheria as clearly as a mountain brook is traced, and still their self-induced blindness will not recognize it, and they meet us with the destructive crusher that we are but "sanitary cranks,"— that sewer gas does not kill, for they and their forefathers breathed it, and it did not kill them; that the water is not foul; the analysis matters not to them, as they use the water and are in good health; that their cellars, yards, and compost heaps do not produce diphtheria or scarlet fever as they have not had either of them.

It matters not what is said, they meet us with the logic that the Irishman did the sanitary officer, who told Pat that the pig and its pen which were at his door must be removed. "And what for?" said Pat. "Because it is unhealthy," answered the officer. "Oh," says Pat, "that is not so, for that pig has been there for more than three months, and never cleaned, and he has not had a day's sickness."

It is with sanitation as all other vital reforms; it requires a complete change of heart, and a verifying of the scripture, "precept upon precept, line upon line— here a little, and there a little."

This may be our last session, but the fact remains, our work is imperative and vital, and life, self-respect, prosperity, and progress all urge us on. Open your eyes to the actual facts in our great State of Ohio, with her three millions of people, and see the mortality that attends her preventable epidemics, and yet what has she given the State Board of Health for our protection?

The beggarly sum of $5000, not enough for the oversight of a single county. Our work is not more nearly done as an organization in looking after the physical, social, hygienic, and vital wefare of our people than is the work of the teachers who look after the spiritual and educational welfare of the people. As long as the mind of man creates, and the heart of man harbors impure thoughts, as long as avarice, selfishness, greed and disregard for the feelings and welfare of others exists, as long as "man's inhumanity to man makes countless millions mourn" there will be an imperative need for organizations of this kind, for general sanitation will never become popular.

Garbage and Night-Soil Crematories ; from a Practical and Financial Standpoint.*

BY GEO. I. GARRISON, M.D.,

Member of the State Board of Health of West Virginia, and Health Officer of Wheeling, West Virginia.

The time has passed when it was necessary to prove by argument the necessity for prompt and thorough removal of all waste materials which are the result of aggregation of people into communities, to insure the greatest amount of health and comfort to the inhabitants thereof. The precise relations of cause and effect, as between filth and infectious or contagious diseases, are now known to the merest tyro in sanitary science. Until within a few years, it was thought sufficient for the disposal of city waste, to discharge it into the water-courses ; and that system has been practiced so long and universally, that our rivers are little less than vast sewers for conveying to the sea all offal of whatever character, from the cities and towns that line their shores. From these filth-burdened sources must a supply of water for domestic purposes be drawn. The pollution of streams is becoming a more serious question every year, and, while some governments of Europe have undertaken its solution, and many States in our own country have enacted more or less stringent laws for the protection of rivers and streams, there has been comparatively little accomplished in the way of relief. So great has been the nuisance in recent years that a great but natural and perfectly justifiable outcry has been raised. As a result of this outcry other means for the disposal of such substances have been sought. It has been attempted to get rid of sewage by irrigation and chemical processes. The effort has been made to dispose of night-soil in a manner other than by throwing it into streams, removing it in barrels or tanks to fields for manurial purposes, where it becomes almost if not quite as great a nuisance as when thrown into the water. It has also been treated chemically and in various ways to remove its offensive odor, that it might be transported to remote distances for like uses. But, when we consider that the average of such substances from each person in a community is about three pounds in twenty-four hours, or one thousand and ninety pounds in a year, in addition to the enormous quantities of garbage and other unwholesome materials accumulating in the same time, we must conclude that either of the above plans is impracticable, or, at least very unsatisfactory for large cities. Experiments have been made, and at several points furnaces have been constructed for the purpose of destroying such substances by heat. This short paper will not permit a description of the various kinds which have been devised in the past twenty years or more. While every one which has been invented, may be capable of burning city offal with varying success, that one which will destroy the maximum quantity at a minimum of time and cost, is the best. The furnace in use at Wheeling combines utility with economy in the highest degree ; hence, I shall confine myself to a description of it, and the system as practiced there. It may not be uninteresting to mention in this connection, the method formerly employed, and the chief cause which led to the adoption of the present system. Briefly, therefore, it was formerly the practice to dump all refuse into the river at the lower end of the city. This plan was particularly objectionable because the intake of the water-works for the city of Bellaire, Ohio, is situated less

---

*Read before the Ohio State Sanitary Association.

than a mile below that point. The people of that city became clamorous, for relief, and justly so. Soon after my election to the position of Health Officer of Wheeling, which was in the early spring of 1885, the danger from such wholesale pollution became so apparent, from the largely increased number of persons sick of typhoid fever and kindred diseases supposed to be the result of drinking impure water, that it was thought necessary to bring the whole matter to the attention of the Council of the city of Wheeling. That body at once determined upon a change of some sort, which should have for its object the relief of the Bellaire people. But, with the tedium which attends reforms of whatever character, their object was not accomplished until nearly two years later, when the furnace which has been in successful operation ever since, was completed.

It is constructed precisely like that of a regenerative, gas-heating furnace found in most of the rolling mills, except that the hearth is basin-shaped, made so to accommodate liquid substances. A low bridge wall is placed in the centre, trans-

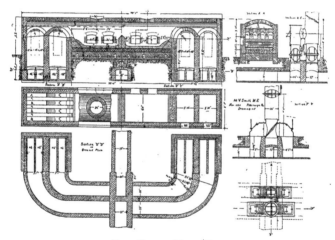

No. 1.—Present and Original Furnace.

versely, to allow greater facility for cremating different substances at the same time. The exterior length of the furnace is 44 feet and 6 inches. Its extreme width is 8 feet and 4 inches, while its height is 7 feet and 6 inches. The main stack, 50 feet high, and a duplicate stack of the same height as the furnace, and connected with the main stack by an elbow, are placed over two semi-circular underground flues, to be hereafter described. At either end are situated two hot-air chambers, which extend the full width of the furnace, 6 feet below the hearth, and occupy 12 linear feet of space; these hot-air chambers are filled with "checker work" and connected with the two flues already referred to, which extend from one end of the furnace to the other in a semi-circle. They are connected at the point farthest from the furnace, with the two stacks by means of "butterfly" valves, which serve also to change the course of the draft. There is another flue which passes under the furnace and at a right angle to it, called the air-flue, and intersects the inner one of the two flues just described at the middle of its course. The fuel used is Natural Gas, and is supplied at both ends of the furnace, so that heat may be applied from either, at will. The furnace is charged through two large circular openings in the crown, large enough to admit the body of a horse; the covers of these openings are shifted by means of cranes under the control of the keeper of the furnace. Air is introduced from the under, while the fuel is introduced from the top portion of the furnace, and heat of such intensity is secured that it would melt the apparatus if left to itself for a few hours.

The substances destroyed are, night-soil, garbage, dead animals, butchers' offal, spoiled meats, decayed fruits, vegetables and fish. The bodies of horses are charged by means of a large crane, also under the control of the keeper. Two men are all that are required to operate the furnace day and night. The ordinance in relation to the crematory provides for the election of a keeper at a salary of $60 per month, and the appointment of an assistant at $1.50 per day, for such time as his services may be required. The same ordinance regulates the manner of collection and removal of substances to be cremated. Contents of cess-pools are not allowed to be removed nor transported by persons except those who may be licensed for that purpose; and they must first obtain from the health office a permit which shall state the name of the person doing the work, the name of his employer, the location of the premises where work is done, the probable amount to be removed and the time of removal. This permit must be conveyed by the licensed party to the keeper of the crematory, who shall fill and sign a blank form on the back, showing date of presentation, name of the person presenting and quantity and kind of substances presented. All permits must be returned to the health office at the end of each week by the keeper. All butchers, grocers, hucksters and green grocers, are required to remove all their offal and garbage to the crematory; all dogs killed by the police, and all dead animals found upon streets, alleys, public or private grounds, in the city, must be removed to the furnace for cremation. The keeper is obliged to record in a book provided for the purpose, the kinds and quantities of substances burned, the names of the persons presenting, and the date of presentation.

Careful examination and study of the operation of the system, based upon the test of more than two years' trial, demonstrates that the following substances can be disposed of in the space of one month, viz.: 1784 barrels of night-soil; 384 loads of garbage; 13 horses or other large animals, and 41 dogs; besides other materials which are occasionally brought to it for consumption. A barrel contains 40 gallons, and 6 represent a ton in weight. 384 loads of garbage represent about 180 tons; 13 horses probably represent 7 tons; dogs and other materials 5 tons more, a total of 489 tons at a cost of about 20 cents per ton. Before the present system was established in Wheeling, the cost of removing contents of cess-pools was $1 per barrel of 40 gallons of contents removed. Now the cost is 75 cents for like service. There should be removed annually, from a city the size of Wheeling (35,000 inhabitants), 12,000 barrels of night-soil. During the months of March, April, May, June, July and August, 1889, there were removed 8,611 barrels.

The following statement will represent the amount saved to the citizens of Wheeling by the new system, and the amount which can be saved to the people of any community in like circumstances. This, however, will represent the saving in cost of removing night-soil only as there is as yet no apparent saving, from a "dollars and cents" view, in the cost of removing garbage.

Let us suppose then, for the purpose of illustration, that 12,000 barrels are removed annually, for the period of ten years, and compare the cost of the new with that of the old system, leaving the question of interest out of the calculation. Then we have something like the following :

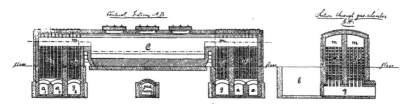

Under the old system, 120,000 bbls., at $1 per bbl., $120,000
   "   new   "   120,000   "   at 75 cts. " $90,000
For salaries, add 12,600   102,600
   The amount saved, not counting cost of furnace, $17,400

The furnace cost originally $2,260
Present building cost 600
Necessary repairs for 10 years 2,000 $4,880

   Which deducted still leaves a margin of . . $12,520

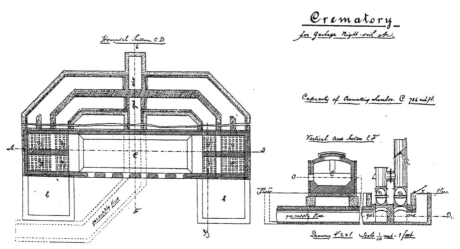

No. 2.—Proposed New Furnace.

Fuel, as an item of cost does not figure in this calculation, for the reason that natural gas does not cost anything for city purposes under the terms of the ordinance granting to natural gas company right of way through streets and alleys of the city. If such results can be accomplished with an experimental furnace, what will one brought to a high state of perfection accomplish? Since the construction of the first furnace at Wheeling, it has been much improved upon. The drawings presented and the following description illustrates fully the latest improved Garbage Crematory. The gas is brought from the coal gas producer by means of the gas supply flue and enters gas valve v^1, while at the same time the air enters by the air door x into air-valve v^2: it is then deflected to the right or left as desired by means of these valves. For purposes of illustration, we will assume that the gas and air are deflected to the right into the flues g and a, whence they are conducted into the regenerating chambers g^1 and a^1; these regenerating chambers are filled with fire brick, forming vertical flues through which the gas and air pass upwards into the combustion chamber M, where they meet and combustion takes place. The flame then passes through the cremating chamber C, which is filled with garbage, night soil or dead animals as the case may be; these materials being put into the cremating chamber through openings in the roof, which are shown on drawing. From the cremating chamber C, the waste heat passes through the regenerating chambers g^3 and a^3, downward into the flues g^2 and a^2, thence into the before-mentioned four way valves, v^1 and v^2, whence it passes up the stack.

(*Note.*—It must be understood that while the gas and air are deflected into the furnace on one side of the valves v^1 and v^2, the waste heat is passing through the other side of said valves into the stack, the valves thus doing double work.)

In passing through the regenerating chambers g^3 and a^3, 90 per cent. of the waste heat is retained by means of the vertical brick flues mentioned above, it being necessary to construct these flues of imported Silica bricks, that being the only material which will stand the intense heat. After operating the furnace as above, for about one hour, the valves, v^1 and v^2 are reversed, thus causing the gas and air to enter at the opposite end of the crematory, and the waste heat to pass out through the regenerating chambers, where gas and air formerly entered.

The regenerating chambers g^3 and a^3 now being at a very high temperature, heat the gas and air as they pass through on the way to combustion chamber m^1, thus producing almost perfect combustion. The gas and air are allowed to enter at this end of the furnace until these regenerating chambers become chilled, when the valves are again reversed, and the gas and air brought in through the regenerating chambers at the other end, which in the meantime have been heated by the waste heat, as previously described. The temperature of the cremating chamber c can be perfectly controlled by means of suitable valves, so that any desired degree of heat is obtainable up to from 3500 to 4000 degrees Fahrenheit, where disassociation of the gases takes place.

In conclusion, owing to the fact that the present furnace has not sufficient capacity to destroy all the refuse of the city, a resolution authorizing the construction of a second crematory has passed both branches of the city council. During a recent investigation with a view to building this second furnace, I ascertained that while the furnace as constructed at Wheeling three years ago would heat but 15 tons of steel in twelve hours, the system has been so improved during that time that the same sized furnace, as constructed to-day, will heat 30 tons of steel in twelve hours, which fact justifies me in saying that I believe an improved garbage crematory, as described above, will consume double the amount that our furnace is now burning.

Further than this, it is practically indestructible, and, with an average annual expenditure of $200 for repairs, will last a lifetime.

The Hygiene of Suicide.

BY HORATIO C. WOOD, M. D., LL. D.,

Clinical Professor of Nervous Diseases, University of Pennsylvania.

The editor of the ANNALS OF HYGIENE has urgently requested me to write him a brief article on the "Hygiene of Suicide." What the hygiene of suicide may be I do not know, nor do I know that I am able to interest or instruct either him or his readers in this matter. But, he is so urgent, that as an old friend I cannot deny him, and after all, most of us are made upon the principle of the Parisian doll —squeeze us in the right place, and the right way, and we squeak.

There are some persons who maintain that suicide is always the result of insanity; this is, however, plainly not the case. Some little time since there came to my clinic at the University Hospital, a man suffering from chronic disease, who said: "Doctor, I am tired of this pain; I have tried all the doctors except you, no one does me any good; I do not believe that there is any hereafter after death, or that I am more than a sheep or dog; I am going to give you two weeks, if you don't relieve me in that time I am going to kill myself." Kill himself I expect he did,—at least he disappeared from the range of our vision. This man was sane, his reasoning logical. We kill a dog to put him out of his pain. If man is as a dog, why should we not kill him, or why should he not kill himself to escape misery?

Lack of imagination, and cowardice together, often lead men to suicide. The fear of the hereafter is the one great deterrent. If a man is to face present exposure and shame, and having little imagination and faith, sees not sharply or clearly the hereafter, he reasons, "I'll take the chances of the future to escape the present."

A vivid imagination, which brings active visions of future punishment before the man, may hold him often, though his reason leads him to doubt the truth of these visions.

The great preventives of suicide in the sane are a pure life, and a strong religious faith. The man who knows in his heart that he has honestly done his best and who believes with his whole heart in a Supreme Being, who will take care of him in the direst extremity, cannot, being sane, take his own life.

After all, probably in the bulk—in the majority of cases—the suicide is insane, and the causes of suicide are the causes of insanity. Blood inheritance may lead a man to commit suicide with such driving power that no religion, nor education, *nor anything*, save physical force, can avert the dark catastrophe.

Wine and women, in other words, vice, is probably at the base of one-half or one-third of the insanity of the world, and even a greater proportion of the suicides. Over-ambition and intensity of desire to climb higher, by the labor which it entails, tends towards insanity. Successful labor, however, has so much of reward in itself that only rarely does it bring complete overthrow, but when the aims have been high, the toil prolonged and incessant, the end disappointment and ruin, then it is that the man overtops himself and falls a mental wreck.

In the case of a recent alleged suicide, many of these elements were present; his face may have been smiling, his manner always self-contained, but in himself the man knew—however honest had been his effort—that he had brought ruin to thousands; and it is very conceivable that this should have kept up a secret strain, of self-accusation, which was capable in the end of overcoming even a strong, clear intellect.

One very important lesson can be drawn from the case spoken of; there is an old and homely saying, when a man's deeds bring penalties, that—" his chickens are coming home to roost." Long sometimes is the day, far off the sunset, but often when least expected, when the history of the strain or the misdeed has almost been forgotten, the chickens come trooping home. Many men die in middle age of organic disease, the outcome of physical and perhaps moral misdeeds of early youth. How many soldiers who went through our war apparently unscathed have since died of diseases, variously named, but all alike in this that they were the result of the strain to vitality, of the ageing of the tissues by the exposures to hardship and the excitement of the war.

Mr. Thomas A. Scott, in early life, was injured by a railway accident; years after he prematurely died, and largely from strain and overwork, but the old wound gaps open first and the brain breaks away, where it had been injured years before. So, may a man take his own life, when struggles and disappointments have become to him memories, nerve tissues, worn and wasted, suddenly giving way, as the mill-dam suddenly breaks, though long it has been preparing for the going.

Constipation—A Cause and Its Treatment.

Dr. A. W. M'Kinney, writing on the above subject in the *Kansas Medical Journal*, among other good points raised, brings out an important one upon the construction and condition of water-closets. "After a residence is built the privy is made of the refuse scraps, and all the carpenter can do is to construct a something that will shield from public view. In addition to ill-construction, it seems that those who use them emulate each other as to who can pollute them most. When we are compelled to use the average privy we feel like condoning the error of constipation, and do not blame any one for dreading to visit a place that might be decent if not pleasant, but is generally loathsome."

There is entirely too much truth in these assertions. All will admit that the disease—constipation—is a very prevalent one, particularly among adult females. It is equally true that its cause often rests in an unnatural habit. It is as natural for a human being to desire, at stated intervals, an evacuation of the bowels as it is for him to fill his stomach with food, and in its natural condition there is no disposition on the part of the lower bowel to refuse to perform its duty. In the lower animals, so far as our observation and experience extend, there is no such affection as habitual constipation. This is so because the receptacle mentioned is always relieved when a desire is expressed, the result being that the bowel is always ready to act when it contains any substance demanding removal. We would not be understood as advocating the immodest adoption of the example set by the inferior animals, but we do mean to say that there is entirely too much mock modesty thrown around this imperative function, and that few resort to it as a pleasure, but as an unavoidable duty. It was prominent among the teachings of the late Austin Flint, Sr., that if so much unnecessary secrecy and so many disagreeable features were not attached to this daily obligation, there would be vastly fewer cases of constipation.

Look, for instance, as has been quoted, at the average country house. The water-closet is built a distance from the dwelling, fifty yards or more, that the house may be protected from the disagreeable odors; its approach is in full view of neighbors and passers-by, and exposed to the pelting rain in winter or the burning sun in summer, as the case may be. The structure is four by six or smaller, open alike to rain and sun, and constantly perfumed with the concentrated essence of rottenness. Arrangements in cities are better, but still far from perfect. There the miserable little stalls in the public buildings, devised for strict privacy, serve as a shelter for the vulgarlarly disposed who take advantage of the seclusion to mutilate the walls with vile writings and drawings and otherwise pollute the place in a manner unmentionable. It might perhaps be better to construct such public places so that they would be more public, and thus compel those who will not be decent alone, to observe decent practices in the presence of others.

As for private dwellings, let the water closet be a comfortable room of ten by twelve, or larger. Furnish it with carpet, wash-basin, towels, table, reading-matter, etc. Let the trap be so arranged that when raised the fact will not be reported through the entire house. If the closet be built away from the dwelling, have its approach protected and pleasant. In short, contrive a room that will not be disagreeable to occupy and bestow not all the good things upon the other less necessary apartments to the utter neglect of this. When such an improved custom becomes general, constipation will become less so.

Look Out for Bees.

It will be well for our country friends, who have a weakness for honey, never to forget a mask when pottering about the bee-hive, for it is related that a bee, belonging to a swarm that a farmer was recently attempting to hive, got down the man's throat and stung him, and the throat swelling very rapidly, he died of suffocation.

Practical Utopias.

"It has been objected (says Sir Edwin Chadwick) that if it were possible to amend communities by Utopias, Utopias would long since have been introduced. Our proceedings—assumed to be Utopian—which I have to recite, are not, however, based upon Utopian ideals, but on "experiences" carefully and separately examined —separately examined as to their assumed and strict application to common conditions. It is no Utopia that death-rates in towns, under the separate system of drainage, have been reduced by one-half through the work of the sanitary engineer alone. It is no Utopia that the death-rate at Rugby, for example, which was one of the towns first treated by our first general board of health, was then twenty-four in a thousand, and is now only twelve. It is no Utopia that at Salsbury the old death-rate, which at the beginning of the century was as high as forty in a thousand is now but about sixteen; or that at Croydon and a number of other places, death-rates of twenty-four in a thousand now average fifteen. These reductions have been effected by the system of "circulation *versus* stagnation," which is yet to be made generally understood, to be by constant and direct supplies of water, by the removal of the fouled water through self-cleansing house-drains and self-cleansing sewers, and by the removal of the refuse—fresh and undecomposed, and unwashed—on to the land.''

THE ANNALS OF HYGIENE,
THE OFFICIAL ORGAN OF THE
State Board of Health of Pennsylvania.

* *

PUBLISHED
MONTHLY.

Subscription, two dollars ($2.00)
a year, in advance.

' The State Board of Health is not responsible for
anything appearing in this Journal except that
which bears the official attestation of the Board,

Address all communications to

The Hygienic Publishing Company,
224 SOUTH SIXTEENTH STREET,
PHILADELPHIA, PA.

EDITORIAL.

Our New Dress.

There is "method in the madness" that has induced us to send our "New Year's greetings" to our friends in the brilliant dress that we have adopted for 1890. Those of our readers who are familiar with railroad signals will at once recognize the fitness of our new cover, while for those who are not we make this brief explanation : In the railroad sign language red indicates *danger*, while white means *go ahead*. Hence do we hope that the cover of this journal may serve as a reminder to those who are thoughtlessly disregarding all the laws of hygiene, that there is danger in such a course, while our white lettering may assure to them the safety of going ahead after they have stopped to reflect on the irrationality of such lives and have familiarized themselves with the teachings of hygiene. Our watchwords, therefore, as indicated by our cover, for the year 1890, will be " DANGER! STOP, REFLECT, and then GO-AHEAD !

The Poor Clerk and The Remedy.
SPECIALISM IN FARMING.

The case recently reported, from England, wherein a young clerk had been, for some time, vainly endeavoring to support his wife and children and keep up an air of respectability on a salary about equivalent to the wages of a day laborer, and wherein the health and mental equilibrium of the wife, finally succumbing to this unequal contest, she finally kills her children and then herself, is not an isolated example of the injurious effects of the artificial lives so many of us lead.

The aversion to nature and to all that is natural, so unnaturally inherent in the mass of mankind, seems to magnetically draw young men and women from the health-giving and peace-producing country, to the disease-breeding and misery-laden city, where so many find not only the tombs of their morality, but the sepulchres of their wasted, useless, and wrecked lives.

It is not the fault of the employer that so many clerks are vainly striving, and inevitably failing, to do what this poor English boy tried to do. It is clearly the result of trying to do that which nature does not wish that we should do. Of course we do not mean that there should be no clerks; they are necessities, and we must have them. What we do mean is that there are some persons who are constituted something after the plan of the patient draught-horse, who seem willing to, and happy and contented when they are, systematically, methodically, day-after-day, working and plodding along; who have no desire or ambition for anything beyond that which they possess. Such a young man, if he is blessed with a wife possessing a similar temperament, will make a clerk who will faithfully work, and in whose family history unsatisfied ambition will never record the history of murder and suicide. But in the case under consideration, and in all those cases of a similar nature, but lesser degree, wherein the desire, the ambition, the struggle for that which is beyond reach, causes physical and mental misery, wherein the health is ruined, marital happiness destroyed, and life made miserable, because the desires born of artificial surroundings cannot be gratified. In such cases, a potent remedy, we believe, may be found in a recurrence to a more natural method of life. Elsewhere,

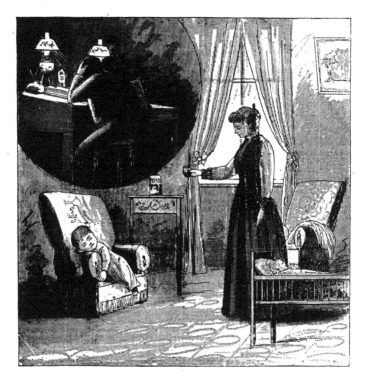

in this issue, we record how all the population of the whole world could be accommodated with standing room in a field ten miles square; in other words, one of the counties in this State could afford space for all the persons now living in the world.

Does this not bring home to us the great disproportion between the size of the world and the number of persons in it, and since omniscient wisdom does nothing unwise, would it not seem that in the design of the universe it was rather intended that each individual should have for his use, rather a few *acres* than a few *inches* of space, as is now the case in our large and crowded cities. Think, for a moment, of the millions upon millions of acres of uninhabited land, holding in its bosom untold wealth, ready to yield it up to him who but works for it. Think of the physical health and peace of mind such toil and such a life would entail. Think of the independence of such a life and then say whether it is not preferable to that of the drudging clerk in the crowded and noisome city.

Of course, we know that the desire for city life and the false idea (false as regards the great majority), that, in the city fortunes are to be made, will ever prove a barrier

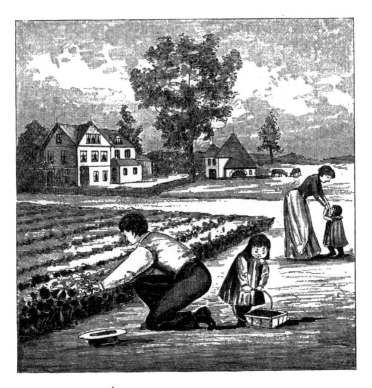

to the general acceptance of the idea we have broached. But, none-the-less, is the abstract idea correct, and he who would be wise would do well to heed it.

To make our ideas somewhat more explicit and, we hope, more attractive, we would suggest a new departure in farming, somewhat akin to that which has, of late years sprung up in the medical profession. It is well-known that the most lucrative branch of medical practice is specialism. A man makes a special study of the eye, the ear, the throat, the nervous system, or the kidneys; he is supposed to be specially well informed on these subjects, and, in consequence, his advice commands specially high prices.

Now, let the overworked clerk secure a little place in the country, which he can rent for much less than he has been paying in the city, and let him apply the doctrine of specialism to farming.

Let one raise chickens, another ducks, another turkeys, another strawberries, still another raspberries, and so on, through all the almost limitless list of the soil's products. Let him devote all his working time, his ingenuity and his experience to the perfection of his particular specialty, and, just as with the medical specialist, his products will command a special price that will make his work remunerative.

The Use of Salicylic Acid as a Preservative.

The general public has but little and the profession, we fear, not much more, idea of the extent to which salicylic acid is being used as a preservative of very many of the foods and beverages now found upon the market.

We have felt, and that most strongly, that it is high time for a most emphatic and unmistakable word of warning to be issued in this connection.

The question is repeatedly asked us whether we consider the presence of salicylic acid in articles intended for human consumption as injurious to health? To this query we can make answer with a gratifying degree of assurance (because we *know* that our reply will not be questioned by any one qualified to give an opinion on the subject), that the habitual ingestion of even the smallest quantities of this drug will have an effect on the human frame that is most undesirable.

Dr. Henry Leffmann, whose opinion will be highly valued wherever his reputation is known, has said, very truly, that the uniform opinion of sanitary chemists is, that salicylic acid is very objectionable as an addition to any form of food or drink, and especially objectionable in malt extracts. This is a point worthy of special consideration. One of the evil effects of the consumption of salicylic acid is a derangement of the functions of the stomach,—it causes indigestion ; at the present time malt extracts are being extensively used in cases of indigestion ; well, then, if a malt extract contains salicylic acid, not only is it the means of introducing into the system that which will prove injurious thereto, but, as Dr. Leffmann tells us, the very purpose for which malt extracts are intended (the conversion of starch into sugar), is negatived by the presence of this acid. Then we may truly say that while any article containing salicylic acid should be absolutely tabooed, when the article happens to be a malt extract there are double reasons why it must not be used.

We are glad to be able to say that all malt extracts are not so sophisticated.

We have more than once taken occasion to observe that hygiene is a science ; that it is, of course, as yet only in its infancy ; but that what we know we *know*, and we know it with mathematical certainty.

For instance, we know that if a man avoids the germs of a particular disease he *cannot* have that disease ; we know that unless the bowels are moved daily one *cannot* have good health ; we *know* that if a man lives on rich food, sooner or later his liver will give out ; so on, we might fill a volume with what we *know ;* but, just as we know many other things, so do we also *know* that salicylic acid is a *drug*, and a powerful one as well ; a drug that no one has any business to consume save under the direction of his physician.

We have said that this acid will derange digestion ; it will cause dyspepsia, which, of itself, is enough to condemn its indiscriminate use ; but we have reserved our biggest gun for our final shot. We have excellent authority for believing that salicylic acid has a very irritating action upon the kidneys, and we have more than once thought that it might not be a flight of fancy to attribute the alarming increase of cases of Bright's Disease to the increasing use of this agent as a preservative in the various canned and preserved articles that now form so large a part of the dietary of the American people.

In conclusion, we assert, as a dogma, that it is very prejudicial to health for any one to consume any article containing salicylic acid.

The Non-Specificity of Disease.

While we have not been exactly ridiculed, yet we have noted the smile of incredulity whenever we have advanced, in the presence of medical men, a theory of which we have been very fond for some years past, namely, the non-specificity of disease. To be more clear, we have long doubted whether there really is a separate and distinct bacillus or seed for scarlet fever, for diphtheria, for measles, for typhoid fever, and so on ; that is to say, whether the one cause did not produce the different manifestations, influenced by the nature of the soil (bodily conditions) in which it may be implanted. Again, given a case of typhoid fever, most authorities of to-day, will claim that it must have originated from a pre-existing case, that the bacillus of this particular disease, derived from a case of the disease is necessary for the development of typhoid fever. This view we have been inclined to doubt, as the result of observation, rather thinking that ordinary organic putrefaction is capable of producing an agency that when introduced into a body where the conditions are present will be capable of causing the disease.

Finding, as a rule, but few sympathizers with these views, we may, we are sure, be pardoned for the feeling of satisfaction we experience, when we find, practically, these same views championed by so high an authority as Dr. Wm. Thornton Parker, of Newport, R. I., who, in the *Medical Record* (December 7, 1889) says :

"It is difficult for some men, myself included, to believe that we have one bacillus for typhoid fever, another for cholera, another for diphtheria, another for scarlet fever, another for phthisis, another for gonorrhœa, and so on, *ad infinitum*, until our collection of these interesting little creatures would rival in number the coins of a numismatist. More easily believed and understood is the paper of Dr. Griffith on the ' Unity of Poison' in scarlet, typhoid, puerperal fevers, and diphtheria, erysipelas, sore throat ; certain forms of diarrhœa and allied ailments, in pleurisy, pneumonia, and pluro-pneumonia, and many other affections heretofore usually considered to be separate and entirely distinct diseases.

Would it not be fair to assume that the unsanitary conditions surrounding the United States ship New Hampshire were sufficient to propagate typhoid fever on board that vessel—without the appearance of the bacillus typhosus to properly start the mischief, according to the scientific theories of some of our modern investigators.

The United States ship " New Hampshire " is an old-fashioned " man-of-war," which, on clear blue water, might have been a safe and healthy home for double the number of men and boys who have lived on her during the past five or six years; but in an abnormal element, *i. e.*, resting in a mud-hole, and surrounded by mud and all uncleanliness, and with tons of fecal matter piled up around her bows, she could hardly have been considered a safe resort for human beings' The fecal element was certainly in the majority here, and the atmosphere, loaded with fecal matter, entered the ports on its death-dealing mission. Her brave old sides of oak, which would have held her gallant crew in safety in the good old days, gave no protection to this new and treacherous foe, when she had been dragged from her normal element into the unnatural and filthy place in which so many of her crew received their death-wounds in the shape of typhoid fever.

It is not my intention to magnify the fact that fecal odor, or the gases escaping from large quantities of decomposing fecal matter, can produce typhoid fever, *but merely to protest against the claim that, given a case of typhoid fever, the bacillus typhosus must have had some influence in its causation.* That many different shaped bacilli can be found in the discharge of patients suffering from various disorders, there can be no doubt. Many admit that a sufficient quantity of these same bacilli may, under favorable conditions, induce disease ; but it seems to me more reasonable to suppose that *decomposition of animal and vegetable matter is more frequently the cause of preventable disease, rather than that the emigration of particular bacilli is to be the principal cause recognizable.*

It is not the intention of this paper to bring forward a theory of odor as the principal causation of typhoid, or to deny the germ of disease which may go from one person to another through the medium of air, water or food, but merely to call for a recognition of the theory of von Gietl, that fecal odor alone—if continued and sufficiently strong—can, and often does, develop typhoid fever, and that this theory has had a very startling illustration in the many deaths which have occurred from the infection received on board the United States ship " New Hampshire."

I believe that true science does not tend toward such a complication of terms and theories that the average mind stands appalled on contemplation, but that knowledge simplifies and makes easy what before seemed incomprehensible ; and that, even as with machinery, the attainment of the more perfect is the employment of the more simple. So, as we advance in medical science, we will discover how much of truth there is to be found in the theory of unity in disease. We have the foul conditions obtaining which I have just referred to, and at one time an epidemic of scarlet fever will result, at another diphtheria, at another more or less severe diarrhœas, and, as in this instance, at another typhoid fever. Filth and health are directly antagonistic. Nature abhors filth, and strives in every way possible to get rid of external or internal waste or foul substance Filth lowers the health, and if it be not destroyed is itself the destroyer of life; but in accomplishing this work, it may do so in many different ways and yet exhibit itself only in one exciting cause or in a combination of causes—foul air, foul water, faul privy vaults, decaying animal and vegetable matter. I believe the time will come when the remarkable exploits of the many-shaped and many-named bacilli will be one of the curiosities of medical literature."

Of course, there is a fascination about this study of the minute, ultimate, particular, specific, if you please, cause of disease ; but, while seeking after such, we must not lose sight of the grand, practical, every-day demonstrable fact that it is filth, or, to put it in less vulgar language, organic putrefaction, that really causes the contagious diseases, whatever may be the special agency utilized by this putrefaction. With Dr. Parker, we are sometimes inclined to think that the wise men of the twentieth century will look back upon our present views in reference to the special bacilli of special diseases somewhat with the same interested but incredulous spirit with which we of to-day are wont to regard the beautiful, somewhat analogous, but delusive theories of Buffon and Bonnet ; theories, which though now disbelieved, yet held captive the intelligence of the eighteenth century.

Seriously, we doubt whether the search after a special seed for each particular disease is any real, true progress. We have always rather held that original sanitary investigation should tend in the direction of ascertaining, if possible, the conditions of the body favoring the reception and development of disease, so that these conditions might be so modified as to render the human being inhospitable to disease.

In the meantime let us keep filth far from us and let us maintain for ourselves and our neighbors that high standard of bodily and mental health, with which disease is incompatible.

A Homely Illustration of the Effects of Boiling Water.

A. Arnold Clark, of Lansing, Michigan, calls attention to the fact that when fruit is canned it is boiled to destroy the germs of fermentation. As the germs of fermentation once introduced into the fruit make the fruit ferment, in something the same way the germs of typhoid fever in the water will make a well man sick with that disease, and as boiling the fruit will destroy the germs of fermentation and save the fruit, just so surely boiling all drinking water will destroy the germs of typhoid fever and save an epidemic.

NOTES AND COMMENTS.

Poisonous Bank Bills.

Some of the employes of the Bank of Switzerland were lately poisoned by handling bank bills. The bills were colored with Schweinfurt green, an arsenical poison.—*Sanitary Inspector.*

The Nature of Arrow Poison.

It would seem, from some recent utterances of Mr. Stanley, the African explorer, that the poison which has proven fatal to so many of his followers is made from ants. The dried bodies of red ants are ground to powder, cooked in palm oil and smeared over the wooden points of the arrows.

School Teachers as Sanitary Watch-Dogs.

By a recent ruling of the Minister of the Interior, of France, the principals of schools are required to immediately give notice of the appearance of any epidemic disease in their schools, and, every three months, a complete report must be made of all such diseases that have appeared during the preceding quarter. Good for France!

Death Comes Cheap in France.

The cremation furnace in Pere-la-Chaise Cemetery, in Paris, is now complete, and the Prefect of the Seine has approved the scale of charges to be enforced thereat. The charge for the use of the cremation furnace is to be ten dollars, which sum includes the keeping in the columbarium of the funeral urn containing the ashes for a period of five years.

Weighty Kitchen Drudgery.

The *New York Medical Journal* thinks that one cause of the ill-health of women is the excessive weight and size of all household or kitchen utensils, boilers, pots, tubs, pails, etc. It says that these were made for men rather than women. Hence, he who reduces these to the proportionate size and strength of women, will have conferred a lasting benefit upon the race.

The Lesson of Munich.

Formerly Munich had a high mortality from typhoid fever. Since Pettenkofer instituted his measures of reform, this fever has become so rare that medical teachers are at a loss to find cases to show their classes. Thus, from being one of the most unhealthy cities in Europe it has become one of the healthiest—all due to the practical application of sanitary science.

Alcohol and Consumption.

It would seem, from the remarks recently made, in Paris, by Dr. Lancereaux, that there is a special reason why those who may inherit a tendency to consumption, should avoid the use of alcohol, for he tells us that by retarding tissue changes, checking combustion and diminishing the appetite, it renders one, so situated, an easy prey to the attack of the germ of the disease.

Germany's Greatest Enemy.

It has usually been considered that France was Germany's greatest enemy, but now we have reason to alter this view, for we have no less an authority than the great Von Moltke for the statement that *beer* is a far more dangerous enemy to Germany than all the armies of France.

Faith-Curing of Contagious Diseases Suppressed.

The Board of Health of Matteawan, N. Y., having encountered a case of diphtheria that was being neglected by some faith-curing practitioners, declared an immediate quarantine, which was maintained by the police. A reputable physician was put in charge of the case, and the child began to improve.

The Drainage of Chicago.

On the 12th of last month nine Commissioners were chosen in Chicago, who are authorized to spend $60,000,000 in constructing a system which will take care of Chicago's sewage and give the city pure water. The Commissioners have the power to employ 10,000 men a year for seven years, within which time the work must be completed.

Poison in Cured Fish.

The Russian Academy of Sciences offers a prize of 5,000 roubles ($2,500) for the best inquiry into the nature and effects of the poison which develops in cured fish. The competition is open to all. The memoirs must be sent in, either in manuscript or printed, before January 1, 1893, and may be written in any one of the following languages: Russian, Latin, French, English, German.

Rubber Bandages for Dyspepsia.

Not to eat them, but to fasten them around the waist. It is claimed, by some good authorities, that a ten-inch wide rubber bandage, applied around the waist and so worn for about one hour after meals, will not only relieve the sense of oppression complained of by dyspeptics, but will cure the trouble as well. Such a procedure can do no harm, and we would advise our dyspeptic patrons to give it a trial.

The Mighty Power of Good Blood.

It would seem that freshly drawn blood has a decidedly deadly action upon disease germs, from which we might infer that blood and disease are naturally antagonistic. We might go still further and inferentially claim that if one's blood be good he will be able to resist the attack of disease germs. Hence, it should be our first aim to have good blood, which we can only procure from the good digestion and assimilation of good food, well cooked, all of which we can have by an observance of the doctrines of hygiene.

Convalescence from Typhoid Fever.

During the convalescence of typhoid fever patients, the *Sanitary Inspector* wisely reminds its readers, the greatest precautions should be taken by the nurses and other attendants against indiscretions in eating on the part of the patient. Carelessness in this direction is very frequently the cause of sudden death, even after the physician congratulates himself on pulling the patient through the disease.

Rain Good for the Complexion.

Don't house your girls in rainy days (says Shirley Dare). Case them in water-proofs and high rubbers, with short skirts and storm hats of serge, and send them out two miles and back for a " beauty walk " in the teeth of the storm. If they can do a block in two minutes they can't take cold, and will come back with a Newport freshness of complexion. When women know how kind rains really are to them they will stop railing at the weather.

Vaccination and Re-vaccination.

In the late epidemic of small-pox in Sheffield, England, among the 81 nurses and attendants who had been recently re-vaccinated, not one took the disease, though they were constantly with the small-pox patients. Among 62 attendants, who had been vaccinated once, but who had not been re-vaccinated, 6 became infected and one died. This is a striking confirmation of the value of vaccination, and of the need of re-vaccination.—*Sanitary Inspector.*

Statistics of Sleep.

Some recent statistics of sleep, though they may not prove anything of importance, are interesting. Students sleep longer and are less tired than other men. The time needed to fall asleep is about the same in all three classes—20.8 minutes for the men, 17.1 minutes for students, and 21.2 minutes for women. In each case, however, it takes longer for those who are frequent dreamers and light sleepers to fall asleep than persons of opposite characteristics.

The Prevention of Consumption.

We really know a good deal about the prevention of consumption, but we know mighty little about the cure after the disease has once fastened its fangs upon a victim. We now know that consumption can be conveyed from one to another by the medium of the expectoration, but not until this has become dry. The consumptive, therefore, has it in his power to prevent himself from becoming a source of danger to his family and friends, if he will avoid promiscuous expectoration ; if he will always expectorate into a little wooden or paste-board receptacle, which can be daily consumed (with its contents) in the fire. Certainly a very simple precaution, entailing but little trouble, yet wonderfully efficacious in its results.

Female Sanitary Officials.

We are glad to learn that a body of five female sanitary police is now established in Chicago, under the appointment of the Commissioner of Health, according to an ordinance of the City Council. The duty of the new female sanitary police is to inspect factories and tenements for the protection of the health of working women. For efficiency and persistency in this kind of work women are far superior to men, and we congratulate the working women of Chicago on this wise provision for their welfare.

Flushing Sewers.

In his report on the Sewerage System of New York City, Mr. Rudolph Hering asserts that some provision should always be made for the artificial flushing of sewers, for he does not believe that rain-storms can be relied upon for this purpose. He thinks that the sudden discharge of a large quantity of water is what we want; deposits become too firmly compacted, he claims, to be carried off by the average storm, while systematic flushing, on the other hand, will prevent deposits from accumulating.

Spontaneous Cow-Pox in Italy.

The Animal Vaccination Committee of Milan has recently had a windfall in the form of a supply of lymph derived from a herd of cattle in which cow-pox had spontaneously broken out. On August 3d the Prefect of Sondrio (Northern Italy) announced that natural cow-pox had appeared in a herd in the commune of Cosio, in Valtellina, at a height of 2,000 metres, near the top of the Tagliata Alp. The eruption had shown itself on the udders on June 27th, and of the eighty cows only four had not been attacked.

Snow is Healthy.

Not to eat or drink, but from some recent researches we would be led to infer that falling snow has a purifying action on the atmosphere. It would seem that in its descent it brings down with it the bacteria that are floating in the air. Of course we must remember that the great mass of bacteria are harmless, but we, at the same time, have the satisfaction of believing that snow will bring down the hurtful bacteria as well. Hence, we would take it that during and immediately after a snow-storm, the atmosphere is unusually pure.

The Late Jefferson Davis.

Of all the prominent figures of war-days, few have so nearly reached the natural limit of human existence as did the late Jefferson Davis, and few have led the natural life that he, for so many years, has followed. Far away from the crowded centres of humanity, communing with nature, in nature's own way, this man has outlived nearly all those who, more than a quarter of a century ago were the men who have contributed most largely to the history of the nineteenth century. Is there not a lesson to be learned from the lives and deaths of these noted men?

How Long to Sleep.

According to *The Sanitary Volunteer*, up to the fifteenth year most young people require ten hours, and until the twentieth year nine hours. *After that age every one finds out how much he or she requires,* though, as a general rule, at least six to eight hours is necessary. Eight hours' sleep will prevent more nervous derangements in women than any medicine can cure. During growth there must be ample sleep if the brain is to develop to its full extent ; and the more nervous, excitable, or precocious a child is, the longer sleep should it get, if its intellectual progress is not to come to a premature standstill, or its life cut short at an early age.

Open Air for Consumptives.

The following remarks, from the Maine State Board of Health, are eminently worthy of being remembered :

" The open-air treatment of consumptives and those who are threatened with the disease, has given much better results than any other. Particularly in Germany, and to some extent in this country such treatment has been systematized in ' sanitaria ' for consumptives. Here the patients have the advantage of a regular life, nutritious food and such exercise as they can bear without fatigue ; but the chief curative agent is an abundance of fresh air. Even in the coldest of winter weather, patients, after a period of gradual habituation, and always guided by the judgment of the physician, pass the whole day walking in the open air, or sitting or lying on resting places wrapped comfortably in blankets. Usually no claim is made for advantages of climate. *An abundance of pure air is the all important thing.*"

Constipation.

We are thoroughly saturated with the idea that a daily out-put from the bowels is just as essential to health as is a daily in-take of food into the stomach. Following up this idea, we believe that very few persons even begin to realize how much ill-health is caused by constipation, and how much good health and happiness would accompany the habit of full, free, daily evacuations from the bowels. Hence do we give prominence to all the accessories that will favor this habit, and we would, consequently, ask careful perusal of the short article on this subject, which we, elsewhere, reproduce from the *Pacific Medical Jouraal.* Read it and heed it.

The President's Message.

Not one word from President Harrison, to Congress, in his recent message, about the necessity for sanitary legislation for *humanity.* His predecessor, Mr. Cleveland, in his last message, did advert to the protection of the health and lives of the lower animals, and we had hoped that, by this time, human life would be thought worthy of executive consideration ; but Mr. Harrison falls behind Mr. Cleveland and even fails to take notice of the lower animals. It is true that he does refer to the necessity of some measures of protection (against accidents) for railway employés ; but not one word about the hundred thousand persons who are annually dying in this country from preventable diseases. Certainly, in these days of sanitary enlightenment, an executive message that fails to touch upon sanitary legislation is like unto the play of Hamlet without the Prince.

A Popular Belief in the Contagiousness of Consumption.

In a paper on the contagiousness of consumption, read at the twenty-fifth anniversary meeting of the Caucasian Medical Society, Dr. Babayeff mentioned the curious fact that among the Georgians the name for consumption is "chlekki," meaning "the contagious disease." When one of their number is found to be suffering from this disease he is at once insolated, and is taken to a hut or tent at some distance from the village. The care of these patients is entrusted to an old woman who carries to them the necessary food and drink, and they are never allowed to associate with the well.

A Good Cologne.

The *Chemist and Druggist* recently offered a valuable prize for the best "*home-made*" cologne. Here is the prize formula, selected from 219 samples:

Oil of Bergamot,	2 drachms.
" Lemon,	1 drachm.
" Neroli,	20 drops.
" Origanum,	6 drops.
" Rosemary,	20 drops.
Alcohol, triple-distilled,	1 pint.
Orange-flower Water,	1 oz.

A Type-writer's Luncheon.

A lawyer of ponderous proportions has been surreptitiously keeping a list of things which his type-writer eats at luncheon. She is in perfect health, robust, pretty, and cheerful. He is suffering from gout and the other effects of overeating. The heaviest luncheon which she ate last week, according to the lawyer, cost exactly eleven cents. It was made up of the following courses: One pear, 2 cents; one Vienna roll, 3 cents; four bananas, 4 cents; one pear, 2 cents." We doubt not that this luncheon would be inimical to portliness, but, at the same time, we can hardly think that four bananas (unless thoroughly well chewed) would be very conducive to good digestion.

The Divine Sanction of Sanitation.

"Our Great Example commanded His first followers to heal the sick and give alms, but He commands us (says Dr. C. G. Wheelhouse, the President of the British Medical Association), and all His followers, in this age, to investigate the causes of all evils, to master the science of health, to consider the question of education with a view to health, and while all these investigations are made with free expenditure of energy and time and means, to work out the rearrangement of human life in accordance with the results they give; and if, instead of undoing a little harm, and comforting a few unfortunates, we have the means of averting countless misfortunes, and raising by the right employment of our knowledge and power of contrivance, the general standard of happiness, we lessen the necessary evils of life, lengthen the term of human existence, wipe out the causes of innumerable griefs and sufferings, make life more endurable and happy, can it be said that we are failing to obey the commands or to undermine the teachings of our great Master?"

A Good Hair Tonic.

If our readers will copy the following formula, which Dr. Bordet recommends to prevent the falling out of hair, they will have a good toilet article at less expense than they have been in the habit of paying:

Carbolic acid	30 minims.
Tincture of nux vomica	2 drachms.
Compound tincture of cinchona	1 fl. ounce.
Tincture of cantharides	30 minims.
Cologne water	1 fl. ounce.
Cocoanut oil, to make	4 fl. ounces.

To be applied to the scalp twice a day with a small sponge.

The Destruction of Mosquitoes.

The Microscope says that Robert H. Lamborn has placed in the hands of Morris K. Jessup, of the American Museum of Natural History, New York, the sum of $200, to be paid in three prizes of $150, $30 and $20, for the three best essays on the destruction of mosquitoes and flies by other insects. It is suggested that the dragon fly is an active, voracious and harmless "mosquito hawk," and that it might, if artificially multiplied, diminish the number of smaller insects. A practical plan is called for in the breeding of the dragon fly or other such destroyer in large numbers, and its use in the larva, pupa or perfect state, for the destruction of mosquitoes and flies in houses, cities and neighborhoods.

The Wonders of Electricity.

One of Edison's chiefs lives in Newark in a house, which is all agog with wires. As one approaches the front gate it swings open and shuts automatically. The visitor's foot on the steps of the porch rings a bell in the kitchen, and also one in the master's study. By touching a button he opens the front door before the stranger has time to knock. An electrical music-box plays during dinner. When the guest retires to his bedroom the folding-bed unfolds by electricity. When he puts out the gas a strange, mocking display of skeletons, gravestones, owls, and other hideous phantasmagoria dances about on the walls, reappearing and disappearing in a ghostly, electrical glare.

The Ideal Physician of the Future.

Two and a half years ago (in our issue for July, 1887), we outlined a plan which we believed, and still believe, would prove much more mutually advantageous both to the patient and the physician than the method now in vogue. Our scheme contemplated the employment of a physician by the year, whose duty it should be to keep us well by advice and to cure us (if possible) when disease did come to us, and for these services a fixed sum per annum was to be paid. The seed we planted has already borne fruit, for we learn that such a custom has come into quite considerable use in New York City. It is an excellent arrangement for the doctor, who can be easy about his income ; and it is good for the patients, as it is clearly to the interest of the physician to keep them as well as possible.

The Water Supply of New York City.

From the *Medical Record* we learn that the report of the State Board of Health on the water-supply of New York City has been made to the Governor, and its details made public. It is a most exhaustive study of the subject, and will be a document of great value in studying the problems of water-supply in cities. The investigation was made under the direction of Professor C. C. Brown and Emil Kuichling, engineers, with the assistance of chemical experts. A full survey of the Croton water-shed, with a detailed description of all the sources of pollution, natural and artificial, is given. It is shown that the Croton water is naturally of pure character, and all the sources of its infection or pollution being now known the problem of keeping the water pure is much simplified.

Cooking by Electricity.

The *Scientific American* says: The Hotel Bernina, at Samaden, has for some time been lighted with electricity, power being supplied by a waterfall. As during the day the power is not required for lighting, and is therefore running to waste, the proprietor of the hotel has hit upon the idea of utilizing the current for cooking when it is not required for lighting, and an experimental cooking apparatus has been constructed. This contains German silver resistance coils, which are brought to a red heat by the current, and it has been found possible to perform all the ordinary cooking operations in a range fitted with a series of such coils.

In a Minneapolis restaurant can be seen in daily operation an electric cook stove invented by an electrician of that city.

The Characteristics of a Locality Without a "Health Service."

A State, city, town, or county without a competent health service has filthy and stifling court-rooms (says Dr. A. N. Bell) ; churches and school-houses with a poisonous atmosphere ; crowded and filthy almshouses and jails, approximating those of the great Howard's time.; factories, shops, and seamstresses' dens of every kind, constructed and conducted without reference to the health of the occupants ; habitual carelessness, cruelty to animals, and numerous " accidents." The highways and the byways partake of the same general condition, extending even into and throughout the households to filth storage in the back yards, food and drink, clothing and habits—all without notice, except a constant dealing with the results, are the characteristics of all such communities.

A Valuable and Unique Business Calendar.

The most convenient, valuable, and unique business table or desk calendar, for 1890, is the Columbia Bicycle Calendar and Stand, issued by the Pope Mfg. Co., of Boston, Mass. The calendar proper is in the form of a pad, containing 366 leaves, each 5⅛ x 2¾ inches—one for each day of the year, to be torn off daily, and one for the entire year. A portion of each leaf is left blank for memoranda, and as the leaves are not pasted, but sewed at the end, any entire leaf can be exposed whenever desired. By an ingenious device the leaves tear off independently, leaving no stub. The pad rests upon a portable stand, containing pen-rack and pencil-holder, and when placed upon a desk or writing-table the entire surface of the date leaf is brought directly, and left constantly, before the eye, furnishing date and memoranda impossible to be overlooked.

Antiseptic Ventilation.

A novel apparatus for filtering and regulating the temperature of air, and, if desired, of sterilizing it, was brought forward at the Worcester meeting of the Sanitary Institute, of England, by Mr. S. M. Burroughs. This apparatus, by means of a revolving fan, blows air to all parts of the building, the temperature being raised in winter by means of waste steam, and cooled in summer by substituting cold water for the steam. The air passes through a coarse strainer to remove dust and floating particles, and, when required, is impregnated with the vapor of carbolic acid, eucalyptol, pinol, etc., by means of a suitable mechanism. It is, of course, only applicable in buildings such as factories, where motive power is obtainable; but where that is provided, it is certainly an effectual and economical method of obtaining forced ventilation.—*Medical Press and Circular, October 9, 1889.*

The Benighted Citizens of Los Angeles.

The wealthy young lady, of this city, who is about to establish a new sisterhood for missionary work among the Indians and Negroes, should have her attention called to the need that exists for missionary work among the evidently befuddled citizens of Los Angeles, California. From the *Journal of the American Medical Association* we learn that this city, of 80,000 people, almost entirely sewerless, is fragrant with the most odorous of smells and ravaged by the terrors of diphtheria; yet the proposition to construct a sewer to the sea has been defeated by a popular vote of the citizens. We would feel inclined to say " God help these poor people," did we not know that God will not help those who help not themselves. In many parts of the city the odor, at nights, from cess-pools is so strong, that it is necessary to close the windows. Hence it would seem that these foolish persons cannot offer the excuse of ignorance of the presence of an evil in palliation of their barbaric refusal to remove it.

The Breeding of Sinners.

The French Government hopes, apparently, by promoting marriages between male and female convicts, to bring back these stray sheep into the fold of morality and good conduct. Arrangements have accordingly been made to facilitate these unions, but physiologists and pathologists must feel sundry qualms as to the expediency of such a course. The physical and moral degradation of many of these social waifs is distinctly hereditary, and a careful moral training (which is not provided for) would, at the most, only modify the tendencies which have brought them within the clutches of the criminal law. The son of a poet is not of necessity a poet, but the offspring of a bawd or an assassin is extremely likely to develop the same proclivities. If even one of the parties to the transaction was worthy of respect, some regeneration might be hoped for, but the association of two hopelessly abandoned bodies and souls is not calculated to improve matters in any respect whatever.

Disease-Ridden Indians.

Indian Agent Jones, of the Berthold Agency, has made application to the Department for a physician who shall remain constantly at the Agency. This request is the result of hurried examination of the health of the Indians. Mr. Jones was recently appointed. He finds that disease runs rampant among the entire Indian community. The Indians at this agency are in a most deplorable condition. In the past their health has been neglected, they have been permitted to roam about the country and, as a result, some members of the tribe have returned to their camps laden with disease, which has spread to nearly every Indian at the Agency. It is understood that the request for a physician has been granted, and that steps will be taken to prevent the further spread of disease among the tribes. The condition of affairs at the agency in the past has not only ruined the health of the Indians, but has been a constant menace to the whites with whom the Indians necessarily associated.

The Multiplication of Bacteria.

As regards the reproduction of the bacteria, many of them can double their numbers every hour when placed in the best conditions for their activity. In such circumstances then, a single bacterium would in twenty-four hours produce no less than 16,777,220. At the end of forty-eight hours the offspring would amount to 281,500,000,000, and would fill a half pint measure—all produced in two days from a single germ measuring $\frac{1}{150000}$ of an inch. Fortunately, however, bacteria can rarely so propagate themselves, they meet with all sorts of drawbacks, and thus in spite of their enormous fertility the survivors are in a general way only enough to keep up a fair balance in nature. The diseases producing bacteria, however, have no claim upon our forbearance, and in these the enormous fecundity we cannot too closely contemplate. Some, like the bacteria of tuberculosis and glanders, propagate themselves slowly; but the great majority of the bacteria causing animal plagues will, in favorable cases, double their numbers hourly.—*Prof. Law, in The Pharmaceutical Era.*

Virchow and the Darwinian Theory.

According to the Vienna correspondent of the *British Medical Journal*, in Professor Virchow's presidential address at the recent meeting of the Anthropological Congress, the Darwinian theory was referred to, and he said that the intermediate link that should bring man and the ape into connection—the proper "prosanthropos"—had been sought for in vain. It was impossible even to determine the descent of single races from others; and it could be asserted that among the ancient races there was none that stood in any nearer relationship to the ape than ourselves. There was no tribe of people in the world that we were unacquainted with; and not one of the known tribes could justly be considered ape-like, appearances common to apes—such as prominences of the skull—being insufficient evidence of relationship. There was evidence that in the course of 5000 years no remarkable changes of type had taken place. This adds to the evidence of the impossibility of the chasm between the highest type of anthropoid ape and the lowest type of man.—*New York Medical Journal*

Your Billions of Ancestors.

" Did you ever think how many male and female ancestors were required to bring you into the world! First it was necessary that you should have a father and mother—that makes two human beings. Each of them must have had a father and mother—that makes four more human beings. Again each of them must have had a father and mother—making eight more human beings. So on we go back to the time of Jesus Christ—56 generations. The calculation, thus resulting shows that 139,235,017,489,534,976 births must have taken place in order to bring you into the world! You who read these lines."

So says the *Weekly Medical Review*, yet such figures needs not frighten us. From them some *anti*-sanitarians might erroneously argue that death is a good thing, in so far that it prevents over-crowding. But from *London Justice*, we learn that all the people now living in the world could find standing-room within the limits of a field ten miles square, and, by the aid of a telephone, could be addressed by a single speaker. So that those who fear over-crowding as the result of the increased longevity which hygiene vouchsafes to us, need not lie awake at night to worry over the matter.

The Czar has had a Cold.

It is one of the penalties of greatness that each "sneeze" should be cabled throughout the civilized world. Therefore do we lay before our readers the fact that the Czar of all the Russias has had a cold. But, in this particular instance, the universality of humanity has overcome the barrier of autocracy and some 40,000 of the Czar's *devoted* (?) subjects have sympathetically had colds at the same time. To be plain, there has been recently, in St. Petersburg, a curious epidemic of influenza, which is spreading to Moscow, and even into far-off Siberia. Among its victims have been nearly all of the imperial family, as well as the occupants of the lowest hovels; the disease lasting three or four days and causing great annoyance. Let us venture to hope that this trifling incident may cause the greatest autocratic tyrant of the nineteenth century to realize that, after all, there is no difference (save an accident of birth) between himself and his very lowest subject, and that it may be the means of "sneezing" some of his nonsenical ideas out of his head, leaving room for the evolution of some sensible, practical, reasonable *republican* reflections.

The Pope Instinctively a Sanitarian.

We have, more than once, ventured the assertion that all really great men are, in practice, if not in theory, sanitarians; that they are so constituted naturally that a natural or hygienic life comes, so to speak, natural to them. They do what nature intends that they should do, because they are not, instinctively, urged to do otherwise. Such persons we might call natural or instinctive sanitarians. Then again we have those who live naturally, not because instinct so prompts, but because wisdom so dictates. In these two classes, we venture to say, if we fairly examine the question, will be found all really and truly great men. The present Pope, Leo XIII, is a remarkable illustration of the results of a natural, simple life. There are few persons in the world, even of half his great age, who possess the clearness of intellect and the capacity for work that he displays. Yet, had he not been careful of his health, he would surely have been in his grave many years ago, for he is not and never has been robust. The frugal, simple, natural life of the Pope furnishes a most admirable example for those who would desire to live long, healthy, happy and useful lives.

BUREAU OF INFORMATION.

The Six Best Sanitary Journals.

EDITOR ANNALS OF HYGIENE :

Will you, through the " Bureau of Information," kindly give a list of what you consider the six best Journals treating upon the subject of sanitary science ? and oblige, W. H. S.

Some years ago a publishing house, in this city, issued a volume of biographical sketches of prominent physicians. In some instances, these sketches were written by the gentlemen themselves, in others, by some ardent admirer. The editor of the work happened, one day, to call upon the late distinguished and lamented Dr. J. L. Ludlow, of this city, and, asking him for a sketch of himself, laid upon the desk before him, (as a sample of what was desired) the biography of Professor Da Costa, as it would appear in the book. Dr. Ludlow (who had a most keen sense of humor) read line after lin until he came to a paragraph which stated that Dr. Da Costa was the "finest clinical diagnostician in this country;" looking up from the page before him, Dr. Ludlow announced that it would be impossible for him to contribute anything about himself to the book. Upon being pressed for a reason, he said, " Well, I think that I am the 'finest clinical diagnostician' in this country; you here say that Dr. Da Costa is; now since there cannot be *two finest,* I will be obliged to stay out of the book." For somewhat similar reasons to those which actuated Dr. Ludlow, we are unable to answer the above query. We think we know, however, which is *the* finest sanitary journal in the country and we are also equally sure the readers of " THE ANNALS " also know. [ED. A. OF H.]

The Effect of Alum on Schuylkill Water.

EDITOR ANNALS OF HYGIENE :

Our Schuylkill water is readily clarified by adding from $1\frac{1}{2}$ to 3 gr alum to gallon, letting stand for ten or twelve hours and filtering through paper. How does water so prepared, compare in quality with boiled water ? The clearest river water we get will deposit some sediment in adding even the smaller quantity of alum. The water thus prepared certainly tastes better and looks better than boiled water and if the alum throws out the bacteria along with the dirt, it certainly would be the better way to prepare it for drinking purposes; also how does it compare microscopically with boiled and with unprepared water ? " IGNORAMUS."

A specimen of water so prepared was forwarded to Dr. Charles M. Cresson, for analysis, and we append his report.

Water " drawn from hydrant and of about average appearance." Part of sample " treated with 2 grains of alum per gallon and after standing over night, filtered."

The results of analysis of organic constituents, expressed in parts to the million, were as follows :

	Free Ammonia.	Albumenoid. Ammonia.	Chlorine.	Sulphuric Acid.
Before treatment and filtration,	trace	0.192	2.139	5.49
After treatment and filtration,	0.083	0.274	2.139	15.62

These determinations show that the result of treatment and filtration was not beneficial to the quality of the water. This is due to the fact that the water was carrying masses of readily oxidizable organic matter which lodged upon the filter, and, becoming oxidized, rendered a part soluble and thus increased the pollution of the water. When the water of the Schuylkill River is free from organic matter in this peculiar condition, the result of treatment and filtration is beneficial to the water, so far as relates to its wholesomeness.

Examination with the microscope, showed that the treatment with alum and filtration, through a paper filter, did not perceptibly diminish the number of cilia and other similar minute organisms, which were quite numerous in the water. CHARLES M. CRESSON, M. D.

City *versus* **Well Water in Erie.**

ED. ANNALS OF HYGIENE:—I have this day forwarded to you twelve samples of water, by direction of the Board of Water Commissioners of this city. It is desired that you make a complete statement of the analysis in the forthcoming number of the ANNALS OF HYGIENE—the official organ of the State Board of Health.   B. F. S.

These samples were forwarded to Dr. Charles M. Cresson, who thus reports :

Waters received from the State Board of Health, marked " Erie, Nos 1 to 12." Locations not given.

Results of chemical and microscopical examinations as follows :

Results expressed in parts per million.

Samples Marked.	Free Ammon.	Alb. Ammon.	Nitrates.	Chlorine.	Remarks.
Erie, Pa., " No. 1,"	0 137	0.055	0.285	1.937	Fair condition for drinking purposes.
" " No. 2."	0.027	0.055	trace	1.772	" "
" " No. 3,"	0.027	0.083	0.171	3.188	" "
" " No. 4,"	0.055	0.165	trace	2.828	" "
" " No. 5,"	0.027	0.083	20.56	17.72	Contains cesspool drainage. Unfit for use.
" " No. 6,"	0.027	0.027	2.742	4.251	Contains cesspool drainage. Typhoid bacillus.
" " No. 7,"	0.055	0.687	2.742	386.3	Contains cesspool drainage. Typhoid bacillus.
" " No. 8,"	0.027	0.055	6.856	8.433	Contains cesspool drainage. Unfit for use.
" " No. 9,"	trace	0,137	0.343	61.93	Doubtful, probably contaminated, and dangerous to use.
" " No 10,"	0.055	0.165	41.136	73.342	Contains cesspool drainage. Typhoid bacillus.
" " No. 11,"	0.055	0.220	8.227	97.094	Contains cesspool drainage. Typhoid bacillus.
" " No. 12,"	0.055	0.083	1 714	103 98	Contains cesspool drainage. Dysentery.

Waters Nos. 1, 2, 3 and 4, are in fit condition for drinking purposes. They contain minute amounts of decaying animal and vegetable matter, but not enough to affect their utility for household purposes. They are to be classed with waters fit for city use

No. 9 is in doubtful condition for household use   I find nothing in it to absolutely condemn it, but indications require that it should be examined frequently for the presence of hurtful material.

Sources Nos. 5 and 8 have been badly contaminated by cesspool drainage and contain sufficient nitrates to forbid their use for household purposes.

Nos. 6, 7, 10 and 11, are sources that should be abandoned at once, as there is evidently free communication with cesspools, and each of them contains large numbers of typhoid bacilli.

No. 12 contains drainage, such as I have found to come from cesspools used by dysenteric cases.

CHARLES M. CRESSON, M. D·

KEY TO ABOVE REPORT.

No. 1, from Channel Piers.
No. 2, from Lake North of Whallons Piers.
No. 3, from Inlet at Water Works.
No. 4, from Water Office.
No. 5, from Private Well, 7th Street between French and Holland.
No. 6, from Private Well, 19th Street between Walnut and Cherry.
No. 7, from Private Well, 431 13th Street, East Parade.
No. 8, from Private Well, —— 4th Street, West of Chestnut.
No 9, from Private Well, —— 2d Street, East of Hospital.
No. 10, from Private Well, 133 8th Street, West of Peach.
No. 11, from Private Well, 15 and 17 7th Street between State and Peach.
No. 12, from Private Well, 405 State Street.

It must be stated that this " key," which was sent, *sea'ed*, to the editor of this journal, was not opened until after the analyses were made, when the seal was broken in the presence of Dr. Charles M. Cresson and the Editor.

This absolutely impartial report adds another strong argument to those already advanced against the use of *well water* in cities.

SPECIAL REPORT.

The Health Exhibition at Brooklyn.

Dr. A. N. Bell, is a veteran Sanitarian, but, better than this, he is a *practical* sanitarian. Dr. Bell believes in *facts* rather than *theories*, in *showing* rather than *telling*, and in pursuance of this wise and *practical* belief, he organized, in connection with the late meeting of the American Public Health Association in Brooklyn, an exhibition of hygienic or health appliances that was not only extremely valuable (as an object lesson), but extremely interesting, as well.

VENTILATION.

The simple device represented in these drawings is well designed to allow the outside air to enter our rooms, without the danger of draughts.

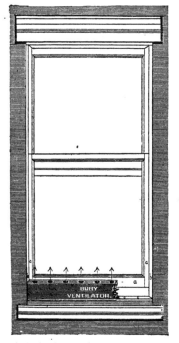 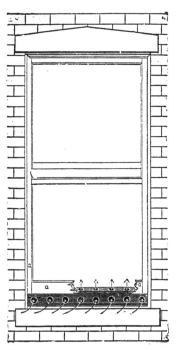

a a. Sash. *b b.* Window jambs. *c c.* Window sill.	*a a,* Sash.
This cut represents the view from within, the Bury Ventilator in operation. It is broken away at one end to show the sash raised above the outer holes to admit the air.	This cut represents the view from without, the Bury Ventilator in operation. The sash is broken away to show the ventilator behind with the fresh air passing in.

THE INFECTICIDE.

"The Infecticide" is a hollow ball, holding concentrated and powerful disinfectants and antiseptics and so devised as to automatically discharge them as needed. This ball is floated in the water-closet tank.

ADJUSTABLE SCHOOL DESKS.

We were much pleased to see on exhibition an adjustable school-desk, where the seat and desk could be lowered and raised independently of each other. This is a great advance in school furniture, for, we can imagine few more detrimental things' than to place a child at a desk, not proportioned to his or her size.

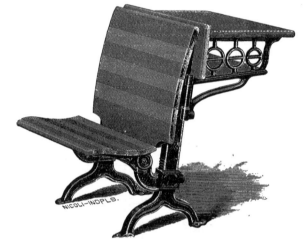

Front View.

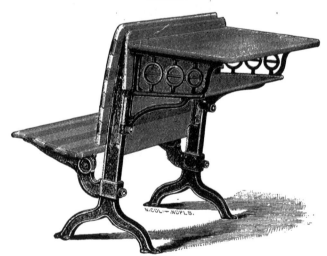

BackView.

STERILIZING MILK FOR INFANTS

Believing in Dr. Bell's idea of *object teaching*, it is our purpose, in this report, as far as possible, to let the various objects speak for themselves to the *eye*, rather than to furnish lengthy, *wordy* descriptions to the *ear*.

Water is poured into the pan or reservoir whence it passes slowly through three small apertures into the Shallow Copper Vessel beneath, becomes converted into steam and rises through the Funnel in the centre to the Sterilizing Chamber above. Here it accumulates under moderate pressure at a

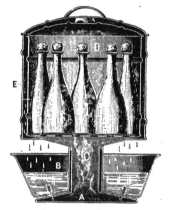 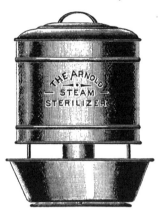

A. Shallow Copper Steam Generator. *B.* Reservoir or Pan. *C.* Steam Funnel. *D.* Sterilizing Chamber. *E.* Hood.

temperature of **212°** F. The excess of steam escapes about the cover, becomes imprisoned under the Hood and serves to form a steam jacket between the wall of the Sterilizing Chamber and the Hood. As the steam is forced down from above and meets the air it condenses and drips back into the reservoir.

It will generate steam from cold water in three or four minutes over an ordinary fire—coal, gas or kerosene. Time required for sterilizing milk—30 to 45 minutes.

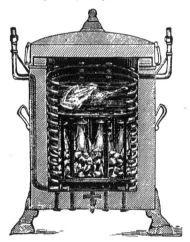

A FAMILY ICE MACHINE.

A most useful apparatus is here represented, by the aid of which those living in the country, where the visits of the "Ice-man" are like unto those of the "angels"; "few and far between," may enjoy the luxury of ice in summer, and can make this ice from water that they *know* is *pure.* As large a block as eighteen pounds of ice can be made with this machine.

THE CARE OF THE LOWER ANIMALS.

There is no earthly reason why the lower animals should not be kept as clean as human beings and, if they were, the food products derived from them would be much more wholesome.

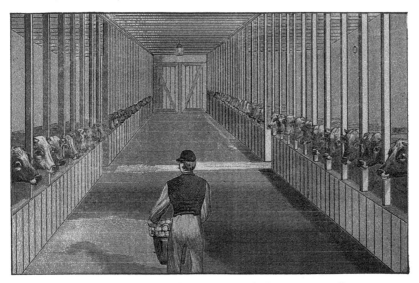

Interior of one of the Echo Farm Jains. "Three o'clock.—Time or Refreshments."

This interior view of one of the "Echo Farm" barns well illustrates the Sanitarian's dream of a *decent* barn, and the cleanliness prevading all parts of this "cow's home" is what should see in *all* out-buildings on *all* farms.

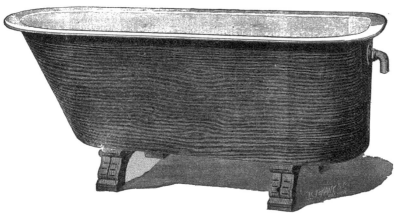

INDURATED FIBRE BATH-TUB.

The material from which this tub is made is a pure wood fibre. It is moulded in one piece under a heavy hydraulic pressure, and without joint or seam. As the rim of the tub is also part of this one piece, there is no crevice where impurities can possibly collect. The material is a non-conductor of heat and cold, adapting it not only for the " Electric Bath," but for retaining the heat in the water, thus greatly increasing the comfort of the bather. The material is the same from which for several years pails and other ware have been made, so well and favorably known throughout this and other countries. The pores of the fibre are filled with a hardening or indurating material, and subjected to a high degree of heat, making them impervious to water and practically indestructible. The outside of the tub in baking, is given a mahogany or rosewood finish, unless it is specially ordered to correspond with the wood-work of the room in which it is to be placed. The rim may be finished either as rosewood or with white enamel, as desired, corresponding with the porcelain tub.

The inner surface of the tub is lined with an imported white enamel prepared expressly for this use. The enamel may be tinted if preferred. This also is subjected to a high temperature, and thoroughly baked into the tub, making a hard, lasting, durable and impervious lining, capable of a high finish, which is easily cleaned without scouring, as it will not rust or absorb.

Throughout the process, nothing in the slightest degree injurious is used, and, with this treatment, the tub will be found to be a luxury, as its surface has a uniform temperature and is never cold.

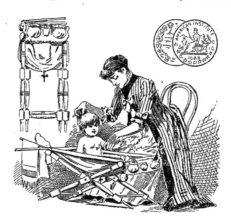

INFANT'S PORTABLE BATH TUB.

A very handy and convenient device is here depicted.

It is made of pure rubber on strong drilling cloth, made especially for the purpose, and folded over a pretty frame made of bamboo, cherry or ebonized wood, of camp-chair design, which can be made larger as the child grows older.

Attached to the bottom of the bath is a hard rubber faucet, for the water outlet. Connected at one end are pockets of rubber, gathered on and neatly trimmed with ribbon—pink and blue—for the reception of numerous little sundries attending the baby's toilet. The other end is furnished with a clothes or towel bracket.

The bath when closed, can be used as a valise in traveling, it having facilities for packing clothing and numerous little articles necessary for the infant's comfort. By placing a board over the frame, it can be used as a bed-side table, to hold a tray, flowers, books, etc. When folded up, the bath is about four inches thick and thirty-six inches long, and can be carried in an ordinary traveling trunk. It is pretty, practical, useful and convenient; which mothers will thoroughly appreciate—giving them an opportunity to enjoy the sweet and delightful pleasure of bathing their own babies, which should be less intrusted to inexperienced hands.

ANTI-SIPHON TRAP VENT.

This Vent fulfills all the conditions sought to be secured by trap vent pipes, and possesses the merit of great simplicity and economy, with *absolute security*.

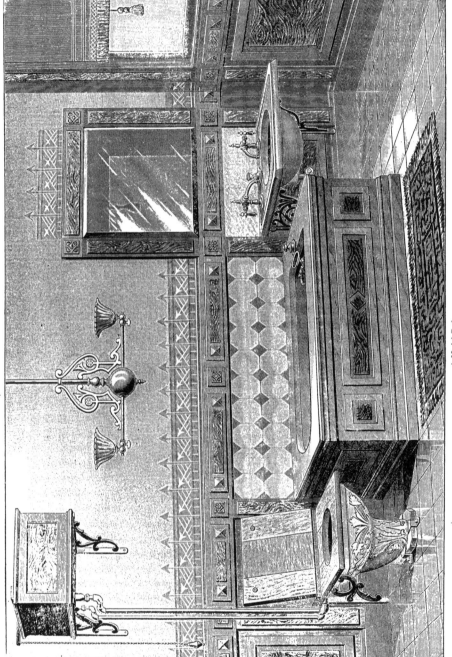

A Model Bath-room.

It admits a free flow of air into the waste pipe on the sewer side of the trap whenever a slight vacuum pressure occurs, *without disturbing its seal.* The air enters through an open thimble extending upward; and the opening is closed by an inverted cup, whose edges dip down into an annular groove containing mercury. (See fig. 1.)

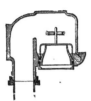

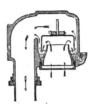

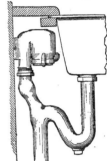

Fig. 1.—Sectional view of Vent with cup in normal position.

Fig. 2.—Sectional view of Vent with cup lifted out of the mercury by the inflowing current of air indicated by the arrows.

Fig. 3.—Showing position of Vent in relation to fixture and traps.

This cup is very light, so that it is lifted out of the mercury and suspended by the inflowing air whenever a partial vacuum occurs in the pipe, as shown in figure 2; but drops back into the mercury the instant the demand for air ceases. The deep seal thus formed, by the mercury around the edge of the cup, furnishes absolute security against any outflow of sewer air.

Practical experience has demonstrated that *each trap must be so vented as to receive on its sewer side an instant supply of air sufficient to meet every demand, without disturbing its seal.*

A MODEL BATH-ROOM.

The cut on preceding page we have introduced, that we may give some idea of how "A Model Bath-Room" ought to look. Plenty of light; spaces under basin and closet open to the air and the eye; instead of being closed receptacles for all kinds of rubbish, as is usually the case; a tile floor, that can be kept clean and withal an air of elegance and style very pleasing to the eye.

PAPER CUPS FOR THE EXPECTORATION OF CONSUMPTIVES.

We have, elsewhere, referred to the necessity for destruction of the expectoration of consumptives, and at this exhibition we were afforded the opportunity of seeing just the device to make this destruction practicable.

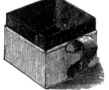

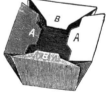

These cups are supported in simple racks, and at least once daily, or more frequently if necessary, should be removed from the rack and thrown into the fire.

WALL PAPERS THAT WASH.

Companionable with "rustless iron" and occupying (by chance, but most appropriately) a position next to it, we saw what we consider an equally great epoch-marking discovery in practical sanitation. As a rule sanitarians condemn the papering of walls, because of the inability to keep them clean, on account of which painted walls are always preferred. So also, after the occurrence of a contagious or infectious disease in a room it becomes necessary to scrape the paper from the walls because it cannot be disinfected. But here we have a wall paper that can be washed, and that with soap, aye, even with a disinfectant soap, and the beauty of it is that this paper looks just like the ordinary wall paper. We strongly commend this paper to every one.

RUSTLESS IRON

One of the greatest practical advances in sanitation, of recent years, we believe, is to be found in the production of the *rustless* iron, shown at this exhibition. Ordinary iron is so treated that it resists oxidation, thus removing the only valid objection that has ever been raised against the use of iron pipes for drainage purposes, namely, that they would corrode and thus become obstructed. The cost of this rustless iron is about 15 to 20 per cent. more than ordinary iron, but its extra durability would soon offset this extra cost.

THE DISPOSAL OF GARBAGE.

The destruction of garbage by fire is now so favorably regarded that it is unnecessary to do more than show the exterior and interior view of a furnace, for this purpose, that was on exhibition.

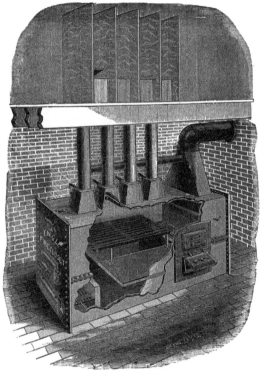

Figure 1. Exterior View of Garbage Cremator

BUTTERINE

Consists of oleo-oil and cream or milk. These ingredients, when churned—the whole being properly salted—give the new food product.

The method of producing oleo-oil is as follows: The selected fat is taken from the cattle in the process of slaughtering, and after thorough washing is placed in a bath of clean cold water and surrounded with ice, where it is allowed to remain until all animal heat has been removed. It is then cut into small pieces by machinery, and melted at an average temperature of 150 degrees until the fat in liquid form has separated from the fibrine or tissue, and then settled until it is perfectly clear. Then it is drawn into raining-vats and allowed to stand a day, when it is ready for the process. The pressing extracts the stearine, leaving the remaining product—known as oleo-oil. It is this article which, when churned with cream or milk, and sometimes with a small portion of creamery butter,—the whole being properly salted—gives the new food product, Butterine.

CHEMICAL APPARATUS FOR HEALTH LABORATORIES.

The laboratory should be supplied with both gas and water, with benches and tables; the gas must be laid on at different points, and the jets provided with burners of different kinds.

Chemical analysis is of two kinds, qualitative and quantitative; the object of the first, as the name implies, is to ascertain the nature of the several component parts of any given compound; that of the second is to determine the proportions or quantities of such components.

The operations of qualitative chemical analysis are easier and occupy less time than those of quantitative analysis; and in many cases it is sufficient to determine the nature of the chemical substance used for adulteration, and not go on to ascertain the quantity present in any article; although, to go thoroughly into the subject of adulteration, this also will in some instances be necessary.

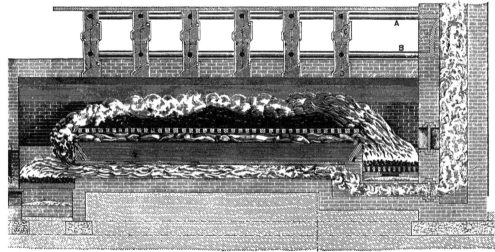

Figure 2. Interior View of Garbage Cremator.

The apparatus enumerated below includes the greater part of that which is required for both purposes.

For drying and evaporating.—A water, a sand, an air, and an oil bath, evaporating dishes of various sizes, and watch glasses.

For weighing and measuring.—A good balance; weights of brass and platinum; a specific gravity bottle, graduated pipettes, flasks, glasses of various sizes and measures, densimeters, as a saccharometer, galactometer and urinometer.

For filtration.—Funnel stands, funnels, and filtering paper.

For pulverisation.—Mortars; a mill.

For distillation.—A still, retorts, and condensers.

For incineration.—Muffles, porcelain and platinum crucibles and dishes.

In addition to the above apparatus, test tubes, a lactometer, thermometer (one not mounted, and having a long range of degrees), a wash bottle, and a drop tube, will be required.

When it is probable that a large number of samples of the same article will have to be examined, and many similar operations conducted at the same time, it is desirable that it should be furnished with series of crucibles, glasses, dishes, etc., of the same size.

Such an outfit was displayed at this exhibition, and, we were told, upon inquiry, that it would cost, with the *best of everything*, about two hundred dollars.

THE KODAK CAMERA.

Not alone as a "plaything" does the "Kodak Camera" possess claims upon our consideration.

It is a wood box, 3¼ x 3¾ x 6½ inches, covered with fine, black morocco, having in one end a lens aperture, on the top a folding key, a cord and a revolving disc, and on the side a button. When not in use it is enclosed in a neat hand-sewed sole-leather carrying case with shoulder-strap.

The workmanship of every part is of the very best, and the instrument will compare favorably with the finest field glass in finish and appearance.

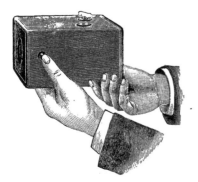 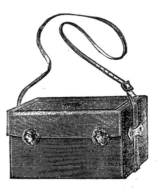

One end of the Kodak box contains the lens and shutter mechanism and the other end the roll holder for operating the band of sensitive film.

The Kodak reduces the ten or more operations, heretofore necessary to make an exposure with detective cameras to three operations, reduces the weight and bulk in the same proportion, and increases the number of pictures that can conveniently be made on one trip from *six* to *one hundred;* and it makes this very decided advance not by any sacrifice of quality of results, but in a way that guarantees a far better average than ever attained under the old conditions.

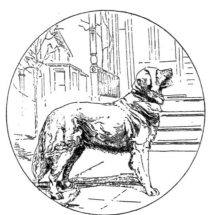

This is the exact size of a Kodak Picture.

It has suggested itself to us that this little apparatus would prove very valuable to Health Officers and Sanitary Inspectors for the purpose of photographing nuisances, and thereby perpetuating, for future reference, that which those so interested might remove from view.

CORONET WATER-CLOSET.

For this closet the inventor claims that, on account of the peculiar construction of the trap, the contents may be expelled by recourse to the simplest means, clogging and freezing are impossible, and the services of plumbers materially diminished.

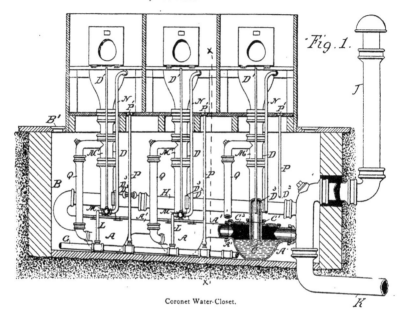

Coronet Water-Closet.

PATENT AIR PURIFIER.

When in operation it is placed preferably near a window. Its case is formed "bureau-like" and is provided with a number of compartments into which are entered a series of filtering webs, which are coated with a suitable absorbent, usually gypsum, which has a great affinity for water and fixes the ammonia in the atmosphere, and through these filtering webs the air is forced. The air is taken in at the window through a hole in the window-strip, A, and passes down a pipe at the rear of the filter case and enters said case below the first or lowest filtering web, illustrated at H. The said filtering webs are so arranged within the case that the air can only escape by passing through them. The air, after passing through the several antiseptics, escapes through apertures in the top of the case and enters the heating chamber proper. This chamber is provided with a lamp for heating the air. The air is here heated to 250° to destroy any living matter that may be contained in the air. While passing through the pipes it becomes cool before reaching the patient, and with an extension, or drum, N, which projects above the chamber, and centrally within this drum is arranged a combustion pipe, which passes through the drum at the top, said pipe discharging the products of combustion produced by the lamp (through pipe M) to the outside of the building at U. To the upper end of the air drum is connected the pure air pipe, F, concealed under the cornice, thence to the head board of the bed, where it is formed into branch pipes, to which are connected flexible tubes, one of which extends to near the patient's head, while the other is of a sufficient length to permit of its insertion beneath any portion of the bedclothes to supply the body with purified air when so desired. Said branch pipes are each provided with a suitable stop-cock whereby the flow of air may be regulated.

Here, we believe, is a " good thing." The inventor claims for it a wonderful potency in the cure of diseases. This aspect we will not discuss, but the moment we set eyes on this apparatus, we felt that we had found the proper way to secure an adequate supply of pure air for our use, when asleep, at night. By the aid of this apparatus the sleeper can be continually breathing the outside atmosphere, warmed to a proper temperature, inaddition to which (and this is a very important point), the tube passing underneath the bed clothes, will keep a supply of pure air constantly in contact with the body, a very great desideratum, as any one will admit, who places his nose to the bed-clothes after a night's rest. We heartily commend this apparatus for the purposes we have mentioned.

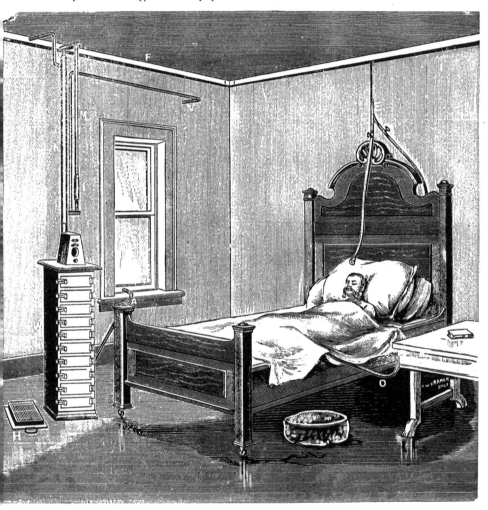

FELT SHOES AND SLIPPERS.

We were much interested in an exhibit of felt shoes and slippers, for it is well known that the human foot is one of the most exposed parts of the body and correspondingly susceptible to external influences. To keep the head cool, and the feet warm, is one of the first laws of hygiene; yet, no part of the body has been more habitually abused and neglected than the foot, without a healthy condition of which general good health is impossible. These All-Wool Felt Shoes are provided to meet this special need.

We reproduce some of these shoes, that our readers may see that a *hygienic* shoe does not necessitate the sacrifice of a *stylish* shoe : for who could want a neater looking foot-covering than is here figured, and if they did want it, WHERE COULD THEY GET IT ?

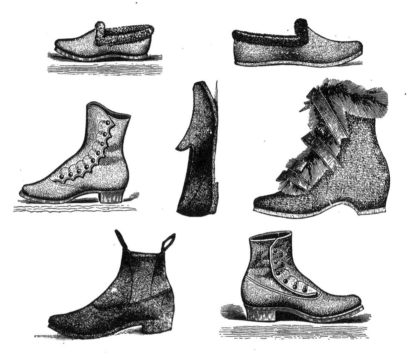

THE SANITARY CLOSET.

The principle of this closet is that of a bottle with a tightly-fitting stopper. The inventor claims that it abolishes the evils of the old privy system. No offensive odor constantly permeates the house. No intolerable smell about the premises at the time of cleaning. No unpleasant odor while the barrel is removed, adjusted, or transported. No exposure to chilling drafts. No pollution of the well and premises.

It is what has been long needed for cottages and country homes ; for villages and towns not having a water supply ; and for every place where the nuisance of a privy or vault has been endured.

Perhaps, the most approved method of removing " night soil " in cities is by transferring the contents of the vault (an unpleasant task) to closed barrels. The Sanitary Closet has all the advantages of this system of clearing, and more :—The time of transferring is saved ; the attendant odor is prevented ; the extra expense is avoided ; the least possible material is handled, only the excreta, and not twice its weight of earth with it.

The constant emptying of open and ventilated vaults into the atmosphere of the city is stopped.

It can be located in any convenient apartment adjoining the house, or in the house itself, or on an upper floor, by extending a pipe to the barrel in the basement.

Local ventilation, where desirable, is effected, as in case of the water-closet, by connecting the bowl with a suitable draft.

Whenever desirable, complete disinfection can be accomplished most easily, because both disinfectant and poison are confined together.

We were very favorably impressed with this device.

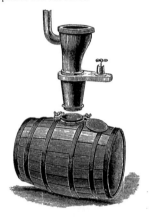

FILTRATION AND PURIFICATION OF WATER.

The system which is here figured claims great economy, because no additional land is required for its introduction, and no reservoir or basin is needed other than what is necessary for the filtration area; and the whole water supply is in constant process of filtration and aeration, and ready for use at all times.

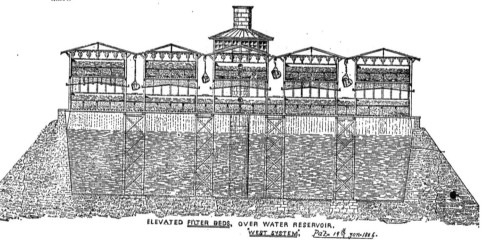

ELEVATED FILTER BEDS, OVER WATER RESERVOIR.
WEST SYSTEM. *Pat. 19th Jan. 1886.*

It has been our purpose in making this report to set before our readers all that was offered to view embodying principles, rather than to make it an advertisement for those who had goods on exhibition, hence we have not noticed the numberless articles for which the owners claimed great merit, but which represented or embodied no special principle. We have reported the exhibition as we saw it, and we have specially commended those devices, which we, ourselves, as the result of our own judgment, would wish to adopt for our own use.

The Foods of Different Peoples.

. Many nations, many dishes! Some articles that are esteemed as delicacies by certain nations are regarded with disgust by others. According to the *Pacific Record* the Turk is seized with violent trembling at the very idea of eating oysters. The American Indians look upon an invasion of grasshoppers as a mark of especial favor from the Great Spirit, and make the best of such a time to lay up a store of provisions for the future. Buckland states that among certain people a mixture of fish, nearly putrefied, and scap-suds is preferred to the best butter. In Canton and other Chinese cities rats are sold at ten cents a dozen, and a hind-quarter of dog is more expensive than mutton or beef. Some of the East Indians eat serpents dried in the oven, but despise the flesh of rabbits. Lizard eggs are a delicacy in the islands of the Pacific, and many people, besides the aboriginies of the Argentine Republic, esteem the flesh of the skunk. Ants are eaten by many peoples, and in Siam a curry of ants' eggs often tickles the palates of the wealthy. The silk-worm is eaten with relish by the Chinese, and a dessert of roast snails is considered a fitting termination of a feast in New Caledonia.

Hon. H. A. Scott on Hygiene.

In the course of an "Address of Welcome" before a recent "Sanitary Convention" at Ludington, Michigan, the Mayor of the city spoke, as follows:

"Hundreds of human lives have been sacrified in searching the Arctics and the Tropics for scientific knowledge; the oceans and the inland seas have been fathomed and made to give up the secrets of their darkest depths; the vast canopy over our heads has been explored and made to furnish us its secrets of science and knowledge; the very surface of the earth, almost from pole to pole, has been dug up and turned over, that its wealth of hidden resources might be utilized by man. The history of the world is conquest after conquest in search of that higher knowledge which shall disclose to us progressive ideas and intelligent thought. And while we may never discover that 'fountain of youth' which has been the bright and shining goal of untold generations, yet with the aid of sanitary science and the minds which have made this science what it is to-day, the people are better prepared than ever before in the world's history to grapple with the causes and to a certain degree prevent many of the diseases to which flesh is heir."

The Fatal "Family Well."

The obtundity of some minds to well demonstrated sanitary truths is something inexplicable (says *The Sanitary Volunteer*). To illustrate: We know of a family, all of whom have suffered for several years from the use of polluted well-water. They have been repeatedly told that the water was responsible for their poor health, but used it just the same. They shut up the house once or twice a year and go away for a fortnight, returning wonderfully improved in health, soon to relapse into their former state of "poor health" through the use of the polluted well-water. Recently, upon the urgent request of thoughtful relatives, they have had the water examined, and it showed a high degree of pollution from both sink-drain and privy. They have now abandoned the use of this water, have greatly improved in health, and are themselves preaching the dangers of water pollution to their neighbors. All this after the same dangers had been pointed out to them for more than ten years with no impression whatever. Sanitarians have learned that if there is anything on earth the average family will defend, till perhaps it destroys them all, it is the family well. It is a pleasure to see that this blind faith is being boldly shaken, and that the dangerous character of shallow wells is being more generally recognized than heretofore.

The Great White Plague.

The "Great White Plague," is what an exchange aptly terms that ever present scourge, consumption. The accompanying diagram from the office of the Michigan State Board of Health represents graphically the relative number of deaths from various contagious diseases in Michigan, as compared with the deaths from consumption:

Consumption.
Diphtheria.
Typhoid Fever.
Scarlet Fever.
Whooping Cough.
Measles.
Small-pox.

About as many die of consumption as of diphtheria, typhoid fever, and scarlet fever combined. And yet how little effort, either public or private, is made to suppress this great white plague. While, when a case of small-pox is learned of by the authorities, there is "hurrying to and fro," and the "mustering squadron" is put "forward with impetuous speed."—*The Health Journal.*

State Board of Health and Vital Statistics, of the Commonwealth of Pennsylvania.

PRESIDENT,
GEORGE G. GROFF, M. D., of Lewisburg.

SECRETARY,
BENJAMIN LEE, M. D.. of Philadelphia.

MEMBERS,
PEMBERTON DUDLEY, M. D., of Philadelphia.

J F. EDWARDS, M. D., of Philadelphia.   GEORGE G. GROFF, M. D., of Lewisburg.
T H. McCLELLAND, M. D., of Pittsburgh.   S. T. DAVIS, M. D., of Lancaster.
HOWARD MURPHY, C. E. of Philadelphia.   BENJAMIN LEE, M. D., of Philadelphia.

PLACE OF MEETING,
Supreme Court Room, State Capitol, Harrisburg, unless otherwise ordered.

TIME OF MEETING,
Second Wednesday in May, July and November.

EXECUTIVE COMMITTEE,
PEMBERTON DUDLEY, M. D., Chairman.   JOSEPH F. EDWARDS; M. D.
HOWARD MURPHY, C. E..   BENJAMIN LEE, M. D., Secretary.

Place of Meeting (until otherwise ordered)—Executive Office, 1532 Pine Street, Philadelphia.

Time of Meeting—Third Wednesday in January, April, July and October.

Secretary's Address—1532 Pine Street, Philadelphia.

Bureau of Registration and Vital Statistics—Department of Internal Affairs, State Capitol, Harrisburg.

State Superintendent of Registration of Vital Statistics—BENJAMIN LEE, M. D.

HENRY LEFFMAN, M. D.,
Analytical Chemist and Expert,
715 Walnut Street,

PHILADELPHIA, Oct. 26, 1889.

MESSRS. EISNER & MENDELSON :

Sirs :—In response to inquiries made concerning the relative merits of the Johann Hoff's Malt Extract, and that sold under the name of Tarrant's Hoff's Extract, I may state as follows :

"That I have, during the past eighteen months, made a number of examinations of the principal forms of Malt Extract in the market, and have among other matters, satisfied myself that the Johann Hoff's Malt Extract, as imported by you, is a Genuine Extract of Malt."

The judgment of the value of a liquid preparation of Malt will be largely based on the percentage of Alcohol, and the presence of any preservative, especially Salicylic Acid. It may be justly said that the less Alcohol found the better, provided its place is not taken by some more objectionable substance. Under such considerations, the Johann Hoff's Malt Extract possesses decided advantages over the preparation sold under the name of Tarrant's Hoff's Extract, in the fact that the former contains three and one-half per cent. of Alcohol, while the latter has yielded in two samples, four and three-quarters, and five per cent. respectively.

Further, I have noted in a number of examinations of the latter article— Tarrant's Extract—the presence of Salicylic Acid, while I have never, in repeated examinations of the Eisner & Mendelson Johann Hoff's Extract, found any trace of such preservative. The effects of Salicylic Acid have been extensively studied, and the unanimous opinion of sanitary chemists is, that it is very objectionable as an addition to any form of food or drink, and especially objectionable in Malt Extract. From some observations made in my own laboratory, and published in the *Polyclinic* in May, 1888, it appears that not only does Salicylic Acid wholly suspend the action of Diastase, to which Malt owes it starch converting power, but that the starch digesting power of the pancreatic secretion is also wholly suspended by it. It thus appears the addition of this body is to render the Extract not only inactive so far as its own function is concerned, but it introduces into the system an injurious substance, and one which interferes with an important function. Sanitary authorities, in various parts of Europe, have given from time to time much attention to the now indiscriminate use of this acid, and have all, so far as I am aware, condemned its employment in any article of food or drink. For this reason, among others as above noted, I am of the opinion that the Genuine Johann Hoff's Malt Extract, as imported by Eisner & Mendelson, is to be preferred. I may say that all the examinations were made on samples obtained in the open market, and in the bottles as originally imported.

Yours,

Henry Leffman. M. D.

Prof. Chem. Woman's Med. Col., and Penna. Col. Dental Surgery,
Food Inspector, Pennsylvania Board of Agriculture.

EQUITABLE
Life Assurance Society

OF THE UNITED STATES.

A comparison of the Statements of the different Companies shows that The Equitable Life Assurance Society of the United States, in 1888, exceeded every other Life Assurance Company in the following important respects. It had

The Largest New Business			$153,933,535
" " Amount of Assurance in force . . .			549,216,126
" " Premium Income			22,047,813
" " Total Income			26,958,978
" " Excess of Income over Disbursements . .			10,129,071
" " Four per cent. Surplus			20,794,715
" " Amount of Surplus Earned			5,067,124
" " Increase in Assurance in Force . . .			66,186,564
" " " " Premium Income			2,932,058
" " " " Interest, Dividend and Rent Income			786,090
" " " " Total Income			3,718,128
" " " " Assets.			10,664,018
" " " " Surplus			2,690,460
" " " " Payments to Policy-holders .			1,821,948

The strength and good management of the Society are also shown by the fact that of all the leading companies it has

The Highest Ratio of Assets to Liabilities . . .	128 per cent.
The Smallest Ratio of Expenses to New Business . .	3.22 per cent.
Assets	$95,042,922.96
Liabilities	74,248,207.81
Surplus (4 per cent.)	$20,794,715.15

The New Assurance Contract of the Equitable Life Assurance Society is a SIMPLIFIED, LIBERALIZED, IMPROVED, FREE TONTINE POLICY. It contains all the advantages heretofore offered, together with many that are new.

For full and exact information, address

FRANK CAMPBELL, General Agent,

P. O. Box 645.   Market and Third Streets, HARRISBURG, PA.

N. B.—First-class Insurance Agents would advance their own interests by corresponding with the undersigned, FRANK CAMPBELL, Harrisburg, Pa.

THE
ANNALS
OF
HUGIENE

VOLUME V.

Philadelphia, February 1, 1890

NUMBER 2.

COMMUNICATIONS

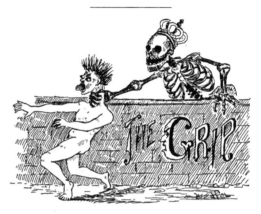

BY SAMUEL G. DIXON, M. D.,

Professor of Hygiene in the University of Pennsylvania.

Epidemic Catarrh, commonly called Influenza, ("fashionable": a secondary signifaction of the word.) The laity have adopted the title "La Grippe," (from agripper, to seize, or from an insect called La Gripper, which abounded in great numbers in France just previous to an invasion of this peculiar malady. It is also called "Creatan" from creat, the chest. The French sometimes call it "Coqueluche," from the cap worn by those suffering from the epidemic. The Germans frequently term it "Chicken disease."

The importance of a full knowledge of this peculiar disease cannot be overestimated when we take into consideration the increased death rate during the prevalence of this disease since the fourteenth century, In fact I have no doubt but that the pestilence related by Homer, which spread through the Greek quarter and lasted but a few days, was this malady. The specific poisoning agency does not of itself often bring about dissolution of the animal tissues, yet it does reduce the vitality of the cells so that they become a prey for other destroying agencies. Cells that otherwise successfully battle against the various pathogenic organisms constantly taken into the system, seem to be robbed by this malady of their resisting powers, and permit the pathogenic microbes to make the tissues their habitat, in which they multiply to untold numbers and disfranchise the rightful occupants. It is in this indirect way that the epidemic Catarrhal Fever causes the death-roll too often double the length of its column.

The malady, now so widespread throughout the world not only attacks man—paying little or no regard to nationality, wealth, poverty, sex, age or temperament or to the conditions surrounding us—but it also attacks the lower animals, such as the horse, cow, sheep, deer, and the swine. It travels hither and thither, without regard to any known lines.

In 1557, the poison seemed to have its origin in Asia, and traveled westward. In 1580, its course was from the East and South to the West and North. In 1782, it first appeared in Canton, and moved westward to Great Britain, while in 1803, its course was from South to North. In 1839 an Influenza visited Chatham Islands, (a group in the Pacific, about 500 miles east of New Zealand.) During that epidemic nearly half the inhabitants died.

It would seem that the points of the compass have little or no influence upon the course traversed by the contagion of this disease, nor does any point seem too far distant for it to reach. The winds and the course of human travel do not seem to entirely govern its wanderings, yet they each must be considered a propelling power. In 1836, two distinct epidemics appeared co-instantaneously, one at Sydney, England, and the other at the Cape of Good Hope. This rarely occurs. History shows that the widespread epidemics usually originate in some one locality, from which they mysteriously take their departure, visiting, sometimes, nearly every inhabited country.

The evidence thus far compiled does not show any positive influence of heat or of its moderate abstraction.

No relation has yet been demonstrated between it and metorological phenomena. From the statistics taken just previous to and during an epidemic it would seem that telluric emanations have little or nothing to do with the cause.

No satisfactory record has yet been made showing the electrical conditions of the atmosphere previous to and during the continuance of " La Grippe." Ozone is irritating to the mucous membrane, and is always found in the atmosphere during a thunder-storm ; from these facts we might suspect the electricity surrounding us of being a predisposing cause of the malady under consideration.

Hygroscopic statistics rather tend to show a relationship between the disease and the damp, foggy weather, so often preceding an invasion of the malady. This is probably only another factor that favors the propagation of some unknown microbe, and at the same time acts as a predisposing cause.

It is possible that several conditions must exist at one and the same time, no one factor being sufficient to form or propagate or disseminate the contagion. Sufficient evidence has not yet been adduced to settle the relation of the germ theory of disease with the origin of this most peculiar epidemic malady.

In 1879, some Doctor of Medicine, I think in Chicago, claimed to have discovered the germ producing the epidemic disturbance. He described it as having the appearance of a nutmeg, with hairs growing from its outer coat. This, however, proved to be but a ciliated epithelium rightfully lining the normal respiratory tract, and not a " Pathogenic animalcule."

Many unsuccessful attempts have been made to discover a microörganism peculiar to the epidemic catarrhal fever now so prevalent in our midst. It may be that the proper culture medium has not yet been found necessary for the existence of the fungus we are in search of. It is quite possible that the spore takes a much longer time to germinate than we have yet allotted it in the artificial culture medium. Our staining processes, used in research for other organisms, may not answer for one peculiar to this malady. If this be so it will account for the numerous failures to detect any microbe in the blood or tissues of those suffering from this catarrh. Our knowledge of bacteriology is still in its infancy, therefore we must be patient and persevering in our work before denying the existence of a microbe peculiar to the present epidemic. We must resist the temptation to be assertive.

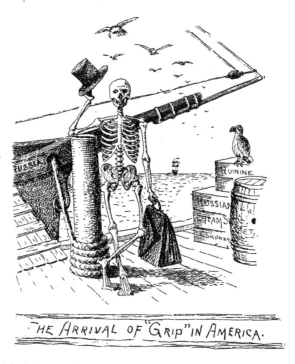

THE ARRIVAL OF "GRIP" IN AMERICA.

The biological research necessary to discover the etiology of the disease under consideration will have to be carried on in the tissues of the body, in the atmosphere and in the soil. It may not ever enter the body, but generate a poison that diffuses through the atmosphere. So general is the distribution of the poison that I must believe that it has the power of reproduction, otherwise it would soon become exhausted.

From the fact that the mucous membrane is mostly affected in contagious diseases, coupled with the fact that the poison in question is particularly irritating to that membrane, I am inclined to again suspect its contagiousness. Diphtheria,

Measles, Hooping-cough, Scarlet Fever, Dysentery and many other maladies that are positively contagious are good examples to substantiate this proposition.

It would be tedious to enumerate all the facts I have collated that tend to prove the contagious character of this and past epidemics of La Grippe, therefore it must suffice to say that my conclusion is that it is slightly contagious.

As the facilities for rapid and more general travel and transfer of merchandise and the mail are increased, so are the labors of the investigator in this regard made more difficult.

An immunity for a time is in all probability induced by an attack of this disease, yet an attack is certainly a predisposing cause to many other ills.

The disturbances in the human system caused by the present contagion are not unlike those related as being present in past epidemics.

The first case that came under my observation was in Paris last August. The patient was a lady about fifty years of age of robust constitution. The disease first manifested itself by a nasal catarrh, a slight bronchitis and much mental distress. She expressed a feeling as if some one was clasping her by the throat. Much headache was complained of, which was so severe that it interfered with sleep. Great weakness of the lower limbs was an annoying symptom. The heart action was feeble and there was a slight rise in the temperature. The case ran a favorable course in four days which was followed by a slow and distressing convalescence. Immediately following this case four other ladies in the same house were taken with a general catarrh. Since the present epidemic broke out in this city, a very peculiar case occurred under my observation in which there was an exaggerated localized hyperæsthesia immediately over both the anterior and posterior heart region.

Many cases are ushered in with a chilly sensation, while others first manifest themselves by exaggerated break-bone rigors, alternating with fever. Others have a long prodrome stage characterized by dizziness, great weakness of the lower limbs and back, followed by diarrhœa and drowsiness. Others again are first characterized by sneezing and marked coryza with a dry, hard cough. Rheumatic pains and mental depression are sometimes the premonitory symptoms. Violent retching is often experienced in the early stage of the disease. Diarrhœa or constipation are generally present. Sweating is a very common symptom. The tonsils and throat are in some cases much inflamed, which inflammation frequently attacks the Eustachian tube and reaches the middle ear, causing ear-ache. The violence of the poison some times would appear to be spent on the mucous membrane of the stomach.

Life is often endangered by heart depression.

We find a feeble heart action in a majority of the cases.

The temperature varies much in different patients.

The onset of some cases is characterized by an irregular chilliness with exacerbations and remissions, giddiness, vomiting, stiffness of the limbs with marked nervous symptoms.

From the great variety of symptoms manifested during the course of this catarrhal fever we must conclude that the Materies Morbi (a certain contagion) is specially irritating to the mucous membrane and that the disturbance becomes a systemic one. This general poisoning lowers the life of the tissues and renders them susceptible to other maladies.

The morbidity and mortality from a great variety of maladies during the present invasion of catarrhal fever go to show its devitalizing characteristic.

A resume would be somewhat as follows :

It takes up its abode both in palaces and in hovels.

Its lines of travel are so diverse and so opposed to all known influences that we are unable as yet to explain its mode of transit.

Meteorology is not known to be a factor in the etiology of this malady.

No unusual telluric emanations seem to precede or accompany the epidemic.

Statistics of the electrical conditions of the atmosphere during an invasion would be of much interest.

Foggy, damp weather frequently foreruns an epidemic.

No microbe has yet been found that is characteristic of this malady, yet we have reason to anticipate its discovery.

It is slightly contagious.

It is the exciting cause that kindles many latent maladies.

It renders the system susceptible to other poison.

Its rapid spread over a vast territory points to the air as one of its carriers.

Death is rarely caused directly by epidemic catarrhal fever.

It grants a very limited immunity from subsequent attacks.

Its onset is sometimes sudden and again it has a long prodrome.

Its active stage averages about four days, during which time a great variety of symptoms manifest themselves, such as sneezing, coryza, headache, nasal and bronchial catarrh, cough, sore throat, earache, vomiting, diarrhœa or constipation sweating, dizziness, pains in the limbs, (muscles, tendons and bones) mental excitement, nervous twitching and delirium.

Convalescence is protracted, and is often attended with great muscular weakness and mental depression, general malaise and irritation of the respiratory tract. During this stage the patient should not be exposed to exhaustion, severe cold or a sudden change of temperature, or to pathogenic microbes. If much care is not observed, consumption, pneumonia or other maladies are apt to follow and terminate in death. A certain number of deaths can be charged to the indiscriminate use of drugs by the laity. It would seem to overlook the fact that a medicine sufficiently powerful to destroy such an intense contagion or to neutralize its poison, or to stimulate the tissues sufficiently to resist or overcome such a potent enemy, also has the power to destroy human life. A layman should never take it upon himself to prescribe. Medicine should only be taken under the advice of the most intelligent and conscientious members of the medical profession.

The great aim of the age should tend toward the discovery of the cause and the means of prevention. It is as difficult to induce the tissues to resume their normal state when once diseased, as to perfectly restore the immaculate sheet that has been once blotted. Preventive medicine points to a higher order of thought than does curative medicine. I think we can safely boast that the era is here in which preventive medicine will take the ascendency. To effectively accomplish this, we must have national sanitary laws governing quarantine and disinfection. The Government should be prompt in taking up this great work. I should think the people would demand it when they stop to think of the vast amount of sorrow,

physical suffering, money and labor that the present epidemic has cost, with the fact that it is quite likely it could be prevented; the question must arise as to the advisability of adding another member to the Cabinet: "Why should we not have a General of Public Health as well as a Secretary of the Interior?

For all we well know that health is man's richest possession, and that disease is man's greatest enemy, and also, that health can be preserved and the causes of disease successfully combatted, the government treats them with indifference.

How active the authorities would be if an English gun-boat ran into one of our harbors and fired upon and wounded a single American citizen, yet an epidemic catarrhal fever has entered into our very midst, wounded and killed, directly or indirectly, hundreds of our citizens, and the Government has treated it with perfect indifference. What would be done by our Government officials should some disease attack the great wheat fields of the West? A commission would be appointed at once to search for the cause and a method of prevention.

The present epidemic has penetrated the very heart of our country, carrying with it suffering and death, and nothing has been done by the Government to investigate its nature and its prevention.

January 14, 1890.

The Ideal Disposition of the Dead.*

BY REV. CHARLES R. TREAT,
Of New York.

It is a strange thing that the time should have come to attack the churchyard in its use for the burial of the dead; but it is really far more strange that the churchyard should have come to be one of man's most deadly foes. This, however, every thoughtful man will now have to admit to be true, and this will make easy what otherwise would have been impossible for a tender or reverent mind.

As a general statement, it will suffice to quote the words with which Lord Beaconsfield denounced the churchyard, in the House of Lords, in 1880. "What is called 'God's Acre' is not adapted to the times in which we live or to the spirit of the age. The graveyard is an institution prejudicial to the public health; and the health of the people ought to be one of the considerations of a statesman. The time has arrived when a safer disposition of the dead should be instituted."

In view of such a statement, and of many more that come readily to mind that have been made in stronger terms, and most of all in view of the fact that the agitation against the churchyard has been maintained for more than a hundred years, it is amazing that this use should die so hard; and, as we survey the past, it will amaze us more, to be compelled to confess, that the churchyard has been made man's foe by civilized and Christian men! The story of this use of consecrated ground is so short that, although familiar, it may well be told again.

In the early Christian centuries, as in the centuries preceding, among men of all religious beliefs and practices, the conviction, both instinctive and founded on

------

* Address elaborately illustrated by stereopticon, before the American Public Health Association, at Brooklyn N. Y., and reprinted from *The Sanitarium.*

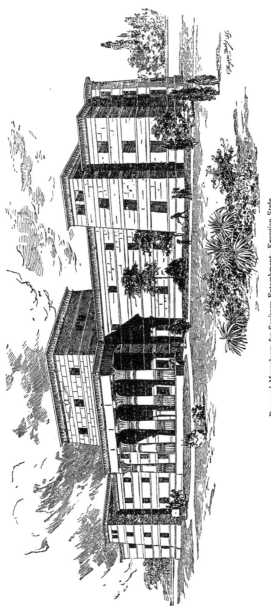

Proposed Mausoleum for Sanitary Entombment—Egyptian Style.

experience, prevailed, that the dead should not be brought into proximity with the living. Accordingly the practice definitely demanded by the "Twelve Tables" became universal, not to bury within a "city" or any group of human habitations. The first step in the wrong direction seems to have been taken at the dying request of the first Christian emperor, who was interred at the entrance of the Church of the Holy Apostles, in Constantinople. The tendency, however, to follow this example, and to secure similar interment in holy earth, was stubbornly resisted ; and it was not until the latter part of the sixth century that burials were permitted within towns or cities, and it was not until the eleventh century that burials were permitted in churches. From this time the custom continued without notable interference, until the latter part of the last century. Then, in that era of tremendous change, the churchyard did not escape. In Paris, the churchyard of the Church of the Holy Innocents was first condemned in the interest of the public health, because much sickness had been traced to the foul stenches that rose therefrom ; and it is worthy of·special notice, as indicating the extent of the danger, that M. Thouret, the official charged with the duty of disinterring the dead, was overcome by the foul air that he was compelled to breathe, and barely escaped with his life from a putrid fever that he there contracted. A little later the grounds about the churches of St. Germain des Pres and St. Eustache were also barred from burial, and the contents of their graves were carried to the quarries that have since become the "Catacombs' of Paris. In Austria, under Joseph II, the ruler of such unhappy methods but of such noble aims and advanced ideas, the burial of the dead within or near to churches was prohibited by law, and this was such an honest enactment that neither rank nor wealth could evade it.

In England, unhappily, the progress of this reform was not so rapid. Bishop Latimer had soundly said, in a discourse upon the restoration to life of the widow's son at Nain: "The citizens of Nain hadd their buryinge-place withoute the citie, which no doubt is a laudable thinge. And I do marvel that London, being a great citie, hath not a burial-place withoute. For no doubte it is an unwholesome thinge to bury within the citie, especiallie at such time when there be great sicknesses and many die together. I think verilie that many taketh his death in St. Paul's churchyard. And this I speak of experience, for I myself, when I have been there some mornings, to heare the sermons, have felt such an unwholesome and ill-favoured savour, that I was the worse for it a while after, and I think no lesse but it is the occasion of great sickness and disease." And it is deserving of mention that Sir Christopher Wren entreated the citizens of London, in rebuilding the city after the great fire of 1666, to put an end to the pernicious practice of burying within their churches and about them, and even within the limits of their city. But these appeals, and many more that were more urgent and more recent, were vain, and it was not until nearly the middle of our proud century that England would listen to the reformer of this crying evil.

In this country, partly because there were few places of large population, and partly because it was an early and general tendency to use cemeteries rather than churches and the grounds adjacent to them, the evils of earth-burial did not manifest themselves so soon or in so marked a manner as in the old world. But there were instances enough to convince the most incredulous that a radical change must be

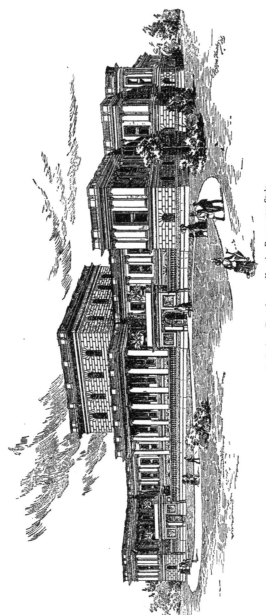

Proposed Mausoleum for Sanitary Entombment—Venetian Romanesque Style.

made. Dr. Ackerly, writing in 1822, thus describes the condition of the burial-ground connected with Trinity Church, New York, forty years before: "During the Revolutionary War this ground emitted pestilential vapors, the recollection of which is not obliterated from the memory of a number of living witnesses." In the same year the *Commercial Advertiser* published an article in reference to the present evils of earth-burial at the same place, in which it was said: "It will be remembered that the graveyard, being above the streets on the west and encompassed by a massive stone wall, and the east side being on a level with Broadway, it results that this body of earth, the surface of which has no declivity to carry off the rain, thus becomes a great reservoir of contaminating fluids suspended above the adjacent streets. In proof of this, it is stated that in a house in Thames Street, springs of water pouring in from that ground occasioned the removal of the tenants on account of their exceeding fœtidness.' At a later date Dr. Elisha Harris brought this telling indictment against the same place of inter-ment: "Trinity churchyard has been the centre of a very fatal prevalence of cholera, whenever the disease has occurred as an endemic near or within a quarter of a mile of it. Trinity Place west of it, Rector Street on its border, the streets west of Rector, and the occupants of the neighboring offices and commercial houses have suffered severely at each visitation of the pest from 1832 to 1854." It seems hardly necessary to add that the foregoing statements are not intended to make the impression that there was a worse condition at the churchyard named than at any other. The truth is, that this only illustrates what was universal throughout the city; and, in proof, it may be cited, among the unsavory recollections of the time, that the sexton of the "Brick Church," Beekman Street, was accustomed to caution the persons standing near, when a body was to be deposited in the vaults, saying: "Stand on one side. You are not accustomed to such smells!" And the sexton of the Dutch Church close by was known to have said that, when going down into the vaults, the candles lost their lustre, and that the air was so "sour and pungent that it stung his nose." Naturally, therefore, it was noted in the public press: "This being the case with all the vaults where dead bodies are deposited and subject to be opened at all seasons, this method of disposing of the remains of our friends is, at the least, an unpleasant and certainly a dangerous one." And the result was to be expected, that the Board of Health should utter their official protest against the continuance of the perilous practice, as they did in 1886: "Interment of dead bodies within the city ought to be prohibited. A vast mass of decaying animal matter, produced by the superstition of interring dead bodies near the churches, and which has been accumulating for a long time, is now deposited in many of the most populous parts of the city. It is impossible that such a quantity of animal remains, even if placed at the greatest depth of interment commonly practiced, should continue to be inoffensive or safe!"

It may now be said: "Yes, this is all true, but we have changed all that! We no longer inter our dead in churchyards or burial-grounds within the limits of the cities. We have provided cemeteries at great distances from our cities and large centres of population, and there the dead can do no harm."

To this the reply is easy and convincing; that, if the dead endanger the living when the population is dense, they certainly also endanger them when the population is sparse. The danger is only diluted. It still exists, and it ought to alarm us

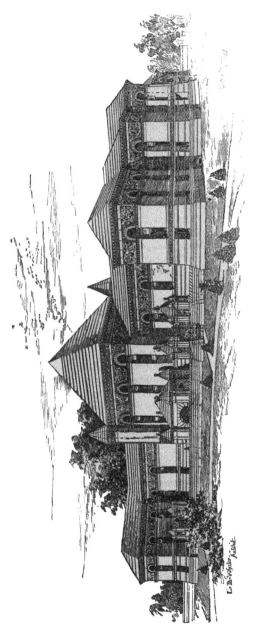

Proposed Mausoleum for Sanitary Entombment—Romanesque Style.

just as truly when a few are imperilled as when many are. As lovers of our kind, as claiming to be humane, we can no more be indifferent to the danger of a few than to the danger of many. True philanthropy has no sliding scale by which to gauge her gifts. And if the evils of earth-burial issue from the facts that a lifeless body is buried in the earth, then these are not escaped and can not be, unless the dead are bnried at such a distance from the living that the living can never come into contact with the earth in which they lie, or breathe the air or drink the water which they pollute. Therefore, the question, as to the effect upon human health of our cemeteries, can be considered settled in the case of all that are not remote from the habitations or the approach of men ; and such cemeteries, as we know, are few, and they are not the cemeteries which lie upon the borders of our great cities.

To strengthen this general position it will be sufficient to quote the familiar but weighty assertion of Sir Henry Thompson : "No dead body is ever placed in the soil without polluting the earth, the air, and the water above it and about it ;" and the testimony of Dr. Holland, who speaks as the opponent of this reform and the antagonist of Sir Henry Thompson, that the best situated cemeteries may be so mismanaged as to become unsafe ; that cemeteries should not be too near dwellings ; that they should not be overcrowded ; that the soakage from them should be carefully guarded against ; and that wells near burial-grounds are unfit sources of drinking water ; and the declaration of the French Academy of Medicine, that the cemeteries of Pére-la-Chaise, Montmartre, and Montparnasse, once suburban now intramural, are the cause of serious disorders of the head and throat and lungs, that result in the loss of many lives ; and to note the experience of Brooklyn, half-girdled with graves, of which the editor of The Sanitarian does not hesitate to assert : "Typhoid-fever is, taking one year with another, increasingly prevalent in Brooklyn, and it is, in our judgment, probably due for the most part to sewage-pollution of the intensest and most loathsome kind—the seepage of graveyards !"

Thus far this subject has been treated as though the only evil influence that a decomposing body could exert would be through the poisonous character of the resultant compounds. Unhappily, the story is only partly told, and greater dangers remain to be revealed.

[*To be continued.*]

Peddlers as Disseminators of Disease.

The danger of peddlers and hawkers spreading infection from house to house has often occurred to me (says the editor of *The Sanitary Inspector*). The new law regulating this business cuts off much of the danger by the exclusion of foreign peddlers from the State of Maine. This class of peddlers was so importunate that it was hard to exclude them from the dwellings of the poorer classes, even if a case of scarlet fever or diphtheria were in the room into which the door opened. An instance of the spread of scarlet fever by a family of hawkers in Scotland is mentioned in a late number of the *Sanitary Record*, but in that case the source of the mischief was more easily traced, because it was found that one of the children of the peddler had scarlet fever.

The Outbreak of Typhoid Fever in Johnstown, Pa.*

BY GEO. W. WAGONER, M. D.

of Johnstown.

At the time of the ever memorable flood of May 31, 1889, there was not, to the best of my knowledge, a single case of typhoid fever in Johnstown. When the mighty rush of waters came, bearing upon its bosom the bodies of its human and animal victims, together with the filth of the miles of territory over which it swept in awful fury, the course of the torrent was held in check by the stone bridge long enough to allow all the organic matter to be deposited over a comparatively small area. In this district the greater proportion of the citizens of Johnstown resided before the flood, and after the work of destruction had been done, the wretched survivors returned to the sites of their former homes and began the gigantic task of making them habitable or building up new ones. They found masses of debris over the familiar places, which appalled by their magnitude, and sickened them at heart when they realized that in the mass were the bodies of their dearest kindred and friends. Over and through it all was a most tenacious mud, from which foul odors arose continuously. In the dark days which followed, the citizens were deprived of many of the common necessaries of life to which they were formerly accustomed ; they were crowded together so that all the comforts of home life were impossible to obtain ; the character of their food was entirely changed ; they were wrought up to the highest nervous tension, and lived with a feverish anxiety which was exhausting in the extreme. And then a persistent, drizzling rain kept the whole valley shrouded in a mist, and added to the intense discomforts of life in this sorely-stricken district. From such a maze of unhappy circumstances it would be reasonable to expect the development of diseases, which would spread with rapidity, and flourish into malignancy, because all the conditions were so favorable. But it is a fact, which deserves to be remembered with profound gratitude, and recorded with feelings of honest pride, that the most virulent diseases did not spring forth to continue the harvest of death among a depressed people, and that those diseases which were met with were mild in character and easily controlled. This satisfactory condition of the public health was not the result of happy chance, but was the legitimate outcome of thorough, persistent and intelligent application of all the principles and methods of sanitary science applicable to the case. The State Board of Health was equal to this unparalleled emergency, and was unrelenting in its efforts until all the gross causes of disease were thoroughly removed. It should not be supposed, however, that there was no sickness in the flooded district. On the contrary, there was enough of an abortive character to indicate what might have occurred had not disinfection been so thoroughly enforced.

The first case of typhoid fever, after the flood of May 31, was observed on June 10, 1889. It was located, however, in Stony Creek township, two miles from the town, in the open country ; several hundred feet above the highest level of the flood and far away from any possible contamination by it. It occurred in a farm-house, and the physician in attendance states there were seven other cases following, which

---

*Prepared at the request of the Secretary of the State Board of Health.

were probably infected by it. The attending physician does not venture an opinion as to the origin of this case, but there is evidence to indicate that there were cases of fever in this neighborhood a short time before the flood. The people used spring water. On June 21st another physician reports his first case, as occurring in the same locality and among the neighbors and friends of the case originating on June 10, 1889. He has knowledge of six cases spreading from his first case. He mentions as the probable cause of the outbreak of fever in this locality, that the farmers stored and washed flooded goods on their premises. But if this were a sufficient cause for the origin of the fever, it should also have developed at an early date in the flooded district, and among the people who were constantly handling the same soiled goods. The earliest date given for the development of a case in the flooded district, positively diagnosed as typhoid fever, is July 29, 1889, two months after the calamity.

Some of the farmers living in Stony Creek township, and who had the disease in their families, were engaged in the dairy business. They all depended upon springs for their water supply. They distributed large quantities of milk to Moxham, a thriving suburb of Johnstown, which was not damaged by the flood, and to which large numbers of the homeless sufferers fled for refuge. The water supply of the farming district does not communicate with that of Moxham. It is a fact that milk was distributed to Moxham from houses in which death had occurred from typhoid fever. On June 21st the first case is reported from Moxham, and the physician has knowledge of six other cases developing in the immediate vicinity. Another physician reports his first case in Moxham as occurring on July 1st, with ten following soon after. Another physician had his first case in Moxham on July 15th, with ten following. Each of these physicians attribute the development of the disease to impure spring water. The water supplied to the case developing on July 1st, was analyzed and found to be full of impurities. It is stated that old clothing and flood goods were washed above this spring and consequently contaminated it with the poisonous germs of typhoid fever. While this may be the fact, yet it seems strange that the disease did not develop at a very early date after the flood, among the hundreds of people who were continuously in contact with the most concentrated filth in the devastated region. It is stated of the case developing July 15th, that the water supply of the family was drawn from a spring located on lower ground and within thirty yards of a neighbor's spring, in which the clothing and bedding of a patient dead with typhoid fever, had been washed a few days previous to the outbreak of the disease in the family. The connection between these two outbreaks seems undoubted.

Four other physicians report their first cases as occurring, one on July 1st, another on July 6th, another on August 11th, and the fourth on September 1st. They were all in widely separated localities, but in each case the patient had been employed at Moxham and drank of the water found there. These facts are very significant, especially when it is remembered that Moxham is a new town, built upon sloping ground, and at that time depending upon surface springs and wells, and surface drainage. These conditions were absolutely unavoidable, however, in a town of such rapid growth as Moxham. The defects are being overcome as rapidly as time and money will allow. Given a community situated as Moxham is, deposit in it the germs of an infectious disease, and it must of necessity spread in all directions.

It is remarkable, indeed, that the disease did not become much more general in Moxham than it did. Three of the four cases which appear to have contracted the disease in Moxham, each became the centre of a new outbreak in their own localities. The home of one of these patients was in a country village two miles from town, and his sickness was followed by that of four other persons. These people used well water. One of the other cases was followed by two more. The third by three new cases. The fourth case infected at Moxham was not followed by any new cases among those in immediate contact with it. The water supply in the two latter instances was drawn from the general system of Johnstown, which proved at all times to be comparatively good.

It seems justifiable to conclude that the original centre of the disease was in the farming community in Stony Creek township, that the flood had no influence upon its development in that locality ; that the germs of the disease were transported in the milk supply to Moxham ; that by reason of the favorable natural conditions of Moxham it spread somewhat rapidly and was distributed from thence to widely separated sections of the Conemaugh Valley. If these conclusions be correct it is quite easy to understand how the disease progressed gradually but surely into all parts of the flooded district. In reply to a number of inquiries concerning the cause, development, location and number of cases treated since the flood, fifteen of the twenty-eight physicians have kindly furnished me with their experience with the so-called typhoid fever. I have also had access to the case book of the Philadelphia Red Cross Hospital, which was established in Johnstown and in which so much was done to aid the sick. From these sources 461 cases are reported with a total mortality of 40. These figures indicate one of two things ; either that the disease was very mild in character and the mortality exceptionally low, or that cases have been included in the list which do not properly belong there. Forty deaths in 461 cases of well marked typhoid fever was a mortality of only 8.7 per cent, while the recognized mortality rate in this country of all types of the disease, is between 15 and 20 per cent. Assuming that all the deaths reported were genuine cases of the fever and calculating the mortality at the lowest recognized percentage, the 40 deaths would be 15 per cent of 266 cases of fever.

There is an honest difference of opinion among our physicians as to the true nature of the disease. One of the reporters states in his reply to my question. "I call it Typho-Malarial Fever ; " and very justly too, for in his series of 40 cases there is only one death. It might readily be conceded that the malarial element must have predominated in the 210 cases reported by seven observers, in which series there were only eleven deaths. The thirteen physicians who did not reply to my inquiries certainly treated their share of the disease, but it is quite likely their experience would have corresponded with the reports received.

But it must not be supposed there was no typhoid fever in the Conemaugh Valley during the past summer. On the contrary, there have been many cases in which the nose bleed, the typical range of temperature, the eruption, the profound prostration, the bowel symptoms, and quite frequently, the hemorrhages resulting in death, all proved beyond controversy the presence of the disease. A large proportion of the cases in Stony Creek township and Moxham were of this character. I believe it can fairly be claimed, however, that the disease was not nearly so prevalent as the public press maintained, or even as the number of cases reported in this paper would seem to indicate.

Another point: these cases were not all in the flooded district. One hundred and ninety were entirely outside of it, and of this latter number, forty-five were far enough away to be located "in the country." In addition to all these cases reported as typhoid fever there was a large amount of sickness treated, which was generally diagnosed as "malaria." This fact would also serve to throw doubt upon the correctness of the diagnosis of typhoid fever in some cases, for a severe attack of "malaria" under such wretched conditions as our people endured, would cause an amount of depression which might justify the term "typhoid" as descriptive of the symptoms, while the patient might be entirely free from the specific poison of typhoid fever.

The majority of the reporters agree that the flood had no direct effect upon the origin of the fever, that is to say, that the fever did not develop solely on account of the flood. They all agree that the great deposits of filth in the valley, the sudden and radical change from the peace and comforts of life, to the depressing miseries of mental and physical suffering, the overcrowding and coarse food, were all indirect factors in the progress and spread of the disease.

There is also a concurrence of opinion among the larger number of the reporters, that the sanitary condition of the valley is fairly good. They remember its condition as the flood left it, and the difference to-day is amazing. They do not mean that the present sanitary condition is satisfactory, for all desire it should be better, and advise the energetic prosecution of sanitary work on the line so satisfactorily followed by the State Board of Health during the Summer. They know there is danger lurking in all corners of the flooded area, and they look forward to future epidemics of infectious diseases with positive dread.

I desire to acknowledge my indebtedness for many of the facts embodied in this report to A. N. Wakefield, M. D., W. E. Matthews, M. D., W. W. Waters, M. D., B. L. Yeazley, M. D., G. B. Porch, M. D., J. W. Hamer, M. D., J. C. Sheridan, M. D., W. N. Pringle, M. D., F. 'i'. Overdorff, M. D., H. F. Tomb, M. D., E. L. Miller, M. D., Horace E. Kistler, M. D., W. J. George, M. D., H. F. Beam, M. D., and the officials of the Red Cross hospital. These gentlemen kindly replied to my questions and gave me the results of their valuable experience, which are here presented for the consideration of the Board.

Form used in obtaining data for the preceding paper:

"DEAR DOCTOR:

"At the request of Dr. Benj. Lee, Secretary State Board of Health, I have undertaken the compilation of facts relating to typhoid fever in the Conemaugh Valley since May 31, 1889. You will oblige me very much by answering the following questions on the enclosed slip and returning it to me not later than December 16, 1889. Very respectfully,

"GEO. W. WAGONER, M. D.,
"*No. 31 Morris Street.*"

Tabular statement of cases of fever occurring in Johnstown and surrounding country during the Summer and Autumn of 1889:

Report Number.	Date of first case.	Location of First Case.	Spread from first case.	Water Supply of First Case.	Total Number of cases treated.	Number of these in flooded district.	Number outside flooded district.	Of those outside, in country.	Deaths.
1	June 10, '89	Stony Creek Township, two miles from town	7	Spring	26	9	17	10	2
2	July 1, '89	Moxham	10	Spring	25	10	15	None.	2
3	July 16, '89	Brownstown, on hill, one mile from town	1	Good (either spring or well)	10	8	2	None.	2
4	Aug. 23, '89	East Conemaugh	Spread to some extent	Well	8	8	None.	None.	None.
5	July 29, '89	Johnstown Borough	4	Well	4	3	1	1	1
6	June 21, '89	Moxham	6	Bad, spring	29	10	19	4	2
7	July 6, '89.	Roxbury, two miles from town	4	Well	46	21	25	10	4
8	Aug. 11, '89	Woodvale	2	Hydrant & spring; first case worked at Moxham	8	5	3	None.	None.
9 Diagnosis typho-malarial	Kept no record of cases treated during June; all work gratis.	....	....	Surface spring	40	8	30	2	1
10	Sept. 1, 89.	Locust Street, Johnstown	3	First case worked at Moxham, water there the cause.	17	6	10	1	None.
11	July 15, '89	Moxham	10	Spring near house.	27	23	4	None.	None
12	July 16, '89	Seventh Ward, Johnstown	50	Hydrant	81	66	15	None.	6
13 Red Cross Hospital	July 29, '89	A large proportion of the cases were workmen in State force.	....	....	53	—	—	—	5
14	June 21, '89	Stony Creek Township	6	Spring	50	20	30	10	10
15	July 1, '89	Grubbtown, worked at Moxham	—	Used water at Moxham	24	14	10	4	3
16	July 25, '89	Conemaugh Boro'gh	—	Hydrant; had been nursing fever patient.	13	4	9	3	2
					461	215	190	45	40

Date of first case, since May 31, 1889,

Location of first case, since May 31, 1889,

Did the disease spread in this locality, if so, how many cases?

Character of water supply in first case,

Your opinion as to cause of the development of your first case of fever,

Total number of cases of typhoid fever treated from May 31, 1889, to date,

Number of these in flooded district,

Number outside,

Number in country,

Number of deaths in your list of cases,

In what manner, in your opinion, did the flood of May 31, 1889, affect the origin, progress and spread of typhoid fever?

Your opinion as to the sanitary condition of the Conemaugh Valley at the present time, and the precautions which should be taken to insure its healthfulness in the future,

The Relation of Climate to Malarial Diseases.*

BY WM. OWENS, Sr., M: D.,

of Cincinnati, Ohio.

Climate, in its modern signification, is defined to be that relation of temperature, heat, moisture, elevation above the sea and meteorological conditions of the atmosphere which impress themselves upon animal and vegetable life.

Malaria is defined to be an earth-born poison, generated in the soil, the energy of which has not been expended in the production of healthy vegetation. This production, it is claimed, is dependent upon and favored by heat, moisture and vegetable decomposition.

It is the commonly received opinion that all so-called malarial diseases do thus originate and cause degeneration of the blood and tissues in those long exposed to their influence.

This definition of climate implies that it depends more upon elevation above the sea, heat and moisture, than distance from the equator, or indication of the sun's rays to the the earth's axis—as formerly accepted. It is found in many portions of the earth, as well as the equatorial regions, that the temperature is much higher at the sea level than it is a few hundred feet above it, in the same latitude. In many locations it will also be found that the diurnal range of the thermometer is greater at the lower level than the higher; and, again, this is because the higher temperature at the sea level may be less liable to so-called malarial diseases than greater elevations quite remote from the alleged causes of these diseases, as we shall see later.

"Malaria," Henry Ward Beecher said, "is a mantle that covers a multitude of morbid conditions." Another writer regards it as a myth, while another affirms that "it is the refuge of ignorance." That as no one has ever been able to define it or describe it, no one has ever seen it or felt it, and no one has ever tasted or smelled it, therefore that which science can not detect by all of her appliances, nor the physical senses discover, however cultivated, must surely be of very doubtful existence. The conditions for the alleged origin of this so-called poison are found around low, marshy lands, sea-coasts, borders of streams, estuaries, ponds, lakes, etc.

It is found that this class of diseases has prevailed with as much violence upon arid barren mountain plateaus, at elevations of eight or ten thousand feet, where rain seldom falls, and on barren rocks, where no vegetation can grow, and where lakes, streams, ponds or estuaries are unknown, as upon low ground. Blanford informs us that malarial diseases are quite prevalent upon the upper Sind and the Indus of India, also upon the whole districts of the Deccan, Guzzerat, Mysore, and Carnatic, most of which regions are from 4,000 to 6,000 feet above the sea. When the monsoon failed for three years in succession, these diseases were most prevalent here. The same is said of the mountains of Ceylon, at an elevation of 6,000 feet these diseases were most virulent. Upon the barren rocky mountains of Hong Kong and the falls of the Orinoco malarial diseases have been notoriously

---

*Read by title before the Ohio State Sanitary Association.

severe. During Wellington's peninsular campaign in Spain, upon the elevated plains of Estramadura, no rain had fallen for two years. The historian says : " The streams were dried up or reduced to rivulets, the grass was burned up and vegetation was dead. The stock had to be driven several miles to water, and much of it died for want of it. Intermittent and remittent fevers prevailed to such an extent that the British army was quite disabled." In our West Indies great heat and moisture prevail with excessive vegetation. The Barbadoes, Bermudas and Bahamas are noted for humidity and vegetable growths. Most of the shores are flat, marshy and hot, being but a few feet above the sea level, which with a luxuriant vegetation constantly undergoing decomposition we would suppose the most favorable possible condition for this class of diseases, and yet we are assured that they are almost wholly unknown here. A British medical officer, who had spent thirteen years at Castle Harbor, Bermuda, informed the writer that his shoes were covered with mildew every morning, and that the atmosphere was constantly saturated with emanations from decaying vegetable matter, and that he had not in all of that time encountered a case of malarial fever on the islands. The Sandwich Islands, as is well-known, are proverbial for the amount of rainfall and humidity, and a most extraordinary vegetation. No malarial disease has been known upon these islands by the oldest inhabitant.

The same may be said of the Friendly Islands, New Zealand and some portions of inter-tropical Australia—great heat, moisture and vegetable growth abound here without the so-called poison.

What, then, is this thing called malaria? Where may it be found? and what its effects?

First,—Negatively. It may *not be found* north of the sixty-second parallel north latitude, nor south of the fifty-seventh parallel south latitude.

Second.—It is not found in any region where the mean annual temperature is below 59° Fah., nor is it found in any district where the daily mean temperature range is below 20° Fah., though heat, moisture and vegetable decomposition may be excessive. If the diurnal rhythm is less than 20° Fah. malarial disease is very rare indeed.

If, then, it be found that so-called malarial diseases are found to prevail extensively and even epidemically in regions of the earth where moisture and vegetable decomposition are quite unknown, as we have attempted to show upon elevated, arid plains and even barren rocks, particularly about the falls of the Orinoco and mountains of Hong Kong, we must conclude that heat, moisture and vegetable decomposition are not essential factors in the causation of these diseases. And again, on the other hand, if we find these diseases quite absent in regions where we have heat, moisture and vegetable decomposition in abundance and even excessive, it must be taken as conclusive also that these conditions do not necessarily cause them, and that there must be some other factor involved which has not yet reached the cognizance of the medical profession or sanitarians. It remains for us to harmonize these facts upon a rational basis and in harmony with material law. It will not be questioned that such morbid conditions as the so-called malarial diseases do prevail in many portions of the earth, but the cause of these is the problem. Where are these diseases found and under what conditions do they exist, may be an interesting point of inquiry. We have shown where they are *not found*, and under what conditions not known to exist. Let us look further, and see if we can find conditions under which they do quite uniformly exist. If we look for a moment at the portions of Italy south of the Appenines, including the Campana, supposed to be the most unhealthy regions of Europe, the days are hot, the temperature often rising to 110° Fah., and falling at night to 60° Fah., rising again during the following day to recede during . the night. These conditions continue to recur rhythmically from May until October, giving a mean diurnal range of from 25° to 50° Fah.

Take again the valley of the Magdalena River in South America, the mercury in the thermometer often rises to 110° to 115° F., during the day, while at two o'clock A. M. it as often falls to 65° 70° F. This condition attains to a greater or less extent up into the interior of the continent as far as Bogota, at an elevation of nearly 9000 feet. A gentleman resident of that city for many years, states that intermittent and remittent fever were quite common there, and that great dampness and mist prevailed during a large portion of the year. In the Mississippi valley and southern portion of the United States the same conditions were present, only in less degree, and quite as bad in the higher and drier regions of northern Texas, and are quite as bad as along the Mississippi or Arkansas, while of our Pacific Coast regions it can be said with safety that a more healthful climate can scarcely be found, and yet from Puget Sound to San Diego there are few places exempt from this class of fevers, and these only by the uniformity of temperature, the mean diurnal range of which is from 14° to 18°* F. In every locality where the range is above 20° F., this class of diseases is found to prevail. The greater the variation, the more prevalent the diseases. This is particularly true of the valleys and plains at the foot of the mountains, where the combined concentrated and reflected rays of the sun raises the mercury to 110° or to 115° F. during the day, and descending currents of air from the snow-capped mountains at night, often reduces the temperature to 60° or 65° F., giving a rhythm 40° 50° 65° F., as has been often observed in some portions of that famous health resort for most other ailments.

The rule will be found to obtain quite generally in all countries and climates that variations of temperature and intensified rhythmical atmospheric conditions go hand-in-hand with the class of diseases called malarial, and that the so-called poison does not exist; that the morbid conditions arising are the product of our own emanations, following a free perspiration during the great heat of the day, and the alternation of the cold at night causing resorption of the exhaled matters during the day ; or, in other words, man is poisoned by his own emanations. Long exposure to these conditions and their frequent repetition, will in time cause blood and tissue changes.

It is a well-known fact that in the inter-tropical regions and on islands in mid-ocean and at other places where the mean daily range of the thermometer is less than 20° F., the diseases called malarial are almost wholly unknown in these places.

---

*San Diego mean is 14°, and Santa Barbara mean, 18°.

Massage and Remedial or Sanitary Movements.

BY WM. A. KERKHOFF,
of Philadelphia, Pa.

It is a well-known fact, that it is better and wiser to prevent an evil, while it is in one's power to do so, than to remedy it afterwards. It is better to prevent disease, by suitable and appropriate means, than to attempt later to cure it, and if necessary to sacrifice habits and tastes for the preservation and enjoyment of good health, it would certainly not be too high a price for the undisturbed enjoyment of a blessing, the absence of which diminishes the value of all other good things in life. All recognize and know the importance of daily out-door exercise for the preservation of health. Walking is not only beneficial to us but a necessity. But experience teaches us that this form of exercise alone is not sufficient for the maintenance of vigorous health, for many eager and conscientious walkers remain both weak and ailing, and become worse and worse in spite of their favorite marching. I do not mean to say that the walking is the direct cause of their debility and sick feeling, rather that this form of exercise does not fulfill all the conditions required for the maintenance and preservation of health and that other means and methods must be employed, especially when we aim to cure disease and debility by exercises. To serve this purpose the exercises used must be estimated and defined beforehand as to their energy, and physiological effects and chosen accordingly.

But in ordinary walking or in driving or riding, the effects are more or less one-sided and vague. The same defects are met with in most forms of labor employed in the various handicrafts, and though varying in their action, they always produce one-sided results.

Gymnastic movements, as nowadays practiced, and as perfected in modern times in all their varied phases, provided again, they are applied strictly in accordance with scientific principles, alone fulfill the conditions of physical labor, when intended for the preservation of health or the cure of disease as preventive or remedial measures.

There is this important difference between hygienic gymnastic movements and those occurring in daily physical labor, that the former have for their sole aim the promotion of health in the human individual, both the movement and the manner of its execution being calculated to subserve this purpose, whereas ordinary labor demands such positions of the body and such movements as will best suit the work, whether they are contrary to health or not, this point being of secondary consideration. As a consequence, the more or less one-sided action belonging to most forms of daily labor, in the long run, disturbs the harmony of the body, so that even working-men often require systematic gymnastic exercise, in order to counteract the injurious influences to which their frames have been subjected by their occupation, and for the same reason hygienic exercises benefit persons leading altogether a sedentary life and having an essentially mental vocation.

In a great measure, it is the possibility of localizing and determining the effects of the movements, which has given to systematic exercises the important therapeutic value they have of late gained throughout the whole medical world, and they are now employed for educational and dietetic as well as for curative purposes. By these means we are enabled to secure the restitution of enfeebled parts to a normal state, for we may ensure to every set of muscles its full share of exercise, and thus produce an all-sided and harmonious general development.

But if we wish gymnastics to be indeed a health-preserving and health-restoring means, then the exercises prescribed should be performed and practiced at least once or several times a day.

To many persons this routine of exercise must be fatiguing or rather impossible, for there are in every large city a great number of people, who, because of their mental exhaustion, physical incapacity, old age, or chronic ailments are unable to undergo any real active physical labor. For such, that form of hygienic exercise called "Massage and Remedial" or "Sanitary Movements" is best suited. It is in consequence of the importance of this treatment, which I have practiced for the last fifteen years in the cases mentioned, and because of its gratifying and remarkable results that I wish to explain the mode of operation.

"Massage and Remedial Movements" secures to a man not only all the advantages derived from ordinary physical exercise, but besides has its own special value. It also combines the advantage that it can be performed upon a chair, sofa, couch or bed, and does not produce the same fatigue as that which accompanies other exercise, and it may be practiced in the most inclement weather.

By massage I mean a variety of manipulations, such as kneading, friction, percussion, vibration and others. These are performed with the fingers and hands upon the living body for therapeutic and hygienic purposes, and are calculated to promote circulation and muscular action.

By movements, I understand both the passive and active movements performed upon the various joints, limbs, head and trunk, such as flexion, extension, rotation, pronation and supination.

In passive movements the operator performs the various movements, while the patient remains inactive, whereas in active movements they are performed with the co-operation and resistance of the patient, through the exertion of the will.

The effect of this combined treatment is very important, as it accelerates and improves the arterial, venous, and lymphatic circulation, eliminates waste products, promotes more pliability and elasticity of the joints, restores muscular power and nervous energy.

Hygienic Warfare.

Since the essence of warfare, as at present managed, is the destruction of life; so, could we devise a method by which life would be saved, we might be justified in calling such a method "Hygienic Warfare." Such a plan, it would seem, was once put into practice by Cabrera, the noted Carlist leader in Spain, who, on the evening before a battle, appeared in the camp of the rival commander and suggested that, instead of allowing their men to kill one another, he and Espartero should throw with dice for the victory. They did so, and Espartero won. Cabrera scrupulously kept his word, and comported himself in all ways as if he had been defeated.

Wells that Cause Typhoid.

BY GEORGE ROBERTS,
Analytical Chemist, of Harrisburg, Penna.

During July of 1889 I was called upon to make an analysis of two (2) wells on adjoining farms near Harrisburg, Pa., where were seven (7) cases of typhoid fever, one (1) resulting fatally. The fact that only those who used these wells for drinking purposes were the only ones who contracted the disease, pointed very strongly to the waters as being impure. The rain and floods of May and June might have been the disturbing agent of these wells, for before the flood sickness of this kind was unknown to the residents of the farms. The wells have been thoroughly cleaned out and in No. 1 was found a *piece of raw beef*, having been hung in there to keep cool during the summer time, the support gave away and dropped it to the bottom. No. 2 well was used every summer as a water supply for a steam thresher and consequently was in better shape than No. 1, the water having been drawn off more often. Below are the analysis of No. 1 and No. 2 wells before cleaning with a sample of Susquehanna River water for comparison.

REPORT IN PARTS PER MILLION.

	No. 1.	No. 2.	S. Riv.
Total Solids	510.0000	240.0000	126.0000
Chlorine	75.0000	28.0000	5.0000
Hardness	180.9484	76.1888	61.9034
Free Ammonia	.0800	.0200	.0400
Alb-Ammonia	.1600	.1200	.1400
Req-Ox, ¼ hour	.1403	.0842	.0000
Req-Ox, 4 hour	.5754	.5684	.5920
Nitrogen as Nitrates	24.9580	13.4179	.0000
Nitrogen as Nitrites	.0045	.0042	.0000

Family Typhoid from Defective Plumbing.*

BY LEWIS H. TAYLOR, M.D.,
of Wilkesbarre, Pa.

An interesting series of cases showing the effect of defective plumbing, is given here in a South Main Street family. The bath-tub, with old fashioned pan closet adjoining, had been leaking from time to time, for the past two years. Had recently dripped down into the kitchen, on to the range and sink directly below. A case of typhoid fever appeared in the Summer or rather Fall, (September 13) in the youngest boy of the family. He was ill in bed two months and did not get out of the house until Thanksgiving day. His mother was taken ill with typhoid fever November 23. One sister, November 29; second, December 4; third, December 5; fourth, December 6; fifth, December 8. The plumbing had been defective for a long time, the dripping had leaked through the ceiling into the kitchen, but it did not make the family ill *until a case of typhoid fever was introduced into the house,* and then after a sufficient time had elapsed, six others were taken in quick succession. We presume the first of the family who became ill in September, contracted the disease as did so many others this Summer, from the water. Boiled water had been used in this family during the Summer, but the boy informs me that he occasionally drank water elsewhere unboiled. Without doubt the latter cases are from secondary infection.

(*Extract from a letter by Dr. L. H. Taylor, Medical Inspector, Wilkesbarre, to Dr. Benjamin Lee, Secretary.)

THE ANNALS
OF HYGIENE,

⁕ ⁕

PUBLISHED
MONTHLY.

Subscription, two dollars ($2.00)
a year, in advance.

THE OFFICIAL ORGAN OF THE
State Board of Health of Pennsylvania.

The State Board of Health is not responsible for
anything appearing in this Journal except that
which bears the official attestation of the Board.

Address all communications to

The Hygienic Publishing Company,

224 SOUTH SIXTEENTH STREET,
PHILADELPHIA, PA.

EDITORIAL.

The Sanitary Significance of Nellie Bly's Trip Around the World.

(Around the World in Sixteen Days.)

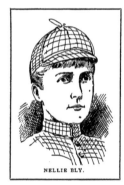

NELLIE BLY.

To our way of thinking, the most suggestive and important feature of the race round the world that has just been completed by Nellie Bly is its sanitary aspect. In about sixty traveling days this young lady covered nearly 24,000 miles of space, moving at an average rate of about 416 miles per day. Circling the globe in this short space of time, brings forcibly before us the fact that the world is not such a very big place after all, and makes us realize how really close together all nations of the world are, after all.

This reflection will suggest to the sanitarian the necessity that exists for what we might call "International Sanitation." The means of intercommunication between all the nations of the world are now so frequent and so rapid that, no matter, comparatively speaking, how good may be the sanitary condition of one country, the neglect of hygiene in another country, formerly remote, because of its inaccessibility. may prove a deadly menace.

We have no reason to absolutely say that disease may not be transported on the "wings of the wind;" and since the wind, not infrequently, blows at the rate of sixty miles per hour, a little calculation will show us that this agency could compass the circuit of the globe in sixteen days. If then the rapidity and means of communication are so favorable to the spread of disease, it would seem to be a universal necessity—in the demand for which all nations alike should unite—that the breeding places of disease, found in certain benighted countries, should be eradicated.

Nellie Bly eloquently asserts that Japan is the most delightful country (outside of our own) in the world, and in the next sentence she tells us that it is the cleanest place imaginable, that everybody bathes daily, and that you can get a delightful shampoo bath, from head to foot, for two cents; while the Chinese, on the other hand, she characterizes as a "dirty-living people," whom one instinctively shuns.

It is worthy of note, in this connection, that HYGIENE is a very live subject in Japan —the people liberally supporting no less than nine journals devoted to this subject.

This unprecedented journey of Miss Nellie Bly has many important results as its justification, but if it tends to rouse and foster a sentiment towards "*international sanitation*," the greatest of all will be found therein.

Renting Unhealthy Houses.

We remember, many years since seeing a diagram, wherein it was demonstrated that the shortest route to a man's heart lay through his stomach. In this *practical* age, it seems to us, the shortest route to the sensitive portion of humanity is through its pocket. It is truly marvellous what enormous reactionary power resides in the pocket of the average individual. Touch the pocket, and he who was, seemingly, as passive as an Egyptian mummy, becomes as uncontrollable as a three-year-old colt. It would, we believe, be almost justifiable were we to so alter our ideas of anatomy as to claim that the nervous system of mankind centred rather in his pocket than in his brain ; certain it is that when we wish to impress the whole individual we can do so more effectually through the medium of his pocket than in any other way.

These reflections are preliminary to a suggestion, which, if acted upon, would mark an enormous stride in the steady march of sanitary reform.

It is a fact, an indisputable fact, that there are, comparatively speaking, extremely few houses that are in proper sanitary condition. The ignorance, avarice or carelessness of the owner is the cause for this fact, as well as the cause of the sickness, misery, and even the deaths that may come to the occupants by reason of the faulty sanitary condition of the house.

To come to the point, as briefly as possible, our suggestion is, that, before renting a house, the proposed tenant should demand from his proposed landlord the certificate of some competent sanitary authority that the house is in proper sanitary condition, so that, in time, it would come to pass that a house, the healthfulness of which was not guaranteed by such a certificate, would be shunned as would the pest-house. By such a plan we would be appealing to the pockets of the landlords and our appeal would not go long unanswered. Is such a plan practicable? Undoubtedly and unhesitatingly, YES. It but requires the demand of would-be tenants for this certificate and it will soon be forthcoming. If some *good* man, who is the owner of large numbers of houses, will start this reform, his fellow landlords will be compelled to follow his beneficent example.

A plan, even more exacting, is now in successful operation in the city of Brussels, in Belgium. When a house is found to be in an unhealthy condition (and such are discovered by systematic inspections) the owner is notified to place his property in good sanitary shape and he is told what it is necessary for him to do. If he neglects to do that which is required of him, those living in the house are compelled to move out, the doors are locked and a *notice posted up that the house is unfit for habitation.* Just think how eloquently this mute notice must appeal to the sensitive pocket of the owner ! Still further, the law of Belgium forbids any one (including the owner) to occupy this house, until its insanitary conditions have been remedied, and, *best of all, it allows the tenant to bring suit against the landlord for damages caused by the inconvenience of this forced removal,* and, such is popular Belgian sentiment, A FAVORABLE VERDICT FOR HEAVY DAMAGES is easily obtained. Here we have the appeal to the pocket, with the expected and anticipated result that the authorities have now only to notify the landlord what to do, and, like magic, it is done. Now for the *practical* result. Formerly the death rate of Brussels was nearly 30 per 1,000, now, it is less than 23; formerly the death rate from zymotic, contagious or infectious diseases was nearly 5 per 1,000; now it is but a little over 1 per 1,000. To put it more plainly, it is easily demonstrable that, by the precautions referred to, nearly 13,000 lives have been saved in Brussels during the last fifteen years, which, in Philadelphia, with its larger population, would have amounted to 40,000 lives; 40,000 more people to occupy houses and pay rent for them,—another powerful appeal to the sensitive pocket.

If every reader of this Journal would demand from his landlord (and urge his friends to do likewise) a certificate such as we have referred to, failing to receive which he would vacate his premises, the custom would soon become universal with the magnificent results above alluded to.

Floods and their Results, from a Sanitary Standpoint.

Arrangements have been completed to hold a Tri-State Sanitary Convention at Wheeling, W. Va., February 27 and 28, 1890.

Representatives will be present with papers and addresses from Pennsylvania, West Virginia and Ohio. The object of the Convention is to consider the question of floods and their results from a sanitary standpoint, and the best methods of managing the sanitary interests of a given community after such a calamity.

Owing to the mutual relations held by these three States with reference to large rivers and the numerous towns in each one of these States, that are annually affected by floods and their results, it has been thought wise to hold a convention for studying how best to manage the sanitary interests of cities and towns so affected.

Every person interested, directly or indirectly, in this important subject is earnestly requested to be present and assist in discussing the papers and add whatever information he can to the solution of these practical and most important questions, affecting as they do the health and lives of thousands of citizens of these three great Commonwealths annually.

Spurgeon's Wisdom.

It is refreshing to occasionally note such true wisdom as that displayed by the Rev. Mr. Spurgeon, who tells us that he has gone to Mentone, *not because of ill-health,* but that he may gather fresh energy and vitality for still better work. To use his own words:

" Many men have been taken away by death, or have been laid aside by failure of brain through not taking rest. It is an economy of time to take off the collar for a little. Our vacation is mainly spent in gathering new subjects for another spell of sermonizing; and when we have been well enough to use in that way, it has enabled us to keep on preaching and printing through the rest of the year."

NOTES AND COMMENTS.

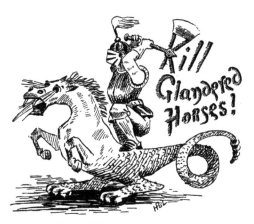

The absolute knowledge which we possess in reference to the causation of disease is, when one stops to reflect, really very great, and were this information universally disseminated and acted upon, the resu t would be astoundingly gratifying. We hold, and always have held, that the people are really very much interested in hygiene, when the subject is properly put before them, divested of scientific technicalities that will always serve to make any subject dry and uninteresting to the general public; but, it is a subject for wonder to us why it is that instinct does not make us all sanitarians. If a man encounters a rattlesnake, his instinct, his impulse, as it were, urges him to kill the reptile, because in it he instinctively recognizes a potency for evil to humanity. Now, why does not this same instinct, at once, suggest the slaughter of a glandered horse, for such is equally dangerous to humanity; aye, more so; because of the more intimate relations that exist between the horse and the man. It is related that a young physician in Vienna was recently inoculating some animals with the pus, or *matter*, taken from a case of glanders, when he, accidentally, inoculated himself; after several weeks of intense suffering he died. Had he bared his arm to the fangs of the moccasin, the fatal result would have been more rapid, but it could not have been more certain. Kill glandered horses; they are menaces to humanity.

How "The Grip" Feels to Some.

T. Bailey Aldrich, who was a recent victim of the grip, compares the sensation to that of "a misfit skull, that is too tight across the forehead and that pinches behind the ears."

Neuralgia and Rheumatism.

All persons with any tendency to neuralgia, rheumatism or sciatica should wear wool next to the skin all the year round. In summer very light weight flannels prevent chills after perspiration.

Convalescence from Diphtheria.

Patients convalescing from diphtheria should be kept in bed, and very quiet, since heart failure often occurs from the slightest exertion, even after the disappearance of all symptoms of the disease.

Sleeping on Pillows.

Do not have too many pillows under your head when you sleep, for such a practice has a tendency to curve the spine, to cause "droop neck," and to interfere with the freedom of the breathing, and the circulation of the blood.—*Sanitary Inspector.*

A Suggestion for the Use of Our Surplus.

Dr. Da Costa, of this city, writing on "The Grip," very wisely says:

"We know nothing of the cause of this disease. It is epidemic, and I think myself that it is feebly contagious. It would be an admirable thing if some of our over-filled treasury could flow into the channels of science, and that a commission be appointed to investigate this disease bacteriologically and chemically. We accept the microbic nature of its origin, but it has not been proven."

Promoting the Spread of Scarlet Fever.

At the Hygienic Congress in Paris, Dr. de Valcour related that a death having taken place from scarlet fever at an hotel in Monaco, the room was relet to another tenant the next day, and he likewise died of the same fever. It was not till a third case of scarlet fever occurred in this room that the hotel was closed and disinfected.

The Relief of Headache.

As a general rule, a throbbing headache, with tenderness and soreness of the scalp, can best be relieved by warm or hot applications continued for a considerable length of time. Whereas, where the head feels full and "bursting," if cold be applied to the head and the heat to the neck, spine and feet, the effect is most agreeable.—*Exchange.*

Where Rests the Responsibility for Epidemics.

If an outbreak of infectious disease occurs in your town, it is rather mean to throw the whole burden of care and responsibility upon the local board of health, especially if your town pays the local board little or nothing for their services. Every person has, or should have, a personal interest in preventing an epidemic; and in lending a helping hand to the afflicted famisy or to the local board of health when needed.—*Sanitary Inspector.*

Saving a Watch.

"If you ever drop your watch in the water," said a jeweler recently, "hasten to throw it into a cup of alcohol or whisky; that will prevent the works from rusting. Two friends were down South fishing lately, and by some mishap their boat was upset, and they were thrown into the water. Both had fine watches and both were forever ruined, because they did not know what to do to prevent their movements from rusting. Just bear this in mind."

A Lesson From Johnstown.

As fire is discovered by its own light and virtue by its own excellence, so must the value of sanitation be determined by its own results. Here we are, now, nearly one year away from the terrible flood that swept Johnstown out of existence, yet the universally predicted "*plague*" has not come to pass. Candor and honesty must surely compel every honest and candid person to freely admit that the present healthy condition of the flooded regions of this State is an unanswerable demonstration of the *practical* utility of *so-called* hygienic *theories*.

The Fall in Farm Values.

It would seem, from the investigations of the Bureaus of Industrial Statistics of several of our States, that there has been, during the last few years, a most alarming falling off in the value of farm land. Many of our leading papers are, editorially, discussing the question and wondering to what cause it should be attributed. We fancy that our editorial on "The Poor Clerk" (in the issue for January), may throw some light not only on the cause but the remedy as well.

Horse Manure in New York.

Is is stated that in New York City the refuse from horses amounts to very nearly 1,000,000 pounds daily. This means nearly 500 tons of the very best kind of manure. Suppose this manure to be worth only five dollars per ton and we have the enormous result of $2,500 per day, or nearly $1,000,000 per year. There is invested in the removal of this manure only $300,000, so that some one must be making a mighty good thing out of the horses of New York.

Hygienic Pride.

Nothing flatters a man (if he be worthy to be called a man) so much as the happiness of his wife, and he is always proud of himself as the source of it. Such pride we would call justifiable or hygienic pride. A man cannot be too full of such pride; it will give to him an even temper; a self-contentment and a satisfaction with his surroundings, that will most favorably react upon his digestion and his sleep. A man who has a pride in the welfare and happiness of his wife and his children is a man who is observing one of the most practical of all the laws of hygiene.

Horse-meat Sausage.

The papers are making considerable of a sensation about the existence of a sausage factory in a town on Long Island, where horse-meat is used in lieu of the ordinary article. Now, let us properly understand this question. There is no earthly reason why sausages should not be made of horse meat, provided the horse is sound and healthy. Of course, deception is always to be condemned and false representation should not be tolerated, but if these sausages are sold for what they are, then there can be no valid reason for the health authorities to interdict their manufacture.

What is the Proper Age for Girls to Marry?

This question being put to some of the most prominent matrons of Washington, by a correspondent of the *Philadelphia Press*, elicited a variety of replies, the most sensible of which was that of Mrs. General Logan, who says that " when a girl meets the man she loves, whether she be eighteen, twenty or twenty-five, she should marry him." He who would arbitrarily regulate the age at which a girl should marry, like the person who would dogmatically assert just how many hours one should sleep, is flying in the face of nature and endeavoring to substitute *artificial* for *natural* laws. Such rules are all nonsense, and are never productive of any good. In this matter of marriage, impulsive love, directed by mature parental reason, should be, and is the natural guide, and he who goes against nature in this respect is very apt to find himself unheeded.

One Cause of Typhoid.

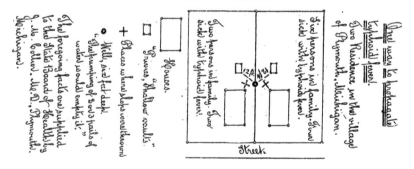

The Art of Getting Drunk.

If the recommendation, made in his recent report by Secretary of the Treasury Windom, should be favorably acted upon by Congress, we imagine that the " art of getting drunk " would be added to the already existing list of arts ; for this gentleman advises that alcohol for use in the arts should be exempted from taxation. Rather let us tax all alcohol and all tobacco (for neither are necessities, as the very fact of the use of alcohol in " art " would proclaim such use a luxury and not a necessity), and since from this source alone, according to Mr. Windom, the government receives annually $37,500,000, let us relieve the national surplus by spending this money in needed sanitary improvements. Let us benefit the masses by the revenue derived from the luxuries of the few, or, better still, let him who will drink pay (for what he considers a pleasure) a mite towards benefiting his fellow-man.

The Increasing Prevalence of Cancer.

The Baltimore Health Department has recently tabulated some statistics which require a word of explanation, because, agreeing with statistics from other parts of the world, they go to show an increase in the prevalence of cancer. It is true that we do have more of this disease now than did former generations, but the reason is interesting, as bearing upon the practical results of hygienic teaching. Cancer is, essentially, a disease of mature life, and its increasing prevalence may be accepted as evidence of the fact that, owing to an observance of the laws of hygiene, more persons now reach a mature age than was formerly the case. For those who value life is it not an improvement to die at *fifty*, of cancer, rather than at *twenty-five* of typhoid fever ? The twenty-five additional years may contain much pleasure and may possess a potent significance for these who are left behind.

Individual Rights *vs.* Public Welfare.

It is a fundamental principle of our government, and one that deeply underlies all the relations of humanity—that individual must succumb to collective rights. A case bearing strongly upon this principle was recently before our courts. It seems that a young man, who was supposed to have small-pox, was removed by order of our local Board of Health, to the small-pox hospital. His disease proved to be measles, but in the hospital he contracted small-pox, as the result of which he is deformed, and he now brings suit against the city for damages. This young man is to be pitied, and his case is worthy of all sympathy ; it is most unfortunate that the mistake in diagnosis should have been made, but we are compelled to believe that it is better, on the principle above referred to, that a dozen men should be mistakenly exposed to small-pox than that one should be allowed to become the centre from which might originate an epidemic that would claim its hundreds or its thousands of victims.

When People Believed In Physic.

The *Tocsin* gives the following particulars relating to the physicking of a patient in the olden times, the good old times when people took physic and plenty of it, firmly believing that it did them good. The individual in question, Mr. Samuel Jessup, died, May 17, 1817, at Heckington. He was defendant in a trial for the amount of an apothecary's bill at the Lincoln Assizes. The evidence at the trial gives the following details : In twenty-one years (from 1794 to 1816), he took 226,934 pills, supplied by a respectable apothecary in Bottlesford, which gives an average of 10,806 pills a year, or 29 each day. In the last five years preceding 1816 he took the pills at the rate of 78 a day, and in the year 1814 swallowed not less than 51,590. "Notwithstanding this," says the *Tocsin*, "and the addition of 40,000 bottles of mixture, besides juleps and electuaries, set out in fifty-five closely written columns of the apothecary's bill, he lived to the age of sixty-five years."

The Sanitary Renaissance of Persia.

It is reported that the Persians have come to believe that the recent European tour of the Shah has unsettled the mental equilibrium of their ruler. This belief has originated from the fact, that actuated by the everywhere evident benefits to be derived from sanitary administration, impressed by what he saw in more enlightened lands, this Eastern potentate has concluded to no longer continue his country as one of the plague spots of the world. He has ordered hundreds of houses to be pulled down, foul slums to be demolished and new streets to be built, while the very latest and crowning proof of his madness is a royal order for the commencement of the systematic sanitation of the Persian capital.

How different are the ideas of different people, and how true is it that we are but creatures of habit, for that which, in this country, we would regard as the highest evidence of intelligence, is, in far-away, dirty, disease-ridden Persia, looked upon as evidence of an erratic mental state.

Double-up the Under-clothing.

Should we have, as we probably will, an occasional day when the thermometer will fall down below freezing point, we will experience much comfort and avoid much danger, if, in the morning, when we find that the temperature has so fallen, we put on *two* undershirts, *two* pair of drawers and *two* pair of stockings. During the old-fashioned winters, when we had one, long, continuous cold spell, it was a comparatively easy matter to dress properly, but in this *Summer-in-winter* weather the sudden and great changes in temperature constitute a serious menace to health, and it is no easy matter to guard against it. Most of us are now dressed for winter, and when a really cold day comes, having accustomed ourselves to the warm days in winter wraps, we are not prepared to resist the onslaught of Jack Frost. The plan we have mentioned, will, if tried some cold morning, give such satisfaction that its practice will be persisted in. It will make a little more washing, but it will prevent much sickness and discomfort from cold.

An Echo from the Plymouth Epidemic.

We are sorry to be compelled to disagree with the decision of the Court in a suit growing out of the typhoid fever epidemic that so frightfully ravaged the town of Plymouth, in this State, a few years since. It seems that a man, who lost two children, brought suit for damages against the water company and he was non-suited, because the Court held that the water company was not responsible for the action of the nurse, who, by depositing the dejecta of a typhoid fever patient on the edge of the stream, thereby polluted the water supply and gave rise to the epidemic. We take it that no precedent has yet been established, but we are quite clear that it should be so ordered, that when the privileges usually given to water companies are granted, they should be, in some way, compelled to protect the water from artificial contamination. Of course it would be too much to ask that they should guarantee absolute immunity against the various freaks of nature, but it seems to us only fair that they should hereafter be required to guard against the gross and palpable pollution of man, of such as occurred in the case under consideration, and that they should be held responsible for the neglect of such precautionary measures.

Crimean Sanitation.

Early in 1855 (says Colonel George E. Waring, Jr.), moved by the most distressing condition of the sick and wounded in the hospitals of the Crimean army, Lord Panmure commissioned Dr. Sutherland, Dr. Gavin and Mr. Rawlinson to proceed to the Bosphorus and to the Crimea, and to take instant measures for the improvement of the sanitary state of those sadly crowded buildings.

The order was issued on the 19th of February. In less than three weeks the work at Scutari was already progressing, and within a month a marked effect was obvious.

Kinglake says: " Then came on a change, which, if only it had been preceded by mummery instead of ventilation and drainage and pure water supply, would have easily passed for a miracle. Down went the rate of mortality. Having already gone down from the terrible February rate of 42 per cent. to 31, it descended in the next fortnight to 14; in the next twenty days to 10; in the next to ·5; in the next to 4; and finally, in the next twenty days, ending on the 30th of June, 1855, to scarcely more than 2.''

This result was achieved by physical changes effected by intelligent engineering.

General Grant in Battle.

The sentimental worship of the soldier is born of our natural admiration for bravery, and it is because of the bravery that he displays in facing dangers, for the common good, that we come to regard him with great respect and admiration. In the case of General Grant, it was his wisdom and bravery that exalted him to the pinnacle of fame. But now we are going to claim (though we do not believe it) that Grant *was not a brave man*, we so claim that we may fight with their own weapons some of those who scoff at hygiene. To the man who says that there is no danger in impure water, foul air, dung-heaps in proximity to the house, rotting vegetables in the cellar, damp and shaded houses; to the man who laughs when we tell of the causes of ill-health, because *he* has been surrounded by such (and maybe his father before him) without any particular appreciable results, to such a man we say that there is no danger in battle, because General Grant, though in many battles, suffered no ill effects therefrom; and since there is no danger in battle, Grant was not a brave man, because he really did not face danger. Our reasoning, of course, is faulty, but not one whit more so than that of the person who argues that there is no danger in insanitary surroundings or customs because he or she does not happen to be among the victims.

Cellar Air.

Cellar air is bad air and not fit for breathing, no matter how clean the cellar is or what care has been taken in cementing it. Cellar air, especially when the suctional power of the furnace is exerted on the cellar, is largely ground air,—is drawn from the soil beneath and surrounding the cellar,—and the air from the ground is very different from the air above the surface. Money expended for supplies of air from pure sources is money put into one of the best forms of insurance.

The fresh-air box, or flue for the furnace of a dwelling house should start from some out-door point where the air will not be liable to pollution, should be as short and direct, and as free from angles, especially sharp ones, as possible, should be tight, preferably of metal or metal-lined, or laid in cement and lined with asphalt, and should be made much larger in cross-section than is customary. For a dwelling house of ordinary size the fresh air inlet should be at least 20 to 24 inches square, we could almost say the larger the better, so that, especially in mild weather, the rooms may be warmed with a large quantity of air of very moderate temperature. This of course, will require a furnace of such construction and with such a setting as to admit of the free passage of the desired amount of air ; conditions which are rather rare in furnaces, but may be found in some.—*Sanitary Inspector*.

Absorption of Tobacco Smoke by Meat, etc.

M. Bourrier, an inspector of the slaughter houses of Paris, has lately reported to the *Revue D'Hygiene* the results of some experiments to determine the influence of the fumes of tobacco on food of animal origin.

Two kilograms of raw beef were minced and subjected to the fumes of tobacco for some time. When offered to a dog of medium size, which had been deprived of food for twelve hours, the dog refused to eat it. Concealed in a piece of bread, it was taken with avidity, At the eud of twenty minutes the dog showed uneasiness and abdominal pain, and uttered plaintive cries. The respiration became noisy and embarrassed, the flanks heaved, the tongue hung from the mouth, the alvine evacuations became abundant, and the animal died in horrible convulsions. Various other kinds of meat, raw, broiled, roasted, etc., were used in the experiments, and with results similar, but varying in intensity. It was found that raw meats, and those which are moist and tender, absorbed the tobacco smoke more readily than others, and that strawberries and raspberries readily absorb the smoke from a tobacco pipe.

The inference which the author would draw from these experiments is, that food which is subjected to the fumes of tobacco smoke, during the process of preparation in factories or other places, may absorb enough of the tobacco poison to become injurious to the health of consumers.—*Sanitary Inspector*.

Poison from Dead Bodies.

An American merchant ship was lying at anchor in Wampoa Roads, sixteen miles from Canton. One of the crew died of dysentery. He was taken on shore to be buried. No disease of any kind had occurred in the ship from her departure from America till her arrival in the river Tigris. Four men accompanied the corpse, and two of them began to dig the grave. Unfortunately they pitched upon a spot where a human body had been buried about two or three months previously (as was afterward ascertained). The instant the spade went through the lid of the coffin a most dreadful effluvium issued forth, and the two men fell down nearly lifeless. It was with the greatest difficulty their companions could approach near enough to drag them from the spot and fill up the place with earth. The two men now recovered a little, and with assistance reached the boat and returned on board.'' Both died, one on the evening of the fourth and the other the morning of the fifth day of a malignant fever, with symptoms resembling plague. The other two men, who were less exposed, were similarly affected, but recovered. Commenting on these facts which are related in "*Johnson on Tropical Climates*," Dr. A. N. Bell, the editor of *The Sanitarian*, very logically says : " That the poisonous emanations inhaled in this case would have been any less dangerous if swallowed with the subsoil water in the vicinity can be surmised by those only who believe inhumation of the dead to be without danger to the living.

Reporting Typhoid Fever.

In Michigan typhoid fever is a disease which the State Board of Health has declared to be " dangerous to the public health," and as such it comes under the law requiring physicians to report to the health officials. Any physician who shall neglect to immediately give such notice, "shall forfeit for each such offense a sum not less than fifty nor more than one hundred dollars." And since October 1, " *any householder* who shall refuse or wilfully neglect immediately to give such notice, shall be deemed guilty of a misdemeanor, and shall be liable to a fine of one hundred dollars, or in default of payment thereof may be punished by imprisonment in the county jail not exceeding ninety days."

The *Medical Age*, October 10, 1889, says that this law applies to scarlet fever, diphtheria, small-pox, and all diseases dangerous to public health, as well as to typhoid fever, and that every case should be reported to the health officer, who is required to promptly attend to the restriction of the disease. The new law makes it a misdemeanor, punishable by fine or imprisonment, for the health officer to knowingly violate the enactment, or for any person to violate the orders of the health officer made in accordance with it. The actual penalty, however, which is incurred is— *Death !* And about one thousand people are lost in this State annually from typhoid fever alone. The saving of a large proportion of these lives is the real reason for the effort, in which it is hoped all people will join.—*Med. and Surg. Reporter.*

The Coming Table Oil.

The use of cotton seed oil as a substitute for olive oil seems to be largely on the increase in this country. For a long time many persons have used it for table purposes when neatly labelled as "*Huile d' Olive*," without a suspicion that it was anything but the best quality of olive oil. We do not believe (says *The Sanitary Volunteer*) in such a fraudulent enforcement of the use of cotton-seed oil, but there is no reason why this valuable food product should not be universally adopted for table use under its proper name. Indeed, the refined oil is being quite extensively used for table purposes, and with the greatest satisfaction. It is used in the preparation of the most delicious and delicate salads, and it is rapidly finding its way into the culinary departments of many households.

In a paper read before The American Public Health Association some four or five years ago, Prof. Monroe said that the chemical composition of cotton oil revealed nothing that interdicted its use as a food, and, if experience proved it acceptable as such, it would be a product of great value to the American people. The proof has been presented. We have in this article a substitute for olive oil, equally as good, and at a price which brings its use within the reach of many who cannot afford to purchase genuine olive oil. So valuable an American product as this ought to be found in every grocery store, neatly bottled, and labelled with its true name, and for sale at a price which, with a reasonable margin for profit, would place it far below the cost of olive oil. We predict that its future use as a table oil will be extensive and satisfactory.

An Incident of " The Grip."

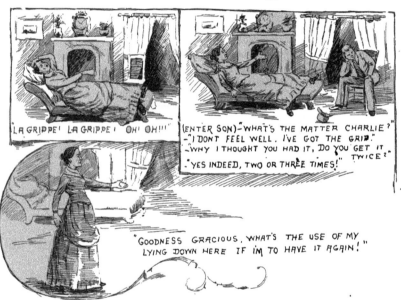

From ife, not the journal *Life*, but *real life*, showing somewhat forcibly the power of imagination, and demonstrating rather forcibly the secret of the so-called " *Faith Cure.*"

Dom Pedro's Common Sense.

It has been frequently said, and with the greatest truth, that the most uncommon sense is "common sense." A moment's reflection will make this truth very evident. The world, to-day, admires Dom Pedro, late Emperor of Brazil, because, in him, it recognizes a most uncommon man ; but it does not quite so clearly comprehend that this very individuality of Dom Pedro is owing to the fact that he is, in an uncommon measure, possessed of the enviable commodity known as "common sense."

When this good man found that a Brazilian Republic was inevitable, he did not, to use a vulgar expression, fall to " crying over spilled milk," but, summoning his " common sense " to his aid, philosophically and placidly accepted that which he knew could not be prevented. His " common sense " told him that " that which cannot be cured must be endured." We question whether there was in the world a crowned head who commanded the universal respect and admiration that was accorded to Dom Pedro; there certainly are few who have attained his venerable age, with a life so full of pleasure and so barren of regrets ; all of which can be mainly attributed to his possession of the blessing of "common sense." Let us all strive for it ; it is not difficult of attainment. It would seem as though the "common sense" of the Emperor had been "caught," as it were, by contagion, by his people, for now we are informed that in the new Republic, a certain amount of intelligence and education will be requisite to entitle a man to vote. No irresponsible, impecunious, lazy, drunken loafer, will there have any voice in the management of that to which he has ailed, by lack of intelligent labor, to contribute. Here we find Brazil setting an example that it would be well for our national health for us to imitate.

Law and Health.

Many people object to laws calculated to govern their customs and manner of living, be they conducive to good health or otherwise, (says *The Sanitary News*). The sentiment of personal liberty so far outweighs the higher demands of civil liberty in their minds that they are blinded to the public good, and are devoted to personal comfort and selfish ends. They protest against almost all agencies that are established in the interest of public health. They oppose inspection, isolation, notification, disinfection, and other means for the promotion of health demanded by sanitation. These persons feel that they have been outraged whenever the law has compelled them to comply with the demands of sanitation. The fact that these laws have been enacted proves that some compulsion was necessary to enforce such rules and regulations as have been promulgated by sanitary science.

It must be remembered that no law was ever enacted to suit the pleasure of the individual. All laws are enacted for the common good of the people they govern. Individual interest, profit and pleasure must give way to the public welfare, and there is no greater public interest than that of health. The individual must comply with its laws, and thus contribute to the general progress of hygiene.

The general experience is that, in cases of epidemics, the most strict enforcement of the law is demanded. Isolation and quarantine are submitted to and insisted on. There is no opposition to the laws governing communities in this regard. Yet the greatest number of deaths and the greatest amount of sickness are not due to epidemics. To the constant, silent progress of insidious diseases which are considered wholly preventable, we find the greatest sacrifices of human life and health. The fatality of an epidemic is plainly observable and its scourge impels men to resort to any preventive measures known. The laws governing health departments and creating their powers are demanded to be strictly enforced. But everywhere disease, not in an epidemic form, is carrying off more victims and endangering more lives than epidemics do. The conclusion is that all laws, creating health departments and defining their powers, should be strictly enforced at all times. An unsanitary state in any community continually produces sickness, and at all times presents the condition necessary to produce epidemics.

Woman's Fatal Clothing.

"Madam, I cannot take your case," said a distinguished medical practitioner, the other day, to a fashionable invalid, after a careful diagnosis.

"But why not take *my* case?" the lady asked in some surprise.

"Because I have had my attendant weigh your garments while I was making the examination," was the frank and most unusual response, "and I find that your skirts weigh fifteen pounds. You have brought on the disease from which you suffer by this manner of dressing, and I do not care to risk my reputation as a physician by treating a patient who will, in all probability, continue to carry such loads."

"This is the first time I ever knew a physician to tell a patient what she should wear," said the visitor, with heightened color. "How many pounds is it lawful to carry, if you please?"

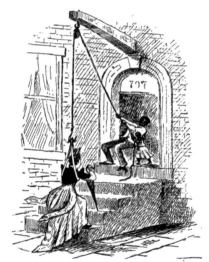

What it will come to if woman's clothing gets much heavier.

"You cannot carry over three pounds with safety; and even such a weight should be suspended from the shoulders."

"How long shall I be obliged to limit the weight of my clothes?"

"As long as you live, madam; for you have so outraged every delicate and sensitive internal organ, so stretched the ligaments which would have been faithful had you treated them well, that you can never exceed this weight with safety."

"Do you think you can cure me if I obey you?" was the next question.

"I can prevent the development of a tumor, which is now imminent, but all the medical science in creation cannot make you strong. But I can help you to help yourself to more health and comfort than you have known for many a year."—
Eleanor Kirk, in Woman's World.

What is Hygiene?

A very extended definition would be required to give its signification in all its applications. In general, it may be said that it covers all the methods that may be needed to seek out and determine the causes of disease, and to formulate rules for their prevention and removal. It may thus be called also, preventive medicine. The progress of hygiene, such as it was, rested for many ages upon an experimental basis; and, indeed, to a large extent, this is still the case. The subject has, however, in later times at least, been studied to considerable advantage, though much remains to be done.

As among the results of the study of hygiene and its experimental investigation, and the application of knowledge thus acquired, it may be mentioned that two centuries ago the mortality of London was 80 per 1,000; at the present day it is under 23. A century ago ships could barely keep the sea for scurvy, while jails and hospitals were, in many cases, the hot-beds of fatal diseases. Now, these conditions are rectified, or at least the means of rectifying them are known. Thirty years ago the English troops at home died at the rate of 20 per 1,000; now their death-rate is less than one-half of this. A knowledge of the causes and modes of propagation of disease being necessary in order to provide rules for its prevention, it is obvious that hygiene must be largely dependent upon the advances made in pathology and the causes of disease; hence the impossibility of any yearly marked progress in former times, by reason of the imperfection of the collateral sciences, and the want of the appliances more recently made available for inquiries of such difficult and recondite character.

Within this century, however, and especially within the last forty or fifty years, it has been possible to follow out the subject on a more strictly scientific basis, and so to lay a foundation at last on which to build a structure which may one day entitle hygiene to a place among the exact sciences.—*Rhode Island Monthly Bulletin.*

Monks as Physicians in the Middle Ages.

Fechin, who figures as the first presbyter named in the Third Order of Irish Saints, according to the famous catalogue given in Archbishop Ussher's "Britannicarum Ecclesiarum Antiquitates," is an interesting example of the circumstance, brought out into strong relief by Montalembert, that the early mediæval monks were the depositories and practitioners of the best medical knowledge of the time. His sphere of activity was mainly in the west of Ireland, and according to Archdeacon O'Rorke, the historian of the County Sligo, leprosy was the disease the saint was most frequently called in to cure. At Fore he was one day begged by a loathsome leper to take him in charge, and Fechin, having carried him on his back to the monastery, left him in the hospital and consigned him to the care of Themaria, wife of King Domnald, who, being promised a heavenly crown in recompense, undertook the unpleasant task. The Queen tended the patient devotedly, and she had her reward; for, so the chronicle runs, "next day, when the saint was going to the hospital, he saw a globe of fire ascend toward heaven from the roof of the building, and on entering the sick-room found that the man they had been nursing, and who had departed in the form of fire, was no other than our Lord Himself—the whole occurrence illustrating the truth of the words, 'Inasmuch as ye did it unto one of these the least of my brethren, ye did it unto me.' In going away the leper left behind a staff and a lump of the purest gold, with directions to the Queen to give them to Fechin, which she did, and the staff became the famous *Bachal Fechin*, with which the saint is supposed to have performed many miracles through life, and which was held in great reverence after his death; but the gold he employed in building hospitals and in other works of charity." Skilfully disentangling this and such like legends from their myth-opæic drapery, Archdeacon O'Rorke accumulates a mass of evidence, corroborated from other sources, which makes it clear not only that the chief, if not the sole, practitioners of Ireland in the seventh century were monks, but that the disease they were most commonly confronted with was leprosy, wrongly supposed to have been first brought into Europe by the Crusaders.—*The Lancet*.

Hygiene and Sunday.

Among the questions treated of at the recent Congresses in Paris, that of the observance of the Sabbath as a day of rest was not the least interesting. The Congress on this subject was presided over by M. Léon Say, who remarked that this rest, which several religions rendered obligatory, is a law of nature, and consequently a law of hygiene, the excellence of which has long been demonstrated, although it is not to be found in all national codes. The resting on the seventh day is of Biblical origin, and the custom of counting the days by seven was formerly the rule among the most diverse races—in India, as among the Celts, in China as well as in Arabia. Now that hygiene has become a positive science, it confirms the moral and material necessity for a temporary rest on the seventh day. The idea was adopted in principle by all the members of the Congress, which received the patronage of two political celebrities—Mr. Harrison, President of the United States of America, and Mr. Gladstone. In a letter which was read publicly, President Harrison declared that he considered that all workers, whether with the hands or with the head, were in need of rest, which alone can guarantee the general observance of the Sabbath. Mr. Gladstone declared that he attributed his robust health and his longevity to his invariable observance of the Sabbath rest. Several reports were presented to the Congress, and physicians, professors, philosophers, and hygienists are in accord on this point. All, without exception, support for workers of all classes and of all ages a weekly day of rest, which should even be made obligatory. It may here be noted that in 1881 this subject was opened to competition by the Swiss Government for a prize, which was awarded to Dr. Niemeyer, of Leipsic. The subject was brillantly treated by Dr. Niemeyer, who observed that the Dominical rest is the first command-ment of hygiene, which should be followed to obtain a peaceful and continued amelioration of society, and in this respect it is as much a rational institution as a religious one. The following is the summary of the conclusions voted by the great majority of the members of the Congress: "Rest on Sunday is possible in varying degrees in all industries. Sunday is the day which best suits the employer and employed, both as regards the individual himself and his family, and it is well that the day of rest should be, as much as possible, the same for all. When the Sunday rest is impracticable for certain reasons, it should be replaced by some other day, so that the workman may have fifty-two days' rest inthe year as equally divided as possible. This rest permits man to produce considerably more and better work, inasmuch as it contributes to maintain his zeal and to restore his physical forces.''—*Lancet.*

The High Death-Rate in Russia.

Dr. Leinenberg, of Odessa, publishes in the *Internationale Klinische Rundschau* a lengthy article on the mortality of Russia, which is full of interest for the statistician. He says that in the number of births alone Russia ranks first of all European States, as they annually amount to no less than 48.8 per 1,000 of the population. The latter would consequently grow with abnormal rapidity if an enormous mortality did not make this impossible. This mortality is, according to Janson, 37.3 per 1,000, while the Statistical Centre Committee reports it at 36.8 per 1,000. As to the causes of such high figures, Dr. Leinenberg points out that they depend largely on high infantile mortality. He states that 104.8 boys are born to every 100 girls, and that amongst the Jews the proportion of boys born rises to 128.9 for each 100 girls. The mortality of boys, as of the male sex in general, is correspondingly greater than that of the female sex, in the proportion of 36.7 to 35.2. Of 1,000 newly-born children 263.4 die before they are a year old. This mortality in the first year of infancy is in the province of Novgorod 281 per 1,000, and in the Rusk dirtrict of the province of Moscow it reaches the figure of 550.8 per 1,000. Even this enormous number has been surpassed by the town of Irbit, which shows a mortality during the first year of life of 560.2 per 1,000. The provinces of Ekaterinoslaw and Wilno are distinguished by the lowest infantile mortality, the figures mentioned in the report of the Statistical Central Committee being 139.7 per 1,000 for Ekaterinoslaw, and 118.9 per 1,000 for Wilno. Comparing the infantile with the general mortality in Russia, the author points to the following two important statistical results: Children up to the fifth year of age form more than one-half of the deaths from all causes. Infantile mortality shows a tendency to increase every year. This great infantile mortality in Russia must be largely attributed to the want of proper diet and of sufficient care, especially amongst the agricultural population. In summer, which is the time when nearly all the children die in the country, the parents are in the fields, leaving their infants at home with no supervision and without sufficient food. This sometimes leads to strange and sad accidents, as in a case mentioned by Giljarowsky, in which pigs devoured the buttocks of a child which had been left alone at home for a considerable period. Griasnoff attended a child which under similar circumstances had been attacked by goats and had lost every finger on both hands. Dr. Leinenberg also goes on to speak of the health of those who have passed the crisis of the fifth year. Of 1,568,315 boys born in the year 1858, only 750,622 were alive in 1879, and when out of this number 272,974 were examined for the purpose of military conscription, 58,824 men—*i.e.,* 21.5 per cent.— were found to be suffering from various incurable or chronic diseases, and had consequently to be returned as unfit for military service, so that of all boys born in 1858, 47.8 per cent. reached their twenty-first year, but only 37.6 per cent. preserved good health.

The Italian Premier on State Medicine.

In his great speech at Palermo on the 14th of October, Signor Crispi gave special prominence to what his administration had effected for the sanitary rehabilitation of Italy. "For four years," he said, "There had weighed on Italians the incubus of an epidemic "—cholera, to wit—"which, besides physical suffering and material loss had induced a moral disturbance, inevitable, perhaps, in a country where hygienic education was still so primitive and so sporadic. It was a prime necessity, therefore, to proceed at once to the sanitary rehabilitation of the State, and we made provision accordingly. We addressed ourselves first to the minds of men, and we prevailed on them to look the enemy in the face as the principal means of overcoming it. With anxious and systematic care we took the sting from present evils, and then we reconstructed laws to obviate their recurrence. Sanitary provisions should impose on the freedom of the individual no restrictions but such as are required for the safeguard of the lives of others. Personal hygiene is on that account one of those salutary measures which we are entitled to exact." In cognate spirit the municipal services were unified and at the same time reformed throughout the Peninsula ; " while," continued Signor Crispi, " we modified the constitution of the Sanitary Councils, so as to insure an earnest and an unremitting surveillance over the public health. We restored to its proper centre—the Home Office—the direction of the seaboard lazarettos, and by furnishing the chief ports of the kingdom with the means of precaution and defence, we established an outpost system to make head against the importation of disease. By degree and by law of favor (*legge di favore*), we assisted the minor communes in carrying out their sanitary rehabilitation—an opportunity of which already more than three hundred have taken advantage. By a modification and extension of the Bill, enacted for the benefit of Naples, the application of which to themselves was craved by some sixty communes, by considerately evoking and approving plans of house-reconstruction (*piani regolatori*) we have brought to the great cities the blessings of effective resanitation." Nor have more strictly medical reforms been neglected. " We have reconstituted," said Signor Crispi, " the whole vaccination service ; we have revised the Pharmacopœia ; and on the frontier towns, as a safeguard against epizootic invasion, we have brought up the veterinary stations to military efficiency. We have wrought, in a word, the practical consummation of that sanitary code whose fundamental idea will prove not the least title to the love and veneration long earned from all Italians—whether surviving comrades, or of future generations—by that soldier of science, of fatherland, and of freedom, Agostino Bertani. Thus we may pronounce ourselves as on the true path of that sanitary redemption for which, not less than the political, Italy was yearning—a redemption of equal necessity, and certainly not less of a blessing. An Italy sound in a physical sense will yield us those vigorous arms which will fertilize her the best—those hardy constitutions which as living ramparts will prove her strongest safeguard." The "youngest of the Great Powers" is to be congratulated on the enlightened legislation set forth in these eloquent periods. It will henceforth be her duty to develop, as well as maintain, the sanitary reforms she has effected, and to justify in this respect the position she has earned in the European State-system.—*Lancet.*

Open-Air Travel in Consumption.

Dr. H. I. Bowditch of Boston read an interesting paper at the meeting of American Climatological Association to show the great value of "open-air travel as a curer and preventer of consumption, as in the history of a New England family." The family under consideration is that of which the author was a member. At the age of thirty-five his father was undoubtedly threatened with consumption, having cough, hemoptysis, anorexia, diarrhœa, and general malaise, with fever and great debility. In this condition he set out with a friend as his companion and driver, in an open one-horse chaise for a tour through New England. After the first day's travel of twenty-five miles he was so much exhausted and had so much bleeding from the lungs, that the friend was advised to carry him home to die. The travelers, however, were both plucky and kept on, and soon every day's travel brought improved health. In this journey he traveled 748 miles, going "down into Rhode Island, thence by the way of Connecticut up through the hills of western Massachusetts to Albany and Troy, and back through Massachusetts to New Hampshire, Vermont and Maine and then to the home from which he started."

The benefit which he derived from this journey had proved to him the absolute need he had of regular daily exercise in the open air. Afterward, under daily walks of one and a half to two miles, taken three times daily during thirty years of life, all pulmonary troubles disappeared. He died in 1838, from cancer of the stomach, one lung presenting evidences of an ancient cicatrix at its apex, both being otherwise normal. He was sixty-five years old—*i. e.*, thirty years after the journey. Dr. Bowditch tells us that his father married his cousin, who, after long invalidism died of chronic consumption in 1834. Notwithstanding the strong predisposing influence to lung disease which would result from such a union, six of their eight children either reached old age or adult life and were married and have had children and grand-children, but not a trace of consumption has appeared in any of these 93 persons.

This remarkable immunity from consumption Dr. Bowditch attributes to the fact that his father, having experienced in his own case a vast benefit resulting from constant, regular exercise out of doors, apparently determined that his children should be early instructed in the same course. Daily walks were required as soon as the children were old enough, and "if any of us, while attending school were observed to be drooping, or *made the least pretence* even to being not '*exactly well*.' he took us from school, and very often sent us to the country to have farm life and out of door play to our heart's content. In consequence of this early instruction all of his descendants have become thoroughly impressed with the advantages of daily walking, of summer vacations in the country, and of camping out, etc., among the mountains. These habits have been transmitted, I think, to his grand-children in a stronger form, if possible, than he himself had them."

Dr. Bowditch adds: "1 submit these facts and thoughts for candid, mature, and *practical consideration* and *use* in the treatment all are called to make of this terrible scourge of all parts of this Union. For my own part I fully believe that many patients now die from want of this open-air treatment. For years I have directed every consumptive patient to walk daily from three to six miles; *never* to stay all day at home unless a *violent storm* be raging. When they are in doubt about going out, owing to 'bad weather,' I direct them to '*solve the doubt*, not by staying in the house, *but by going out*."—*Sanitary Inspector*.

Dangerous Dried Fruit.

Good housewives are often tempted, in visiting groceries, with the attractive dried apples and other fruit (says the *Monthly Bulletin of The Iowa State Board of Health.*) This is especially true of the laboring class, who are unable to indulge in the luxury of the more expensive preserved fruit. Public attention is called to the danger from dried fruit, suggested by Dr. Joel W. Smith, of Charles City, who has given the subject extensive investigation. It is a lamentable fact that a very large proportion of the food supply of this country, both dried and preserved, is put upon the market for purely speculative purposes, regardless of all hygienic considerations.

Danger from bleached dried fruit is hardly suspected, yet the use of such fruit is not without risk. Fruit is now bleached by all the larger evaporator establishments and by many others. This is well understood by those in the trade and by grocers, but hardly known by most consumers. Bleaching is done by exposing the green fruit to the fumes of burning sulphur in the evaporator, or, quite as often, before it is placed in the evaporator, the time of exposure to sulphur vapor varying with the degree of whiteness desired.

The practice has only become general within a few years. Most grown people recollect the advent of very uniformly white dried apples in 50-pound boxes. There was soon such a craze for the "nice white fruit" that nearly every evaporator company felt compelled, by the increased price of such fruit, to adopt the bleaching process. It is now applied to all kinds of fruits. (It had been to hops to some extent years previously.)

Are bleached dried fruits ever poisonous? Germany answers that they are, after repeated chemical examinations of American evaporated dried apples, zinc— poisonous in very small quantities—being found to such an extent in the samples, that all such fruit was ordered destroyed, and a decree issued forbidding future importations unless accompanied by a chemist's certificate that each lot or invoice was free from injurious substance. Such action—as there is no competition with such fruit—may well set the American public to thinking, and better to some action against the bleaching of fruit. Greater and uniform whiteness is the chief recommendation of the practice and against it are the losses and dangers from the bleachings. No farmer thinks his hay is improved when bleached by as innocent agents as sunshine, dew and rain.

The zinc found by German chemists is evidently from the zinc-coated or "galvanized" iron trays used in many if not most of the evaporators to hold the fruit while drying. Some sour fruits may act slightly on zinc, but it is chiefly from the burning of the sulphur, which causes the formation of sulphuric acid, and this acid in contact with water and air—as in an evaporator—is oxidized or changed to sulphuric acid—known also as oil of vitirol—and though in a very weak form, it readily acts upon zinc, as is shown in telegraphic and other galvanic batteries.

If not always poisonous, careful tasters know that bleaching always injures the fruit flavor. This is probably why so many people have lost their former relish for dried fruits. Grocers who realize these things, now find it almost impossible to longer obtain unsophisticated dried fruits. Canned fruits, though more expensive, are now often preferred to the uncertain dried fruits; while the latter, if pure, should and would be preferred over average canned goods, as safer and more economical, especially for distant points. Bleaching and tampering with fruits is calculated to greatly injure if not destroy, this important industry, which should now be only in its infancy. These views help explain the "over-done" evaporator business of 1888.

The quality and even the variety of well-known fruits, if unbleached, can often be told by the looks and by the taste when cooked, but when bleached those made from good and poor fruit, all look and taste alike.

If consumers of dried fruits will insist upon obtaining honest, healthful unbleached fruit, or none at all, such self-preservative action, added to that of the German government, will soon correct such a fraud as the useless and injurious bleaching of fruits,

The Psychology of Epidemics.

Every epidemic carries in its train curious exaggerations of many well-recognized characteristics, and these frequently call for appreciation and for treatment almost as much as the disease in which they originate. Perhaps one of the most striking of these mental perversities is to be found in the idea that the epidemic is to be treated by "common sense," or by nostra which have been largely advertised, or by specifics which are known to the laity mainly through their frequent mention in the daily press. Those suffering under this delusion feel that it is wholly unnecessary to seek skilled assistance, and they boldly dose themselves with remedies of whose power and properties they are absolutely ignorant. In Vienna it has already been found necessary to forbid the sale of antipyrin, except under doctor's prescriptions, as no less than seventeen deaths were attributed to stoppage of the heart's action owing to overdoses. The freedom with which the prescription of this remedy has been assumed by the public has long since been viewed with anxiety by the medical profession, and frequent warnings have already fallen upon deaf ears; and yet it is to be feared that if the epidemic of influenza should spread, many more examples of recklessness will have to be recorded. It is serious enough to cope with an epidemic and its sequelæ, without having matters complicated by ignorant and reckless experimental therapeutics.—*Lancet, Jan. 4, 1890.*

Cholera and Europe.

The epidemic of cholera which has for so many months been raging in the valleys of the Tigris and Euphrates and the interior of Mesopotamia, has also made considerable inroads into Persia. Reports of the epidemic having crossed the western boundary of Persia have been heard from time to time, but it has now been announced to the Faculty of Medicine, of Paris, that there has been an alarming increase of the disease in Central Persia and on the Turko-Persian frontier, and that the inhabitants are fleeing towards the north. All those who can afford the journey are trying to reach the Russian ports on the Caspian. Remembering that this is the route into Europe which the cholera has so frequently taken, the announcement must be regarded as one of great gravity.—*Med. and Surg. Reporter.*

NOTES ON "THE GRIP."

The Late Epidemic

Has made the young doctors dance wlth joy, while the older ones wish they had never been born; and the specialists are a little in doubt, but expect something later from the wreckage.

A Royal Prophylactic.

A report, which is probably a foolish canard, is cabled from London to the effect that the Prince of Wales always wears a sachet filled with frankincense next his skin as a preventive of infection, and attributes his freedom from influenza to its virtue. The Princess of Wales and her daughters wear similar sachets.

Mixed Pathology.

"What do you mean by la grippe, Count, in France? It seems such a strange name for a cold in the head." "Yais, Mees Hartingtonne, eet ees singulaire. I sink ze grippe in America is a sort of—of—vhat you call a handshake—n'est ce pas? And pairhaps zat has somesing to do vith vhat you call ze malair—ze shakes? C'est la même chose, pairhaps."—*Harper's Bazar.*

The Home of the " Grip."

Dr. Edward M. Buckingham, of Boston, sends to the *Boston Medical and Surgical Journal* a letter from Mr. F. E. Rand, formerly of the Caroline Islands, a group lying about six thousand miles southwest of San Francisco. The writer says that in these islands an epidemic closely resembling the present influenza always appears twice a year, in January and August. This disease attacks nearly everybody. How about hay fever there?—*Medical Record.*

A Humor of " The Grip."

In Germany a railway flagman at the crossing at a small station thought he had the grip when all the other employés of the road were getting leave of absence for the same cause, and applied to the company's doctor to be examined. The doctor could not spare the time to stop at such a small place, so he telegraphed to the flagman to be standing beside the track when the train went past, with his tongue out, and he would examine him on the fly. The flagman dutifully stood with his tongue out all the time the train was slowly passing his station, and the next day the company received from passengers a dozen complaints of the impertinent conduct of one of its employés at that station.

The "Grip" in Paris.

At a discussion before the Academy of Medicine, Professor Sée stated that the epidemic, in his opinion, was a special form of catarrhal fever. Professor Potain made measurements of the spleen in patients affected with influenza, and he remarked an augmentation in the size of that organ, a fact tending to prove that the malady is the result of a true infection. One curious circumstance brought to notice is that those addicted to alcohol do not take the disease. The doctors have therefore recommended their patients to use warm alcoholic drinks. Unfortunately, on the strength of this prescription, the public have been indulging in these drinks to such an extent that in three days, iucluding Christmas Day, no less than one thousand five hundred persons were arrested in the streets of Paris for drunkenness. Of this number, at least one thousand two hundred stated, in defence, that they were simply following the treatment prescribed for influenza.

BUREAU OF INFORMATION.

Trees on Streets and Highways.

EDITOR ANNALS OF HYGIENE:

As chairman of an important committee, I am endeavoring to obtain all possible information upon the subject of proper streets and highways in modern cities.

Our streets now are as follows:

The movement is to narrow the main driveway to thirty-four instead of forty feet and put a grass plot of three (3) feet wide along the tree line. Street paving is very destructive to trees when so very near, etc.

Are we right in our projection as to leaving a proper space for drive—as to the well-being of the tree—the beauty of the continuous grass plot and the *sanitary* result incident to such a street construction over the other. Is not the tendency of new cities in this direction, and will not all the considerations incident to the best development warrant an abandonment of the old and the adoption of the new idea herein contemplated, if it can be called new.   J. A. P.

SCRANTON, PA.

We would incline favorably towards the proposed change, from a sanitary point of view. We have a very high opinion of the value of trees in our streets, as an actual factor in increasing the heathfulness of a locality, in addition to which we believe that a sight so pleasant as such a street would be would produce upon the mind of the beholder an agreeable sensation, that, reacting upon the whole system, would be most favorable to health. We cannot say positively as to the effect of close paving on the life of the tree, but we have seen many large, thriving trees, planted in our cities, where the paving encroached very closely upon the trunk of the tree.   ED. ANNALS OF HYGIENE.

Purgative Milk.

EDITOR ANNALS OF HYGIENE :

I send you a bottle of milk for examination. Will you be kind enough to let me know if there is anything injurious in it for a child two years of age to take as a nourishment ?

My object in asking this information is that my child has been taking this milk for the last six months and during that time has been troubled with looseness of the bowels almost continuously, and after calling the milkman's attention to the fact he acknowledged that he had colored his milk with dandelion.   W. N.

The admission of the milkman is sufficient answer that this milk does contain an injurious foreign matter. A very powerful drug is made from dandelion; a drug that, in appropriate cases, will have a most beneficial action, but an article that would prove very injurious if given, indiscriminately, to young children. The practice of putting dandelion into milk to give it a "*good rich color*" is not uncommon and it is a practice that cannot be too strongly condemned.

ED. ANNALS OF HYGIENE.

The Abatement of Nuisances.

To a subscriber, living at Ardmore, Pa., who asks how the attention of the State Board of Health can be secured to a supposed nuisance, prejudicial to health, we would reply that a complaint signed either by the authorities, or, in lieu of this, by ten (10) reputable citizens, directed to Dr. Benjamin Lee, Secretary State Board of Health, 1532 Pine Street, Philadelphia, Pa., will be promptly followed by the visit of an Inspector. If this official finds the complaint well founded he so reports to the Board, and an order at once issues for the abatement of the nuisance.—[ED. A. OF H.]

SPECIAL REPORT.

State Board of Health and Vital Statistics, of the Commonwealth of Pennsylvania.

PRESIDENT,
GEORGE G. GROFF, M. D., of Lewisburg.

SECRETARY,
BENJAMIN LEE, M. D., of Philadelphia.

MEMBERS,
PEMBERTON DUDLEY, M. D., of Philadelphia.

J. F. EDWARDS, M. D., of Philadelphia.   GEORGE G. GROFF, M. D., of Lewisburg.
J. H. McCLELLAND, M. D., of Pittsburgh.   S. T. DAVIS, M. D., of Lancaster.
HOWARD MURPHY, C. E. of Philadelphia.   BENJAMIN LEE, M. D., of Philadelphia.

PLACE OF MEETING,
Supreme Court Room, State Capitol, Harrisburg, unless otherwise ordered.

TIME OF MEETING,
Second Wednesday in May, July and November.

EXECUTIVE COMMITTEE,
PEMBERTON DUDLEY, M. D., Chairman.   JOSEPH F. EDWARDS, M. D.
HOWARD MURPHY, C. E..   BENJAMIN LEE, M. D., Secretary.

Place of Meeting (until otherwise ordered)—Executive Office, 1532 Pine Street, Philadelphia.

Time of Meeting—Third Wednesday in January, April, July and October.

Secretary's Address—1532 Pine Street, Philadelphia.

Bureau of Registration and Vital Statistics—Department of Internal Affairs, State Capitol, Harrisburg.

State Superintendent of Registration of Vital Statistics—BENJAMIN LEE, M. D.

State Board of Health of Pennsylvania.

FOURTEENTH REGULAR MEETING.

The Fourteenth Regular Meeting of the Board was held at the Supreme Court Room, Harrisburg, November 13th, 1889, at 9.30 A. M.

Present :—Dr. J. F. Edwards, Dr. G. G. Groff, Dr. P. Dudley, Dr. J. H. McClelland, Howard Murphy, C. E., and Benjamin Lee, Secretary.

In the absence of a President the Board was called to order by the Secretary.

On motion Dr. J. F. Edwards was called to the chair.

An order of business presented by the Secretary was adopted as the order of the day.

The Secretary announced that since the last regular meeting .the term of Dr. David Engelman, as a member of the Board, had expired, and the Hon. Samuel T. Davis, M. D., of Lancaster had been appointed by his excellency, the Governor, to fill the vacancy.. The office of President was therefore vacant.

Nomination of a President *pro tem.* being in order, the Secretary nominated Dr. Geo. G. Groff, and there being no other nomination, it was on motion resolved that the Secretary be instructed to cast a single ballot for Dr. Groff as President *pro tem*. This was done and Dr. Groff was declared unanimously elected, and took the chair.

The minutes of the twelfth regular meeting held at Pittsburgh, May 30th, 1889, were read.

•Mr. Murphy moved that in order to preserve the continuity of. the record a note be appended to the minutes stating that the occurrence of the Johnstown flood, prevented the chair from calling a final session as was contemplated. The resolution was carried and the minutes approved.

The minutes of the thirteenth regular meeting held at Johnstown, July 10th, 1889, were also read.

Mr. Murphy suggested the following correction, that in the motion authorizing members to employ a typewriter, in preparing reports, the words " and stenographer " be introduced.

Dr. Dudley suggested the following correction, that the statement made by Dr. Van Kirk, be amended to read " that the conveyance of scarlet fever to Fredricksburg, Ohio," and "not the death of the child," " was due to the carelessness of the child's parents." These suggestions were adopted and the minutes approved.

The minutes of a special meeting held at Johnstown, September 27th, 1889, were also read and approved.

The Secretary then presented his report, which included the following items :

1. Annual report. (See THE ANNALS OF HYGIENE for December, 1889.

The Secretary read his fifth annual report to the Board. It was accepted with the thanks of the Board, and ordered to be transmitted to his excellency, the Governor, together with the minutes of the Board for the past year, as the annual report of the Board. It was further ordered that such portions of it as related to the work of the Board in Johnstown, and the other flooded districts, be printed and published in a separate monograph.

The Board then adjourned to 2.30 P. M.

SECOND SESSION.

The Board reconvened at 2.30 P. M., when the report of the Secretary was proceeded with, as follows :

2. Report of the work of the Board in Johnstown subsequent to the meeting of the Board, September 27th, 1889, by Benjamin Lee, M. D., Secretary.

The proposal to withdraw the State forces on the 30th of September had called forth such serious remonstrance from the citizens of Johnstown, that after consultation with his excellency, Governor Beaver, it had been decided to permit the special work of opening the choked mouths of sewers and freeing the channel of Stony Creek River from obstructions to the flow of sewage and drainage to be continued for a few days, without reorganizing the general work on streets, cellars and yards. This was successfully accomplished to the great satisfaction of the people, and on October 10th, a final report was addressed to his excellency, declaring the nuisance abated on and after October 12th, in the name of the Board.

The report was accepted, thereby endorsing the action of the Secretary in declaring the nuisance in the Conemaugh Valley abated.

3. Second annual report of the State Pharmaceutical Examining Board of Pennsylvania.

The Secretary presented the second annual report of the State Pharmaceutical Examining Board of Pennsylvania, and suggested that it be inserted in the Board's annual report. The suggestion was adopted.

4. Meteorological report for the year ending November 1st, 1889.

Resolved that abstracts of the reports of the Pennsylvania State Weather Service, with maps, be published in the annual report, as suggested by the Secretary.

5. Report on insanitary condition of Mexico, Pennsylvania, through flood. By C. B. Dudley, M. D., Medical Inspector, Altoona.

It appeared from the report that a large quantity of grain and other material was fermenting, and in bad condition and threatening the public health. The Secretary had sent disinfectants and instructions, and had notified the Governor of the need of assistance at this place.

The report was accepted.

6. Suggestion for a hospital for infectious diseases with crematory. By L. M. Davis, M. D., of Lancaster.

Dr. Davis had been for some time perfecting a quarantine hospital and crematory, so arranged that all air infected by patients should be destroyed, and isolation perfected.

The Secretary had replied and had referred plans and letters to Surgeon General Hamilton, of the U. S. Marine hospital service.

The report was accepted, and the Secretary was instructed to obtain cuts and plans for publication in the annual report.

7. Report of smallpox at Canonsburg. By J. Guy McCandless, M. D., and medical inspector J. R. Thompson, M. D., of Pittsburgh.

Dr. Thompson had vaccinated the persons in the hotel where the case originated, had disinfected the bed linen, etc., and fumigated the rooms. He also distributed the disease circular No. 8, in the district. No other case occurred.

The report was accepted.

8. Report of inspection at Millerstown. By Medical Inspector Paul A. Hartmann, of Harrisburg.

Dr. Hartmann reported there were nine slaughter houses in the town, all of which were found in a bad condition, to which he attributed two cases of typhoid fever. He further reported the town to be without sewerage, nothing but surface drainage being provided for, all kinds of filth were exposed. He had given directions for all insanitary premises to be cleansed. He also recommended the removal of the slaughter houses outside the town.

The report was accepted, but that part relating to slaughter houses only was approved.

9. Report on flooded districts on West Branch of the Susquehanna River. By Wm. Leiser, Jr., M. D., Medical inspector.

On instructions from the Secretary, Dr. Leiser had made a thorough search for dead animals along the streams, from Montgomery station to Georgetown; Penn's Creek, through Snyder and Union counties; Middle Creek through Snyder county; White Deer and Buffalo Creeks through Union county; a total distance of one hundred and fifty miles, and had found and burned the carcasses of fifty-eight animals. He further reported that the people in the districts had formed local boards and were placing the towns and villages in sanitary condition.

The report was accepted, and the action of the Secretary and medical inspector were approved.

10. Report of smallpox at Glen Lyon. By L. H. Taylor, M. D., of Wilkes Barre, medical inspector.

Dr. Thompson reported the disease to have been contracted on board a canal boat below Shicks-shinny. The patient had been promptly removed from the boarding house where he resided, in which were twenty people, to a pest house erected specially for the case, and which was properly isolated. Those exposed were vaccinated, and no other person took the disease.

The report was accepted.

11. Report on typhoid fever at Dry Run. By R. L. Sibbet, M. D., of Carlisle, medical inspector.

Dr. Sibbet reported that on instructions from the Secretary, he had investigated the typhoid fever epidemic at Dry Run, from which it appeared that eighteen of the cases arose from the use of water from one well, into which human and animal excrement, which was deposited near by, found its way. There were ten wells in the village, only two of which contained water fit for domestic purposes. In the valley there were about sixty cases of fever. He had addressed a communication to the people living in this valley, advocating the adoption of stringent sanitary precautions; had condemned the use of water from several wells; distributed circulars on prevention of typhoid fever; and had strongly urged them to obtain an act of incorporation as a borough, in order to take organized action for the protection of the public health.

The report was accepted, and referred for publication and the action of the inspector cordially approved.

12. Report on inspection of the old bed of the Pennsylvania canal at New Florence. By H. F. Tomb, M. D., deputy medical inspector.

Dr. Tomb stated that he had found the water in the canal to be stagnant, and generally in a foul condition. From six inches to about two feet of mud of a putrid nature, was found in the bottom of the canal; the weeds on the banks and surface shut out the sun. There was a bad odor from it, and many cases of malarial fever were attributed annually to its insanitary condition. He stated that the canal had been in this state for some years, and suggested remedies for the abatement of the nuisance.

The Secretary had addressed a communication to Mr. T. T. Wierman, chief engineer of the Pennsylvania canal, on the subject. He had replied promising that the matter should receive immediate attention.

The report was accepted, and the action of the Secretary and the suggestions of the deputy inspector were approved.

13. Report on typhoid fever at Wilkes Barre. By L. H. Taylor, M. D. medical inspector, and Benjamin Lee, M. D., Secretary.

An alarming outbreak of typhoid fever had prevailed during the summer months at Wilkes Barre. Up to October the total number of cases reported had exceeded six hundred and fifty, and many cases it was suspected, had not been reported. In his report Dr. Taylor stated that nearly all the cases were those of persons using the Laurel Run water. He had made an exhaustive examination of the sources of supply of this water from the mountains, and had discovered opportunities for contamination. The Secretary had subsequently made a personal inspection of the streams, and verified Dr. Taylor's observations. The reservoirs had since been thoroughly cleaned. In addition to this, wells had been sunk on the opposite side of the river, to obtain water by percolation from the river.

The report was accepted and referred for publication.

14. Report on case of glanders, at Mt. Gretna. By Benjamin Lee, M. D., Secretary.

The Secretary reported that in August, he had received a telegram from Veterinary Surgeon Huidekoper, stating that there was a glandered horse at Mt. Gretna, and asking for instructions, as he had used his best efforts to get instructions from the Secretary of the State Board of Agriculture, but unavailingly The secretary had replied, giving instructions for the horse to be shot. His Excellency, Governor Beaver, at this period visited the camp, and concluded that the animal might safely be quarantined.

The report was accepted.

15. Report of Inspection of Susquehanna and Nittany Valleys. By George G. Groff, M. D.

Dr. Groff reported that he had first visited Williamsport, and found it in fairly good condition, the people having cleaned the streets, and taken other sanitary precautions.

He then visited Jersey Shore, which he found in a very bad state. The streets were covered with mud sixteen inches deep; the whole town being covered with this deposit from the flood. The walls of the cellars were reeking with wet and slimy matter, and generally everything appeared in a condition detrimental to health, the people seemingly being unable to help themselves.

Tioga was next visited. The flood had also deposited here mud and rubbish, nine or ten inches deep, in the cellars, and the district had been under water, but the inhabitants had cleaned up the place to a great extent.

Lawrenceville was also found in a bad condition, but the flood had not been felt so severely here as at Tioga.

The Health Officer at Lock Haven, reported that that town had been cleaned up and was in good condition.

The Nittany Valley was next visited. Here in some of the villages, the destruction to life and property by the flood had been nearly as severe, in proportion to the population, as at Johnstown. Everything was in bad shape, and there was evidence of great suffering.

Renovo had entirely recovered. The flood had stopped at drift wood, and no help was needed there.

Huntingdon had felt the flood severely, but very little remained in bad sanitary condition there except the slaughter houses.

Punxsutawney was also inspected. It had been flooded, but was in fair condition.

At Huntingdon, it was found that a manufactory located there had filled up numerous hollow places in the streets with wood-bark, impregnated with sulphuric acid, which was not perhaps injurious to any great degree.

The condition of Jersey Shore and Tioga, was declared insanitary, and a nuisance, and Dr. Groff had suggested that assistance be given to the people in these towns, and that inspectors be appointed to supervise these valleys during the summer. The secretary stated that he had reported the conditions thus detailed, to his excellency, the governor, who had sent money to the districts mentioned as requiring help, and that he had himself, supplied disinfectants and circulars. Dr. Holloway had been instructed to keep a strict supervision of the towns in the valley.

The report was accepted.

16. Report of Inspection at Kilkenny. By Wm. B. Atkinson, M. D., of Philadelphia, Medica' Inspector.

Dr. Atkinson reported that acting on instructions from the secretary, he had inspected Kilkenny and found nuisances from manure heaps, wells and imperfect drainage.

The secretary had given instructions for the abatement of these nuisances, which had been attended to.

The report was accepted.

17. Report of Inspection at Phillipsburg, Centre County. By G. G. Groff, M. D.

Dr. Groff reported that cholera infantum at this town, with a population of three thousand, was very severe. He had examined the water supply, which appeared to be excellent. He attributed the sickness to hot days and cold nights, and had freely distributed the circulars on the care of infants. The flood at this place had proved a benefit in thoroughly cleaning the streets.

The report was accepted.

18. The secretary had prepared an explanatory circular letter on the establishment and formation of Local Boards of Health, in Pennsylvania, which he now read.

The letter was approved and ordered to be printed as read.

19. Report of Inspection at Hulmeville. By Wm. B. Atkinson, M. D., Medical Inspector.

Dr. Atkinson reported finding twenty-six pigs in the pens of a slaughter house, which were being fed on blood, and slaughter-house offal. There was no floor to the pen and the drainage ran on the ground.

The secretary had given instructions for the pen to be removed outside of the town; the place to be cleaned up, and the proprietor to cease feeding swine on slaughter-house offal.

The report was accepted, and the secretary's action approved.

20. Report on typhoid fever at Nanticoke. By L. H. Taylor, M. D., Medical Inspector.

Dr. Taylor reported that the disease had been confined to two families, who used water from one well. On analyzing samples of this water, it was found to be contaminated, and on instructions from the secretary, the use of this water was forbidden.

The report was accepted, and the action approved.

21. The secretary reported that sometime in August, some of the principal residents of Muncy complained that a company intended to construct water-works to supply that town with water, from a source which would render it liable to pollution, and dangerous to health; and to construct a dam in connection therewith, which would be a menace to the people living in the valley below.

Dr. G. G. Groff had made a thorough examination of the sources of supply. He reported the proposed pool, or reservoir, to be in a narrow gorge, and that in his opinion, a sufficient constant supply of water could not be maintained without a dam fifty feet in height. The proposed sources of supply were from eleven springs in the immediate neighborhood, but owing to the excreta from privies, drainage from kitchens, and other liquids from several farms, passing into the streams which flowed from these springs, he regarded these sources of supply as dangerous. Neither could the drainage from these farms be diverted into other channels, owing to the conformation of the surface. He considered that a serious epidemic might be caused by the use of this water, should a case of fever occur in any of these farm-houses, and further, that the proposed dam would be a constant menace to the people living in the valley.

Other sources of supply of a purer nature, were open to the company, but the one contemplated was the cheapest.

He recommended the Board to advise the Borough Council, in the interests of the public health, not to accept this source of supply.

The secretary stated that he had received several communications in favor of the proposed scheme, and requesting the board not to interfere. Such works were, however, often speculative schemes, got up by persons living at a distance, who were quite indifferent as to the quality of the supply, as they were not compelled to use it.

After considerable discussion it was resolved that the report of Dr. Groff be accepted and approved, and that the authorities of Muncy be notified that the proposed supply is, in the opinion of the board, liable to be impure and injurious to health, and that the board, therefore, advises them not to accept it.

22. Report on disinfection of clothing and household effects at Rankin. By J. R. Thompson, M. D., Medical Inspector.

The secretary read a communication from the Braddock Wire Company, stating that the premises of one of their tenants who was under arrest, was required, but the furniture and effects were in such a filthy condition as to be a nuisance. On investigation, Dr. Thompson found the facts, in the main, as reported, but declined to destroy the furniture. He had disinfected the linens, woolens, etc., by boiling, and taken such other precautions as rendered the premises and effects sanitary.

The report was accepted, and action approved.

23. Report of inspection of Trout Run. By E. D. Payne, M. D., Medical Inspector.

Dr. Payne reported that his investigation led him to conclude that an epidemic of typhoid fever at this place was caused by the June flood washing out the privy vaults, and thus contaminating the wells. The discharges from former cases of typhoid had been emptied into these vaults without being disinfected. He had instructed the people to clean and disinfect their cellars, and have their premises placed in sanitary condition. If this supposition were correct, it would show that the typhoid germ might retain its vitality for many years in a suitable soil.

The report was accepted.

24. Report of inspection as to cause of dysentery at Danville Insane Asylum. By Benjamin Lee, M. D., Secretary.

By request of Dr. Shultz, the superintendent, who reported a large number of cases of dysentery at the Asylum, the secretary had made a careful inspection at this institution. Samples of the water used, were sent to Dr. Cresson for analysis, and found to be contaminated. He considered it possible that that portion of the suction-pipe supplying the drinking water, which passed beneath the bed of the canal might leak, thereby contaminating the water with that of the canal.

Just prior to this inspection, Dr. Shultz had made arrangements, on a grand scale, to boil the whole of the drinking water of the establishment, by introducing super-heated steam from the boiler into a series of large, air-tight, iron cylinders, and at once the cases began rapidly to diminish.

The report was accepted.

25. Report of inspection at Lock Haven. By G. G. Groff, M. D.

At the request of several residents, Dr. Groff had inspected Lock Haven, it being reported that there was much fever and other sickness there. He had called upon the health officer and several others, principally physicians, and while some thought that there was an unusual amount of sickness, others considered that there was nothing serious to be apprehended. He had visited the reservoir, the water of which appeared clear and wholesome. Unless there was pollution of water from the farms as its source, he was unable to account for the typhoid, fever prevalent. There were at present one hundred and forty-four cases of fever at Lock Haven.

At Renovo and other places, the water supply from the mountains appeared pure, and yet there was much sickness in these places.

Mr. Howard Murphy considered that we had no more uncertain or dangerous sources of supply than mountain streams, unless they were protected by the purchase of considerable tracks of land on both sides of them.

The report was accepted.

26. Report of analysis of suspected waters from Butler, Pennsylvania. By Charles M. Cresson, M. D.

Dr. John E. Byers, had reported the prevalence of typhoid fever at Butler, which was attributed to impure water. He submitted samples for examination, one of which was found to contain typhoid excreta. The secretary had reported the fact to Dr. Byers pending a more complete analysis and examination.

The report was accepted.

27. Report on diphtheria at Gallitzin. By C. B. Dudley, M. D., Medical Inspector.

Dr. Dudley reported that another severe epidemic of diphtheria, had been ravaging Gallitzin. He had visited the district on October 9th, and again on October 15th, and found the outbreak serious. He attributed the disease to insufficient and impure water supply, lack of cleanliness, and want of drainage. He had called a meeting of the citizens, and pointed out the necessity of a stricter regard for cleanliness; had distributed the board's circulars, and taken other precautions. The epidemic was now abating. Much support had been received from the Catholic priest, Father O'Riley.

The report was accepted, and the action of the inspector approved.

28. Report of inspection at Confluence. By C. L. Gummert, M. D., Medical Inspector.

The inspector reported a serious epidemic of typhoid fever at this borough, and an entire absence of precautions to prevent its spread.

The secretary stated that Dr. Gummert had endeavored to form a Local Board of Health, at Confluence, but owing to a dispute between the resident physicians, this had not been fully accomplished. Dr. Gummert had approved a health officer, which action the secretary had disallowed, as he considered the inspector had exceeded his powers, and those of the board. He had requested Dr. Gummert to urge the council to assume the responsibility, as it legally belonged to them alone.

The report of the secretary was accepted, and his action approved.

29. The secretary reported that at the request of the authorities of Allegheny, he had recently inspected Butcher's Run, accompanied by Dr. J. R. Thompson and Dr. J. H. McClelland, Health Officer James Bradley, and several of the sanitary committee of the city council. The difficulty with which the city had to contend, was that the run lay partly in an adjoining township, and beyond the reach of its ordinances.

They carefully examined the entire uncovered portion of the run from its source, and found the stream polluted by sewage, garbage, and butcher's refuse, and he had forthwith condemned it as an unqualified nuisance, and advised the construction of a sewer as the remedy, and had notified the property-holders in the township to do their part in abating it, under a penalty of $100.

Dr. McClelland stated that since this action on the part of the Secretary, the authorities had given instructions for the covering of the stream by a properly constructed sewer.

The report was accepted, and the declaration of the Secretary sustained.

30. Report of Inspection at Berwyn. By Howard Murphy, C. E.

Mr. Murphy reported the stream complained of to be badly contaminated by sewerage from a hotel. The water was unwholesome, in fact poisonous, and the drainage a nuisance. The hotel authorities had given assurance that they would endeavor to abate the nuisance, and he suggested that further action be postponed, until their engineer, General Russell Thayer, could mature this plan.

The report was accepted. and recommendation adopted.

31. The Secretary reported that accompanied by Drs. J. H. McClelland and J. R. Thompson, he had recently inspected the Rider Garbage Furnace Company's furnace, at Allegheny. He found the furnace destroying garbage at a rapid rate, and was informed by the fireman that it was fully capable of destroying all the garbage the city furnished.

The claim made by the company is that no fuel is necessary, except just at the first heating up of the furnace, but he found coke being used in the grate in front. With that exception the furnace appeared to be performing its work inoffensively, and in an efficient manner.

The report was accepted.

32. On the same day the Secretary had examined the abattoir at Herr's Island, which was found very complete, clean and well ventilated. The animals were strung up by the heels before being stunned, and the jugular vein and arch of the aorta being at once severed, the blood drainage was very thorough. The disposal of filth and refuse was dealt with in a very efficient manner. An essential feature of this establishment was the profitable disposition made of every portion of the animals. The absence of any offensive odor in every part of the building was remarkable. The Secretary believed it to be the most scientifically constructed abattoir in the country.

The report was accepted.

33. Report on Transportation for Medical Inspectors.

The Secretary reported having communicated with the Philadelphia and Reading Rail Road Company on this subject. A satisfactory reply had been received. Dr. W. B. Atkinson had been appointed an employee of the company, and for future inspections would travel free where it was necessary to use the company's lines.

The report was accepted.

34. Nomination of Medical Inspectors.

The Secretary proposed the formation of a new district comprising the counties of Cambria. Westmoreland, Indiana and Armstrong, to be named the " Conemaugh District."

The motion was carried.

The Secretary nominated Dr. W. Matthews, of Johnstown, as Medical Inspector of the Conemaugh District. The nomination was confirmed and Dr. E. Matthews was declared duly appointed.

35. The Secretary presented his requisition for stationery and supplies received for the year, from the Secretary of the Commonwealth.

It was ordered to be printed.

36. Financial Report.

The Secretary presented the financial report, showing the expenditure for the year ending

The report was approved.

37. The Secretary reported that the number of written communications received by him during the year had been seventeen hundred and thirteen (1713), and the number sent by him, nineteen hundred and ten (1910). The total number health circulars and forms distributed, was twelve thousand seven hundred and eighty two (12,782). Of this number three thousand four hundred and seventy (3470), were distributed at Johnstown and the immediate neighborhood in connection with the flood of May 31st.

The distribution of the Third Annual Report was then detailed, showing twelve hundred and fifty-one, (1251), copies to have been distributed up to the present time. The total number of Compendiums of the Law, relating to Public Health and Safety, distributed during the same period, was one thousand and eighty-two (1082).

The additions to the library during the past year, were reported to be, of books, one hundred and sixteen (116), and of pamphlets, one hundred and thirty-one (131).

The report was accepted.

The Board then, on motion, adjourned to meet at 8.30 P. M., at the Bolton House.

The Board reconvened at 8.30 P. M., when the Reports of Standing Committees being next in order, were presented as follows :

Report of Executive Committee.

Dr. Pemberton Dudley, Chairman, reported that this Committee had held four meetings during the year, when accounts, amounting to $ and covering vouchers numbered to had been examined and approved.

The report was accepted.

Report of the Committee on Registration and Vital Statistics.

The Chairman, Dr. Lee, stated that he expected to have an interview with the Secretary of Internal Affairs to-morrow, with regard to registration of marriages. The Register of Physicians was in the printers' hands.

The report was accepted.

Report of Committee on Preventable Diseases, and Supervision of Travel and Traffic.

Dr. J. F. Edwards, Chairman, stated that he had a report in preparation. He solicited permission to place it in the printers' hands for publication in the Annual Report.

The statement was accepted, and the desired permission granted.

Report of the Committee on Public Institutions, and School Hygiene.

Dr. J. H. McClelland, Chairman, stated that in plumbing and ventilation regulation of schools there was great improvement. Substantial progress in heating these buildings was also being shown.

The report was accepted and ordered to be published.

Report of the Committee on Adulterations, Poisons, Explosives and other Special Sources of Danger to Life and Limb.

Dr. Pemberton Dudley, Chairman, reported that as a result of the limited means at the disposal of the Board, little or no expenditure of the funds had been deemed prudent, especially as during the past year unusual demands had been made upon the resources of the Board. When the means and facilities at the Board's command would warrant it, a more energetic policy would be pursued.

The report was accepted.

Reports of Special Committees came next in order.

Dr. J. F. Edwards, Chairman of the Committee oppointed to inspect the towns in the flooded regions of the West Branch of the Susquehanna, reported that the committee had visited Jersey Shore, Tioga and Lawrenceville, all of which were found to be in fairly good state as regards sanitation—they having apparently recovered from the effects of the flood with the assistance rendered by the State, and their own energy; and the committee now recommended that the declaration declaring these places a nuisance be withdrawn.

The report was accepted, and the recommendation adopted.

The appointment of Standing Committees for the ensuing year being in order, the President decided that the committees should remain the same as last year, except that Dr. S. T. Davis be substituted for Dr. George G. Groff, as Chairman of the Committee on Sanitary Legislation, and as a member of the Committee on Registration.

New business.

Dr. J. H. McClelland having been accredited as a representative of the Board during his recent visit to Europe, presented a report on an examination of the mode of purification of the water-supply of Antwerp, Belgium. In investigating this system, Dr. McClelland stated that he had received the cordial support and coöperation of Colonel Stewart, the American Counsul at Antwerp, formerly of Pittsburgh, who introduced him to Mr. E. Devonshire, the chief-engineer of the water-works. The process consisted of bringing the water into forcible contact with small pieces of iron, and was described at length. (See ANNALS OF HYGIENE for December, 1889.)

The report was accepted, with the thanks of the Board, and referred for publication.

The Secretary then presented bills to the amount of $1439.74, covering vouchers Nos. 281 to 304, inclusive, which had been audited and found correct by the Executive Committee.

They were read, and on motion, approved.

Mr. Howard Murphy moved that the meetings of the Board be held in Harrisburg, in future, at four o'clock in the afternoon.

It was carried.

On motion of Dr. P. Dudley, it was resolved, that the President and Secretary be a Committee to prepare a resolution expressing the regret of the Board, at the severance of Dr. David Engelman's connection with it, and to forward such expression of regret to Dr. Engelman.

Dr. J. F. Edwards, presented the report of himself and the Secretary, as delegates to the recent Annual Meeting of the American Public Health Association, in Brooklyn.

It was accepted.

The Board then, on motion, adjourned *sine die*.   BENJAMIN LEE, *Secretary.*

THE
ANNALS
OF
HUGIENE

✳

VOLUME V.

Philadelphia, March 1, 1890

NUMBER 3.

COMMUNICATIONS

" Water."*

BY R. HARVEY REED, M. D.,
Of Mansfield, Ohio,

City Health Officer, Mansfield, Ohio; Member American Public Health Association, American Climatological Association, American Medical Association, British Medical Association, National Association of Railway Surgeons, Ohio State Medical Society; Honorary Member D. Hayes Agnew Surgical Society, Philadelphia, Texas State Medical Association, Texas State Sanitary Association, etc.

I trust the members of the medical profession will pardon me for directing my attention to the people instead of my professional peers in the preparation of this address.

My only excuse is that I take it for granted that there is not a doctor in this audience who does not know as much about this simple subject as I do, while the people, you must remember, have not had neither the time nor the opportunity to study the problems that cluster around the water they drink, and which play such an important part in their health, long life and prosperity.

Geographers have long since informed us that about three-fourths of the earth's surface is covered with water, while physiologists tell us that about 60 per cent. of the human body is made up of the same compound of oxygen and hydrogen.

I believe it was Landois who said "water is of the utmost importance in the economy, and it is no paradox to say that all organisms live in water; for though the entire animal may not live in water, all its tissues are bathed by watery fluids, and the essential vital processes occur in water; a constant stream of water may be said to be passing through organisms," and hence it hath been truly said that "the most important substance used as food is water."

We have now two general axioms before us:

First.—That nature has furnished us with an abundant supply of water.

Second.—That in our physical organization, water holds the controlling stock.

From this it would be reasonable to argue, on the basis of supply and demand, that if the wants of our system are large, and nature's supply very greatly in excess of this demand, that we should have very little to worry about.

*The President's Address, delivered before the First Annual Meeting of the Tri-State Sanitary Association, held at Wheeling, West Va., February 27 and 28, 1890.

But the chemist comes up and tells us that water is not only a powerful, but *general* solvent, that it dissolves to some extent nearly everything with which it comes in contact, so that it is *never* found chemically pure in nature.

Even rain, as it falls through the atmosphere, dissolves and washes out the particles of dust and organic matter that are constantly found floating in the air; it absorbs the oxygen, carbonic acid, ammonia and nitrogen in its descent from the clouds to the earth; hence we speak of the freshness of the air after the grateful summer shower.

Our farmer friends often brag of the purity of their springs; yet these are all modified by the character and constituents of the soil through which their supply percolates on its way to these natural fountains; the same may be said of wells which are only artificial springs and are governed by the same laws.

Rivers play an important part in the continuous forces that join the oceans below to the clouds above, yet their waters are subject to the same laws of dissolution and absorption, as the former; and thus we might go on from the lakes to the ocean, the ocean to the clouds, and from the clouds back to the ocean again, seeking for pure water, until wearied and disgusted, we exclaim with the Psalmist of old, " There is none of them good; no, not one."

But I hear some one ask, if all this is true, how does it come that we have been drinking water from some of these sources for years and years and are still alive?

I answer, simply because you have not *imbibed* enough of these impurities to kill you; or, perhaps, you have been blessed with a constitution sufficiently strong to eliminate them from your system as fast as you have forced them upon it.

Again, a water may be far from being chemically pure and yet not be dangerous, or even injurious to the human economy.

Then the question naturally follows, What kind of water *is injurious*, and what kind *is not?*

I will answer the first proposition of this question by saying that all waters containing decomposed organic material is injurious, and the more they contain the more dangerous they are; again, waters containing certain minerals, such as salts of lead, mercury, antimony, arsenic, etc., are injurious, and if they are contained in any quantities they are even dangerous.

To the second proposition of the above question I will answer, that pure distilled water stands *par excellence* above all; next to that, boiled rain or spring water, then follows ordinary pure rain water, good spring or deep well water, from uncultivated soil, or insoluble rocks, such as granite, quartz, or spar.

You will observe that we have not included the so-called mineral waters, which usually contain the salts of magnesia, soda, iron, sulphur, etc., and with the exception of these may be very pure; for the reason that such waters belong to the domain of the therapeutist, whose duty it is to prescribe them according to the disease of the patient; for it is not supposed that any healthy person wants to be continually taking medicine, whether in the form of a mineral water or pills, and especially in a food, which constitutes 60 per cent. of his whole physical organism.

In going back to the first axiom, it may seem somewhat paradoxical when I say that usually *a city's water supply is one of the most perplexing problems the city authorities have to deal with.*

The fact that it requires 60 per cent. of water as compared with all the food taken to complete and keep in a healthy condition the human economy, saying nothing of its multiplicity of other uses, demands that this supply be not only *bountiful*, but of the purest character possible.

On this fact depends a city's health, and to a certain extent its low mortality, both of which are prime factors in the prosperity of a given commonwealth.

Wells sunk in a city, no matter how pure they are at first, or how deep they penetrate the earth, are bound to become contaminated in time with organic matter; and not only correspondingly injurious, but absolutely dangerous, whether they reach rock, or only penetrate the soil or clay above.

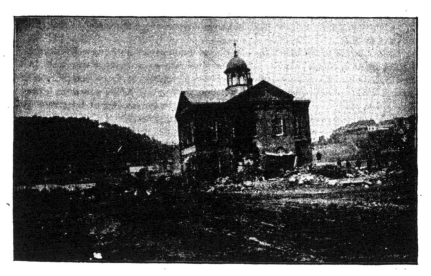

Public School Building—Johnstown.

The soil of any city soon becomes an immense mass of organic filth; sewerage of all kinds penetrate it as water does a sponge, until wells which, when dug, were in the country and yielded a bountiful supply of good, wholesome water, but when surrounded by a city become simply the receptacles of percolations through this mass of organic filth and corruption; especially is this true in cities using the old-fashioned privies for their "night soil," in which cases the original and previously harmless soil is perforated like the lid of a pepper box, with these intolerable slums of seething corruption, from whose foul receptacles ooze with every rain the juices of these sickening masses, befouling the soil wherever they touch, until they find exit in the *wells* of the city, because they are deeper than the former, and thus by the law of gravitation are the natural outlets for all this liquid filth.

Even wells drilled deep in rock are not exempt from this source of contamination. I remember a case occurring in my own city where a family was being severely afflicted with typhoid fever. Inquiries were made as to the probable cause ; the well was suggested. Oh no, it could not be that ; they had the finest water in the city ; their well was deep, and nearly all of it in rock ; their water was crystal clear ; had a delicious taste, and was beyond suspicion. It was finally decided, however, to pump it dry, and go down in it and seè if it needed cleaning.

When this was done nearly a foot of slimy " night soil " was found in the bottom of this same well, whilst from a crevice in the rock was found a constant stream of the same, busily keeping up the supply from a large privy some 75 or 100 feet distant, which vault was driven into the same strata of rock, whilst the solutions of this " night soil " had found their way, through the laws of gravitation, into this well, even carrying with them much of the solids to this receptacle, thus contaminating what was supposed by the *family* to be the " purest water in the city."

There is not a city in our land in which this or similar cases cannot be multiplied by the scores.

Nor do the cities stand alone in the pollution of wells. Only a few days ago I was called in counsel with a neighboring physician, whose practice was chiefly in a rich farming district among the " Richland Heights," to see a case of typhoid fever. When I arrived at the house I found that out of a family of seven all had been sick with typhoid fever, with one death, and the last member of the family was not expected to live (and has since died) with this terrible disease ; besides the suffering they had endured, saying nothing of the risks of life, in addition they had lost an aggregate of over sixty weeks of valuable time, saying nothing of doctor's bills and associate èxpense.

I had been called in counsel with the same physician in the same family when the first case of this series of typhoid fever cases broke out, and made a sanitary survey of the premises, with a view to discovering the cause.

They lived in a healthy farming district, among the hills, with ordinary farm surroundings, with a dry yard, cellar and house. There had been no typhoid fever in the neighborhood for miles around ; but I found a shallow well, which the family bragged on for its excellent quality of water ; and when its virtue was even suspicioned, they at once avowed its innocence, and argued that they had used its water for years, and they had had no trouble of this kind before, and besides, " it was the finest water in that neck of the woods."

On examining the surroundings of the well, I found a smoke-house close to the well under which the chickens had roosted, whilst a short distance from that was a chicken-house, with an earth floor which was covered with hen manure, and beyond that was a garden which was heavily manured every spring ; all these lay in close proximity to this well, and in a favorable position for drainage into the same.

An unusually wet season had favored the percolation from these various sources in finding their way into this well ; the water of which contained large quantities of chlorine, showing the presence of organic matter, also large quantities of free and albumenoid ammonia.

I condemned this water as unfit for use ; but my warning was not heeded by the family in time, and the result was a most terrible scourge of continued sickness, with the loss of a mother and a son, besides over sixty weeks of time lost, and other expenses, before they had atoned for the violations of the sanitary code.

I could multiply these cases by the scores resulting from both springs and wells of this or any other county in our State, were such necessary; but it would be useless to waste your time and weary your patience with such repetitions when a word to the wise *ought* to be sufficient, to convince you of the dangerous character of well and spring waters, when subject to pollution from organic filth, which depth does not guard against, as was proved in the case of the Ludlow-Lane well, near Liverpool, England, which was 443 feet deep, yet was fouled by percolations from cess-pools.

We will now turn our attention to the next most frequent source of water supply to cities—the rivers and lakes.

If wells are fouled under circumstances much more favorable for a pure water supply, what must be the water supply from our rivers, which are used as the natural sewers for all sorts of the *foulest* of the *foul* of organic filth!

Ah! but some one says that running water purifies itself. Don't you believe it. The old theory that "filthy water becomes pure by running over half a dozen pebbles," has long since been proven false, and without foundation.

It is true that organic filth, whether in solution in a running stream or elsewhere, gradually oxidizes, and to a certain extent loses it poisonous character; yet this oxidation is so slight as compared with the immense quantities of organic matter dumped into our rivers from all sources, that it cannot under any circumstances be relied on for safety, from a sanitary standpoint.

Just imagine the Mississippi River purifying itself, when eight cities alone dumped 152,675 tons of garbage and offal, besides 108,250 tons of "night soil," and 3,765 dead animals into this open sewer in one year; or the Missouri River, when only four cities furnished its waters with 36,000 tons of garbage, 22,400 tons of "night soil" and 31,000 dead animals in the same length of time. Oh! what a delicious decoction of organic filth with which to slake the thirst of mortal man, and breed pestilence and disease?

In referring to the above pollutions of the Mississippi and Missouri rivers, Dr. Kilvington, of Minneapolis, says: "No theory of self-purification of running water will dwarf the magnitude of this sanitary crime."

Follow the Mississippi River from its source in Lake Itasca to its delta in the Gulf of Mexico, and count the cities and towns that have multiplied along its banks and estimate their aggregate population, each one of which use this for their natural outlet for all their filth—saying nothing of the refuse from the thousands of boats that traverse this great water-course—and then estimate its utmost capacity of purification, and you will soon be engulfed in a sea of the darkest sanitary despair.

The same may be said of ALL our thickly populated rivers, where the cities and towns *above* furnish their neighbors *below* with a daily supply of the foulest of their filth; while the cities and towns *below* have been, and are still drinking of this diabolical mixture, with only here and there a sanitarian to molest them or make them afraid.

For an example of the results of this awful sanitary crime, I need only refer you to the terrible epidemic of typhoid fever which occurred to your next-door neighbor (Bellaire) only a few years ago.

In the report of the Rivers' Pollution Commissioners on the Domestic Water Supply of Great Britain they say:

"River water, usually in England, but less generally so in Scotland, consists chiefly of the drainage from land which is more or less cultivated. When it is *further* polluted by drainage of towns, and *inhabited* places, or by the foul *discharges* from *manufactories*, its use for drinking and cooking becomes *fraught with great risk to health;* a very large proportion of the running waters of Great Britain are either at present thus dangerous to health or are rapidly becoming so."

The truth of the above findings was proven true in the "Queen City of the West" only a few years ago, which paid the penalty of drinking polluted river water by the deaths of scores of her inhabitants from typhoid fever, and hundreds of cases of continued sickness from the same disease.

In our own city we paid the penalty of our sanitary sins, while we supplied our city with water from a filthy creek which ran near-by, by numerous deaths from typhoid fever annually, together with scores of cases of sickness, with all their suffering, loss of time and unnecessary expense, from this same cause.

But since we have supplied our commonwealth with water from ten deep artesian wells (drilled in an unpopulated tract of land just north of our city), whose fountain head is believed to be in the Allegheny Mountains, and whose purity, after repeated chemical analyses by our State and other chemists, has shown our water supply to be exceptionally free from organic filth and a water of unusual purity; typhoid fever has almost vanished from our midst; our last annual report of the health department showing but one death from that disease in the city and that party used water from one of our many old wells, which are all more or less polluted with organic filth.

Lake waters, although less liable to the same percentage of contamination per 100,000 parts than river water, owing to its increased bulk to the same linear space of bankage, is not by any means free from organic filth, especially where they are densely populated.

To prove this, we need only refer you to the long series of water analyses of Lake Michigan at Chicago, and Lake Erie at Cleveland, and Lake Ontario at Ontario, Canada, which speak for themselves in unmistakable tones to the observing sanitarian.

It is true that the farther you recede with your intake from the shores of densely populated lake districts, the less organic impurities you will find ; yet it is not always practical to put the intake of a city's water supply beyond the *possible* contamination of organic filth, which is swept hither and thither by constant currents and counter-currents, besides being lashed about by frequent storms.

When the water supply of a city is affected by floods and freshets—which is usually the case when taken from a river and often the same when supplied by a lake—we have still another source of contamination which severely affects the public health, from this great troubling of the waters, which in their fury dissolve and wash out immense quantities of accumulated filth, which is pumped up in our water pipes during the floods, and that often require weeks to wash out, after the freshet has subsided.

You will now, no doubt, realize, if never before, the truth of the assertion I made in another part of this paper, "that usually, a city's water supply is one of the most perplexing problems the city authorities have to deal with."

Dr. Henry B. Baker, the eminent secretary of the Michigan State Board of Health, once said, "When a fire breaks out in a village every person considers it a duty to give a general alarm, and especially prompt notice of it to the fire department; and all citizens co-operate for the speedy extinction of the fire." If this were not done the *property* in the village would be quite generally endangered by the possible spread of the fire; but when the city authorities endeavor to improve your city water supply in order to prevent the spread of sickness and disease among your fellow-men, do they always receive the support and co-operation of the people as in the case of the fire? Do you ever find the people jumping out of their beds in the middle of the night and rushing half dressed to their fellow-citizens' support on account of

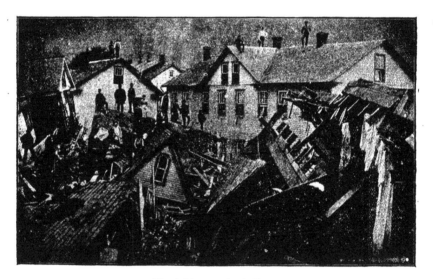

View in Johnstown after the Flood.

sickness? Not much: when it comes to that they fold themselves snugly in their "little beds" and sooth themselves to sleep by repeating the question "Am I my brother's keeper?" The taxes are already too high; we can't afford to have any more money spent in improving our water system, which is good enough for us, just to satisfy some "sanitary crank" in his exalted notions about a purer water supply.

'Tis thus they weigh out life and health, the real bone and sinew of a city's prosperity, against taxation; and by their howling they so intimidate the average councilman, who holds his office by the franchise of his countrymen, until he in turn really weighs out *life* in the balance against the chances for *re-election* at the next political contest.

. The people must learn the force and practical meaning of the good old adage that "Public Health *is* Public Wealth," before these obstructions to sanitary progress can be effectually removed.

They cannot expect the officers of their city to go far in advance of public opinion in the enactment of ordinances which require financial support to insure their execution; especially when opposition to public opinion means the political decapitation of the authorities who dare to thwart it.

Did you ever stop for a moment to think what your police force costs your city annually? Ah! but you say we *must* have a police force. What for? To protect the lives and property of our city. Why, sir, you would not be safe an hour in any large city in our land were it not for our police force.

True, we must have a police force and they must be paid good salaries and be efficient officers, and see that the law is executed, for the protection of our lives and property—just what we must have health boards for; and yet show me a city in the land that allows its health department more than a mere fraction of the financial support it appropriates to its police force for precisely the same thing—the protection of the lives and property of its citizens.

But some one says, What has a board of health to do with the property of a city? I will do like the Yankee—answer your question by asking you another—and ask you, what the property of a city would be worth were its citizens continually unhealthy and dying off by the hundreds from the effects of pestilential disease, as compared with a city blessed with a low mortality and the continued good health of its citizens?

You, the people, must learn that money judiciously expended for the protection of the lives and health of a city is always well invested, which will never fail to insure you a paying dividend.

Just think of it! Chicago, the great metropolis of this nation, pays a thousand dollars a day in support of her health department, and considers its money well expended, which, in return, yields a lucrative profit to that great commonwealth.

We have discussed briefly the importance of practical liberality in the support of the sanitary interests of a city, because this is one of the first considerations in the establishing or improvement of its water supply, which in time plays the leading rôle in the great drama of protecting the lives and health of its citizens.

We have tried to show you that notwithstanding water was one of the most liberally-supplied constituents of our food, and that we require more of this compound to supply the necessities of our bodies than any other, yet it is one of the most easily adulterated compounds we use in our daily *menu*, and less frequently found in a good, wholesome condition than almost any other product used in our daily bill of fare.

This brings us to the practical question proposed by the poet, who said

> "The River Rhine, as is well-known,
> *Washes* the City of Cologne;
> But, oh! ye gods and saints divine,
> Who then shall wash the River Rhine."

To the first proposition of this question I will answer, stop washing the filth of your cities in the River Rhine, and to the second proposition I will say, first, filter the water you use from the River Rhine, and second, boil it before you use it.

In regard to the first part of the poet's question, permit me to say, that in Ohio we have the following law, which, if put in force, would cover this proposition completely:

It says that "Whoever puts the carcass of any dead animal, or the offal from any slaughter house or butcher establishment, packing house, or fish house, or any spoiled meats, or spoiled fish, or any putrid animal substance, or the contents of any privy vault, upon or into any lake, river, bay, creek, pond, canal, road, street, alley, lot, field, meadow, public ground, market space, or common, and whoever, being the owner or occupant of any such place, knowingly permits any such thing to remain therein, to the annoyance of any of the citizens of this State, or neglects or refuses to remove or abate the nuisance occasioned thereby, within twenty-four hours after knowledge of the existence of such nuisance upon any of the above described premises owned or occupied by him, or, after notice thereof in writing from any supervisor, constable, trustee, or health officer of any municipal corporation or township in which such nuisance exists, shall be fined not more than fifty dollars nor less than one dollar."

Our law goes on still further and says, "Whoever intentionally throws or deposits, or permits to be thrown or deposited, any coal dirt, coal slack, coal screenings, or coal refuse from coal mines, or any refuse or filth from any coal oil refinery or gas works, or any whey or filthy drainage from a cheese factory, upon or into any of the rivers, lakes, ponds or streams of this State, or upon or into any place from which the same will wash into any such river, lake, pond or stream, shall be fined in any sum not more than two hundred nor less than fifty dollars."

The question now arises, What shall we do with all this daily accumulation of filth? I answer, utilize it on a sewage farm if possible, which should be located where it will not affect the public health. If this can't be done, then cremate the garbage rather than throw it into our rivers and lakes.

But, you say, both of these are expensive luxuries and will greatly increase our taxation.

Suppose they are; are you going to weigh out life against taxation? Are you going to allow our rivers to become poisonous streams, dealing out sickness and death from their source to their mouths, simply because it will cost you a few dollars to keep them clean?

No city or county can afford to do this. Life is too valuable, sickness too expensive, and death too terrible to allow our citizens to be slowly poisoned by throwing our garbage into the streams, simply because it is a convenient and cheap method of disposing of it.

This has become a momentous question and the time is near at hand when it must be stopped by the enactment and enforcement of rigid federal laws, if in no other way.

But, you say, while the *garbage* of cities increases the filth of our rivers, yet their waters are impure at best.

This being the case, what are we to do for good, wholesome, potable water? I answer, where it is possible to secure an artesian well supply that is practicalty pure and wholesome, by all means do so, taking care to locate your wells in an uncultivated, unpopulated district.

When this can be accomplished pump your water directly from the wells into your mains without any intervening reservoir.

In this way your water will be free from organic filth, of an even temperature, winter and summer, and free from the effects of rains and floods. If this cannot be done, however, and you must depend on a river or lake for your water, then you should subject your city water to a process of precipitation and filtration, and thus remove the sedimentary products that are always more or less present in river and lake water.

In order to make it absolutely safe from the poison of typhoid fever, and free it from the possibility of producing enteric irritation, all potable water should be boiled, as I do not consider any filterer proof against typhoid fever germs.

Under no circumstances should you trust the well water of our cities, which are all more or less contaminated with organic filth, and never free from the possibility

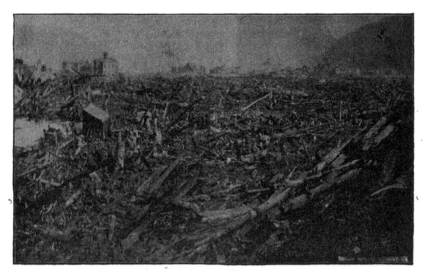

The Jam near the Stone Bridge—Johnstown.

of organic poison|; especially is this true in cities which have not adopted and enforced the dry closet system.

Ladies and Gentlemen : I have already detained you longer than I expected when I first commenced this address. My only excuse for doing so is the magnitude and importance of the subject I have endeavored to present to you this evening.

If I have been plain and outspoken on this subject, you will pardon me on the ground of my interest in a theme that involves the life and health of my fellow countrymen.

And now, before closing, allow me to thank you for your interest and attention to this vital subject ; also, allow me to thank my fellow sanitarians for the honor they have bestowed, by electing me the President of this Association ; and, finally, if what I have said or done has aroused any one of you to the importance of this great sanitary problem, I will feel that my labors have not been in vain.

On the After-Dangers of Floods : Their Nature and Remedies.*

BY E. D. PAYNE, M. D.,
Of Towanda, Pa.,
Medical Inspector to the State Board of Health of Pennsylvania.

In case of a flood, after the waters have subsided, after the dead have been gathered in and disposed of, after the driftwood and carcasses have been burned, there is still work for the State Boards, demanding the exercise of sound judgment, large discretion, and not a little labor.

This work may not take the public so readily, nor produce so profound an impression on the public sense as that which precedes it, but it is not less important, and in many ways, requires greater care and more constant vigilance. The first is like fighting an open enemy who constantly presents his front; the latter is fighting no less an enemy, but one that lurks in ambush, who strikes in secret, who is invisible and intangible, and yet whose blows are none the less deadly. We are struck with horror at the rush of the waters, the giving way and sweeping down the stream of large buildings, the piling of wreck on wreck, the struggle and agony of men, women and children fighting for their lives; a feeling of awe and dread takes possession of us, and he must be strong of heart and steady of hand who dares make an effort to save life. The after-fight with disease and death requires different qualities; moral courage now takes the place of physical; a keen eye, a pleasant and persuasive tongue, a firmness in enforcing commands, which in many instances must appear like requests, some knowledge of disease and its derivation, some knowledge of State law, a moderate amount of that quality of mind which dares assume responsibility.

The waters have not only carried death and destruction in their path, but they have left behind broken sewer pipes, emptied vaults, wells deluged with waters holding in solution or suspension the filth of the flooded district. The walls of houses have a deposit of filth adhering to them, and the cellars are filled to greater or less depth with slime and mud. The weather is hot and sultry, or becomes so before the situation is rectified. Nor is this all ; poor or scanty food and improper clothing assist in depressing the system and rendering it an easy prey to disease in one who has been demoralized by the catastrophe, and breathes in with his sleep the foul odors which surround him.

Under these conditions it is not unreasonable to say sickness may be expected —sickness of the most deadly type, that known as filth disease, from which comes fevers, specific and non-specific, fluxes without fever, adynamia, that peculiar form of the mucous membranes which is accompanied by a train of symptoms

> " Variable as the shade
> By the light quivering aspen made,"

and which we call malaria, perhaps, because we do not know what else to call it.

Not only this, but the place becomes a centre of infection ; the breezes catch up the germs and float them in the air to other localities ; the waters carry them

---

*Read before The Tri-State Sanitary Convention, at Wheeling, W. Va., Feb. 27 and 28, 1890.

down the streams to some point where an economic water company thinks filters bring additional expense without additional safety; and many accept the dispensations of Providence without a thought of fighting against them.

Kind friends come to nurse the sick, and carry away infection to some point where each becomes a new centre of it. People, actuated by various interests or simple curiosity, do the same. Public funerals are held where the simplest services and quietest interments should only be allowed.

The first question in this respect is, Do the conditions justify the statements above made? To my mind they are so plain as to need no supporting argument. I think the specific nature of certain diseases is so universally accepted among scientific men, and that in any one case of a specific disease it has had for a parent the same form of disease, that an apology is needed in such a meeting as this, for introducing the question; and I only do it, and give some illustrations, as a basis upon which to build my statements as to the nature of the duties of the State Boards after floods, and the duties of citizens in co-operating with them.

Strange as it may seem, I have known instances in late years of a physician in large practice, telling the families under his care that they need not take pains to isolate the children sick with scarlatina—conveying the impression that scarlatina was a mild form of scarlet fever, and giving that name to those cases which appeared in a mild form; that it often appeared to but one child in a family; that in very many instances persons were exposed without contracting the disease. I will add to this statement another, viz. : That within the past few years, I have known otherwise intelligent members of the community to take the same position, and not only laugh at the efforts of the physicians to establish good quarantine and good hygienic surroundings, but to do so honestly, and honestly regard the efforts to produce disinfection as one of the fads of the day—one of the popular crazes to be met.

It is a matter for congratulation that the great daily papers have given space to science for the furtherance of the new ideas. The country papers take up the subject, and, not to be thought to be behind the new ideas, reproduce the subject until it reaches the quiet valleys and distant hill-tops. A great change has taken place in the minds of the people in a few years.

So long as we could only say, "I believe that certain diseases which are ordinarily called 'catching,' are the result of the reception into the system of a germ, which produces the disease," we were at a disadvantage; for we were immediately told to produce the germs. If asked what it looked like, we could not tell.

We were laughed to scorn, if a case of diphtheria, scarlatina, measles or typhoid appeared in a community as the first case, and no apparent connection existed between it and any other. Unpleasant experience may have been had with the itch. Did they not *know* they " got " it from another? Had they not actually put a "magnifying glass" over the ascarus and seen it? They know they must not come in communication with smallpox, but exactly why they did not know. They know that in case of scabies they need not fear if they did not come in contact with it. But in the case of variola they know that they must neither come in contact with it nor in communication with it; but why, they didn't know. They could understand contagion, but not infection.

This, however, they did know; that contact with scabies did not produce variola, and that communication with variola meant something more serious than rubeola; that exposure to the mumps, which they know to be "catching," did not mean to them a case of scarlet fever.

In other words, they were able to demonstrate that like always produces its like, and that exposure to disease did not mean that the resultant might be any one of a dozen forms, as individual characteristics and environments might decide. They also knew that to " take the breath " in a case of mumps, meant an attack of the disease, if they had never had it before. But why did not taking the breath from an ordinary cold produce mumps? Evidently, because they thought a certain something was conveyed in the breath of one sick with the mumps to the healthy individual. How many stopped to consider that that certain something must be of material substance and form, we probably will not know.

So, when we come to consider the matter, we do not wonder that investigators have been hunting for and trying to identify this individual certain something which when passed from one individual to another always reproduces itself and its attendant phenomena. It is more than thirty years since Prof. J. K. Mitchell taught his class that he had seen so many instances of apparently healthy husbands or wives sickening and dying of tuberculosis in a short time after burying a tuberculous spouse, that he had come to believe that one contracted it from the other; and, though mildly indulged and mildly chaffed, he taught that, in his belief, the time was coming soon when the germ theory of disease would prevail. It is more than twenty years since Dr. J. H. Salsbury hunted for and thought he individualized the germs of a number of diseases. I knew of these men long before I heard of Pasteur or Koch. *En passant*, let us honor the names of our countrymen who, though hunting after truth sometimes fail to find it, as much as we would those of foreigners who though they often think they find some new thing are frequently shown it is no new thing at all.

For myself, I as firmly believe that any infectious disease is the result of the reception into the system of its own specific germs as I do that any plant that grows in my garden is the result of its own specific seed; and I would as soon expect a pumpkin or a squash to spring up where I had planted a potato, depending upon soil and climate to determine which should appear, as I would typhoid, diphtheria or smallpox to proceed from a germ common to all. More than that, I would as soon expect a plant to grow where I had put the ground in the best possible condition for its growth but had planted no seed, as I would a specific form of disease to appear, no matter how favorable the circumstances for its appearance, if the specific germ of that disease had not found reception in the individual.

When asked why do not all persons exposed to specific poison contract the disease represented? I ask, in reply, Why do not all seeds of the vegetable kingdom germinate? Why do not all bullets fired in battle kill? Why do some fuses fail to explode a bomb?

I should feel that I was unwarrantably encroaching on your time in this discussion, but for two reasons. If the germ theory of disease is not true, then is your labor in vain. In case of a flood an engineer with his gang of men; a cartman, with his gang; a scavenger with his gang; and an emergency committee, to distribute food and clothing, would answer every purpose. But; believing it true, I use it as a basis for the consideration of the dangers which are likely to arise after a flood. I will illustrate by some examples : A number of years ago scarlet fever appeared in a family in this town. The child was confined to an upper room, where she passed through the disease and made a fair recovery. A year from that time, a young lady came to visit the family and was put in'the same room, and on the ninth day came down with the disease.

Six years ago, my own little child was attacked with scarlet fever. There was no other case in town, so far as I could discover. She had certainly not been exposed in any known way. But in a town sixteen miles north of us, the disease existed in an epidemic form, and a strong north wind blew for a number of days.

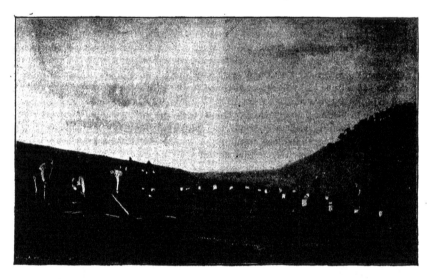

The Cemetery on the Hill. The last Resting Place of the Victims ot the Flood at Johnstown.

A few years ago diphtheria appeared in a family of West Franklin, this county ; immediately after, a large number of cases appeared in the neighborhood. Its appearance was inexplainable until it was found that a female relative of the first family had passed through this town, and had slept with a child that had sore throat.

A number of years ago the nurse girl in a family in this town was called home to help care for her sister's children, sick with scarlet fever. On arriving home, she went into an unoccupied room, completely changed her clothing, and helped care for the sick. When ready to come back, she went to the same room where she had left her clothing, took a bath and put on the clothing she had worn there. When she arrived at the house where she was in service, the youngest child was delighted to see her. He climbed into her lap, put his arms about her neck, and was fondled. Nine days after, he sickened with scarlet fever. The other children had had the fever previously, and did not take it. It seems probable to me that though the nurse had taken what she thought were good cautionary measures, she had carried the germs in her hair, and, during the fondling of the child, he had inhaled them. I think the reason why in each of these cases the same form of disease was reproduced, was owing to the law long ago given by the Almighty, when he said, Go forth and multiply, each after his own kind. Neither do we grow grapes on thorns, nor figs on thistles.

To proceed with the statement of the nature of the work to be undertaken by State Boards after floods, I would say it is manifestly their duty to protect the country from the influence of specific diseases. When I say the country, I speak advisedly; for if the flood of May of last year, is any criterion, disease might be scattered far and wide, but for prompt action. The waters bring to the surface and distribute over large sections, all the filth that has been hidden for years. This was not only the case in the Conemaugh Valley, but in the counties of Lycoming and Tioga, in this State, and the Southern Tier of New York.

In reference to the germs of specific disease, I will argue no farther, except to say that I am not aware that the period of viability or ability to reproduce its like has yet been determined for any of them. I have cited a case of scarlatina, which shows the germ to be active after it had apparently lain dormant for a year. How many germs of scarlet fever and diphtheria are packed away in family closets to be brought out and be the origin of sporadic cases, we shall probably never know.

That the action of floods, in bringing to open exposure all these germs, is different from any other action I cannot see. I have cited a case to show that the germ of diphtheria can be carried for miles after transient exposure. During an inspection at Trout Run, Lycoming Co., last year, I demonstrated to my own satisfaction that the flood had washed out a vault in which typhoid dejecta had been deposited at least four years previously, and that the water holding in suspension these germs had flooded a section of a town, where water was supplied to the public by driven wells and that the people so supplied had contracted typhoid.

But we will leave the question of specific germs, and inquire whether the waters that simply hold in suspension earthy matter—often foul smelling and disgusting—can, without containing specific germs, produce disease. I do not hesitate to say they can. But I would differ from those who say the form of disease would depend upon personal characteristics and environment. I do not believe this world was made by chance; I do not believe a tree or plant springs up by chance; and I do not believe that any form of disease appears by chance. Certainly these non-specific deposits will produce disease, but not specific disease. The mucous membranes will be affected; resulting in nausea, vomiting, diarrhoeas and dysenterys. The nervous system will be affected; producing malaise, general prostration, adynamia and malaria. Fevers will result, but they will be of an ephemeral or simple continued type, and in no instance will either of them reproduce itself in a fresh subject unaffected by the conditions which produced it in the first.

I would say then, that the first duty of State Boards under such circumstances was to take possession of all such flooded districts, and by the judicious use of its inspectors, ascertain the precise conditions which obtain. These inspectors should be clothed with authority to enter upon any and all premises and find out the exact conditions; and these they should minutely report to the Board or its Executive. I would say the first remedial measures should be to prevent the use of any water that was suspected of contamination. I would next direct attention to the food supply, inspecting all that was offered for use.

Next the clothing that was brought out of their own closets, where it had been stowed away, and that which came out of all the closets in the land, offered them for use, should receive attention ; and all that appeared musty or long disused should be disinfected. This could all be preliminary to or go on at the same time as the general cleaning up, and would be the most effectual guard against infectious diseases. Next in order would come a thorough cleaning of houses, cellars and premises. This should be as thorough as possible. The simple pumping out of cellars and washing of their walls should not be sufficient. They should be washed and re-washed until all appearance of slime is gone. Then they should be washed with disinfecting solutions, until all odors and suspicion of filth was destroyed, and finally left with lime washed walls and lime distributed on the floors to absorb the moisture.

But what shall be done with the sick cases as they arise? I would say they should be immediately taken charge of by the Board and treated by its own agents, who would make daily reports. Immediately separate each infective case from its surroundings, place it under the care of a physician of the Board, and care for it by the Board's trained nurses. To this end, I would have erected so many small hospitals as might be needed.

They need not be expensive. Abundant experience has shown that cheap board structures, properly situated, built only tight enough to keep out the storms but not to keep out the air, are the safest and afford the largest percentage of cures in infective diseases. Costly and substantial structures—no matter how perfect the system of ventilation, fall far behind these in warm weather. The well-to-do man would fare far better in such a structure than in his well-appointed home. I would also have a separate structure for each specific form of disease, if practicable, so that no person might be exposed to an infectious disease other than that he already had.

I would say further, that not only should these measures be under the control of the Board, but that all voluntary assistance that was not ready to place itself at the disposal of the Board and under its system of rules, should be warned off. Such an occasion is not the one for gaining cheap fame or reputation, It may make better newspaper items, but it will not meet the emergency so speedily, grasp it so firmly, or overcome it so readily.

All voluntary contributions and State appropriations should also be placed in the hands of the Board. Food, clothing, medicines and supplies of all kinds should go into the store-houses of the Board, for distribution, and not subject to the indiscriminate misuse and waste they might have if each man who brought supplies insisted on being able to say on going home that he distributed them himself.

Finally, this scheme would involve the necessity of a greater appreciation on the part of the several States of the necessity and usefulness of these State Boards, and the legislatures should place at their disposal such funds as would make their usefulness effective.

Immediate Disinfection of Debris of Floods.*

By M. HOWARD FUSSELL, M. D.,
Of Manayunk, Pa.

It is with diffidence that I, a humble practitioner of medicine, presume to speak before a body learned on sanitary matters, upon a subject in which you are experts and I a novice.

No one, however, can pass through the experience that was the lot of the workers in Johnstown, after the memorable flood in 1889, without having decided impressions made, and consequent opinions.

It is to be devotedly hoped that there does not exist another such death-trap on the surface of the globe as existed at Johnstown before the 30th of May, 1889.

But as the cause of that great disaster was not heeded by the few who recognized it, and not known to many, so there may be many other places just as perilously situated, and though no such great emergency may arise, it behooves us to profit by the lessons learned in the valley of the Conemaugh, in order to apply that knowledge in the lesser emergencies constantly occurring. Just here I wish to add my testimony to the praise of the State Board of Health of Pennsylvania.

Few persons recognize the heroic work done by Dr. Benjamin Lee, its secretary, and by his associates. But for the energetic and wise measures adopted by Drs. Lee and Groff, who were in immediate charge, it is as certain as fate that a great pestilence would have followed the horrible flood.

The survivors of the flood were paralyzed by their unparalleled misfortune ; they apparently did not think of the great danger that would certainly arise from the thousands of decaying bodies of animals : their whole thought naturally centered on the recovery of the bodies of the dead human beings. Into this chaos of thought and action came Lee, Groff, and their associates, instituting, promptly, measures for the destruction and disinfection of the carcasses, and thus saved the whole country from what might have been a terrible epidemic.

The writer did not reach the scene of the disaster until early in the morning of the the fifth day. By that time the Secretary and Dr. Groff had taken measures to clear the banks of the river below Johnstown, and had begun to form the Sanitary Corps of Johnstown.

Vast numbers of dead and decaying bodies lay exposed everywhere about the acres of *debris*, and hundreds more were buried in the wreck, with putrefaction somewhat delayed but none the less certain.

The great question presenting itself to Dr. Lee and his associates was *how* to rid the town of these sources of danger. The resources at hand were limited, sadly limited, but in the course of twenty-four hours after the Chief Deputy was appointed the corps was in good temporary working order.

The first necessity here, as it must be in all emergencies, great or small, was efficient assistants.

I think that when it is at all possible, the assistants should be medical men, or men trained in sanitary work.

An ordinary doctor certainly should have better ideas of the dangers of filth than an untrained individual.

*Read before the " Tri-State Sanitary Convention at Wheeling, W. Va., Feb. 27 and 28, 1890.

The ordinary man will view with composure the decomposing carcasses of hundreds of brute animals, and still more complacently masses of decayed vegetable matter, while he is filled with horror at the sight of a decaying human body. The reason of this is self-evident of course; but while the fact remains it would certainly be unsafe to put such an individual in charge of a disinfecting corps, for fear he would likely allow the many animal bodies to go without destruction, while he buried or carried to a morgue the one human body.

Therefore, those in charge of the disinfecting corps should be physicians when it is possible.

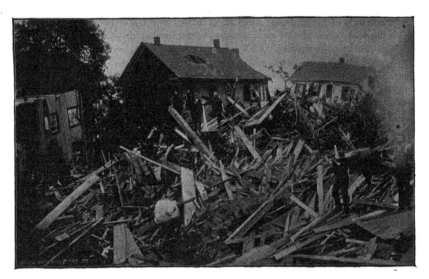

View in Johnstown after the Flood.

It seems almost trite for me to write that the bodies of animals should be destroyed and not buried; yet I found in many instances gangs of men busily engaged in burying the carcasses of horses, instead of destroying them. The region to be disinfected should be divided into districts, and a medical man placed over each. The smaller the district the better and quicker the work will be done.

The equipments of the disinfecting corps need be but simple. A rope is a necessity, axes and shovels are needful, but in a dire emergency can be dispensed with.

The choice of disinfectants then comes up, and I take it that they can be divided into fire and chemicals. Fire to be used when it is at all possible; chemicals in the few instances where the bodies and other decaying objects cannot be burned.

When it is possible, each corps should consist of the chief and twelve men. That number of men I found to be amply sufficient to take the body of a large horse any reasonable distance, and over any sort of surface.

The corps starts out armed with a rope, axes and shovels where obtainable, chemicals if possible, and the means of producing fire. If it is possible to obtain it, each corps should carry as large a quantity of rosin as convenient. Everything should be burned when it is practicable.

If a large animal is found covered up deep in the *debris*, one of two plans can be adopted. Either a certain section of the *debris* can be separated from the rest, and fired as it lay, while the remainder is protected by the use of water ; or the animal can be removed from the *debris* and burned on a clear spot.

It is in very rare instances that the latter cannot be done ; the wreck can be cleared in order to allow approach to the body. A rough path of boards laid over the pile of wreckage, all the twelve men can easily slide the body over this to a place where the pile will not be fired.

With my twelve men I in one instance removed the bodies of five cows from the porch of a house, in the centre of one of the wards and conveyed them several hundred yards to a place of safety, this was done in about four hours.

The bodies can be burned by simply covering them with wreckage and setting fire to it, a good blaze over the body for eight hours, will certainly destroy it, and the blaze can be kept up by leaving one or two men in charge with orders to keep piling on the fuel.

If rosin can be obtained it is a good plan to cover the body thickly with it and then place the burning materials. This however I do not consider a necessity.

Human bodies should of course be removed for burial and wherever it is possible a special corps should be detailed for that duty.

Besides the bodies of men and animals there will always be quantities of beds and bedding, vegetable matters of all kinds, which are prone to putrefaction.

One of the most difficult tasks the inspector will have to perform will be the destruction of these latter articles. Beds, soaked, foul odored and certainly useless, will be lugged into the cellars and garrets of the inhabited houses to be dried. This of course must not be permitted and many tongue lashings will the inspector receive who presumes to destroy what the poor loser considers useful to himself.

In this, however, as in all other matters must the inspector's judgment come into play, and he must not allow his kindly feelings to overcome his disinfecting sense.

I wish to emphasize my thoughts upon the use of fire. Fire is the most certain, swiftest disinfectant in our possession, and for that reason alone should be used where at all practicable.

There was a strong movement on foot in Johnstown to burn the wreck, which was overcome by the officers in charge of the town.

Two objections were offered to this :

First.—That many human bodies would probably be burned.

Second.—That valuable property would be destroyed.

The same suggestions and the same objections are likely to be raised in the event of any great flood.

Doubtless many bodies would have been burned, but, personally, I would much rather think of the body of one near to me being burned in an act to protect health, than I would of its being exposed and becoming a source of danger to others.

Many of the bodies recovered later are sure to be unrecognizable, save by wearing apparel or some peculiar marks, and it must be but a melancholy satisfaction to possess a body out of all semblance to a human being, not to speak of the one dear to us.

I am quite sure that thousands of dollars and weeks of valuable time, together with much of the comparatively slight sickness that existed after the flood at Johnstown, would have been saved, by the early firing of the worst parts of the wreck.

One week after the flood, existence in the centre of parts of the wreck was almost unbearable, and must have been detrimental to the health of the survivors.

Firing of sections of the wreck would have been perfectly practicable with but little loss of valuable property. A certain area could have been separated from the rest by means of alleys cut through, and firing of the rest of the town could have been prevented by the concentration of the fire engines on this one point.

In this way masses of wreck, that it required days to clear up by hand, would have been cleared in hours. A clear saving of money and perfect immunity from danger of disease.

If the orders were given by the authority of the State Board and by means of the fire, good property destroyed the owners of that property could recover from the insurance companies.

Of course such wholesome firing could apply only where there were masses of useless wreck, and not to blocked up streets with valuable buildings on either side.

Instances will arise where some body or mass of putrefying substance cannot be removed from the drift to be burned, and when prudence on the part of the inspector or positive orders from higher civil authorities prevents firing of the wreck as a whole. Such cases must be met by the free use of chemicals.

Copperas, powdered as finely as possible, or a saturated solution of copperas may be freely used. The first should be used where the body is not permeable to water. The latter where the mass is more or less porous.

In this manner a large mass of decomposing matter may be made innocuous for a considerable time.

Bromine is certainly a good actual disinfectant as well as a deodorizer. A foul mass sprinkled with a moderately strong solution of bromine will remain innocuous for several hours.

Bichloride of mercury can be used, in strength of 1 to 500. Whenever enough of this solution can be brought in contact with the mass it is needless to say that the process of putrefaction at once ceases.

Solutions of carbolic acid can of course, be used with the same effect as bichloride of mercury and possibly with less danger.

In any case where disinfection in this manner is used the disinfecting substance must be applied daily, or oftener, for obvious reasons.

In order to facilitate the work of the disinfecting corps, it will be well to have additional inspectors to search for places that need disinfection, and report to the chief of the corps, in order that he may go at once to his work of disinfection, and not spend his time in searching the drift.

To summarize: *First.*—The flooded district should be in charge of the executive officer of the Board of Health, where such a board exists, or under a medical man of wide experience.

Second.—It should be divided into as many districts as practicable.

Third.—The chief of each district should be a medical man, or one trained in sanitary matters.

Fourth.—All putrefying masses should be at once buried or disinfected.

Fifth.—Where practicable, the drift should be burned as it lay.

I have spoken often of the flood in the Conemaugh, because my sole practical experience consists in my labors after that flood, and because such a text has never before been given to any sanitary convention, and, it is to be devotedly hoped will never again occur.

The Sanitary Surprises of the Flood of 1889.*

BY J. B. KREMER,
Of Harrisburg, Pa., Secretary of The Flood Relief Commission of Pennsylvania.

The thoughts which I have gathered together at this time must be considered as coming from a plain business man, and formed from that standpoint, rather than from one whose line of thought and general experience is in the sphere of diseases, their causes, and the methods for their relief. Indeed, I feel strangely out of place in a convention of Physicians, and I attribute the honor of a position in your programme entirely to my active connection with the distribution among the sufferers in the recently flooded parts of our State, of the most magnificent charity the world has ever seen. This work extended over many counties, along many waters, and afforded me an opportunity of seeing, under varied phases, the havoc wrought, and the consequent results, by this most powerful element when it had broken away from its natural bounds, and I have been much interested in noting the different effects produced in the several localities which suffered most severely.

After the first great cry from the nation, of horror, at the merciless destruction of life, and the outburst of sympathy for those whose friends and kindred had been swept away, and after food was provided for those cut off from all sources of supply, the thought of the people seemed to turn at once to the care of the living—as to their sanitary surroundings. The profession, as well as the laity, expressed great fears for the health of the towns and cities which had been submerged, and, the calamity occurring at the opening of our summer season, for the effect which the decomposition of animal and vegetable matter might have upon the people whose water supply was in part received from streams flowing through the valleys most seriously suffering from loss of life. The attention of those who were selected to actively have part in the work of relief was thus early directed to this element of danger, and, as far as possible, at the suggestion of members of your profession, disinfectants were sent to the flooded districts, but beyond this no steps were taken, and having had no experience, no suggestions were made by the relief commission having in view the · prevention of disease.

*Read before the Tri-State Sanitary Convention at Wheeling, W. Va., February 27 and 28, 1890.

Being prepared, therefore, for a possible call upon the fund contributed for general relief, by reason of an epidemic, I have been greatly surprised that though the conditions of the several districts varied much, yet in no one of them, except only in the case of Lock Haven—to which reference will be made again—has there been directly chargeable to the overflow of the waters any large increase, either in the death-rate or in the number of cases of sickness of the character anticipated, and in some cases, very seriously overflowed, both the sick and death-rate have been lower than the average. That this statement is warranted I think there is no doubt; my information being received from the committees, who, in their several localities, acted with the Commission in relieving the wants of their neighbors.

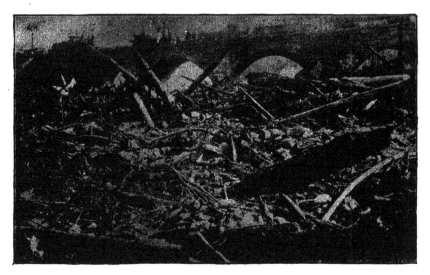

The Jam at the Stone Bridge—Johnstown.

On the Susquehanna River, the cities of Clearfield and Renovo were in part submerged, but from waters coming from higher points on the river, rather than from a sudden rising in their vicinity, and the same may be said of Tioga, Lawrenceville, Jersey Shore, Williamsport, parts of Muncy, Marysville, Milton and Harrisburg, and, the waters subsiding, there was left behind a comparatively small amount of residuum. This is true, also, of the towns along the Juniata river, Huntingdon, Mapleton, Lewistown, Mifflin, Newport and Duncannon, while Lock Haven—which seems to have been within easy distance of an extraordinary rainfall—was left when the waters receded with a layer of mud, the character and quantity of which could only properly be appreciated by personal observation. Some of these towns have a partial sewerage system, while others have but surface drainage; cesspools were washed out and the contents, mingling with the waters, must certainly have formed part of the sediment left by the receding waters. In some cases cellars were cleaned with scrupulous care and sediment was removed to a presumably safe distance from dwellings, while in others only the most necessary work was attended to in removing mud from the cellars, and the deposits from them and from the streets were used to fill up low places in the house yards and lots of the citizens. It is true that directly within the current rushing through these towns the water had in one respect a beneficial effect, as it thoroughly cleaned its course and left the streets and yards in better condition than before, and this was especially the case in the many small settlements which suffered severely along the smaller streams, where in many cases, an entirely new surface soil is presented, the old having been washed away ; but the parts of towns most severely affected were those away from the direct current and covered only by the quiet, backed-up water which receded as slowly as it had advanced. In some of these towns disinfectants were rather freely used, in others to a limited extent, and in others not at all; except as individuals may have used lime about their own premises.

The conditions being thus present to which we have been accustomed to attribute certain forms of disease, viz. : general inundation, thoroughly soaked plastered walls, moulding paste on wall papers, a deposit of mud mixed with decaying organic matter, which was not only about but within the dwellings—in some cases in every dwelling in the settlement—and which, as it dried in concealed places, under floors and within wall partitions, became a part of the breathing atmosphere at every agitation, and with all a summer of exceptional dampness, and with less than the usual amount of sunlight, had we not reason to be surprised at the general freedom from disease ? Lock Haven—to which reference has been before made—as having to a greater degree than other towns the conditions requisite for the full sway of malarial diseases, after passing through the summer without trouble, was visited in the late autumn with a low type of fever which threatened serious consequences. By many this was attributed to the causes above mentioned, but it is more than probable that these had, if any, only a modifying effect, the prime cause being of an entirely different origin. But on this, I presume, some of your members have formed an intelligent opinion based on personal investigation.

While surprised at the record of the settlements on the Juniata and the Susquehanna, we yet more wonder when we consider the condition in the Conemaugh Valley. Here were all the conditions present in the other localities, but in vastly greater degree. Deeper water, standing for a longer time ; a greater amount of sediment, and mixed with it car-loads of flour, meats, and provisions, the contents of all the storehouses of a large city, with their various kinds of animal and vegetable matter, and this for months, under a burning sun, being stirred up and carried through the streets on hundreds of wagons ; to say nothing of the bodies of animals and of human beings, who even to this time are being found almost daily, and in many cases within a few inches of the surface of the ground. Add to this the changed conditions of living ; from comfortable homes to tents and shanties, or still worse, crowding to many times their proper limit, the dwellings of their more fortunate neighbors ; from comfortable beds to sleeping, for weeks in some cases, on the floors or on the ground ; from a home table to meals, which though abundant, yet from the lack of facilities were but illy prepared ; and to all this the terrible physical and mental strain to which the whole population had been subjected and which rendered them less able to withstand or to throw off the attack of disease. It was not a surprise that knowing of these conditions, physicians from all parts of our

State and from some of our neighboring States, hastened there to give the benefit of their skill and experience to the many who would most likely require their assistance; but it is a surprising thing that the records show but little, if any, greater mortality in this valley than is usual, and that the number of cases of sickness of the character referred to has not been greatly in excess of that of other years. Here disinfectants were used, of kinds innumerable, in quantities marvelous, and in cost—as I learned when the bills were presented—stupendous, and the contributions from the various makers and dealers may have nearly equalled the purchases. They were used in every way, carted from house to house and left in abundant quantities, carried by the workman to their places of labor, placed in, on and under everything in the valley, and even sprinkled on the street from watering carts; they were everywhere, they permeated the atmosphere, and a traveler from Johnstown, could always be known by the foul odor he carried away on his clothing.

Can the good health, or rather the freedom from the feared epidemic of the citizens of this valley be attributed to this free use of lime, chlorides, *et al ?* If so— and both science and experience seem to affirm it—this to the laity is again a surprise, and the facts should be so heralded that a greater faith in this form of preventive would be made to possess the minds of the people generally.

A practical suggestion may here be made for the consideration of your body. When casting about for information as to what best could be done for the several settlements in the flooded districts, I failed to find such specific directions as to the various kinds of disinfectants, and how and in what quantities they should be used, as was desirable. True, each maker accompanied his product with "full directions," and the Commission was besieged with offers of all kinds from manufacturers for the introduction and use of their particular preparations, but we had no code of rules for the guidance of individuals, whether in town or country, as to the best use to be made of the materials which might be most available to them. Such rules, in popular form, may be in use, but we were at least unfortunate in not finding them.

In looking, then, to the future care for submerged districts, it would be well for Boards of Health to prepare in advance circulars or hand-bills, giving in plain terms full directions for the use of the various disinfectants, and particularly for the benefit of farmers and residents in small villages, information as to the use of such articles as would be most nearly within their reach when it is not possible to send to them the more powerful preparations. They should have information concerning the advantages of the use of the more simple articles which are available in every neighborhood. These rules or instructions should be kept in quantities, and at once sent to towns and villages and mailed to isolated individuals when the necessity might arise.

Believing, as I do, that the general good health of the Conemaugh Valley was made possible only by the free use of such means, and that, whatever other causes may have assisted, their use was an important factor as to the other places mentioned, it is very necessary that not only should such information be given as suggested, but that promptly, and in the most liberal manner, through properly organized channels. A supply of the disinfectant which may be judged best for the purpose, should be sent to the places requiring aid; for it must be remembered that at the time of such calamity the people affected are least able, for many reasons, to help themselves, and that charity is the best which is dispensed at the time of greatest need.

"The Destruction of our Forests the Chief Cause of the Floods that have Devastated our Country."*

By C. F. ULRICH, A.M., M.D., A. A. Surgeon U. S. Marine Hospital Service, Wheeling, West Virginia.

Our country has lately been ravaged by extensive and disastrous floods. The great flood of the Ohio Valley in 1884, with its attendant destruction of property and, in many instances, of life, will long be remembered. The subsequent overflow of Wheeling Creek and other streams, with its wholesale destruction of bridges, carrying away of houses, and the drowning of entire families, will not be soon forgotten. But the climax of this series of calamities was reached by the horrible disaster of Johnstown, in 1889, the horrors of which will be related in song and story long after the present generation shall have been laid in the dust.

The question naturally arises, "Must these things be? What is the cause? and Can they be prevented?"

There are, no doubt, various causes working together to this end, the discovery of which requires a thorough knowledge of meteorology, which the busy practitioner is unable to attain, and which must be left to the special student of that department of science,

But there is one cause—in my opinion the chief one—that lies near the surface, and that every one, learned or unlearned, can easily understand. It is the whole-sale destruction of forests, as it has been practiced for the last hundred years. This cause has been recognized in Europe, and is well understood there, as shown by their forest laws and the care taken of the original forests, as well as the continual planting of new ones.

This is not only a cause of floods, but also of their opposite—of droughts ; the two complementing each other.

It has often been remarked that floods and droughts are of much more frequent occurrence now than they were in the earlier history of the country, and surprise has been expressed at this fact.

Our rivers, in former times, afforded a highway for thousands of boats, great and small, being navigable the greater portion of the year. Now we either have the channels so shallow that no boat of any size can run, or the stream overflows its banks and cannot be satisfactorily navigated on that account. The principal reason of this difference is the reckless and wanton cutting away of the forests that once covered our land.

Let us see how this cause produces such disastrous effects.

When the rain falls upon a dense forest, a large portion of it is retained by the foliage, which prevents it from reaching the ground so rapidly as it does in an open country. We all have experienced this when, caught by a sudden shower, we made for the nearest large tree that was in sight and took refuge under its spreading boughs, where we were comparatively safe from the rapid gush of waters.

The ground, protected by trees with heavy foliage, is soft and spongy, rendered more so by the annual fall of leaves which decay and combine with the soil.

---

*Read before the Tri-State Sanitary Convention, at Wheeling, W. Va., February 27-28, 1890.

Now, when a heavy rain falls, it is first delayed, as I have stated, by the foliage, so that it does not come down with such force and rapidity, but strikes the ground softly, enabling the spongy soil to absorb a large portion of it and give it off gradually. This finds its way into the streams with sufficient slowness to enable the stream to carry it off without overflowing the banks ; for we all know that streams overflow because the water rushes into them faster than it can be carried off.

On the other hand : Denude a certain extent of country of its forests, and the ground is baked hard on the surface by the heat of the summer sun. When the rains fall with force and in large quantities, the water rushes with tremenduous rapidity down the naked mountain sides, washing deep gullies as it goes along, carrying with

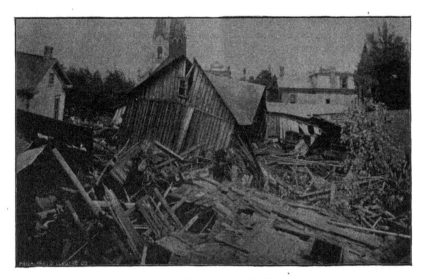

View in Johnstown after the Flood.

it whatever there may be of soil, which is no longer held together by the roots and radicles of the trees, depositing it in the valleys or carrying it to the mouths of the large streams, thereby obstructing navigation.

Let us take, for example, the great Ohio Valley, in which we are all so much interested. Suppose, instead of the wholesale destruction of forests which has been practiced during the last century, the valleys and hilltops had been put in cultivation, while the steep hillsides had remained covered by the original forests ; only the largest trees being cut out as the timber was needed, or those beginning to decay removed to make room for the young and vigorous trees to grow and spread out. What would be the condition of things at the present time? The country would present a more beautiful appearance ; the climate would be more equable ; there would not be such extremes of heat and cold ; our spring rains would not result in disastrous floods ; nor would our summers be rendered almost intolerable by such awful droughts. Look at the countries bordering on the Mediterranean Sea, once the garden of the world; producing fruits, grains and flowers to delight the eye and make glad the heart of man; where arose, bloomed and grew to perfection the highest civilization and culture known, at that time, to the human race. What is it now? Mostly a barren waste, with naked rocks and arid, unproductive soil, where the inhabitants can scarcely earn a livelihood. The causeless, wanton and wicked destruction of the forests, promoted and encouraged by the Mohammedan religion has done the greater part of this work. The beautiful forests, cultivated by the Hellenic races, the groves, sacred to their divinities, used to beautify and adorn the land, have been leveled by the ruthless vandalism of ignorance and superstition, until the inevitable consequences followed; a succession of droughts and floods; the former rendering the land unproductive; the latter washing away what good soil there was; thus permanently ruining the land and converting much of it into arid wastes.

The final result of this was that the countries, subjected to these changes, were reduced to poverty; such of the inhabitants as were willing to work, emigrating to other countries; while the indolent portion of the population, better satisfied because there was nothing to do, remained, earning a precarious livelihood, by preying upon tourists and antiquaries. Thus, what was once the Eden of the world and the home of civilization and culture, is now almost a barren desert, inhabited by a people not far removed from beggars and robbers. A similar result will inevitably follow in our beautiful and fertile Ohio Valley if the vandalism of the wanton and causeless destruction of our forests is persisted in. Already as you descend " La Belle Rivière," the beautiful Ohio, in one of our palatial steamers, you see the bald hillsides, shorn of their beautiful and health-giving forest-coverings, seamed with gullies and ravines, which make them most unsightly to behold and utterly unfit for cultivation. In the long summer, without rain, the whole face of the country is parched up, the crops are poor, the people look discontented and unhappy.

When at the close of winter the snows begin to melt and the rains to fall, the gullies become rapid brooks; the ravines are converted into mountain torrents; the creeks are changed to great streams, and the rivers are transformed into inland seas. Houses are swept away; the accumulated comforts of a lifetime are annihilated in a few hours. The damage does not stop here. What is it that makes the " Father of Waters," the great Mississippi, so much higher than the country through which it flows, necessitating the building of expensive levees? Why is it that millions of acres of fertile land are inundated by crevasses, or breaking through of these levees, and the labor of years destroyed in a day, preventing those lands from being culti-vated as they should be and making them a desert waste? It is because the tributa-ries of that great stream, unprotected by forests, wash all the soil of the lands through which they flow, into the Mississippi, thus filling it with alluvium, raising its bottom higher and higher, compelling its waters to rise above the level of the adjacent lands, and where unprotected by levees, causing it to spread over the land, rendering it useless for cultivation and unfit for human habitation.

Down at the mouth of the Mississippi there is accumulated such an immense mass of this alluvium that the government has been compelled to expend many millions of dollars in the construction of jetties to keep open the navigation between

New Orleans and the Gulf of Mexico. I merely make incidental mention of this; the subject being the floods in the Ohio Valley. The final result of these oft-repeated calamities is, that 'the inhabitants of these beautiful and fertile valleys become discouraged by so often losing the fruits of their labor, and cease to improve the land, refusing to expend their energies on what will only be destroyed by the next great flood. The cultivation of the land will grow less and less; and civilization, instead of marching on, ascending higher and higher, until the wildest imagination of the enthusiast has been surpassed, will retrograde and mankind will revert to his original barbarism.

What is to be done to prevent this calamity? Cease to destroy the forests where they yet exist; replant them in places where the greed and ignorance of mankind have annihilated them; enact forest laws as they have in Germany and other European countries; plant new forests where they never existed before; plant willows on the banks of your streams to prevent them from being washed away; plant groves in the immediate neighborhood of your cities;' in short, foster trees wherever it is possible. Cultivate the valleys and the undulating highlands; leave the precipitous, untillable hillsides and mountains with their beautiful and health-giving forest coverings, presenting us with the ever-varying picture of foliage, of delicate green interspersed with white and pink blossoms in the balmy springtime; the varying shades of rich deep green affording a pleasant shelter from the burning summer sun, and the lovely variegated autumn foliage toward the end of the year. We will then have an abundance of land under cultivation; an equable and temperate climate; a sufficiency of moisture, even in mid-summer; moderate spring rains falling in such a way as to enable the rivers to carry off the water without flooding the country, and destroying the results of man's labor, but simply to improve navigation and add to our commerce.

The inhabitants of a country thus blest will be contented and happy. Receiving the full benefit of their efforts, they will be stimulated and encouraged to labor still farther, adding to their comforts, beautifying their homes, educating their children and bringing them up in habits of industry, economy and virtue; thereby improving the human race until the wildest dreams of the speculative philosopher are more than realized; the world becomes an Eden and the Heaven which has been so variously described by religious dreamers, is to be found in the beautiful mountains, valleys and plains of our lovely planet.

Emergencies.*

BY A J. GRAHAM, M. D.,
Of Peoria, Ill.

We understand by an emergency, that which calls forth immediate action; an instance or an event that springs upon us unawares, often, too, at a time when we may be least prepared, if not wholly unprepared to meet it.

These emergencies are of usual, of every-day happenings, seemingly they momentarily confront us, some of a minor, others of a most serious nature.

---

*Read before The Tri-State Sanitary Convention, at Wheeling, W. Va., February 27 and 28, 1890.

In reality a man's life-work consists in battling with emergencies, with reverses and with calamities. He cannot hope to pass through this world without coming in contact with them. They are liable to confront him in moments of prosperity as well as in times of adversity. None are exempt, the rich and the poor are sufferers alike, and at divers times nations have been known to tremble under and monarchs to be prostrated by them.

If they have no other mission, it may be said they serve as a test scale, upon which a man is placed and weighed for what he is worth, and with many it is " Mene tekle uphàrsin." His success, however, in battling with and emerging through them, depends upon his experience, knowledge, his decision of purpose and in the exercise

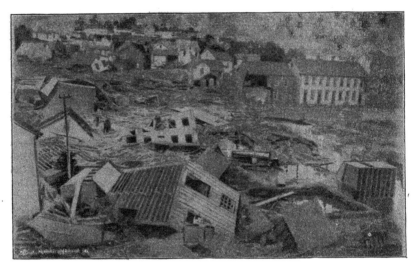

The work of the Flood.

of sound judgment, and of profound, coolness. In the history of all important undertakings these traits of character, the two latter in particular, have been exemplified as the reliable, and with strict adherence to them it is remarkable, and oftentimes one feels surprised at the degree of success attained, though in attaining it he may have had to labor under the most adverse circumstances. With every appliance and convenience at hand to work with, it is not always then a true test of one's ability. The test comes when calamity comes. When an emergency exists, and unexpectedly he is called upon to meet it, with, perhaps, comparatively speaking, nothing at hand, excepting his own bare hands to meet it with.

In considering this subject, then, we draw valuable lessons as we study the conditions, magnitude and surrounding circumstances under which we are liable to be placed. In studying it from a sanitary standpoint, as is our brief, but special aim, we must deal practically, lay special stress upon practical work, whereby the greatest degree of proficiency may be realized, in the least possible space of time. Under such circumstances, but little time or opportunity is there for speculating or theorizing. Systematizing is a necessity, but undue delays are hazardous. . What is to be done must be done with promptness, or else the golden opportunity is lost, and one' is left to suffer the chagrin and mortification of a failure.

The emergencies liable to confront sanitarians are most perplexing, and embrace complications that often tax the mind to its utmost endurance. His is to skirmish and to battle with the most formidable and treacherous of foes—"pestilence"— upon which the eye of public safety ever rests with grave and nervous suspicion. To the indifferent this may seem impractical, an idle waste of time and a useless expenditure of means, but the close and studious observer of the origin, development and fatal course of epidemic diseases can see differently, can readily understand the sanitarian's worth, and his close alliance to the best interest of public welfare. It is not to be presumed, however, that though under the most favorable circumstances he is capable of obliterating epidemic diseases. This would be superhuman, but the experience and actual results of past instances are conclusive that he often has it in his power to prevent or to suppress the same, by due and timely destruction of materials liable to produce the germ. This, then, is the object *per se* of the sanitarian and opens before him an inexhaustible field for speculating, theorizing, as well as for practical and protracted labor, and he can hope to succeed as he is best able to draw his plan of operations from theories long and well established. Thus we see the necessity of the study, and the worth of a mind richly stored with knowledge ; knowledge that may be utilized and reduced to practice at will, thereby the better qualifying him to meet the imminencies of the most trying moment. The condition or cause for operation presents a specific, also a general aspect. The specific lies in the germ itself. To discover and to trace it to its origin is a duty most incumbent. This once accomplished the great burden is removed, and the pest short-lived. But here we are confronted by a most complicated, uncertain, if not hopeless task.

The analysis of well water, sinks, cesspools, etc., has often, it is true, revealed the secrets of typhoid and kindred diseases, but the secret of the more wide and rapidly spreading epidemics seems to be as much a mystery to the scientific world to-day as it was thousands of years ago, and irrespective of the great advance in science, seems to run the same fatal course as has been so characteristic of its history. Thus as the last, if not the only hope of success, he is driven to consider the general condition, as it lies before him—a vast field to explore, to renovate and to relieve of all substances liable to produce danger. Then the magnitude of sanitary work is plainly to be seen, and in the emergency of flood-time nothing is more liable, in fact most certain, to confront the sanitarian. The uncontrollable floods are upon us at an unwarned moment, regions are devastated, towns, villages and cities submerged. The open country a sea of back water, cesspools, etc., overburdened with the garbage, sewerage, filth and refuse of the flood track, to decompose, to diffuse and to contaminate the air with its poisonous germ, and to meet this condition, is to be embarassed and harassed by surrounding circumstances most discouraging.

So gigantic an undertaking requires equally as gigantic means at command. This is seldom in readiness—oftentimes unavoidable—and he is master of the situation as he is best constituted to grapple with and to surmount difficulties. The floods of 1889 in the Susquehanna and Conemaugh valleys are illustrative, and demonstrate beyond a question the value of sanitary work. Though surrounded by the most trying and embarrassing circumstances, yet it can be truthfully said the great emergency was most heroically met, the threatening pestilence abated, and the world's history left to record no greater, no. more distressing calamity, no greater undertaking, and in fine·no more complete and successful results attained.

Some of Johnstown's Lessons.*

BY BENJAMIN LEE, M. D., Ph. D.,
Of Philadelphia,
Secretary of the State Board of Health of Pennsylvania.

The State Board of Health of Pennsylvania has firm faith in the value of Sanitary Conventions, believing that they subserve these two useful purposes : *First.*—The improvement of the sanitary conditions of the city in which the meeting happens to take place, by leading the citizens to seriously consider the particular evils which threaten the health of the community ; and, *Second*, the more general, and perhaps more important object, of educating public opinion as to the necessity for sanitary reforms,' and thus acting by reflection on the Legislatures of the several States, and leading them to pass the necessary measures to initiate and carry out such reforms.

On the thirty-first day of May, last, the Board was holding such a convention in the "Iron City." If the Board had stationed a hand-organ with a monkey in front of the hall in which its sessions were held, and posted a placard stating that the Brown-Séquard Elixir would be administered free of cost, the meetings would have been thronged ; but, as it had no higher aim than to teach the good citizens of Pittsburgh how many valuable lives might be saved every year, and how the general longevity might be increased by the adoption of certain simple rational rules of living, and of civic administration, the many admirable papers which were presented were read to meagre, though intelligent and deeply interested, audiences. It must be allowed that there were special reasons, which made the attendance smaller than it might otherwise have been. Much of the time it rained copiously. The Allegheny River was rising rapidly and becoming turbulent, and on the second day, the immense mass of wreckage which it swept along excited universal interest and drew crowds to the shores and the bridges to watch anxiously for indications of human habitations and loss of life. The suspense was not long. Rumors of wash-outs on the Pennsylvania Railroad were soon followed by the more definite report that the mountain city of Johnstown had been partially destroyed by flood ; and the following morning, which was Sunday, left no room for doubt that a disaster without parallel in the annals of the country had been caused by the bursting of a dam, and that no figures under thousands would be adequate to count its victims. The State Board of Health at once set itself to work to avert the dangers to life and health

---

*Read before the Tri-State Sanitary Convention at Wheeling, W. Va., February 27 and 28, 1890.

which, in the past, have invariably followed wholesale drownings of men and domestic animals, and destruction of homes. In these efforts it was supported to the fullest extent by the Chief Executive of the State, who did not hesitate to assume the risk of the immense burden of a loan of $400,000 to meet the expenses of the gigantic work, when it was found that the State Treasury could not be drawn upon for the purpose. With what success it labored, the health conditions of Johnstown during the following Summer must be the witness.

When the Board was first established, four years ago, it issued an address to the people of the State defining what it felt to be its scope, its duties and its responsibilities, in the course of which the following language occurred. "In an immense

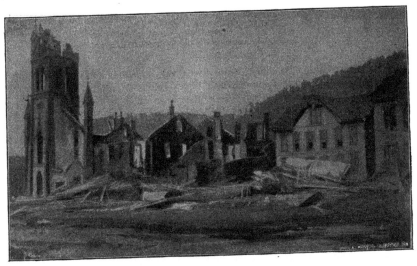

The wrecked Catholic Church, Johnstown, Pa.

territory like our own, larger than that of most of the nations of Europe, with its great diversity of surface, its lofty mountain ranges and its vast forests, wonderful opportunities exist for sanitary engineering on an immense scale,—determining in what directions water-sheds shall be encouraged and in what diverted, to what extent private corporations are to be allowed to jeopardize the health of large sections of the country by obstructing natural water-courses, for the purposes of manufacture or navigation ; deciding how far certain forests act as natural barricades against devastating winds, and should therefore be left untouched by the axe, in order to maintain a permanent average rain-fall, and thus avert droughts, cyclones and floods, and how far others interfere with the circulation of healthful breezes, and may therefore be with benefit removed." This was but one of the many neglected functions of State Government which it felt that it might properly be called upon to assume in the absence of any other authority charged with its performance.

If there was ever a State in which self-government was pushed to the verge of absurdity, in which affairs are allowed to manage themselves in a happy-go-lucky sort of way, every man for himself and the devil take the hindmost,—that State is the great, the venerable Commonwealth of Pennsylvania. Hence, three great evils have been allowed to go entirely unchecked in her mountain regions :

First.—The reckless destruction of forests, leaving the mountain sides bare and denuded. From this, two results : The substitution of cataclysmal downpours from the clouds for the gentler rains which characterize well-wooded countries, and the almost instantaneous passage of this water into the large water-courses, in place of its absorption by the foliage and roots of the trees of large forests.

Second.—The construction and maintenance of large dams without proper governmental oversight ; and,

Third.—The encroachment of manufacturing and other companies on the beds of streams, thus rendering them too narrow to allow storm waters to escape, and making devastating floods a thing of course. In the light of Johnstown's disaster, to the production of which all three of these conditions contributed, this utterance of the Board seems almost prophetic. But it was as it was in the days of Noah. The warning fell on heedless ears. "They did eat, they drank, they married and were given in marriage, until the day that the flood came and destroyed them." To most of those who took the trouble to read the address, these suggestions undoubtedly seemed wild and impracticable, and it will probably be many a long year before these three most evident of Johnstown's lessons will be sufficiently well learned to lead to such legislation as shall render a repetition of Johnstown's calamity impossible. But, given a similar calamity, what are some of the lessons which she can teach us out of the bitterness of her experience?

Next to that of food and clothing, provision for which it would be impossible to make in advance, the want most urgent, and that which interfered most seriously with the rendering of relief during the first two weeks following the disaster, was that of bridges. Communication with the different portions of the flooded district was well-nigh impossible. For several days, two small, leaky skiffs were the only means of transporting food, laborers, coffins and corpses to and from the Pennsylvania' Railroad station and the ruined city. The first really substantial relief to this painful embarrassment was that afforded by the United States Engineer Corps, who came bringing boats for the construction of pontoon bridges. The thought naturally suggests itself that a pontoon train should form a portion of the equipment of the Militia of each State, and that an Engineer Corps should be established which should be drilled in the construction of such bridges, with the same regularity that characterizes the instruction of other arms of the Militia service in the life-destroying branches of the art of war.

The second great need was that of shelter. Like Robinson Crusoe on the desert island, having obtained the wherewithal to cover their backs, and stay the cravings of hunger, these unfortunates had to look about them for habitations. The comparatively few houses which were left in a habitable condition were crowded to repletion. Many of them contained the remnants of four or five families in addition to their ordinary occupants. Under these conditions it required the utmost vigilance on the part of the Board to prevent the occurrence of the diseases which are known to accompany overcrowding. This want was measurably met by the Flood Relief Commission in the purchase of ready-made houses from the West, designed for persons forming temporary camps. It was difficult, however, to obtain a sufficient supply of these on short notice, and they had to be brought a long distance. It would be a wise move on the part of State Legislatures to procure a considerable number of such portable dwellings, and keep them stored at different points, to be ready for immediate use in such emergencies. In the event of the occurrence of epidemics they would serve an admirable purpose as hospitals. The Engineer Corps might also be instructed in the most expeditious manner of putting them together. Being comparatively inexpensive, they could be burned after being used by patients with contagious diseases.

The third difficulty which confronted the State Board of Health was the absence of·any local sanitary authority or organization. There was no nucleus on which to form a sanitary corps. The whole machinery had to be created *de novo*. But for the prompt arrival and intelligent assistance of the sanitary police of the cities of Pittsburgh and Allegheny, the task would have been much more perplexing. The services rendered by these officers in house to house inspection, and in the distribution of disinfectants, and in instructing the new recruits of the corps in these duties, cannot be too highly estimated and contributed largely to the prevention of sickness. Pennsylvania is one of the few States which still lag far in the rear in the matter of sanitary organization. Her Legislature makes no provision for the establishment of Boards of Health in any places having less than ten thousand inhabitants or not possessing a city charter. In several instances where the Board sent disinfectants to flooded villages the inhabitants refused to remove them from the cars, and there was no local authority of any kind to make the proper use of them. The dream of the State Board of Health, as expressed in the address above referred to, that " there shall not be a hamlet in the entire domain of the State without its regularly constituted health officers " is apparently as far from realization as ever.

Such organization would also obviate to a great extent another obstacle with which the Board had to contend, viz., the difficulty of obtaining recognition and compelling obedience on the part of local subordinate officers. Johnstown was like a place in a state of siege. *Ex tempore* policemen, armed with ball clubs, muskets, shot-guns and pistols, and decorated with a rude tin star, seemed to spring out of the ground at every turn, like the dragon's teeth sown by Cadmus, and made it very uncomfortable for one not well supplied with passes from the half dozen officials who ruled in the different sections of the devastated region. The delay thus caused was often a serious interference with the conduct of business. To avoid this I adopted the following device. In the Pennsylvania Railroad Station, which was one of the first established morgues, and the floor of which was covered with nude bodies of both sexes and all ages, I fortunately found a can of black paint and a brush designed for marking freight. Tearing a strip from a roll of white muslin, in which the dead were being hurriedly enwrapped, I painted on it the words " Sanitary Corps," and pinned it to the front of my hat. This worked like a charm, proving pass-word, countersign and open sesame to the most obdurate guard. The suggestion that occurs to me in this connection is this : That in each State there should be adopted a uniform for sanitary officers, or, at least, a sanitary badge which would at once be recognized by all who saw it, in all places and under all circumstances, as conveying authority, and entitling the wearer to proceed to the |performance of his important duties without hindrance. The value of such a provision was made strikingly apparent upon the arrival of the uniformed sanitary police from Pittsburgh. The people at once manifested confidence in them and listened respectfully to the suggestions and orders, while they had been inclined to be suspicious of the motives of the un-uniformed men, and to resent their interference, and the special constables rarely stopped them.

No one who was present in Johnstown before and after the time at which the State Militia were commissioned to assume control of operations for the abatement

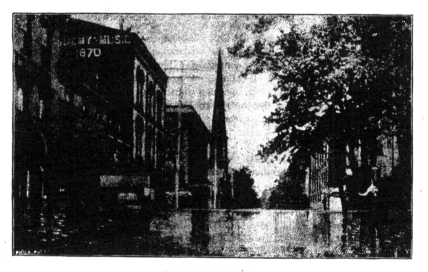

Pine Street, Williamsport, Pa.
The water up nearly to the second floor, and rushing through the street at the rate of ten or twelve miles per hour.

of the great nuisance, under the supervision of the Board, could have failed to notice the immense change for the better which at once took place when General Hastings assumed command. Order out of chaos, a sense of security, as contrasted with a feeling of apprehension and uneasiness, amounting almost to a reign of terror—more work done and better done, with fewer men at work, because more thorough system prevailed, the work was more intelligently arranged and the authority was centralized. Johnstown will ever be a monument to the efficiency of the National Guard of Pennsylvania—a body of citizen soldiery, existing not simply on paper and fit only for parade, but ready to take the field at a moment's notice, perfect in all its departments, prepared not only to repel invasion or repress riot, but to undertake the management of a great work of relief, requiring very varied attainments of administration. It is not too much to say, and it is saying very much, that the Guard, from the General in command to the lowest subaltern, proved itself equal to the emergency. The annual encampments, introduced of late years, have undoubtedly been the principal factor in familiarizing both line and staff with the routine duties of camp life and administration. The value of a well organized militia is, therefore, one of the important lessons of Johnstown.

But how did the guard come to be upon the scene? What justification was there, in a time of profound peace, in the absence of rebellion or riot, in defiance of the express provisions of the State Constitution, for placing a military force with the entire General Staff of the State in control of a territory, as large as some European principalities. It was simply because the Legislature, yielding to the importunities of certain sanitary cranks had, a few years before, had the wisdom to create a State Board of Health. This Board possessed the authority to declare the conditions existing at Johnstown, and in the valleys of the Conemaugh, Kiskiminitas and Allegheny Rivers a "nuisance prejudicial to the public health," and to call upon the Chief Executive of the State to furnish men and means for its abatement. Without this declaration the State would have been powerless to interfere, unless extra constitutional measures had been resorted to. The presence of the guard at Johnstown was a striking exemplification on the grandest scale, of the truth of the proposition contained in the address of the Board referred to in the opening to this paper that, "It is no empty figure of speech, by which we call disease a public enemy. It requires to be met with organized resistance, and this resistance must be directed by a responsible head. When pestilence threatens, that head must be clothed with powers analogous to those of a general when the foe is at the gates. Sanitary Law, in place of Martial Law is then proclaimed; and what are, in times of general health, recognized as sacred rights of person and property, are sternly set aside. When such emergencies arise, the Board confidently looks to the sound sense and self-control of the people to lead them to submit cheerfully to whatever temporary inconveniences it may be deemed necessary to impose." Such absolute powers the Board exercised at Johnstown. Such sound sense and self-control were displayed by the people of Johnstown under the most trying circumstances, leading them to acquiesce in restrictions, which may have appeared to them harsh and unnecessary. Whatever, therefore, may have been the faults, failures or shortcomings in the administration of the Board during its period of occupancy it may at least be credited with having taught the lesson, and it is the last to which I shall advert, that a State Board of Health is the only constituted authority which can legally cope with such an emergency, and that its powers in the premises are ample and supreme. Rarely has the truth of the motto of the Board, which has also been chosen as that of this Convention, received a more triumphant vindication. Let it be the rallying cry of the Sanitarian.

"SALUS POPULI SUPREMA LEX."

Sanitary Convention at Norristown.

At a recent meeting of our Board it was decided to hold a Sanitary Convention some time during the month of May in Norristown, an invitation to this effect having been received from the local Board of Health. In our next issue we will furnish further particulars.

Some of the things we Eat and Drink.*

BY PROFESSOR JOHN A. MYERS,

Of Morgantown, W. Va.

Director of the West Virginia Agricultural Experiment Station.

It will scarcely be expected upon an occasion of this character that I should deal with the more theoretical questions involved in protection from diseases incident to the use of unwholesome and adulterated food and drink. The greatest good, I apprehend, to be derived from meetings of this character is in the stimulation of the growth of a sound and uncompromising public opinion upon sanitary affairs. With this in view, I desire to touch upon several matters connected with our food supply, which I am confident should receive the serious consideration of all good citizens.

There is a suspicion abroad'in the land that much of the food offered in the markets is adulterated ; that it contains foreign substances which, either immediately or remotely, affect the health of the people. It has been shown that there are two causes leading to this :

First.—The avarice of the manufacturer or dealer.

Second.—Their carelessness or their inability to avoid the introduction of poisonous substances in preparing certain articles of luxury.

By far the greater amount of adulteration of food and drink is caused by the profit that it gives to the manufacturer or dealer.

The art of adulterating lard or butter, olive oil, cheese, beer, syrup, honey, confectionery, wines, vinegar, flour, baking powders, spices, cocoa, chocolate, coffee or tea so as not to be readily detected necessitates, in many cases, the employment of scientific skill. The separation of lard and beef fats into their several ingredients so that they may be employed for the adulteration of other articles of food, necessitates the employment of the highest kind of chemical skill, and it is only when this technical skill is employed that this adulteration becomes an important factor in the commercial transactions of the country. Many of the adulterations in the market are not harmful to the health, but are simply a species of fraud practiced upon the purchaser, the profits of which are divided between the dealer, and the manufacturer of the spurious goods. Our hotels will not allow it to be known that they are using oleomargarine upon their tables and in their kitchens, and our fancy grocerymen take as much pains as possible to conceal the fact that they are selling artificial butter for the genuine article. The milkman who waters his milk is not nearly so dangerous as the milk dealer who removes the cream and adds lard or oleo oil to the skim milk, and sells it again for the genuine article. I do not know that butter made with a strong admixture of oleomargarine by a skillful and careful manufacturer is worse than country butter containing the accumulated extracts of badly washed milk vessels and milk contaminated by the foul odors of the kitchen where it may be kept standing, or of cow stables where the animals may be kept. In the one case, it

---

*Read before the " Tri-State Sanitary Convention," at Wheeling, W. Va., February 27 and 28, 1890.

would be considered as adulteration. In the other case, public opinion would consider it as necessary impurity. Cheese fattened by the addition of lard, oleo oil, or cotton-seed oil, which would be considered as adulteration, is perhaps a better article than cheese from which the cream has been extracted by the dishonest cheese maker. Beer sweetened by glucose and flavored with malt and hop substitutes, and preserved by antiseptics, some of which may be dangerous to health, and certainly none of them conducive thereto, may be relished by some, but surely the great mass of beer drinkers would prefer to have an unadulterated, straight, genuine article.

When a man comes into a store and calls for syrup, he would much prefer to get the article called for to artificial glucose, and when he asks for honey, he wishes honey rather than glucose or cane sugar, and when he goes into the confectionery he would prefer to have the genuine sugar sweets to the artificial glucose to which starch artificial essences, poisonous pigments, terra alba, gypsum and other matter intended to impart weight, flavor or color have been added.

When a man calls for vinegar, he does not wish 'diluted sulphuric acid, and when he calls for flour or bread, he does not want it loaded with mineral matter or alum.

When a man wishes to buy baking powders, he prefers the genuine article to starch or alum, and if he buy spices, he does not wish flour, starch, turmeric or buck-wheat hulls. Cocoa and coffee are none the better for their adulteration with sugar, starch and flour ; and coffee is certainly the worse for having introduced into it chickory, peas, rye, corn, wheat, beans, coloring matter and 'grains of clay. Tea containing exhausted tea leaves or leaves of other plants to which artificial indigo, prussian blue, turmeric, gypsum, soapstone and sand have been added certainly is not as wholesome as the genuine article. Canned goods into which antiseptics have been introduced, or into which metallic poisons have fallen, are not used if known, and pickles turned green by the salts of copper, while admired for their color, certainly do not strengthen the digestive system of any man.

It is, however, not so much the question of fraud upon the public that I wish to reach at this time as the question of danger to health. If men will submit to being regularly and systematically swindled when ample means of protection can be provided at a nominal cost, I do not think that it is a matter of any special concern. It was Barnum, I believe, who said that the American people love to be humbugged, —they really enjoy a moderate amount of it—and I presume few could speak with more certainty upon this point than Mr. Barnum. But the American people do not enjoy being shot at from ambush, and being stabbed in the dark or waylaid at night. Murder and robbery in any community, if unpunished by the courts, is very likely to be suppressed by vigilance committees. But public sentiment has not been educated to that point which will prevent the grocer, the butcher, milkman or saloon-keeper from slowly poisoning our health and sending one after another of our dear ones to their long resting place. If the butcher were to stand in his shop and occasionally shoot a member of your family, public opinion would sustain you in training a well loaded Winchester rifle upon him, even if the law failed to reach him. But he may poison your whole family, and frequently does do it, by supplying meat infected by trichinæ, tape-worm, the germs of tuberculosis, and other diseases which may be traced in many cases most directly to meat supplied from diseased animals.

What would·the public say if he were to poison that meat with arsenic which, in many cases, would only be a little more prompt in its action, not more certain in its results.

If such be the condition of affairs at the butcher shop, what shall we say of our milkmen? The milkman who skims his milk and then waters it is a saint, and deserves a front pew among the most pious, compared with him who brings the milk of diseased cows—such as those suffering from tuberculosis, ulcerated udders, diseased joints or swollen glands, or from cows fed upon the decomposing swills and slops of various manufactories, or waters his cows with water ladened with all of the disease germs flourishing in sewage. There should be very stringent laws passed and enforced

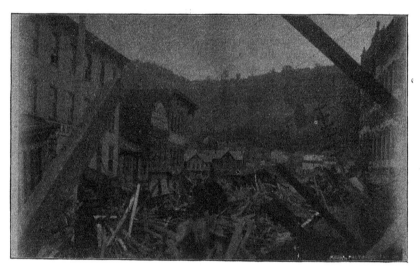

Main Street, Johnstown—After the Flood.

against this class of citizens who deal out death at the rate of eight cents a quart to our children. What do they care if a few children die of diphtheria, scarlet fever, typhoid fever, or have their blood poisoned by the germs of consumption. The great problem is to secure the eight cents a quart, and have as many quarts as possible.

I look upon public opinion that is so misguided or so lethargic as not to suppress daily crimes of the character hinted at as very much to be regretted.

Time will not permit me to notice more articles of food. I will next touch upon the water supply, and in this, I strike a fruitful source of disease and death.

Science in the hands of the chemist and microscopist may do much to indicate the causes of typhoid fever, enteric diseases and malarial complaints; but until public opinion is developed to such a point that our people will no longer permit their drinking water to be contaminated by sewage, and their homes poisoned by sewer gas, and the foul odors of decomposing garbage piled in all of the neighbors' back yards, and in all of the alleys of the city, science cannot do much. What cares the average ward politician whether the springs, wells, hydrants, cellars, back yards and commons in his ward, or all over the city are polluted, and the water drank by the people and the very air breathed by them is rendered foul with the refuse of the city, so long as a few of his political henchmen may be permitted to shirk their work, thereby making a few dollars a month more than they would if the work of cleaning the city were honestly and thoroughly done. What is the difference to him if the death rate of the city rises to 50 or 100 per 1,000 so long as public opinion will not force the proper officers to do their duty.

What magnificent economy it is to bury 50 or 100 of your population because some one raises the cry of too much expense to clean the city—too much expense to suppress the sale of unwholesome food—too great injustice done to the poor butchers, grocers, saloon-men and milk-men—too heavy expense to dispose of the citizens' garbage. Away with such economy ! Away with such politics ! Any sensible man in this country is willing to be taxed if you convince him that the money is being judiciously expended for the good of the public. If he does object, he will find himself in the minority, and I believe Mr. Reed says that the majority must rule in this country.

Scientific men, I think, have shown beyond doubt that many of the diseases to which our race is subject are contracted from the animal food supplied to our people, either as meat, milk, butter or cheese. It was stated last year upon the floor of the United States Senate that statistics showed that 500,000 children die annually in our cities in this country from the use of diseased milk. Dr. Laws states that in some country districts of New York can be shown large herds of cattle with 90 per cent. subject to tuberculosis.

In the case of consumption, Villemin, Janewaw, Toussaint, Koch and others have carried on exhaustive series of experiments, demonstrating beyound doubt that the Bacillus Tuberculosis can be readily communicated from one animal body to another. Koch and his assistants have isolated the Bacillus Tuberculosis and after cultivating it through successive generations for months in blood serum, found in every case where the purified Bacillus was introduced into the circulation of healthy animals, the disease was reproduced.

Galthier has demonstrated that this Bacillus retains its activity at temperatures ranging from 18 degrees below freezing to 108 degrees Fahrenheit. That it resists the action of water, desiccation and strong pickle, so that it may occur even from the use of corned beef or dried beef from animals infected with this disease. Lydtin states positively that it may be taken into the lungs through the inspired air, or into the digestive system with food or water. Ballinger produced tuberculosis in pigs by feeding them for a long time on milk from tuberculous cows. But why should I continue to cite experiments which have demonstrated beyond reasonable doubt the fact that a large share of the incurable diseases are spread among our people by the use of animal food containing the disease germs which develop and multiply in the human body until it literally swarms with them.

The Bacillus may and generally does attack the lungs and lymphatic glands, but is, by no means, confined to these organs. These germs may even enter through a wound as reported by Taschering in " Reports of the Progress of Medicine " for 1885, where a young woman became infected from some of the sputa raised from the lungs of a consumptive patient accidentally getting into the slight wound in her finger which had been cut upon the broken vessel containing the sputa.

It is more than probable that where children are fed upon the milk from tuberculous cows serious intestinal disturbances may occur.

Looking at the question of adulterations from a commercial standpoint, it occurs to me that it makes no difference to this meeting whether sugar, coffee, milk, bread, butter, cheese, canned meats, pepper, spices, pickles, chocolate, tea and every other article dealt in by the grocery-man or the liquor merchant is adulterated to a greater or less extent. If people are willing to pay full price for half quality of goods and be swindled in the value of their purchases, anywhere from two per cent. to fifty per cent., or more, without protest, and without any attempt at correcting the evil, we need not bother ourselves about it at a Sanitary Convention. On the other hand, it becomes a matter of great interest to us when we find the health of the community menaced by these adulterations, and when we find the adulterations consist of indigestible or poisonous matter, or when the food products are injuring the health of the people by reason of diseases propagated or spread thereby, then it is proper for us to enter our most vigorous protests. I do not believe that men should be permitted with impunity to undermine the health of a single-fellow being, whether it be the infant nursing at the bottle or the old man tottering on the grave. I am disposed to resent a man's setting a death-trap for me or for my family, either intentionally or ignorantly, and I believe that some system of protection to the public should be inaugurated that will suppress the traffic in adulterated groceries, diseased meats, unwholesome and contaminated milk, and check the constant tendency to poison the water supplies of our great cities by sewage and city wastes being dumped into our rivers. Vigorous and positive laws should be enacted and enforced against every one who jeopardizes the health of innocent and unsuspecting fellow-citizens by the sale of any manipulated product whatever.

We are likely to be met by three flimsy arguments in urging a measure of this kind :

First.—One class will oppose it on the ground of expense. There is a class of people who would be willing to suppress every measure toward the protection of the health of a community, and would be willing to see hundreds of people die from the effects of bad sanitary conditions rather than spend a few hundred or thousand dollars of the public funds in suppressing or removing the exciting causes of disease.

Another class will oppose it on the ground that it increases the office-holders in the community, and anything that will give the party in power political patronage they argue should be suppressed, no matter how much good may result to the community or what great benefits may be derived from the inauguration of proper sanitary reform.

Then we have a third class, who oppose measures to regulate anything of this kind, because they are themselves engaged in selling or in manufacturing the articles complained of. They have money to back their pretensions. They wear the garb of respectable citizenship. They conspicuously regret very much that the health of so many people should be endangered by these adulterations, and that it is now almost impossible for persons to secure pure articles of food. But they say, " Shall we raise the price of our food products by compelling our manufacturers and dealers to sell pure articles? They tell us that the price of milk will have to be raised, and the price of butter, cheese, meat, sugar, and all of the groceries in the market would have to be raised if the manufacturers were not permitted to adulterate them so as to compete with one another. Think of it. They are persistent and noisy in their declarations that every man should be permitted to buy and sell anything that he wants to, and can we, say they, in this great country, afford to assail the personal liberties of men who are engaged in carrying on the commerce of this country? They want no more class legislation, and set up the claim that an adulterated article, if not actually injurious to the health, should be permitted to be sold whether the purchaser is aware of the character of the article or not. Their argument is to reach the pocket of our citizens and through that pull a veil over the keen eye of reason.

But what shall be done? Can public opinion be so stimulated that the people will rise in their might and adopt measures to suppress these evils? Are they willing to bear the expense of having these manufacturers and dealers in adulterated goods detected and prosecuted, and the business suppressed? Are they willing to have adulterated milk and milk from diseased cattle destroyed, and the men who produce and sell it punished? Will they sustain the health officers in making regular inspections of the dairies in this and other communities and suppress these hot-beds of disease? Are our people willing to have the animal products offered at the shambles inspected, and the diseased, adulterated and spoiled goods destroyed, and the men who knowingly deal in them fined or otherwise punished? Will the public opinion of this city sustain the health officer or Board of Health (I suppose it has a Board of Health) in suppressing the cause of diphtheria, scarlet and typhoid fevers, and all that long line of diseases induced by the contamination of the water supplies and the failure to remove the refuse of the city and to properly control the sewerage. Why not authorize the proper authorities to secure the proper scientific skill to detect and suppress these evils.

There is a tremendous responsibility resting upon our citizens, and it is hoped that what has been said in reference to the adulteration of food, to the spread of disease, to the suppression of the sale of such articles, to the enactment of laws and their enforcement, may receive the most serious consideration of the citizens of the States represented in this Convention.

Our Grip Illustrations.

Dr. Samuel G. Dixon fears lest some of our readers may hold him responsible for the illustrations which appeared in connection with the article on " The Grip," in our last issue. In this connection we would therefore say, that for those, as for all illustrations that have or that may in the future appear in our journal, we assume the responsibility, unless an explicit statement to the contrary is made by us. Dr. Dixon had nothing whatsoever to do with these illustrations.

Flood Debris Dangerous to Health, and How to Dispose of It.*

BY SPENCER M. FREE, A. M., M. D.,
of Beechtree, Pa.
Inspector to the State Board of Health of Pennsylvania.

Should I remark just here at the commencement of this address, that all the time, money and thought that has been expended in the endeavor to prevent epidemics after floods, has been time, money and thought wasted, I should make a statement that would cause criticism if it did not even evoke sympathy in my behalf for exhibiting such lamentable ignorance of these important events in the history of the world.

Yet, if I made such a statement it would be much nearer the truth than the opposite one would be.

For, from the deluge down to the present time no authentic account has been given of any epidemic disease (unless malarial diseases be regarded as epidemics) caused purely by the materials left by floods, and not more properly and truthfully traceable to other causes.

To properly understand the topic proposed for discussion we must enter a little into the subject of definitions. Therefore, by "flood debris dangerous to health," I mean, those materials, local and foreign, (from some other place) which are left in any locality after the disappearance from it of water that has submerged lands not usually coursed thereby, which materials directly or indirectly prevent the parts of the human body from freely performing their natural functions—in other words, from being healthy.

A brief glance at the history of water floods, which are the ones to which our discussion is limited, shows us that they are not unusual occurrences. Nor are they trifling accidents in their immediate or in their remote results. If we begin with the deluge and accept the account of it as given in Genesis, both the results mentioned above are incalculable. Quite certain is it that no serious epidemic disease or serious disease of any kind followed this flood, although all conditions were favorable to such an outbreak.

Sanitary science was not so well understood then as it is at the present time, nor was disinfection so thoroughly practiced.

In fact, so far as the reports show, the people knew nothing of either of these subjects, hence no serious diseases occurred, or this convention would not be a necessity—not even a possibility.

These destructive agents are not confined to any country or locality. Europe, Asia, Africa have all felt their terrific power. Our own beloved land has time and again been called to mourn the loss of life and property consequent therefrom, but never before to such great degree as in May, eighteen hundred and eighty-nine, in the beautiful valley of the Conemaugh.

Colin, in his "Maladies Epidemique" relates that it is said that the Arabs caused the death of over 12,000 of the inhabitants of Bassora by sickness, by making the river to overflow. But it is not shown that this is a true historical fact, nor can any information be obtained as to the kind of disease.

---

*Read before The Tri-State Sanitary Convention at Wheeling, W. Va., February 27 and 28, 1890.

In 1748 the Dutch compelled Austria to quickly make terms of peace by inundating their country, but the sicknesses following the disappearance of the water compelled a second inundation.

No accounts are obtainable as to the character of the diseases, but from the fact that they were ended by the second inundation we conclude that they were malarial in origin.

Great increase in the amount of sickness at Strasbourg, following the flood of 1824, is recorded, but it is definitely stated that it was entirely due to malarial diseases.

In China, where floods are frequent and severe, causing annually the loss of thousands of lives by drowning, very little sickness of any kind follows.

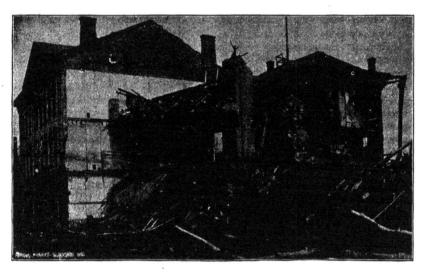

A Specimen of Flood Work.

In India, where floods and inundations are also frequent occurrences, they are not followed by epidemics. Dr. C. R. Francis, Surgeon-General of the English Army in India, says that " no unusual sickness follows these inundations."

In this country the lower Mississippi furnishes one of the most fruitful fields of study, as inundations are very frequent.

The subject has been thoroughly investigated by Prof. Chaille, of New Orleans, and his conclusions are " that floods are not injurious but beneficial, by covering up the soil and cleansing the streets."

New Orleans is probably the most afflicted city in the United States as regards floods and inundations.

Its peculiar situation renders it subject to overflows from both the river and lake. Since its founding, in 1718, there have been no less than seventeen severe floods, and although yellow fever is epidemic, and cholera has been frequent, neither of these diseases have been worse after floods.

Only once, in 1846, were dysentery and bowel troubles increased. The flood occurred in May; the dysentery in July. It also prevailed as badly in districts not flooded. Other causes seem to have had greater action than the debris of the flood.

The worst flood ever known, in 1849, when the city was covered with filth forty days. No bad effects on the health of the city were found.

In 1856 the streets in the lower district were covered several feet deep for over a week, and no ill effects.

In 1871 eleven thousand people were flooded out, and one observer states that the district in which these people had their houses "presented the appearance of an offensive and putrid cess-pool," the contents of cess-pools, sinks, stables, garbage, dead animals, and all the usual materials consequent upon floods were found throughout the city in abundance, but the health continued good.

Not even malarial diseases were more frequent. In 1871 the deaths from malarial diseases were but thirteen to the thousand, while in 1870 they were twenty-eight to the thousand. In this year disinfection was practiced.

In 1881 an overflow of a similar nature occurred and said to be fully as bad. No disinfection was practiced, yet we find Dr. Holt, one of the sanitary inspectors, saying: "As the water receded I carefully inspected the ground and was struck with the increased cleanliness of the district." The event would seem to suggest an overflow as a providential sanitary measure.

Thus we find we must look elsewhere than to New Orleans to find proof that flood debris is responsible for epidemics of disease. The investigation has been made carefully for the whole lower valley of the Mississippi and the only increase is found in malarial diseases; but as this is not found after all inundations and as it is found in years when no overflows occur, there is certainly room for doubt as to the cause being due to the results of the overflows.

The Johnstown flood of 1889, so terribly destructive of life and property, covered the Conemaugh Valley for miles with all manner of flood materials, and dead bodies. No epidemic (at any rate of a serious nature) has followed The bowel troubles and dysentery were not much greater in amount than usual, and when the subjects of food, houses, clothing, mental condition, etc., are considered, we do not feel that the flood-debris is very much, if at all responsible. Indeed the surprise has been expressed by many sanitarians, and by many more who are not of this class that so little sickness prevailed immediately after the flood, and that so little has developed since that time.

How much this may be due to the speedy supply of food, clothing and shelter, that was furnished the unfortunate people; the prompt, thorough and long continued sanitary measures instituted by the State Board of Health; the rapid removal and destruction of the vast amounts of debris and dead bodies, no one can say. But while giving all praise to these measures and to those who so nobly and so self-sacrificingly labored in these causes, we must when viewing the question as honest searchers after truth, confess that the natural tendency was the same here as in other places and times, not to have outbreaks of diseases after floods.

Any one who saw the condition of things at Johnstown could not deny that all manner of flood materials were present in great amount, and that if they are dangerous to health, that the health of the city and valley was in constant jeopardy for a long time. The fact that in the presence of all this threatened danger the health maintained itself almost unharmed, argues that the danger was not so great after all.

It was very clearly brought out in the celebrated Lennox trial that many mistakes existed in the human mind in reference to the relations existing betwen floods, inundations, overflows, stagnant water, swamps and diseases, especially in reference to the former as causative agents of the latter.

Hirsh, in his great and admirable work, the "Hand-book of Geographical and Historical Pathology," teaches that the diseases which are commonly expected to follow floods namely, the acute infectious diseases—such as typhoid, yellow fever, cholera, scarlet fever, etc., are not influenced to any noticeable extent, if at all, by them.

The most frequent diseases for which floods are directly responsible are the malarial ones. The debris is not alone responsible however. There must be three things present before malarial diseases develop ; a soil that is wet, but not submerged ; an amount of organic matter, especially of a vegetable nature ; a moderately high temperature.

Any of these conditions wanting will prevent the development of malaria. Floods therefore by bringing organic matter and by saturating the soil, predispose to malarial complaints, and these are the ones to be looked for and prevented rather than the acute infectious ones.

Having hastily and rather superficially (because time will not permit an exhaustive investigation) examined flood and flood materials, and having found their general effect is not toward the production of ill health, let us look at some of the specific forms of debris and see their dangers.

Air is temporarily affected by dust, which by invading the mucous surfaces, causes bronchitis, coryza, etc. This promptly disappears of itself—needs no special plan for removal. Odors soon fill the air, especially if much animal matter is decaying. This has no harmful effect other than producing nausea, and preventing labor for the removal of debris. This can be overcome by the free use of deodorizers, such as bromine, chloride of lime, carbolic acid, etc.

Dampness, another effect on atmosphere, is dangerous, in its tendency to produce catarrhal affections, rheumatism and pneumonia. This slowly disappears if warm sunshiny days follow, but numerous fires are to be recommended.

Water—the stream itself—is not dangerous unless used as a source of water supply, and not then if it is a large body of water. By this I mean that it is not any more a source of danger than under ordinary circumstances ; but admitting that all streams used as a water supply are dangerous, the water from which should be boiled before being taken into the system.

As a matter of fact the water used at Pittsburgh showed a better chemical analysis just after the May flood of 1889 than it had shown before. What its bacteriological conditions was I do not know.

Springs and wells are injured, temporarily at least, by the large amount of foreign matter introduced, which is most likely not beneficial to health, for many stables, pig-styes, water-closets and their contents have been brought with the flood.

There is but one way that is cheap and easily applied for the removal of this danger and that is boiling before taking into the system. The sooner that people will learn that the only perfectly safe water under all circumstances is boiled water, the sooner an important disease-bearing element will be removed.

Foods—I refer to those remaining in houses and stores that have been wet, in many cases have been lying under the water for some time. They are dangerous. They may contain germs of disease carried from some neighboring houses or cess-pool, which, taken into the system, may reproduce itself. Hence, though it may be apparently economical, it is dangerous, and may prove in the end very expensive.

It is possible that an exception could be made in the case of foods that can be thoroughly washed and boiled before eating, such as beans, potatoes, etc. Much better, however, to err on the side of safety and destroy all such things by fire or by burying them deeply in the earth, than to use them and get sick.

Houses that are left standing are dangerous. They are partly filled with mud, etc., the carpets, furniture, clothing, etc., are saturated with mud and water.

The furniture can possibly be cleaned, as also carpets, clothing, etc., by thoroughly washing and drying and then thorough fumigation with sulphur or by subjecting them to high temperature for a long time.

The safer plan is to destroy them by fire ; for no one knows but that some germs of scarlet fever, diphtheria, small-pox, or other diseases may be in them, and when dry, will float in the atmosphere and be taken up by the inmates of the house.

The cellar floors should be cleaned of mud, thoroughly washed in water, then in solution of bichloride of mercury and dried by heat and lime. The walls should be scraped clean, and washed with bichloride solution or with some other one equally good. Such houses are unfit for immediate habitation, and should not be lived in until they have been renovated and are thoroughly dry.

I need not stop to enumerate the diseases liable to occur by immediate occupancy. In the same category with dress goods I would put muslins, clothing, etc., from stores. By subjecting them to thorough washing, drying and fumigating processes, they may be made safe. But the fact remains that perfect sanitation is destruction by fire.

Accumulations of debris in the streets and yards, such as boards, trees, lumber, houses of all kinds, etc., can best be destroyed by fire. They may not be dangerous to any great extent, and are not, so long as they are wet, but, like furniture and clothing, when dry, they may give off the germs of disease to the atmosphere, which in turn imparts them to those inhaling it. The mud or dirt can best be disposed of by dumping into holes, and sprinkling well with lime.

Hay and straw are dangerous, when wet, we are told by some authorities. Especially is this true of straw. It will produce measles. The Surgeon-General of Pennsylvania has written on this subject, claiming that such is the case, and that he has demonstrated it on several occasions when in the State militia encampments. These materials can easily and effectively be destroyed by fire.

Decaying vegetable and animal matter. We saw some time ago that these, especially the former, are, in the presence of moisture and heat, fruitful sources of those numerous and varied symptoms which, for want of better knowledge, we call malaria. Decaying animals are not the great source of danger that many think. Before decomposition sets in bodies are dangerous, in that they may transmit contagious diseases which they had at the time of death ; but after decomposition has been well established they are, in all probability, free from danger, as the germs of decomposition destroy those of disease. Hence, if removed immediately after the flood, and any suspicion rests of contagious disease, the bodies should be wrapped in sheets, soaked in bi-chloride solution, and burned or buried at once. Either burying or burning is a safe plan for disposing of animal matter, but fire is preferred as the more effectual.

Driftwood, which usually is present in large amounts, can be used to burn up what materials are to be thus destroyed. When the flooded stream is small, the drift and animal and vegetable matter can readily be collected by means of a brattice

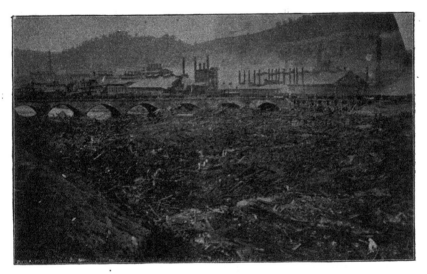

The famous jam at the Stone Bridge, Johnstown.

across the stream. It allows nothing but very small drift to pass, so that all materials can be collected at this point and destroyed, thus protecting places below.

Floods will continue to increase in frequency and severity, so long as the destruction of forests continues. As sanitarians, we should, therefore, use every effort to stop the cause.

Our duty in regard to the flood itself, is to faithfully teach the specific dangers, and how to avoid or control them. But this is not all. We should also endeavor to correct the false impressions concerning the general tendency of floods to cause great epidemics of disease.

By this means we shall get rid of that abnormal mental condition which is so important an etiological factor in disease, and keep the people in such shape that they can calmly and intelligently meet the specific dangers and successfully overcome them.

Sanitary Jurisprudence.*

BY HON. J. B. SOMMERVILLE,
Of Wheeling, West Virginia.

" *Salus populi est Suprema lex* " is a most suggestive and appropriate motto for an association, one of whose objects is the consideration and discussion of the subject of " Sanitary Jurisprudence." This term is a comparatively new one, though it is one which if not strictly technical, is destined soon to become so. We of the legal profession have been provided through the skill, energy and ambition of our brother practitioners of the present and former generations, with numerous works on Medical Jurisprudence, seeking to apply the principles and practice of medicine to the determination and settlement of questions arising in the courts of law out of the relations of sex, the infliction of physical injuries and the like, but no one amid all the ranks of legal authorship—already crowded to overflowing—has attempted a systematic treatise on that branch of modern jurisprudence which aims to prevent the contraction and spread of disease, and to preserve the public health. This is a new and fruitful field. It opens up new avenues of thought and presents splendid inducements for the display of ability, learning and zeal. It is a subject of the greatest practical importance, and one which presents a dual aspect to the gentlemen of the medical profession. While they constitute the only class of individuals who possess sufficient knowledge and skill to enable them to successfully deal with the various methods of preventing diseases, they at the same time constitute the class who have the greatest interest in concealing the knowledge of such methods from the general public. And I pay the highest possible tribute to the humanity and philanthropy of the medical profession when I say that with all their interest in preventing an investigation of these subjects, they have not only inspired such investigations as have been made, but have actually made the investigations themselves. The common law—that great conservator of the rights and interests of individuals—it is true, recognized both the right and the duty of the Courts to exercise their jurisdiction and powers, to some extent, for the preservation of the public health; but, compared with our modern notions on these subjects, the jurisdiction and powers of the Courts over them, as measured by the common law, was scarcely more than nominal, and extended but little, if any, beyond the power of preventing and abating such nuisances as injuriously affected the public health. The great march of progress of the human race has, in a great measure, carried the questions pertaining to the preservation of the public health from the judicial to the legislative department of our governments, both State and National. The Courts, always extremely, but in the main properly conservative in their character and constitution, have dealt rather too cautiously with these questions to suit the vigorous and energetic leaders of modern thought and action, and to meet the demands of modern times; and hence it is that these leaders have looked for their remedies to the less conservative and more aggressive legislative tribunals. The first instances of this which are to be found in the mother country, to which we are indebted for so many of our laws and institutions, are the statutes of 51 Hen. III, to prevent the sale of unwholesome provisions; 1 Jac. I, to prevent the spread

---

*Read before the Tri-State Sanitary Convention, at Wheeling, W. Va., February 27 and 28, 1890.

of the plague by preventing persons who were afflicted with it from associating with others who were free from it, and 26 and 29 Geo. II, providing for the *quarantine* of vessels sailing from infected countries. The Congress of the United States, as early as the 25th day of February, 1799, showed its recognition of the importance of the health laws of the various States by enacting, among other things, that the *quarantine* and other restraints, which shall be established by the laws of any State, respecting any vessels arriving in or bound to any port or district thereof, whether coming from a foreign port or some other part of the United States, shall be observed and enforced by all officers of the United States in such place. 1 Story, U. S. Laws, 564. These provisions, somewhat enlarged upon, are still to be found upon our Federal Statute books. Revised Statutes, U. S. S., 4,792.

The instrumentalities through which the greatest influence is to be exerted in the direction of sanitary legislation, outside of the public and general discussion of these questions, are the legislatures of the various States. And the great *desideratum* in this direction is to perfect, unify, and harmonize, as far as possible, the legislation of the various States upon this subject. This will, of course, have to be done gradually and under great difficulties, and many and great perplexities will have to be met and overcome. The two leading questions to be considered in this connection are :

First.—How far should the legislature go in enacting laws to protect and preserve the public health ? And

Second.—How far can it go, in view of the limitations on legislative power fixed by organic law ?

The first is a question of policy and expediency which addresses itself to the enlightened judgment of the legislature.

The second is a question of law which addresses itself to the courts. As a matter of policy merely, the legislature can not safely go far in advance of the sentiment of the general public on these questions, and this is especially true in this country in which the government derives its power and authority, at least theoretically, from the consent of the governed. All progress in this direction has been and must continue to be comparatively slow, although much has already been accomplished. Prior to the twenty-fifth day of March, 1882, the only legislative enactments to be found upon our statute books in the State of West Virginia, on the subject of the public health, were contained in Chapter 50, of the Code of 1868. They were taken bodily from the Chapter 197, of the Code of Virginia of 1860, except that the word " free," was stricken out of the statute by the legislature of West Virginia to make it conform to the new order of things produced by the great civil war, and the consequent abolition of slavery. They consisted of two sections. The first provided against the sale of diseased, corrupted and unwholesome provisions, and was modeled after the English Statute of 51 Hen. III, already mentioned. The second provided against the fraudulent adulteration of anything intended for food or drink, or of any drug or medicine, with any substance injurious to health. I am unable to state just when the first effort was made to secure additional legislation in this State, but I had the honor to be a member of the House of Delegates during the session of 1877, and at that session a bill was introduced in the House by Dr. M. S.

Hall, of Harrisville, Ritchie County, which was known as "House Bill No. 70," and was "A Bill to establish a State Board of Health." House Journal, 1877, page 318. The measure met with very decided, not to say violent, opposition, and finally both it and its devoted author became the victims of a humorous but cruel joke. Section 4 of the bill provided that "It shall be the duty of the State Board of Health to revise and control the State system of registration of births, marriages and deaths." One of the members of the House at that session was Judge James H. Ferguson, of Charleston, known all over the State as a legislator of great experience, ability and shrewdness. The Judge was the recognized leader of the House, and at the same time the implacable enemy of the bill, and when it came up on its second reading he

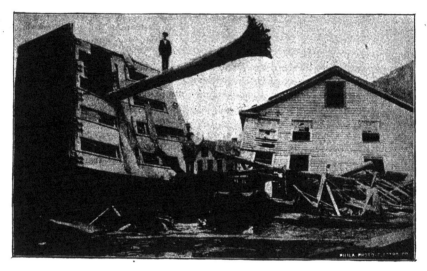

One of the Marvels of the Flood.
A forest tree driven through the second story of a house, and two heavy freight cars carried half a mile from the railroad.

moved to amend Section 4 by striking out the words "of registration." The House, perhaps without perceiving the effect of the amendment, voted to strike the words out, upon which Judge Ferguson called for the reading of the section as amended. You can better imagine the frame of mind in which the patron of that bill, who was naturally an impulsive and irascible man, found himself, than I can describe it to you, when Col Peyton, Clerk of the House, in a loud musical voice with which some of you are perhaps familiar, read; "It shall be the duty of the State Board of Health to revise and control the State system of births, marriages and deaths." It is needless to add that after this amendment had been made the bill was indefinitely postponed, many of its friends and supporters, including your humble servant voting to postpone. But the friends of sanitary legislation were not discouraged by the result of their efforts, and continued to agitate and discuss the question at each subsequent session of the legislature, until, at the session of 1882, success crowned their efforts, and an act was then passed, which, with the subsequent amendments made thereto, has been pronounced by competent judges to be one of the most thorough and complete sanitary codes,to be found in any of the States. This statute is so familiar to the members of the medical profession of this State, that for me to attempt to give a synopsis of its provisions would be a work of supererogation. An examination of its provisions will show how far the legislature of our State has deemed it expedient to go in the line of sanitary enactments. We have certainly taken a great step in advance, and yet no one who has given the matter due consideration, will say we have gone too far or too fast. Great progress has also been made in other sections of the country. And it can scarcely be doubted that, as the world progresses, and the subject of health—so essential to the welfare, happiness and prosperity of the human race—receives its due share of attention, still greater efforts will be made to secure its inestimable blessings by legislative enactments. There is one question remaining to which I have already referred, and which I now desire to briefly discuss, and with the discussion of which I shall bring this paper to a close, and that is: How far can the legislature go in the enactment of sanitary laws without trenching upon the limitations which have been placed upon its power by organic law? It may be laid down as a general rule in the construction of statutes that the legislature of any of the States of the Federal Union, has the power to enact any law which is not prohibited by the constitution of such State. Coley on Con. Lim., 168, *State* vs. *Dent.*, *25 W. Va.*, 8-9. In the case of *Osburn et al* vs. *Stanley et al*, 5 *W. Va.*, 85, the Supreme Court of Appeals of this State held that "While the legislature is governed by the spirit of the Constitution, theCourts can not declare an Act of the Legislature invalid, unless its invalidity is placed beyond a reasonable doubt. A reasonable doubt must be solved in favor of the legislative action, and the act be sustained. The Courts must be guided by the express words of the Constitution and not by its supposed spirit. Whenever an Act of the Legislature can be so construed as to avoid conflict with the Constitution and give it force of law, such construction will be adopted by the Courts."

With these general rules to guide us, let us take a hasty glance at some of the adjudicated cases on the subject. In the case of the *State* vs. *Dent*, already referred to, the point was sought to be made that Sections 9 and 15 of our sanitary statute, are unconstitutional and void, because they are in conflict with Article X, and with Section 1 of Article XIV of the Constitution of the United States, and also with Sections 1, 2, 4, 10 and 11 of our Bill of Rights, Article III of the Constitution of West Virginia. These sections of the health law prescribe certain qualifications for the practice of medicine and penalties for practicing without complying with those requirements, and it was contended that they were in conflict with certain fundamental principles of government recognized by the Constitutional provisions referred to ; but the Court held, Judge Green delivering the opinion, that there was nothing either in the Federal Constitution nor in the Constitution of this State to prevent the Legislature from enacting these sections and that they were therefore perfectly valid. And the reasoning which the Court applies to these sections would seem to apply with equal force to the entire Act. Indeed this may be regarded as a leading case on the general subject of the constitutionality of sanitary legislation, and shows that the Courts will, in general, uphold such legislation unless it is in clear conflict with some provision either of the Federal Constitution or the Constitution of the State by which it is enacted. Judge Green, in his opinion in this case, cites a number of cases from different States, which, in a greater or less degree, sustain the conclusions reached by our Court of Appeals. An interesting and instructive case arose a few years since in the State of Iowa, and was finally decided by the Supreme Court of that State. I am indebted for a report of this case to the kindness of Dr. G. I. Garrison, the worthy and efficient Health Officer of this city, and Dr. J. M. Shafer, of Keokuk, Iowa, who has taken a commendable interest in everything relating to the preservation of the public health. The case involved the power of local Boards of Health to prohibit hog-pens, a very practical question, and one which, with many others of a similar character, may arise at any time, in the enforcement of the various provisions of law in the several States of the Union relating to the health of the general public.

The Mayor and aldermen of the city of Cedar Rapids, pursuant to an act of the General Assembly of the State of Iowa, appointed a Board of Health for that city, and the Board of Health thus appointed adopted and published a regulation in the following language : " There shall not be kept or maintained within the city of Cedar Rapids any hog-pen or enclosure wherein swine are kept and fed by the owner, lessee or occupant of any property therein, save and except such pens as may be used for purposes of commerce only, and all such pens used for purposes of commerce shall be kept clean, and the owner, lessee or manager thereof, shall see that the same do not become nuisances in any respect." The city thereupon passed an ordinance providing a penalty for violations of the regulation thus adopted. One E. B. Holcomb was prosecuted for and convicted of a violation of this regulation, and appealed to the Supreme Court of the State, where the only question raised was, that the regulation of the Board of Health was void, because it amounted to an unreasonable restriction upon the rights of individuals. The agreed facts in the case showed that the city of Cedar Rapids had a population of 15,000, and the Court says in its syllabus in the case : " A regulation adopted by the Board of Health, and enforced by an ordinance providing a penalty for its violation, prohibiting hog-pens, except for purposes of commerce, in a city of 15,000 inhabitants, can not be said to be void for unreasonableness, even though it thereunder becomes a misdemeanor to keep in such city a clean and inoffensive pen with only one hog therein." *State* vs. *Holcomb*, *68 Iowa, 107*. The Court says in its opinion (and this is the vital question to those who are interested in upholding sanitary laws) : " The Board had the authority to establish such reasonable rules and regulations as in its opinion would preserve the health of the inhabitants of the city. The only question, therefore, is, whether the regulation is reasonable. It is said that "while ordinances which unnecessarily restrain trade or operate oppressively upon individuals will not be sustained, yet such as are reasonably calculated to preserve the public health are valid, although they may abridge individual liberty and individual rights in respect to property."

Dillon on Municipal Corporations, Sec. 320, and *Commonwealth* vs. *Patch*, *97 Mass., 221*, are cited in support of the decision, and part of the language of Judge Dillon is quoted. A singular typographical error appears in the report of this case, which I received through Dr. Shafer. In the statement of the facts, the Court is made to say: " The defendant maintained in the corporate limits a pen in which was kept one hog, *and* for the purpose of commerce." With this statement of facts, the decision of the Court was wholly unintelligible, but an examination of the official report of the case (68 Iowa, 107) shows that the language of the Court was: " The defendant maintained in the corporate limits a pen in which was kept one hog, *not* for the purpose of commerce." This, of course, removed the difficulty. Had I more time I should like to go further into an examination of these questions, but

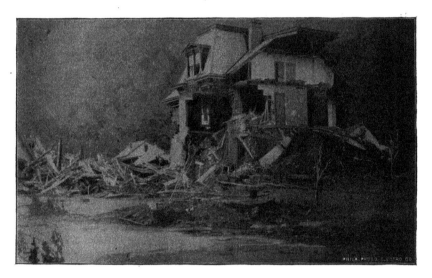

One of the handsomest residences in Johnstown, as it looked after the Flood.

what has already been said is sufficient, I think; to show that the Legislature of every State of the Union has the right to enact such laws for the preservation of the public health as are not prohibited by the Constitution of such State, or by the Constitution of the United States, and that when either a State or local Board of Health has been created by legislative authority and clothed with the power of adopting rules and regulations for the accomplishment of the objects for which it was created, it may adopt, and the Courts will enforce, such rules and regulations as are reasonably calculated to preserve the public health, although such rules and regulations may abridge individual liberty and individual rights in respect to property.

THE ANNALS OF HYGIENE,
.THE OFFICIAL ORGAN OF THE
State Board of Health of Pennsylvania.

The State Board of Health is not responsible for anything appearing in this Journal except that which bears the official attestation of the Board.

✳ ✳ PUBLISHED MONTHLY.

Subscription, two dollars ($2.00) a year, in advance.

Address all communications to

The Hygienic Publishing Company,
224 SOUTH SIXTEENTH STREET,
PHILADELPHIA, PA.

EDITORIAL.

Our Flood Issue.

We have devoted the whole of this issue to the papers that were read before the "Tri-State Sanitary Convention," recently, at Wheeling, W. Va., because by so doing we have been enabled to lay before our readers, in compact form, a mass of not only extremely valuable, but, at the same time, *unique* literature.

When the terrible floods of last spring suddenly confronted our State Board of Health, they offered to us a problem, as yet unsolved ; they presented to us conditions such as had never before, in the history of the world, confronted any sanitary authority.

We had no precedents to guide us in our work ; we were compelled to call to our aid the general principles of sanitation, and, with these as our foundations, to meet special conditions, as they presented themselves, so to speak, to the best of our ability. It speaks volumes for the fertility of resources of those in charge of our sanitary work that these varied and unprecedented emergencies were intelligently and effectually met and combatted.

The outcome of our several months' work in the flooded regions of this State has been an accumulation of most vitally valuable knowledge, and it was with a view of crystallizing and making available this information that the "Tri-State Convention " has convened.

Should, unfortunately, such terrible problems ever again present themselves to the sanitary authorities of any State or locality, they need but to turn to the pages of "THE ANNALS OF HYGIENE" for March, 1890, to find recorded therein the plans and methods by which the dangers to health and life that always follow floods were successfully battled against by the sanitary authorities of Pennsylvania in the spring and summer of 1889.

The Danger to Health From Flood Debris.

We have devoted this issue to the papers read before the tri-State Convention, and we, therefore, publish the paper read by Dr. Spencer M. Free, but we feel that we cannot let this paper go forth without a most emphatic word of dissent from the views therein expressed.

To argue that, because disease did not follow the Johnstown flood, there is no danger to health in flood debris, partakes, to us, of the nature of fatalism and seems somewhat akin to the reasoning of the authorities who, once upon a time, abolished a most efficient local Board of Health, because *as the health of the town was good there was no need for such a board.* We have not space, in this issue, to controvert Dr. Free's arguments ; we merely wish to utter a word of warning against, what we are forced to consider, the heresies that he utters.

"Swapping Gum."

The practice of chewing gum has become very widespread. It is not a very elegant habit; to many it is positively repulsive; and there are sources of danger, too, that should not be overlooked. A case in point was related to us a few days ago. Diphtheria broke out in a family in East Des Moines. After the child had recovered, and the clothing and all the exposed articles were fully disinfected, the parents, with the convalescent child, visited some relatives in the country. The indispensable chewing gum, like Satan, went also—in the mouth of the little child. Prompted by generosity it allowed its country cousins—two children—to chew also the gum previously chewed by the visiting child. In three or four days, without any other known source of infection than the chewing gum, the two children were simultaneously stricken down with diphtheria in a most serious form. It would be hard to imagine a more successful mode of propagating—distributing the disease. It would be a great deal safer not to chew the stuff at all, but if it must be done to satisfy the demands of a weak head and a depraved appetite, our advice is don't. "swap" gum—don't chew anybody else's gum, nor allow anybody else to chew yours.—*Iowa Monthly Bulletin.*

State Board of Health and Vital Statistics of the Commonwealth of Pennsylvania.

PRESIDENT,
GEORGE G. GROFF, M. D., of Lewisburg.

SECRETARY,
BENJAMIN LEE, M. D., of Philadelphia.

MEMBERS,
PEMBERTON DUDLEY, M. D., of Philadelphia.

J. F. EDWARDS, M. D., of Philadelphia.	GEORGE G. GROFF, M. D., of Lewisburg.
J. H. McCLELLAND, M. D., of Pittsburgh.	S. T. DAVIS, M. D., of Lancaster.
HOWARD MURPHY, C. E. of Philadelphia.	BENJAMIN LEE, M. D., of Philadelphia.

PLACE OF MEETING,
Supreme Court Room, State Capitol, Harrisburg, unless otherwise ordered.

TIME OF MEETING,
Second Wednesday in May, July and November.

EXECUTIVE COMMITTEE,

PEMBERTON DUDLEY, M. D., Chairman.	JOSEPH F. EDWARDS, M. D.
HOWARD MURPHY, C. E..	BENJAMIN LEE, M. D., Secretary.

Place of Meeting (until otherwise ordered)—Executive Office, 1532 Pine Street, Philadelphia.

Time of Meeting—Third Wednesday in January, April, July and October.

Secretary's Address—1532 Pine Street, Philadelphia.

Bureau of Registration and Vital Statistics—Department of Internal Affairs, State Capitol, Harrisburg.

State Superintendent of Registration of Vital Statistics—BENJAMIN LEE, M. D.

THE
ANNALS
OF
HUGIENE

VOLUME V.

Philadelphia, April 1, 1890

NUMBER 4.

COMMUNICATIONS

Co-operation between Boards of Health and the Temporary Authorities Developed by Sudden Local Crises.*

By A. J. MOXHAM, of Johnstown, Pa.,
Chairman of the "Citizens' Flood Committee."

The matter to which it is my purpose to briefly call your attention was suggested to me by the following extract from the Annual Report of the Secretary of the State Board of Health of Pennsylvania, Dr. Benjamin Lee, for the year 1889:

" Arriving at Morrellville, about a mile and a half below Johnstown, by the first morning train, General Hastings and Mr. A. J. Moxham, Chairman of the Local Committee, were at once conferred with, and the headquarters of the Board established in the same room with those of the Committee, in order to avail ourselves of telegraphic, mail and messenger service, as well as to be in constant communication with the Committee. The Chairman of this Committee, as well as Mr. J. B. Scott, of Pittsburgh, who on the fifth day of June, having been elected by the representatives of the various boroughs as Director, with absolute authority, assumed the reins of power, while naturally enough not recognizing fully the authority of the Board, were very ready to avail themselves of its assistance in all matters of sanitary precaution and police. To the latter gentleman, especially, the Secretary desires to make his acknowledgments for his constant readiness to co-operate with him in all such measures, and his intelligent appreciation of the necessities of the situation from a sanitary standpoint."

To those who know the Christian-like patience and unselfish devotion of Dr. Lee to the cause of the suffering at Johnstown, during the days of her trouble, there is conveyed a lesson in these words. To me, personally, they came with somewhat of a shock and the reproach that somehow I had (unconsciously perhaps) been false to my trust in the early days of our trouble, in not co-operating to the fullest extent possible with the doctor's early efforts. In those early days the difficulties encountered were such that mutual co-operation and help counted for more than on ordinary occasions.

*Read before the Tri-State Sanitary Convention, at Wheeling, W. Va., February 27 and 28, 1890.

To those who, like myself, know the difficulties and dangers of the situation of the first few days, the remarks suggest nothing short of ignorance in that such invaluable co-operation as could be offered by the State Board of Health was not grasped with a willing hand, and looking back it has seemed to me that if in those days there was any lack of the appreciation of the authority of the State Board it conveys a lesson, and one that we should profit by in cases of future trouble. That we were "very ready to avail ourselves of the assistance of the Board in all matters of sanitary precaution and police" goes without saying. It was simply a case of necessity. We were ready to avail ourselves of anything that could help the problem ; but that the authority of the Board was not properly recognized simply means that we were not intelligent enough to avail ourselves of its help to the extent that we could have, had this authority been duly recognized.

Those who went through the Johnstown Flood troubles from the beginning, realize that the difficulties of existence in the first few hours were infinitely greater than in the ensuing hours; that the problem of the first day was infinitely greater than that of the second day ; and that the conditions of the second month can scarcely be compared to those of the first.

It was, so to speak, the problem of a patient jumping, not from convalescence to the full strength of health, but from the crisis of the disease, first to convalescence, and then to health.

In those early days, not merely had those of us who were able to think at all to look ahead and anticipate the wants that were to come, or the dangers that might be precipitated by carelessness or lack of thought, but this had to be done at the time when the necessities of the survivors, and the chaos into which everything was thrown, rendered it almost an impossibility to take care of the present, let alone to think of the step that was to come.

In the first organization of the Citizens' Committee we needed a location for each of the sub-committees. Some form of table was a necessity. The debris supplied us with an unlimited amount of lumber out of which a table could be made, but it had not left us tools with which to make that table. Although within three squares of us, in the remnants of what had been a furniture warehouse, we knew these tables existed, it took us many hours to climb the debris and get the tables over those three squares.

Each table needed a sign to guide the throngs that pressed into headquarters, to the proper committee. Paint-brush and paint were something not to be had, nor in the early hours was ink available. We used a blacking-brush to paint the signs, and blacking was our paint, and in some of our early records blacking was the substitute for ink.

Some badge was necessary for the police force organized, and tomato-cans furnished the material ; and so through the list.

While we found difficulties in these little nothings, people, who thought they were going to starve, had to be reassured ; drunkenness had to be controlled and stopped ; robbery had to be put an end to ; the recovery of dead bodies attended to, and preparation made for the digging of their graves. The distinction between what was easy and what was hard was swept away. There was nothing easy ; everything was hard.

It was a case analagous to a surgeon having to suddenly care for a dangerous operation, bereft of his instruments, his liniments, and still more, the assistance of his fellow-men.

I speak here of our first days. As stated, each succeeding day the conditions changed, as in the nature of things they had to change, with increased rapidity for the better. As a mathematician I would put it in the form of a formula, that our conditions of existence improved as the square, if not the cube, of the time elapsed. This being so, what but ignorance could have permitted on the part of the authorities any indifference to that help, which, of all help, was most valuable; or, of that experience, which, of all experience, would guide us best. The authorities, from the first moment, were cognizant of the great danger to public health that existed. The State Board of Health (if my recollection is correct) reached us either Sunday evening or Monday morning. The day previous (Saturday) and all day Sunday, large forces of men, that could be badly spared from other work, were engaged with teams that were taken away from the distribution of food, and ropes and tackles and other appliances that were in sore need for pulling away the debris to recover the dead, in pulling out dead amimals to some point of safety and burning them. The first day over fifty-seven carcasses were thus destroyed; the second day a larger number; so that the authorities were certainly in that frame of mind which would appreciate the help to be given by the State Board of Health, and until I had read the extract quoted from Dr. Lee's report I was under the impression that we not only availed ourselves of all that he could do for us, but that we did so with more than a grateful heart, and if there was any failure to appreciate the authority that was brought to us by his presence, it was because we did not know it. If we were in ignorance, others are apt to be so in similar cases, and it behooves us to seek some means to remove the possibility of its recurrence. How can this be done best?

From the nature of things all great catastrophes change the normal conditions of men. Anything, be it what it may, that interrupts, even for a very little, the continuance of the regular motion of the machinery of civilization, may produce incalculable disaster to humankind.

Speaking generally, it is not realized that were the productive current of every-day life to be held in check for even a few short hours, the evil results would take days, if not months, to remedy.

In the presence of such catastrophes man is governed less by his reason than by what may be termed instinct. While perhaps the usual form of organization may be gone through in the shape of appointing of committees for this, that, and the other, the real truth of the matter is that the situation is inevitably controlled by *one man power*. Not only in the case of the chairman—say of the Citizens' Committee, which is generally evolved from such troubles—but also in the case of each sub-committee.

The emergencies become so rapid, and prompt action so necessary, that without stopping to discuss the problem as a matter of logic, the instinct of the mass prompts it to obey blindly every order issued by the parent committee; the parent committee by the same instinct obeys blindly, and without discussion, every order issued by its chairman. There is no time for discussion. And so with the sub-committees.

Indeed, if I had this problem to face again, I would urge the appointing of committees of *one*, and would not burden it by the farce of ordinary organization.

It may also be taken for granted that such a catastrophe as that of the class we are dealing with must first be grappled by the survivors on the ground, and that therefore any State Board of Health reaching the scene of trouble will find something in the form of organization awaiting·it.

I take it that these conditions may be assumed to be normal. Now, with these conditions, in what way in the future can our State Board of Health best secure that proper recognition of its authority which will render it most useful to the cause? It seems to me that there is a simple method, and one perhaps worthy of thought.

We all remember the moral conveyed in the old adage about changing horses while crossing the stream. A sudden and total change of organization would at least involve great loss of time, when perhaps every minute is pregnant with results.

This method is, that the first representative of the State Board of Health who has arrived on the scene should make a formal request that the Board of Health should find room in the existing organization as one of the committees. By this means the organization would drop into the groove of a recognized and absolute authority without a particle of disturbance of existing conditions, and without the loss of a moment's time. The conditions being that of *one man power*, the authority will be absolute.

Great as is the power of such Boards of Health in most cases, it is, in the face of such calamities as we are dealing with, *a power on paper* until incorporated into active work. By this means it becomes a power in fact, and it has at its command that co-operation of the one man, whoever he may be, that has been evolved as representing the authority of the people at such junctures. I take it that we cannot permit such considerations as the question of loss of dignity to influence our discussion of the matter, because we are dealing with a condition of affairs in which dignity as such is non-existent, and by the time that affairs improve to such an extent as to permit the entry of this consideration, in all probability the Board of Health will be master of the situation to the full extent of its real powers. I do not take it that there can be any clash of authority.

Believe me, gentlemen, that at such junctures a man feels very small. Let his courage be what it may; let his abilities be unlimited, he feels in the first grappling with such a problem very weak, and very helpless, and if there ever is a time when man becomes unselfish, and when petty jealousies are utterly swept away it is at such a time as this.

In my control of affairs at Johnstown I endeavored from the first to follow a consecutive plan. I find in my notes made at that time the following abstract of what demanded attention first.

First.—Doctors.

Second.—Police.

Third.—Food.

Fourth.—Shelter.

Fifth.—Burial of the Dead.

Subsequent events added much to the list, but they were not in writing. Had I to write that list again, it would be read as follows :

First.—Brains.

Second.—Doctors.

Third.—Police.

Fourth.—Food.

Fifth.—Shelter.

Sixth.—Burial of the Dead.

In other words, the problem is greater than the mental power of any one man, and brain power is therefore that man's weakest point. Where can the brain power capable of dealing with such problems as these be more readily found than in an organization whose duty it is to deal with the problem of death, and what can be more certainly taken for granted than that the usefulness of our State Board of Health will always find at headquarters a vacant place awaiting its arrival? It may appear that we are harping on a little thing, and so in ordinary conditions, perhaps, it may be called a little thing—the mere technicality of how one organization shall approach another—but so far from being a little thing, does it seem to me, that I would even urge that in addition to the request for a direct representation in whatever organization exists, a telegraphic notice, if possible, should precede the arrival of the Board's representative, and such notice should state clearly his authority and power.

Remember, that while you as a body know full well what these powers are, and their efficacy, it is notoriously the fact that the public at large give themselves very little concern as to the peculiar nature of any of our State organizations, and that, in all probability, the very men who can co-operate best with the Boards of Health, are men who know very little of their scope or power.

Speaking for myself, I must confess that until circumstances forced me to look into it, I was in absolute ignorance of the facts.

Experiences in Sanitary Work.*

By GEO. W. WAGONER, M. D.,
Late Deputy Medical Inspector, Johnstown, Pa.

The propositions which I shall attempt to present are based upon the sorrowful experiences following that deluge of horror and death in the Conemaugh Valley, Pennsylvania. It may be possible that no such calamity may ever occur again in our generation, for this one presented all the combinations of wretchedness, misery, destruction and death that the wildest imagination could picture, and in it can be sought precedents for action in all future emergencies. With thousands of my fellow-citizens of Johnstown I have drained the cup of sorrow to its bitterest dregs. With them I have passed through the fearful ordeal and its horrors are buried deep into our memories. In a few short hours our peaceful valley was changed into a dismal hell, out of which came tales of agony that excited the sympathy and pity of the civilized world. The charitable of all nations furnished relief in every possible way, or, God knows, we should still be in that terrible ooze and slime, the most miserable of mankind.

----

*Read before the Tri-State Sanitary Convention at Wheeling, W. Va., February 27 and 28, 1890.

The problem presented to our people and to those who hurried to our aid on the day following the destruction was an appalling one. A city blotted out of existence, and on its site a deposit of debris of amazing proportions and a character most dangerous to health; the terrible fact that all over the valley were scattered the bodies of thousands of victims; the survivors who had been swept through the jaws of death and were now huddled together on the hillsides, heartbroken, impoverished and utterly hopeless of the future. Their only thought was of the dear ones who lay still in death somewhere in that awful filth. The civil officers did not assert themselves and assume the authority which all would have gladly obeyed. In the dreadful emergency a leader did appear in the person of A. J. Moxham, a clear-headed citizen whose dignity of character, energy, determination and scrupulous justness, inspired all with confidence in his ability to organize the terrified people. He called to his aid a few men of similar character who dared put aside their own griefs in the interest of the public. With heroic energy these men met the unparalleled emergencies of the first few days. They supplied food for the hungry, and protected the poor remnants of property from the hands of the brutal vandals. They encouraged the depressed people and commenced the herculean task of clearing away the wreck. With profound sympathy they sought out the dead and provided means for their decent burial. They evolved a system to bring order out of the horrible disorder, which was the germ of all the future successful plans. All this work was done upon the personal responsibility of Mr. Moxham, and when it was planned no one had reason to believe that the charity of the world would provide a fund to meet the heavy charges of such an undertaking. It is this fact which makes the actions of Mr. Moxham and his committee assume heroic proportions. It is needless to recite in detail the different steps by which the management of affairs passed into the hands of the State authorities. It is sufficient to know the latter soon appreciated the magnitude of the calamity and the extraordinary means required to counteract its baneful influences upon the public health. Dr. Benjamin Lee, Secretary of the State Board of Health, hastened to the devastated regions and unhesitatingly declared the conditions prejudicial to health and public nuisances. This action opened the coffers of the State and provided the means for conducting the most extensive sanitary work of our age. At the sacrifice of his private interests, Dr. Lee devoted his entire energies to the management of this work, which will ever be the most noble monument of his ability as a scientific sanitarian. The power vested in him was used most judiciously; he exercised it with determination and energy, yet with such sympathy and discrimination that it proved the richest blessing our suffering people enjoyed. From the first moment when the officials of the State Board of Health arrived on the scene, the strictly sanitary work began. Men were sent out over the entire region with strong disinfectants and with directions to destroy by fire all dead animals. While this was being done a system was formulated by which the work could be continued with accuracy and all possible speed. The flooded region was divided into districts, each of which was placed in charge of a Medical Inspector, who was also supplied with men and material to do the work he found necessary in his district. By daily reports the central office was kept informed of all the work done from day to day and the condition of the people in each district. From these reports the executive officer directed the work and met emergencies as they arose.

As Medical Inspector of one of the districts, my experience has convinced me that one of the most important duties devolving upon a health officer in any such calamity is that of careful and repeated inspection of each particular house, its surroundings and occupants.

This duty was constantly kept in mind, and while all the other and varied work incident to sanitation was in operation, competent agents were traveling from house to house, outside the flooded district, in which the survivors were concentrated, inquiring into the health of the people; examining the cellars, outhouses and the methods of disposing of the kitchen slops; giving directions how, when and where to use disinfectants and making reports of everything coming under their view.

They examined the streets and alleys outside the flooded districts and reported when they were becoming filthy. Part of my force were thus employed in a large territory which had not been touched by the water, but in which was gathered all that had been saved from the ruins. This territory was kept in a good sanitary condition, and during the months through which the work continued not a single case of infectious disease developed. This gratifying result could only have been attained by making use of the knowledge gained by thorough inspection.

Another matter of extreme importance is the supply of disinfectants. The supply should be of such liberal proportions as to meet any possible requirements. To make their use general they should be furnished free of charge, and even then I found many people would neglect to use them, or use them in too small quantities. This difficulty was overcome by hauling the disinfectants along the streets, taking a supply into each house and in many places applying them directly where needed. To further accomplish this desirable end fifteen places were fixed in my district where the disinfectants could be procured by any resident who would take the trouble of walking a few steps for them. At each place there was a barrel of Bromine Solution, and a gang of laborers were kept going from one to another, filling the barrels and sprinkling the streets and alleys by means of the common sprinkling cans. In this connection I desire to bear testimony to the excellence of Bromine as a disinfectant in all open places. A solution of proper strength can be handled safely and is certain in its action. It removes foul effluvia by destroying the germs of decomposition and does not mask a bad odor by substituting a worse. It was commonly remarked during our operations that everything smelled fresh and sweet after our gang of sprinklers passed along a street or alley. There were used in my district about 20,000 gallons of the solution of bromine during our operations.

Another important point was the cleaning of houses and cellars and the removal of debris. By a legitimate enlargement of the circle of sanitary endeavors, this class of work easily falls within it. The health of people can never be assured so long as they are living over a cellar which contains a flood deposit of mud, or when the house is surrounded by filthy debris. As a rule the people do not realize the danger of such surroundings, and it becomes the duty of the Health Officer to warn them, or, better still, to remove the deposits at the earliest opportunity. They are always rich in animal and vegetable particles, and under the proper conditions of heat and moisture afford all the essential elements of a breeding place of poisonous germs. This danger was recognized early by our Board and every available means used to counteract it. · The people were urged to throw the mud and filth out of their cellars, when the Board would have the mass disinfected and removed to a place of safety. But many people were unable to do even this, when the Board, as a matter of necessity removed the deposits and disinfected the premises. The removal of the debris and deposits of mud and sand was done by contractors working under the supervision of the State authorities. Before any particular piece of work could be done for an individual, an application had to be filed with the State engineer in charge of the work; he would then direct one of his subordinates to examine the locality and report as to the necessity of it. The application was then referred to the Health Office, and from there it was referred to the Medical Inspector, in whose district the premises were located. It was then the duty of the inspector to visit the locality and report to the Health Office its sanitary condition. The Health Office would then inform the State Engineer of the inspector's decision and he in turn would direct the contractors in accordance with it. All this circumlocution may have been necessary and therefore desirable, but after all it was a circumlocution that kept many applicants in suspense for days and weeks, and resulted in gangs of laborers moving about over the town doing jobs here and there, while all around was work that could have been pushed straight forward. I was of opinion at the time and am still, that the supervision and direction of the Medical Inspectors was all that was needed or required. In theory the Health Office and its Inspectors were the final authority that made the performance of any and all work done by the State, legal, and it did really appear that the work could have been done quicker and cheaper without the intervention of the numerous officials, their clerks and staffs, and all the other trivialities hung on for the sake of dignity and show.

It would certainly be proper for the State to have time-keepers and clerks to look after its interests, but there was no pressing necessity for a complete military establishment, whose business it was to secure authority from a few medical inspectors and then see that their orders were executed. The Health Office should have had direct and immediate control of all the contractors, and have been responsible to the State for the proper performance of its duty. It seems to me that this is one of the great lessons to be learned by the Conemaugh flood. That health officials should not only be expected to give opinions and advice about great public nuisances, but they should have the power to direct and control the means used to abate them, and thus be alone responsible for their advice and actions.

The disposal of the dead during times of great disaster is a question of immense importance. Our feelings of humanity and pity prompt us to make every effort to have the victims buried decently and in the ordinary manner. The controlling idea seems to be to get the bodies out of sight in the shortest time possible, and from a sanitary point of view it is a just and proper one. But while the public interests are being cared for in the disposition of the dead, the wishes and feelings of the surviving friends should also be respected, and every means furnished them for the identification of their dear ones. The management of the Conemaugh Valley morgues was somewhat crude during the days immediately following the flood. It was the rule, from which there were few exceptions, that when a body was brought into the morgue no one was expected to examine it for the purpose of identification until all the clothing was cut off and cast away, the victims hair cropped close and flung into the garbage pile, all articles of jewelry removed, the body washed, laid out upon a board covered with a sheet, and numbered. Then the friends searching for their dead were allowed to wander among the bodies, straining their eyes to catch some familiar feature or mark which had not been obliterated by the morgue attendants. If one found a body which bore some fancied resemblance to a loved one and sought out the so-called description list, he was rewarded by finding the most meagre and trifling details, which served only to aggravate. When the work of removing the dead from the temporary burying grounds to Grand View Cemetery was undertaken, and the people were again given an opportunity to examine the bodies and compare them with the morgue records, it was found that the bodies of many victims did not correspond in any particular with the descriptions attached to what purported to be their number in the morgue books. In many cases the bodies and numbers were hopelessly mixed. When all the distressing circumstances surrounding the horrible tragedy are remembered, many mistakes can be excused ; but if there was any one duty, the perfect performance of which would have touched the hearts of the survivors, it was the one which made the identification of victims reasonably easy and certain.

I think it is safe to assert that if the clothing and hair had not been removed from the bodies, hundreds who are now occupying unknown graves would have been identified, to the intense relief of their sorrowing friends, and be laid away in spots ever hallowed by the tears of those whose only relief is to mourn in bitterness of spirit.

It is certainly true that when the bodies were brought into the morgues they were covered with mud, their clothing torn, and their bodies bruised and battered. But notwithstanding these facts it still remains equally true that the paramount duty of the authorities was to prepare the bodies so identification would be easy, and not to make presentable corpses of them.

God knows water was plenty with us then ; the mud could have been washed off, and in the torn clothing and drabbled hair would have been found evidences of the identity of the body which never could be found in the distorted faces and mangled limbs of the victims. The experiences of a search for the bodies of nine of my immediate family justifies me in speaking with positiveness upon this subject. Even now, months after the calamity, the bodies which are unearthed are almost invariably identified, and entirely by means of the clothing.

These considerations make it evident that everything which might serve to identify a body should be left upon it, even if by so doing the corpse does not present the conventional appearance that most people deem so necessary.

Among the sanitary lessons taught by the great Conemaugh flood, I believe the following to be the ones of distinct value : Repeated and thorough inspection of a district, and the application of the knowledge thus gained; persistent disinfection ; the speedy removal of all filthy deposits ; the concentration of power and responsibility in the hands of the Health Officer, and the abolishment of all cumbrous extra-official authority; and, finally, the preservation and burial of the dead in the condition they are found, as nearly as a proper regard for decency will allow, always bearing in mind, however, that identification of the dead is one of the chief objects to be aimed at.

The Floods as they Affect the People of South Carolina.*

By W. D. CLINTON, M. D.
Of Lancaster, S. C.

The idea has suggested itself to my mind that perhaps, as a general thing,, from pride in our Association, and in the desire to present something worthy of it, we are too apt to think that our papers should embody something original, or should reach the dignity of elaborate essays. But since entering the study and practice of medicine, I find there is not much of original thought for one to produce, for we are studying and combatting with the same diseases that your fathers had to fight against. Now, since there are men here to represent the sanitary condition of the three States, and men who were successful practitioners before I knew there was such a thing as medicine in the world, or before I came into the world, I feel highly honored and grateful to God and man that I should be appointed by our worthy secretary to have something to say. In accordance with these views I desire to cast in my mite by having a few words to say concerning the floods as they affect the people of South Carolina. Having been born on the soil, drank of her water, and breathed her healthy and unhealthy air, it is with much pleasure that I speak of her. South Carolina, as you are doubtless aware, is in the alluvial belt of the United States, which has not the natural surroundings that you have here. No lofty peaks of mountains are to be seen which gives power to the rivers as you have here ; but there is a flat plane, which is quite often covered by water and debris, which is brought there from other parts of the State. In this we find a great deal of animal and vegetable matter which finds its way into the wells, springs, and reservoirs of the State. Then it is that the germ of disease begins its work and especially the one which is called bacillus malaria. It is this disease which rises in the garb of its kingly power and sways its sceptre over the State, rebellious to the power of all the antipyretics. Thus it works its way and has its sway until summer, with her hot days and sultry nights, compels it to seek a refuge in the swamps which are covered by water. There this bacillus remains dormant until the fall season brings back reinforcement for the poisonous germ which has made its home in the swamps, wells and springs, then it is that it bursts forth in the power of its might and shakes the very foundation of the medical skill. Though this bacillus is severe, yet there is one thing in its character to be admired and that is this : it has no respect for persons ; it goes into the rich man's house though surrounded with all of the luxuries of South Carolina, and having everything to make him happy, yet this germ comes upon him and gives him the same kind of a shake as it does the herdsman, who attends to his goats, or the beggar, who wanders in search of his bread. Even the Governor in his place is shaken by the same malady. Hence, we find it in one phase a noble disease. Nor less so is the dreadful disease of typhoid fever, which is ushered in upon the people living in the districts which are fooded by the Cataba, Lynces, Congree, Waterree, Ashly and Cooper Rivers. This germ finds its way through the floods of said rivers into the springs, wells and reservoirs. It is thought there that it is found in the vegetable as well as in the animal kingdom. The working of this germ or bacillus, as Dr. Klebs

---

*Read before the "Tri-State Sanitary Convention at Wheeling, W. Va., Feb. 27 and 28, 1890.

calls it, is different from the one in malaria. It seems to flourish most in hot weather and dry autumn. This disease enjoys good weather when it spreads its wings and feasts on the bodies of the people of South Carolina. Though it seems to think more of the rich and the intelligent than the poor; it is the poor people who are the victims of this malady. In all ages and in all parts of the State, since I have had the chance to read of the course, effect and cause of the disease there have been able, scholarly and refined physicians striving to find a remedy to kill the germ. It floated in the hearts and minds of the medical fraternity of the State. They have depicted in ever glowing colors the rise and progress of this disease and the incentive, which has given a better understanding to their labors in combatting this dreadful disease. And now they are diving into the Klebian doctrine and striving for the saving of mankind. Though the flood has brought the disease upon the people and in it the germ is sown, but by a united effort of the medical profession they keep it abated, and in some cases they drive it from their patients, though leaving them emaciated and weak, yet they rally and get back to their former powers. This disease seems to have a great desire for the colored man and poor white man of South Carolina. Since they work in the lowlands, on the rice and cotton farms, they seem to be more subject to the disease than those who are seldom seen in the lowlands. These are not all of the diseases which we find affecting the people of South Carolina through the influence of the floods. Acute dysentery is found, in the most flooded parts of the State, to be more severe just after a flood. It is one of the dreaded epidemics of the State. The cause or germ has not been discovered yet, but from observation we find it at its highest pitch just after a flood. It was observed by the profession during the year 1876, there were very few floods and no cases, comparatively, of dysentery; but in the year 1884, when the rivers spread and watered the country for miles, it was then seen that dysentery created much havoc in the State. Most all of the farmers suffered from the attacking arm of dysentery—not only man, but the cattle, were affected by the water. Now the Medical Society of the State is searching for a remedy to combat successfully the different diseases as they may arise from flooded districts. They are striving to uproot the firm foundation of the different diseases caused by the flood in that State and hunting remedies to kill all of the germs which may arise to baffle the skill and judgment of the young practitioner.

They are laying a firm foundation, worthy to be emulated by those who are to take up the mantle of the profession as they yield to the power of time. It is a great pleasure to me to see the old physician standing on the wall and calling to the young man to come up here. We know they did not, neither could they prevent the flood; but they did successfully combat the effect which the flood produced. Now they can look back over a well-spent life, and read to their delight the record of the past.

There is no set time in South Carolina for the districts to be partly covered by water, for most any hard rain will cause the rivers to overflow. In some parts of the State all of the debris, including animal and vegetable matter, is burned with the idea of killing the germs; but they are like the ghost that will not be downed.

Having been greatly benefitted by this Association, I thank you for the honor conferred upon me.

Domestic Hygiene.*

By J. Y. DALE, M. D.,
Of Lemont, Pa.

I have the honor of appearing before you this evening in response to a kind invitation, for the purpose of reading to you a paper on " Domestic Hygiene."

Hygiene may be briefly defined as " the art of preserving health," and you may readily suppose it to be a subject so vast in extent that hours might be spent in the consideration of any one of its numerous divisions. In this paper I can touch on but a few general topics relating to the prevention of disease.

Cicero said, " In no way does man approach more nearly to the gods than by giving health to his fellow man." There are two ways in which physicians perform this god-like function ; *first*, by successfully treating the sick ; and *second*, by trying to keep those who are well from getting sick. Prescribing medicines for the sick is popularly supposed to be the only business of a medical man, but in treating almost any case of illness a portion of his advice must of necessity pertain to hygienic management, such as proper food, clothing, ventilation, rest, exercise, etc. ; and in case the patient has a contagious disease, suitable precautions must be ordered to prevent its spread, which are for the welfare of other members of the household, or of the community ; so that every physician, according to his ability, is perforce more or less of a sanitarian, and must employ such means as he is acquainted with, or are at his command, to prevent the spread of all kinds of diseases.

It will thus be seen that not only has a physician duties to his patient, and the patient's family, but also to the public at large ; and it is absolutely necessary for him, if he wishes to perform his whole duty, not only to be competent to treat the sick, but also to understand the most approved methods of preventing disease.

We have all heard of the ounce of prevention that is worth a pound of cure. Nearly all the disease in the world is preventable, and one of the first steps in prevention is to find out the cause, and if that can be done, to remove it, if possible.

When we once know what it is that produces any given disease we are in a position to study the means of destroying, or of avoiding, this cause. On this account it will be profitable for us to have at least a general idea of the manner in which some of our commonest and most fatal diseases originate. Much progress has been made during the past few years in this direction, and it has been proved conclusively that cholera, splenic fever, lock-jaw, cholera-infantum, typhoid fever ; and rendered probable that most other infectious, contagious or epidemic diseases, are caused by a specific vegetable germ, which finds its way into the body.

These germs are the lowest, simplest, and most minute form of plant life, so small as to require the most powerful microscope to make them visible, and being so transparent that even then they can only be seen readily by being stained or colored.

Let me try to explain to you, however imperfectly and briefly, something about these plants or germs, the scientific name for which is *bacteria* or *microbes*, as those that cause disease are most commonly called.

*Read before the Farmer's Institute, at State College, Pa., January 9, 1890.

We often see the seeds of thistles and other plants floating in the air, and this is one method by which they are carried from place to place. One of the worst weeds that farmers have to contend with, the Canada thistle, is distributed in this manner, and it has been so widely spread over the country that few farms in Centre County are free from it. It is so well known an evil that our Legislature has enacted laws making it a punishable offence for any one to allow Canada thistles to run to seed on his premises.

We need acts of legislation to limit the spread of seeds infinitely worse than those of any visible plant that grows ; and physicians all over the State for years past have sent petitions to the Legislature, and urged, by every means in their power, the passage of laws that would help to protect the people against contagious diseases; but it takes a long time to accomplish such a work, and our great commonwealth, in this respect, is far behind many other States of the Union.

The air that is near the surface of the earth, the water, and the soil, contain countless numbers of these little bacteria of many different kinds, and also their seeds, or spores, as they are called. Many of them are not only harmless, but they are of very great service to us. They come in contact with everything that is exposed to the air, and whenever they find suitable conditions for their growth they multiply with incredible rapidity, causing the destruction of what they live on, so that all fermentation or decay that takes place in any vegetable or animal structure is probably owing to them. In this way they assist in bringing about the more or less prompt decomposition of every organized substance, or anything that ever had life, and render such material capable of being again used for plant food. It is also believed that it is due to their agency that any seed the farmer sows is enabled to germinate.

Fresh meat exposed to the air in warm weather soon becomes tainted from this cause, so that it must be salted, smoked or thoroughly dried, to keep it from spoiling. When our wives put up fruit or vegetables air-tight they exclude these little bodies, and not only must the air be kept out, but the material to be canned must be thoroughly boiled, to destroy any that may be already contained in it, or they will soon begin to grow, and cause the contents of the can to ferment, or, as it is commonly expressed, to "work." Great heat or prolonged boiling will kill all bacteria, but freezing does not seem to have a damaging effect on them.

Heat, moisture, and a proper soil, are as necessary for the growth of these plants as for any other kind—and in any sort of filth they increase very fast. Wherever the harmless kinds grow the best, there are also found the conditions for the prompt growth of many of those that are harmful or poisonous to man, and this is an extremely important fact that should never be lost sight of.

As before mentioned, it has been proved beyond question that several diseases are directly caused by the entrance of these minute bodies into the system, where they find a soil, or the conditions favorable to their development, and during the course of their growth they produce such disturbances as to cause sickness. Judging from what has been proved, the great probability is that every contagious and epidemic malady that the human frame is liable to is caused in the same manner.

It has been ordained that every tree and herb shall yield seed after its kind, and this is equally as true of the plant, which is so small that hundreds can live in a single drop of water, as it is of the mighty oak. Each one of these little spores or seeds will bring forth a plant after its own kind, just as surely as will corn or wheat ; and as far as is known at present, each different disease is caused only by a certain plant or germ. During the process of growth in the body these little plants are believed to produce a chemical substance that is highly poisonous, and which, being absorbed and carried throughout the system in the blood, gives rise to the various symptoms of the special disease.

The way to prevent such diseases, or at least to lessen their frequency, is to attempt the destruction of these plants or germs wherever we suspect them to be found, and by every means in our power to prevent them from getting into our bodies. Consequently whenever they are in a state of active multiplication, as in a case of sickness caused by them, all due precautions should be observed. In grave germ diseases, like small-pox, scarlet fever, or diphtheria, this is especially necessary. It does not come within the scope of this paper to enter into details for the management of such cases, as full information ought to be always furnished by the physician in attendance ; or it will be found in the circulars issued by the State Board of Health, and which have been widely distributed over the country. Isolation of the patient, and prompt destruction by fire, or careful disinfection of everything contaminated, constitute the main features of prevention.

When death results from any such disease, the funeral should be strictly private ; and after either death or recovery the apartment occupied by the patient, with all its contents, ought to be thoroughly disinfected.

The proper use of disinfectants in the sick room is no doubt of great service in destroying disease germs, but they should never be allowed to take the place of cleanliness and ventilation.

If a domestic animal dies of consumption, rinderpest, hog-cholera, chicken-cholera, or any similar disease, the best and safest way to get rid of the body, instead of burying it, would be to burn it ; indeed, this is the proper method of disposing of human remains ; and as the population of the world increases, the safety of the living will probably demand the cremation of the dead. The carcass of even a large animal can be effectually burned without a disagreeable odor by thickly covering it and the ground around it with rosin, over which should be piled sufficient wood, and fired. This plan was used successfully at Johnstown last Summer.

No living thing can continue to live and at the same time be food for another plant or animal. Our lives are a constant warfare against these minute organisms, and the most terrible wars of the world sink into insignificance in comparison with the deadly work wrought by these silent, invisible and ever-active agents of destruction. Look at the frightful ravages produced by the plague that formerly prevailed so extensively, and which, in the fourteenth century killed twenty-five million people in Europe in four years' time ; or, by an epidemic of cholera, yellow fever, by small-pox before it was brought under control through vaccination, to say nothing of local epidemics of scarlet fever, typhoid fever, measles, diphtheria, of malaria, consumption, and dozens of other diseases. An example on a grand scale of a disease probably caused by a microphyte or microbe, is presented by the late pandemic of influenza. On the steppes of Russia, or some other favorable locality, this plant found the conditions so suitable for its rapid development, that it multiplied into countless myriads, and finally gained sufficient volume and elevation to be carried by the upper wind currents over continents and oceans, raining down abundantly everywhere into the surface strata of the atmosphere, and being breathed into the air passages, caused the disease in prince and pauper alike.

Do not understand me to say that every time any of these microbes get into our bodies we are bound to have the special disease they are capable of producing; if this were so, there would be no chance for any of us to live in comfort. Without doubt we all many times take them into our systems, but either they do not find the proper material for their growth, or for some other reason we are able to get rid of them without their doing us any harm. Good health, if I may be allowed a Hibernicism, is the very best preservative against disease.

We can hope great things from the advancement of science, and in the future possibly inoculations against all infectious diseases may be successfully practiced from germs that have been subjected to repeated cultures, and weakened enough to be safely used for this purpose, while yet retaining sufficient activity to exhaust from the system the special material necessary for their growth. One attack of most of the contagious diseases, from chicken-pox to small-pox, is a protection against the same disease in the future, and this is probably due to the cause mentioned, that the one crop has permanently exhausted the soil, so that a succeeding one cannot grow.

I can give you in one word the secret of nearly the whole art of hygiene, and that is *cleanliness*, which we are told is next to godliness. By cleanliness I mean not only the absence of what we commonly call dirt, but the broader definition which includes everything impure or unclean. Clean living and right thinking are a protection, physically and morally.

The observance of the rules of personal and domestic hygiene was made a religious duty by the Hebrews, and the Old Testament contains many valuable precepts relating to the preservation of health, which we would all be the better for following. To this day the Jews do not suffer from many of the maladies that prevail in the countries where they live.

There are certain things that are very essential to health, such as pure air to breathe, pure water to drink, pure food to eat, and a pure soil to live on.

There is no excuse for farmers not eating the most wholesome and finest quality of food, because they have access to the very best that the country affords, having the first choice of good meat, fresh eggs and milk, and ripe fruit and vegetables. I can testify from personal knowledge that many of the farmers' wives and daughters in this community cannot be excelled as cooks and housekeepers. Indeed, women generally are the best sanitarians; and there can be no doubt that much disease is prevented by the very thorough cleaning that our houses get every spring and fall, however much we may grumble over the discomforts we have to undergo during the process.

Pure water is one of the most important of all the essentials to life and health, and the more thickly settled a country is the more difficult it is to procure. Theoretically rain-water contains the fewest impurities, but this depends much on the means of collecting and preserving it. If the roofs of buildings are thoroughly washed by rains before the water is run into perfectly clean cisterns, through properly constructed filters, and all needful precautions taken to prevent the entrance of bugs, flies, worms, snails, etc., the water will be sufficiently pure, but how many of us do this? Surface and subsoil waters are often very impure, so that springs and wells may be sources of disease. No privy, manure pile, or other filth should ever be within a hundred and fifty feet of a well, and the further away the better. Wells ought to be carefully cleaned at least twice a year, and the same precautions are requisite as with cisterns to keep out insects, toads, rats, etc. It is not desirable to have trees near a well, as the roots will find their way into it, loosen the soil, and form natural drains from the surface. The greater the depth from which water is obtained, as in artesian wells, the less likely it is to contain disease germs or filth; but the objection to such water is that it generally holds so large a percentage of lime and other minerals in solution as to make it very hard. A pleasant taste and a clear color are not sure indications of purity. Sometimes the most sparkling and refreshing water is loaded with chlorides and other poisons. Whenever we have reason to suspect the purity of our water, it should always be thoroughly boiled before drinking.

Many people think that freezing purifies water, but this is a mistake. The safest plan is never to take ice from water that is not good enough to drink. The germs of typhoid fever have been found uninjured after remaining in solid ice for more than three months.

There is no greater nuisance, or more active breeder of disease in a civilized country, than the ordinary privy. The health of every community would be improved if it were utterly abolished. Disease germs often multiply in filth, and this is particularly true of those that cause typhoid fever, and no more favorable conditions could be selected for their growth than in a privy vault. The contents of a privy will ooze through the soil, and find its way into a well or under-ground water course. For this reason all privy pits, cesspools, or sewerage into the crevices of rocks may be a source of danger, because no human foresight can determine whether this worst of filth may not get into water and cause disease, possibly miles away from its point of entrance. In this portion of the State the limestone formation is cavernous, and when the roof of a cavern falls in it makes a sink-hole; instances of which can be seen in this immediate vicinity. In such localities geologists tell us there are underground water-courses, which will often account for the absence of surface streams. The configuration of the surface of the ground gives no indication of the directions of these subterranean channels.

Every privy vault should be emptied, the contents disinfected, the hole filled with earth, and a dry earth-closet substituted, which can be easily and cheaply made by any one capable of using a saw and hammer. If used with ordinary care and cleanliness, it will be free from smell, and cannot fail to give good satisfaction. Instead of dry earth coal-ashes may be used, and, when the receptacle is full, it can be emptied on the manure pile, which it will help to enrich. The dry earth system has the sanction of the highest authority, for the men of Israel, in journeying through the wilderness, were directed to carry a paddle, with which to dig and cover their discharges.

In this part of the country we should be specially interested in having a pure water supply, because the poison of typhoid fever, which usually gets into the system through the stomach, is most generally introduced by means of water. This, as you all know, is a very common disease hereabouts, but being preventable, it ought to be as rare as small-pox. It prevails extensively in the late summer and fall, because then there is the most decaying filth of various sorts to be found—yet I meet with it in every month of the year.

For the general welfare every householder must be a sanitarian as far as his own premises are concerned. Unfortunately we are all more or less at the mercy of others from a sanitary point of view, so that the greatest care in personal hygiene will often not protect us from the faults and ignorance of our neighbors. After an epidemic of any serious disease people are very apt to screen themselves by calling it a mysterious dispensation of Providence, which is little short of blasphemy, when, as is too frequently the case, it may be owing to the most flagrant violation of well-known sanitary laws.

There is a common saying that every generation is growing weaker and wiser. However, it may be about our wisdom, it is a mistake that we are not as strong physically, nor as long-lived, as were our ancestors. On the contrary the average duration of human life is increasing, and not only do many people still live beyond the three-score years and ten allotted to man, but by our improved methods of living many reach a green old age, and make useful citizens, who, under former conditions would not have survived infancy. The race is not always to the swift, nor the battle to the strong. Living in a frugal, simple, natural manner, will enable even a person of delicate constitution to enjoy life, and perform a full share of work.

In that happy time in the future, when the laws of health shall be fully understood and carefully followed by every one, disease will vanish from off the face of the earth, and then, barring accidents, every individual will live long enough to die of old age, and doctors' bills will be unknown.

The Prevention of Consumption.*

BY A. ARNOLD CLARK,
Of Lansing, Michigan.

Dr. Baker said that he would speak only a few moments, and yet during the few minutes that he was standing upon this platform, some two or three citizens of the United States—men and women filled with happy, hopeful dreams—men and women to whom life is joy, have surrendered their lives to this Destroyer. I have here a diagram accurately drawn to scale, showing the relative number of deaths from different diseases, and from this you will see that every time one person dies in Michigan from small-pox forty or fifty die from consumption. And yet, though there is no disease which causes so many deaths, there is no disease about which scientific men know so much and which they could so easily prevent if the people only knew.

DEATHS IN MICHIGAN, 1886-87.

Consumption.
Diphtheria.
Typhoid Fever.
Scarlet Fever.
Whooping Cough.
Measles
Small-pox.

*Read before the Vicksburg (Mich.) Sanitary Convention.

A great change has come about recently in opinion as to the relative parts played by heredity and the germ in the causation of this disease. Though the lungs of children of consumptive parents may have a lower vitality and less resisting power, the cause of the disease is known to be a specific germ, and 999 cases out of every thousand are communicated from person to person, and it is these cases which we must prevent. Where does consumption generally first appear? In the lungs, because the germs of consumption are carried to the lungs in the air which we breathe.

Dr. Baker alluded to the fact that the germs of consumption have been found on the walls of rooms where consumptives have been. These experiments have been conducted by Dr. Cornet, of the Berlin Hygienic Institute. He found that the sponge scrapings from the walls of rooms inhabited by consumptive patients, inoculated in guinea pigs, produced consumption in those animals.* Sponge scrapings from the walls of rooms where no consumptives had been did not, on inoculation, produce consumption in the guinea pigs. Now, how did the walls of those rooms become contaminated with the germs of consumption? Not by the breath from the consumptive patient. Guinea pigs have been placed in a rubber sack and they have been breathed upon two hours a day for six weeks by consumptives without contracting the disease.† So, the danger is not in the breath.

Cornet found that where consumptives had invariably expectorated in cuspidors filled with water, the dust from the walls of the room showed no germs ; but where the sputa had been allowed to dry on the floor, the germs had risen with the sweepings and covered not only the walls but the pictures, dishes, the bed, and everything in the room —so virulent, as to produce the disease sevaral weeks after the patient had left the room. It is then from the dried sputa of consumptives that this great foe of the human race scatters its seeds. This is proved beyond question. These germs have been found repeatedly in the sputum, in the dried fly-specks on the windows of rooms inhabited by consumptive patients, the flies having fed upon the sputa.

Animals feeding on the sputa of consumptives die of consumption. Dr. Cagny‡ tells of a young consumptive who took care of a large number of fowls, and who amused himself by coughing for the amusement of the chickens, which

GREEDILY DEVOURED THE SPUTA.

Many of the chickens died of consumption, and the germs of consumption were found in the dead chickens.

Consumption has been produced by inoculating with the sputa, by swallowing the sputa, by breathing the sputa. The disease has been transmitted to cattle, pigs, sheep, rabbits, rats, mice, dogs, monkeys and men.

---

*Zeitschrift für Hygiene, Vol. V, pp. 191-331. See also references to this subject in London *Lancet*, May 19, 1888 ; Phthisiology Historical and Geographical, pp. 275-277 ; Fourth Annual Report State Board of Health, Maine, 1888, pp. 199-212 ; also, *Buffalo Medical and Surgical Journal*, June, 1889, p. 639.

†Experiments by Graucher, mentioned in Centralblatt für Bakteriologie and Parasitenkunde, Vol. V, p. 289. Similar experiments with similar results were made by Cadeac and Mallet on rabbits. Revue D'Hygiene, Vol. X, p 255.

‡Transactions of Congress for the Study of Consumption, Paris, Vol. 1.

When Tappeiner was causing dogs to
BREATHE THE PULVERIZED SPUTA OF CONSUMPTIVES,
a robust servant of forty laughed at the idea that consumption could be caught in this way. In spite of warnings he went into the inhaling room, breathed the sputum dust, and got the consumption just the same as the dogs. In fourteen weeks he died of consumption.*

Thousands in Michigan every year do unconsciously just what this man did consciously and willfully ; and when we think of the ten thousand consumptives in Michigan who every hour in the day are expectorating along our streets and even on the floors of public buildings, post-offices, churches, hotels, railroad cars and street cars, when we think how these germs are being dried and carried into the air by every passing breeze, by every sweeping, and how they are capable of producing the disease six months after drying, when we think of the miscellaneous crowd sleeping in hotel bed-rooms, when we think of the close, unventilated sleeping car, with hangings and curtains so well calculated to catch the germs, and where, as some one has said, the air is as dangerous as in those boxes filled with pulverized sputa where dogs are placed for experiment ; then, when we remember that a man's lungs are a regular hot-house for the growth and multiplication of these seeds of consumption, is it any wonder that one citizen in every seven dies of this disease? And if a human life is worth anything to the State, is it any wonder that the State spends money to hold such conventions as this, where the people may be told how they may destroy these invisible yet almost invincible germs swarming in the air we breathe.

DESTRUCTION OF THE SPUTA.
Now, the object of this discussion is not to make you afraid to breathe, but to make you so dread the sputum from consumptives as to insist on its destruction. Every person after coughing a month or so and raising sputa, should have a microscopical examination of the sputa both for his own comfort and for the public safety. No consumptive should be allowed to expectorate on the floor or street, and all sputa should be disinfected or burned. The disinfection of the sputa has been recommended by the American Public Health Association, by the Michigan State Board of Health and by many other Boards, and if it were universally carried out there would be two or three thousand less deaths in Michigan every year.

But you say that you have not the consumption, you cannot go around seeing that your neighbor disinfect his sputa, are there no
PERSONAL PRECAUTIONS
which you can take ? Yes ! It does not follow because we breathe the germs of consumption that we will get the disease. Our lungs may be so healthy and vigorous that the germs will not find a congenial soil. Dr. Trudeau's experiments show that when animals are inoculated, if they are kept in good sanitary surroundings, the disease is sometimes arrested. So post-mortem examinations show that a great many men and women are attacked by consumption sometime in life, and they recover from it. They have such good food and air and their lungs are so healthy and vigorous that the tubercular process is stopped. Consumption never attacks wild oxen, but it

Buffalo Medical and Surgical Journal June, 1889, p. 637. Dr. Gautier, a French physician, in similar experiments, accidentally breathed the sputum dust and contracted the disease. Science, Vol. XIII, p. 162.

is a great catch for tame elephants and pet canaries, for foreigners who try to accommodate themselves to the food and habits of another race. It yields a higher death-rate in the closely crowded cities, in the great industrial centres, than in the open country. One-half of all the deaths which occur in States' Prisons are from consumption, and Ziemssen says that imprisonment for fifteen years is equivalent to sentence of death by consumption. Any environment which weakens the system or irritates the lungs simply

HARROWS THE SOIL

for the easier cultivation of the seeds of consumption. It may be the irritating dust from a factory, or it may be only a hard cold. All of these unfavorable conditions you may avoid. You may strengthen the body in every possible way. You may go further: Without considering the question at length, it is known that consumption is a very common disease in cattle, and may be communicated to man by the milk which he drinks and the flesh which he eats. Now, you may boil all the milk which is suspected, to destroy the germs, a meat inspector may destroy the flesh of all tuberculous animals, and all of this will do good. But more important than all this, more important than anything else—let me emphasize again in closing—the disinfection of the sputa. The consumptive should do this for his own good, because, when he continues breathing the germs of consumption from his own sputa,

HE CONTINUALLY RE-INFECTS HIMSELF,

and thus diminishes his chances of recovery. But more than this, the people should demand it for their own safety. It is more important than to fortify our bodies. It is better to kill the germs before they commence trying to kill us. You have probably heard of the Irishman who swallowed a potato bug and then swallowed Paris Green to kill it. If a battle must go on with the germs of consumption, I prefer it to go on outside of my body, and the place to take the germs at a disadvantage is in the sputa. This plea for the disinfection of the sputa may seem a rather prosaic and commonplace recommendation with which to close a long speech—something like those long column articles in the newspapers, which picture the horrors of some disease and close with an innocent little line at the bottom, "Use Warner's Safe Cure." But when I look at this diagram, more eloquent than words, when I think of the thousands who every year are cut off in the prime of life, I sometimes feel that a man could not have a better epitaph written over his grave than this:

He Taught Consumptives to Destroy Sputa.

Every day in the week and every hour in the day one citizen in seven is giving to every passing current and to the four winds of heaven those seeds which surely mean a wrecked ambition and an early death to some fellow creature. Every hour in the day that great "reaper whose name is Death" is gathering with his sickle where we, in our ignorance, have sown the seed. And yet a nation which has spent thousands of dollars studying the diseases of peaches and pears, a nation that has spent thousands of dollars to protect its fish and the young seals of Alaska, has never given a dollar for the study or prevention of consumption in men. If Jefferson and the signers of the Declaration were right, and the first object of government is to guarantee to all men the enjoyment of life, surely that work is highest and noblest whose object it is to prolong the lives of millions and to endow those lives with health and strength.

Bismarck as a Sanitarian.

BY THE EDITOR.

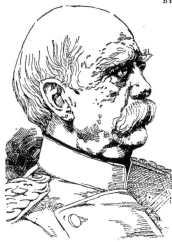

There are two kinds of sanitarians—those who observe all the laws of hygiene, or of nature, and by so doing secure for themselves good health and long lives; and those who, by observing only some of these laws (combined with the inheritance of a robust constitution), secure such an amount of vigor that they are enabled to do with impunity that which would prove very injurious to others. To this latter class belongs the great Bismarck; but it is a class of exceptions rather than of rules, and it is not a class from which we should draw our deductions. Bismarck, in his personality, is as peculiar and as unique as in all of his other attributes. If we are to believe the current reports, he drinks and smokes enough to kill a dozen ordinary men; but then we must remember that he is not an *ordinary* man. Old General Patterson, of this city, who died a few years ago at the age of over ninety, was a man who ate and drank almost, we would say, without limit. Meeting him (when he was fully ninety years of age) one morning in market, a gentleman, who happened at the time to be talking to Dr. Joseph Leidy, of this city, remarked: "What a wonderful old man General Patterson is;" "He is not a *man*," replied Dr. Leidy, "he is a *phenomenon*." So might the sanitarian truly say that Bismarck is a *phenomenon*. But there is a strong lesson to be drawn from Bismarck's life—while we must admit that he is very fond of art, so far as liquor and tobacco are concerned, we must note, at the same time, that he has an all-consuming love for nature, for from his youth he has always been a fervent admirer of the country, and even of late, in spite of his years and bodily infirmities, his chief pleasure has been to get away from his office for a day's sport in the woods with his dogs and gun. It was during a stay at Varzin that the painter Lenbach caught on the face of the Chancellor, who at the time was watching the flight of a flock of wild fowl, the fine expression which makes his portrait in the National gallery of Berlin the finest one that has ever been painted, and it was this same one that the artist recopied when Leo XIII asked for his likeness. "Believe me," said his wife, one day when speaking to a diplomat about her husband, "believe me, he takes as much interest in a turnip as he does in all your political questions."

Because of this love for nature, has nature rewarded Bismarck with the ability to withstand, to a certain extent, the evil influences of art. But, who can say that had this man been even more natural—had he avoided that which we all know to be injurious—he would not have been a greater man, even, than he is. It is a well-recognized fact that alcohol and belligerency are very closely allied, and since most of Bismarck's fame has been derived from the sword, may we not suppose that his habits may have had something to do with his bellicose spirit? Bismarck is a diplomat of exceeding acuteness; might he not have been even more acute had he been guided by nature rather than have been influenced, as he must have been, more or less, by the alcohol within him? and would not his fame have been even greater than it is, had it been procured solely by diplomacy, rather than, mainly, by the force of arms? Evidently, he, himself, thinks so, for he tells us that his career has given very little satisfaction to himself personally and won him very few friends; he has not added to the happiness of himself, his family, or of any one. One of those who heard him say this suggested that he had made a great nation very happy. "Yes," he replied, "but how many other nations have I rendered unhappy? But for me three great wars would never have taken place, 80,000 men would not have been killed in battle; fathers, mothers, brothers, sisters, and wives would not have been plunged into misery. I have settled all that with my conscience and with my Creator; but I have reaped very little, if any, happiness from all that I have done. The only things it has yielded me are various anxieties and griefs."

There is one thing certain: the irritability and fretfulness, which are prominent traits of Bismarck's character, and the gout and indigestion from which he suffers so much, may be honestly ascribed to his habits. Hence, then, do we find in this great German, a queer contradiction; a love for nature that has enabled him to partially multiply the evil effects of art, and a love for art that has antidoted the workings of nature; so that we find the resultant production of a great man, but less great than he might have been; a strong man, but an imperfect man; a man who, had he wholly communed with nature, might have approached very closely to perfection.

The great sanitary lesson to be drawn from the life of the late German Chancellor is that a vigorous, out-of-door, active, natural, life will so brace a man as to help him to withstand the evil influences of hygienic negligence in other respects; but, from this exceptional example we must not argue that we can all do, with impunity, that which this phenomenon has done, for we may rest assured that where one Bismarck would survive, 999,999 ordinary mortals would succomb.

Physical Development as an Aid in Society.

We are all rather familiar with the fact that, as a nation, the Germans are magnificent specimens of physical development. It has been this careful attention to the physical aspect of their humanity, as much as anything else, that has made Imperial Germany, physically speaking, the foremost nation of the world. Reading recently of a ball in New York City, we had brought home to us the fact that this thought for physical development is not confined to the male portion of the German populace. "There," said a young man after completing a waltz, "Well, I got back." From where? he was asked, "From Paradise, I guess," he replied, "for I have never in my life danced with a woman more graceful than that magnificent-looking German girl whom I have just escorted to a seat." The girl in question was a tall, splendid young woman whose very manner gave evidence of that perfect health, that delicious grace and that absolute control of every muscle and nerve which alone can be the result of a magnificent physical development.

THE ANNALS OF HYGIENE,

THE OFFICIAL ORGAN OF THE
State Board of Health of Pennsylvania.

The State Board of Health is not responsible for anything appearing in this Journal except that which bears the official attestation of the Board.

❈ ❈

PUBLISHED MONTHLY.

Subscription, two dollars ($2.00) a year, in advance.

Address all communications to

The Hygienic Publishing Company,
224 SOUTH SIXTEENTH STREET,
PHILADELPHIA, PA.

EDITORIAL.

Walking.

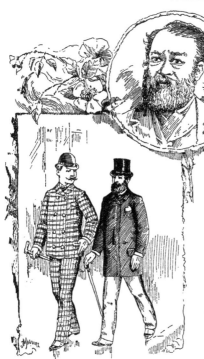

Jay Gould and his son, George, find the " poor man's medicine " better than any that his millions can buy.

From the daily papers we learn that a year or more ago Jay Gould was such a sick man that he was comparatively rarely seen in Wall Street ; to-day he is, practically, as well and as clear, mentally, as ever, and Wall Street knows him as of old. Jay Gould's millions afforded him the opportunity of consulting the most distinguished physicians in this and other countries, and he was not obliged to deny himself the most expensive drugs (indeed he could have lived on gold, had he been so ordered), nor was any system of treatment too costly. Yet, the sought-for health was not procured.

What, then, produced the change from Mr. Gould (as we see him in our vignette), a miserable, dyspeptic, worried, anxious-looking man, unable to attend to business ; to Mr. Gould, as we see him walking up Fifth Avenue with his son ; his countenance placid, his step springy, his mind free from worry, with all its old-time acuteness restored. It was the *" poor-man's medicine "*—walking ; for Mr. Gould, himself, tells us that outdoor exercise has done more to build him up anew than all the medicine his physicians have prescribed. A regular afternoon task for him is to walk from the Western Union Building to his home above the Windsor Hotel. George Gould always accompanies him on these trips. The two start out about four o'clock, and walk at a pretty rapid pace.

The great feature about what we might call the " Gould Restorative " is, that it is so cheap that it is within the reach of every one ; the streets of our cities and the highways and by-ways of our country are the common property.of us all, and our legs are our own. Hence we require neither permission nor money to enable us to avail ourselves of this great curative or preventive agent.

We firmly believe that if every human being would make it an absolute rule, with which nothing should be allowed to interfere, to walk at least five miles every day, be the weather fair or stormy, we would hear much less of sickness. Walking, as an exercise, as a life and health preserver, is incomparably superior to any and all other forms of exercise, and this fact is, we fear, not sufficiently appreciated.

We are quite clear in our idea that everyone who is well (that they may keep so), and those that are unwell (that they may regain their health), should give more thought and practical attention to this form of exercise, which is as accessible to the pauper as it is to the millionaire.

The Danger to Health in Flood Debris.

We had not space in our last issue to point out wherein we thought that Dr. Spencer M. Free was in error in giving expression to the views with which he begins his paper, which we there published, hence we were obliged to content ourselves with a general expression of disapproval of his propositions.

Thinking over the effect which his article may have upon the minds of our non-professional readers, we feel called upon to more specifically point out wherein we see the heresies, already alluded to, and this we do with no personal feeling, holding, as we do, the highest respect for Dr. Free, as a sanitarian, but, thinking that with Dr. Free, as with the greatest lights of the world, in all ages, human nature is not perfect, and we are all liable, at times, to fall into error.

As we take it, the general idea that would be gathered from Dr. Free's paper would be that the generally accepted notion that there is danger to health in flood debris is erroneous ; for, comparatively few persons, we imagine, would give sufficient importance to Dr. Free's parenthetical qualification of his general assertion (tenth line) "*unless malarial diseases be regarded as epidemics ;*" now, we understand malarial diseases to include all diseases that are produced by bad air (*mal-aria*) and since Dr. Free is willing to exempt diseases caused by *bad air* from his sweeping assertion, that epidemic disease is not caused by flood debris, then do we come down to the proposition with which all will agree, that flood-debris will not cause *specific* disease, unless the *specific* germ be contained in this debris ; and, if this is what Dr. Free means, then no one will differ with him, but, if he does so mean, it is unfortunate that he has not so expressed himself. Unfortunate, because he leaves the impression upon one who reads the first paragraph of his paper that bad-air diseases are not worthy of thought ; that the time and money expended for their prevention has been wasted.

We must remember that in time of great floods, such as that in the valley of the Conemaugh last summer, the contents of cess-pools will be disturbed and will be carried great distances to be deposited in new localities ; now, for instance, if the germs of typhoid fever have previously existed in one or more of these disturbed cess-pools, it is more than likely, it is almost certain, that, by their transportation into the water supply of a locality they will be the cause of an epidemic, and what has been said of typhoid fever is equally true of all specific diseases.

So much for *specific, particular* diseases ; we are ready to agree with Dr. Free that floods *per se*, will not originate them *de novo*, but we, uncompromisingly, hold that floods may be the means of conveying from an obscure, isolated and, compara-tively, harmless locality, a few germs into a thickly settled vicinity, wherein, being offered by the flood debris a condition favorable for their rapid multiplication, they will produce, in reality, an epidemic of a specific disease.

So also, these specific germs, multiplying in the flood debris, may, when dry, be wafted into the atmosphere, producing a *mal-aria* that contains the specific germs of specific diseases.

But, it is when we come to the evil influence on health of the inspiration of air and the drinking of water contaminated by the results of organic decomposition that we mostly wonder how Dr. Free can assume that the money and time spent in the prevention of this influence have been wasted.

According to the most reliable estimates there were 6,000 dead human bodies, 1,000 horses, and 1,000 cows, together with an almost innumerable quantity of smaller domestic animals, (in addition to large quantities of groceries and vegetables,) deprived of life and subjected to the conditions of putrefaction, in the immediate vicinity of Johnstown on the first day of last June. We would, probably, not be guilty of exaggeration were we to assert that, at this time there were nearly *2,000 tons* of dead and putrefying organic matter, the emanations from which were poisoning the atmosphere, and the drainage from which was poisoning the streams that flowed into the water supplies of remote localities.

Will any one assume that *2,000 tons* of putrefaction, confined in a small space, would not prove injurious to health, and that the money spent in its removal and destruction was money wasted. But, Dr. Free may say, "All I claimed was that floods do not cause ' *epidemics*,' and by an epidemic I mean the *unusual* prevalence of a *specific* disease." Granting this distinction, we think we have demonstrated how, while a flood may not originate a *specific* disease, it may yet transport and multiply its cause, so that an epidemic is the result ; and we also remind Dr. Free that the usual, popular interpretation of " *epidemic* " is not that given above, but that the word is popularly used to designate the unusual prevalence of sickness, whether the same be due to a *specific* cause or to the more general and less accur-ately defined influence of bad air, and that in speaking before a Sanitary Convention of to-day, we are supposed to be addressing the masses, and not the professional mind, which fact greatly modifies the sense in which our expressions will be received.

So, then, we have done with the question as to whether the conditions after a flood are favorable to disease, believing that they are most favorable wherever the life of organic matter has been destroyed thereby, to the production of *bad air* diseases, and that they are very liable to transport and multiply the causes of *specific* diseases.

Now for Dr. Free's historical arguments, and, to begin at the beginning, we will take the " Deluge," as he has done. Dr. Free says: " If we begin with the deluge and accept the account of it as given in Genesis . . . quite certain is it that no serious epidemic disease, or serious disease of any kind followed this flood, although ALL *conditions* were favorable for such an outbreak." Unfortunately, for the tenacity of Dr. Free's first historical argument, one very important condition was wanting, for *there was no one left on the face of the earth* to be afflicted by disease, save Noah and his seven companions, who (in addition to the fact that they were favorably located, on the top of a mountain, to escape the influences of the putrefaction going on around them) we must believe were under the special protection of the Lord, for it would be hardly reasonable to suppose that after having, *by his special intervention,* saved this handful of his creatures from death by flood, the Almighty would permit them, a few days later, to die of disease as a result of the flood.

Dr. Free then goes on to quote several instances wherein history *does record* unusual sickness following floods, *questioning, however, their accuracy,* and tells of some cases wherein the reverse *appeared* to be the case, but in these latter instances he fails to say one word about the *possible unreliability of the reports.*

Finally, while Dr. Free devotes one-half of his paper to the effort to prove that there is no danger of epidemics in flood debris, he devotes the last half to telling us how to avoid these dangers. If, then, Dr. Free really believes what he says in the first part of his paper, why should he advise all the trouble and expense that he recommends in the latter part. It seems to us, as a correspondent has expressed it, that this paper of Dr. Free's contains in its latter half a thorough refutation of the heresies to which utterance is given in its earlier parts.

Let not this paper give wrong impressions. It is an established fact that organic putrefaction is inimical to human health ; hence, when floods produce a great accumulation of such putrefaction, they *must,* in a general way, prove dangerous to health ; while, as we have shown, there is also the power in, and liability of, floods to transport and multiply the seeds of, and thus to cause a veritable epidemic of specific diseases.

Take Time to Eat.

The opinion that hurry in eating is a prolific cause of dyspepsia is founded on common observation. The ill results of "bolting" the food have been attributed to the lack of thorough mastication, and to the incomplete action of the saliva upon the food. Two-thirds of the food which we eat is starch, and starch cannot be utilized in the system as food until it has been converted into sugar, and this change is principally effected by the saliva. But there is a third reason why rapidity of eating interferes with digestion. The presence of the salivary secretion in the stomach acts as a stimulus to the secretion of the gastric juice. Irrespective of the mechanical function of the teeth, food which goes into the stomach incompletely mingled with saliva, passes slowly and imperfectly through the process of stomach digestion. Therefore, as a sanitary maxim of no mean value, teach the children to eat slowly—and in giving this instruction by example, the teacher, as well as the pupil, may receive a benefit.—*Sanitary Inspector.*

NOTES AND COMMENTS.

The Unnecessary Education of Children.

There is a strong moral in the story related of the mother who was unable to help her little child in deciding as to whether the *Putamayo* joined the *Amazon east* or *west* of the confluence of the *Maranon* and *Ucayle* rivers. Shifting the scene to a period some twenty years later we find this child, now a mother, asking *her* little child, who is struggling helplessly with the geographical problem that is troubling her, what it is. Upon learning that her daughter is endeavoring to locate the *whereabouts* of the river Amazon, the mother, after considerable reflection, tells her that she thinks it is somewhere in Africa or Asia, but she really forgets which. The mind, in the brain of this woman is the same mind that years before was endeavoring to solve the problem already referred to in relation to this self-same river, the very locality of which, in mature years, she is unable to decide, owing to the fact that since her school-days she has had no special reason for thinking of the river Amazon. So is it with very much of the knowledge which our little children are compelled to acquire by our present system of school education, knowledge that will be of no earthly practical use, either in a material or æsthetic sense in after life. Does it not seem somewhat ridiculous to force our children to fill their minds with knowledge, that, as we have said, can never be of any special service to them; and further, when we reflect that in very many instances we are imposing upon these children tasks that by their magnitude must prove more or less injurious to the health of the child. Does it not seem cruel, or we might even say, brutal, because while we must admit that much, as we have said, of this learning will never be of any practical use, we cannot, at the same time, help but admit that there is nothing, absolutely nothing whatsoever, that will be of so much use to the child in after life as good health.

Ventilate Closets and Wardrobes.

After you read this little paragraph put down the journal for a moment and open your closet or wardrobe door, and if your sense of smell is as accurate as it should be, you will be prepared to believe us when we say that the average closet and the average wardrobe does not receive the ventilation that it should have. Remember that the dead tissue from the surface of your body clings to your clothing, and that when you put soiled clothes into your closet or wardrobe you are putting away with them small particles of identically the same matter that you place six feet under ground in a coffin when you bury a corpse. That is to say, in the former case you have particles of organic matter undergoing decomposition, so small, it is true, that they are invisible to the naked eye, yet none the less there; while in the latter case you have a large accumulation of particles undergoing decomposition; such a great accumulation that it becomes obvious to our sight. However, the result is the same in both cases, the difference being one of degree and not of kind; hence, since we have dead organic matter undergoing decomposition in our wardrobes and closets, does it become very necessary that we should allow a pure atmosphere access thereto?

How to Get Pure Milk.

We have elsewhere in this issue taken the ground that the remedy for adulteration is to be found rather in the education of the people than in legislative enactments. We find now our City Board of Health endeavoring to secure municipal legislation looking towards a proper inspection and supervision of the quality of the milk offered to our fellow-citizens. While this is unquestionably a move in the right direction we cannot but feel, as we have elsewhere said, that no system of inspection, however stringent it may be, will accomplish the purpose until the masses appreciate the importance of, and are unanimous in their demand for a pure and wholesome supply. We would feel tempted to ask, in the event of this effort for legislation becoming a reality, *who will inspect the inspectors?* Again, is it at all a matter of

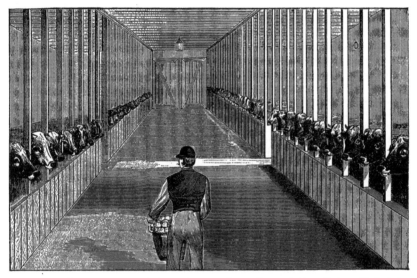

possibility that any system of inspection can be so thorough that all the milk being brought into the city will be subjected to it? Of course, we are not arguing against the value of the system of inspection, which we believe to be a step in the right direction, but we are utilizing this agitation for a purer milk supply to point the idea we have that the truest and best way of securing such a supply is first to educate the people who consume the milk to the importance of purity, and secondly, to bring about the realization of the responsibility resting upon them, to those who are producing the article. We are heartily in accord with those who say that healthy cattle and cleanly farmers are the prime requisites. We have taken occasion before to say, and now most emphatically reiterate this statement, that there is no reason why a barn in which cows are housed should not be kept as clean and sweet and pure as is usually kept the refrigerator in which we are accustomed to preserve the milk derived from these cows until ready for use ; such a barn as our illustration depicts will be the home of clean and healthy cattle, who will furnish clean and healthy milk.

Art Could Supply What Nature Lacked.

Clara Belle, writing from New York to the *Philadelphia Press*, and commenting upon the difference in appearances that are observed in members of the same family, tells of an extremely handsome actress whom she had recently seen on the stage of a New York theatre, and then goes on to say that looking towards a box in this same theatre, she saw two girls, sisters of the actress, without a grain of beauty to serve for both of them. They were absolutely without a particle of physical attraction, and the writer felt called upon to marvel that the same parentage could have produced such a creature of beauty and such marvels of homeliness. As we read, the thought was forced upon us that the contrast in personal attraction between these sisters must be the source, frequently, of annoyance to the homely ones. Then followed the reflection that art, (that is to say, *true art*, by which we do not mean the use of cosmetics, frizzes and appendages innumerable,) that art could so aid these homely girls as to make them wonderful specimens of attractive womanhood. What we mean is, that while nature had denied to these girls, as it has denied to very many, the attractions of a beautiful face and a fine figure, that art, that is to say, a system of physical development which each and every girl has it absolutely in her own power to procure, could metamorphose naturally homely girls into those, who, because of this very beauty of physical development would become attractive; aye, extremely so, because no one can resist the irresistible attraction of a healthy, well-developed, physically perfect woman.

A Wise Duchess.

It is related that the Duchess D'Uzes of France, being greatly impressed by the physical development of English women, has returned to her native land fired with the ambition of making the French women equal to those of England. In accordance with this idea, she has started lawn tennis clubs and rowing clubs and walking clubs, and is endeavoring in every way to make the French women interested in physical development.

The Influence of Boiling Water.

We are accustomed to be told that the most impure water will be rendered pure by boiling, and that in this we have an absolute safeguard against the dangers of water containing disease germs. Now while it is true that boiling will kill the germs of disease, yet the fact has been brought to our notice, by so high an authority as Dr. Chas. M. Cresson, that while boiling kills the germs of a particular disease, it yet, in reality, renders the water more impure than it was before, because, by the very death of these germs, dead organic matter is allowed to remain in the water which it pollutes by putrefaction. Hence, while boiling is a most excellent precaution against the occurrence of typhoid fever or similar diseases when we have occasion [to think that the germs of these diseases exist in the water that we drink, yet we must remember that this boiling does not purify the water; it simply removes from it the specific power to produce a specific disease.

Fagin and Beaconsfield.

Between the lowest depths of human misery, degradation and villainy, as typified in Dickens' wonderful creation of Fagin, the Jew, to the highest pinnacle of fame, of brilliancy and of historical reputation, as personified by Victoria's creation of Beaconsfield, the Prime Minister of England, there would seem to be an insurmountable barrier. Well, when one reflects over the real personality of the óne and the fancied individuality of the other, does not a thought suggest itself to us that between the two there is an extremely close relationship? The pre-eminent trait in the statesman, Beaconsfield, was undoubtedly his ability to read human nature, (as it is with all the great statesmen and political leaders of this and every other generation,) so also, the glaring point in the character of Fagin, as depicted by Dickens, the trait that made him the king among criminals, was his ability to penetrate the hidden thoughts of his associates. Had Fagin turned his energies in the direction of statesmanship, rather than that of villainy, would he not have possessed all the attributes necessary to have made him the Prime Minister of England? while, on the other hand, had Beaconsfield directed his natural talents towards the acquisition (in an illegal way) of the property of others, would he not have equaled in rascality, in villainy, in sublime and diabolical perfection, the crafty Jew? All of which goes to make us think that, after all, we are, each and every one of us, much less the creatures of circumstances and much more the creatures of our own creation than is usually believed and admitted by the majority of persons; from which we are led to draw the inference that a man can mould himself much as he wills, and that when we hear one say, "I cannot control my emotions," we should rather say, "you *will* not control them." You fail to recognize the power within you; you are allowing your emotions to control your will. The will, just as the muscles, becomes strengthened by exercise, and he who would approach as nearly as possible to the perfect man must so develop his will by use that he will have it ever ready to control his entire nature. The man whose life is regulated by his will, rather than by his emotions is the man who is leading a thoroughly rational life, and he who leads a rational life is leading a natural life, and he who leads a natural life is, in the highest sense of the term, a sanitarian. To make our thought a little clearer: Was not Beaconsfield the statesman and Fagin the thief rather because of the *will* than of the natural inclination? Have we not all within us a dormant will power that, by exercise, we can so strengthen that it will be our controlling power, and, with such, can we not mould our lives as we will.

Poison in Greenbacks.

It seems to be an admitted fact, disputed by no one, that there is real danger to health in the manufacture of our paper money as at present carried out. The green color on the back of the notes is produced by arsenic, and we are told that it is not uncommon for those working with these notes to have an unpleasant, unsightly eruption of the skin, caused by this drug. Would it not be just as easy to make these notes some other color, and are we justified in continuing the green color when we know for a fact that it works an injury to those who are employed in the manufacture of this money?

Bismarck's Gout and the World's History.

It may seem strange to assert, yet we do so, with the sanction of science, as expressed in the language of Dr. A. Jacobi before a recent meeting of the Medical Society of the State of New York, that very much of the modern history of the world has been made by the good or bad digestion and the gouty constitution of the Great Bismarck. The most conservative of men and the greatest of intellects are more frequently influenced by emotions than one generally imagines. And it is a fact that a man's words and emotions, his sentiments, his thoughts, his reflections and the actions resulting therefrom, are very much influenced by his physical condition. Old Dr. J. L. Ludlow, of this city, used very often to illustrate the intimate connection that existed between a man's stomach and his brain, by comparing these two important organs to the two ends of a dumb-bell, while the nervous connection or communication between them he likened to the shaft. When we see an infant thrown into convulsions because of some indigestible article of food in the stomach, and when we understand that these convulsions are due to a disordered condition of the brain, we can readily understand how intimate must be the relations between the stomach and the brain. So that, just as the great mind of Bismarck, as influenced by the condition of his liver, or his stomach, or his kidneys, or his gout, has so impressed itself upon, has so influenced the history of the whole of Europe, so, in a lesser degree, will the lesser mind of an ordinary individual impress itself upon his personal history, just as it may be influenced by his physical condition. Could we but fathom the whole working of the many causes of domestic infelicity, we would be surprised to learn how much dyspepsia and biliousness has had to do with marital unhappiness. How often does one say, "I wonder what could have caused the unhappiness in the family of so and so. They seem so devotedly attached to each other; he has wealth and everything that wealth can give to make life happy, yet they seem very miserable." In not a few of such cases the non-observance of the laws of health would be found, upon critical examination, to be at the bottom of the trouble. A man whose vital machinery is not in good running order will be a disagreeable man. To a certain extent he will be an irresponsible man; that is to say, he will do and say certain things which, were he in a condition of health, he would not do or say. To this extent, therefore, is he irresponsible. On the other hand, the healthy man, and by a healthy man we mean one whose every function is properly and naturally performed, the healthy man will be not only a pleasure to himself, but the source of pleasure to all who come in contact with him. Looking at the matter from this point of view, realizing how great will be the influence upon our personal history and upon the history of those near and dear to us, of the condition of our health, does it not seem as though it should be not only our duty, but our pleasure as well, to familiarize ourselves with the rules of health and to observe them.

————————

The Streets of New York.

New York has 574.88 miles of streets to clean, and there are collected half a million cubic yards of street-sweepings and one and one-half million cubic yards of garbage and refuse yearly, at an annual cost of about one million dollars.

To Be Prepared for Emergencies.

From Berlin we learn that a great sensation was recently created by the sudden receipt of an order from the emperor for all the troops present in the garrison of the city to march at once to a certain point. The people were almost panic stricken until it was learned that the manœuvre was simply one of the military surprises inaugurated by the emperor to test the efficiency of the garrison to repel a sudden attack by an enemy. We all know that every day, at noon, in most of our engine-houses, an alarm is sounded, simply for the purpose of keeping both human and brute employees in a state of efficiency when the time for action may arise. So, we take it, it should be with sanitarians. As it is, we wait until the emergency arises, and then, after the horse has escaped, lock the stable-door. We would like, for awhile, to see such a man as the Emperor of Germany, possessed of all the power that he now enjoys, at the head of a sanitary corps equally subject to his orders as is the German army. Such a force, with such a head (of course on a much smaller scale) should be found in every community—a body that should be so well organized and so efficiently officered that it could never be taken by surprise at the advance ot the greatest enemy of mankind, namely, disease; a force so well disciplined and so well understanding how to successfully meet the foe that the community might feel safe in its hands. But we almost despair of such an ideal condition, because, for its full result, it would be necessary that every individual should be a member of this corps. The public are too apt to consider that they have paid (very poorly paid) sanitary officials, who guard the health of the community; and, having provided for the appointment of these officials, and contributing to their pay, they feel that they have themselves nothing to do with the preservation of the health of the community, but that this duty should be left to those who are paid for attending to it. One might just as well say that, since a city has a well organized fire department, he need not bother himself to take any precautions whatsoever to prevent his house from taking fire, relying solely upon the fire department for his protection. After the fire has started the department may control its spread, but its existence will not prevent the inception of the fire. Neither can the most efficient sanitary official always prevent the inception of an epidemic, though with the hearty co-operation of every individual he may effectually prevent its spread after it has once started. It is a fact that everyone must learn for himself that in this matter of sanitation in the question of the preservation of health, each man must look to it for himself. Of course, we must have a sanitary organization in order that the general sanitary condition of a locality may be looked after, but, at the fear of repetition, we must say that, in order to accomplish the greatest results, each and every individual must be himself a sanitarian.

Consumptive Prisoners.

It is a step in the right direction that has been taken by the California State Board of Health, who have asked the judges, before sentencing a criminal to State Prison, to have the county physician make an examination of his physical condition. If he is consumptive, or there is any tendency thereto, he is to be sent to a special prison, wherein all possible precautions against infection are to be instituted.

Religion and Hygiene.

It must be extremely gratifying to the mind of the sanitarian when he sees a tendency towards the recognition by the masses of the fact, that is already truly familiar to him, that hygiene really is, as it should be, a most intimate part of religion. In the minds of most every one there is an inherent respect for religion, so that when we come to look upon hygiene as a part of religion so will there be an inherent respect for and observance of the teachings of hygiene. That hygiene is rapidly coming to be regarded as a part of religion we daily see evidence, but rarely more marked than when we read, in the *Cumberland Presbyterian Review*, the following :

" This is above all ages the dispensation of clean homes and cultivated tastes. Woe betide the Church that has failed to realize this truth, and to keep step with the people. Our young people are taught in our public schools the God-given principles of hygiene and refined tastes, and they will certainly seek pleasant and tasteful surroundings in the public assembly. David could worship God anywhere, but he was peculiarly ' glad ' when his feet turned towards the sacred Temple on Zion's Hill, which was unsurpassed for external loveliness. God has always been jealous about the cleanliness and order of His house. Dirt and disorder will certainly retard the worship of any Church. If every congregation would scrupulously obey the divine injunction—' wash and be clean '—we should have more living organizations and fuller sanctuaries."

Cooling Off Between Sweats.

Reading, recently, an account of the employees of our gas works, we note a paragraph] wherein it is stated that the workmen, after being extremely overheated by their proximity to the furnaces, are in the habit of going out to the river bank to cool off. We have seen this same process of " cooling off " between sweats on our trans-Atlantic steamships, wherein the men, stripped to their waists, engaged for hours down in the hold of the ship throwing coal into the furnaces, will, upon the first opportunity, hasten to the deck, still stripped to the waist, and expose themselves to the strong wind of mid-ocean that they may cool off. If these same men were to come up and drink a pint of laudanum, the suicidal element would be more patent to the eye of the observer, but it would be none the more effective in producing its results. We cannot too strongly condemn the practice, so common among those who work in an extremely warm atmosphere, of thus suddenly " cooling off."

The Hygiene of the Rebellion.

In a recent issue we had occasion to note that the physique of the American was steadily improving, and was equal, if not superior, to that of most of the nations of the world. One of our readers, commenting upon this observation, said that he believed, strange as it might seem, that this fact was indirectly due to the influence of our great rebellion. That the martial spirit that was developed in the breasts of the children of that time, who are the men of to-day, caused them to become so much interested in drilling, in walking, in athletics, in training, and in all that pertains to the physical life of a soldier, that it has bred up a race of men superior, physically speaking, to those who had been the outcome of many previous years of peaceful existence.

Sanitarians and Alarmists.

We dislike ever to be compelled to differ with the always admirable words of the *New York Medical Record*, but we feel compelled to have a word about some remarks published in that journal recently, wherein the position was taken that sanitarians are too much of alarmists ; that is to say, that by pointing out to the public the dangers to health lurking so universally in food and drink and air and clothing and pretty much everything that goes to make up the sum total of life, that, by so doing, they are antagonizing rather than enlisting ,popular sentiment. "Men are willing to· be scared a little," says the *Record*, "but they will not allow themselves to be scared too much." Now we take it (speaking absolutely and positively for ourselves, and we think, correctly for our co-workers) that it is not the intention of sanitarians to alarm any one, but in point of fact, our effort is continually to point out what we might term sanitary perfection, if you please, and to indicate that the nearer one approaches to this ideal the better for him will it be. We do not believe that any man was ever made a sanitarian by fear, such a result being, in our opinion, the result of conviction ; therefore, when ,we point out the dangers to health that undoubtedly do exist universally about us (for we all know that disease-breeding agencies are everywhere, we all know that life is a constant struggle against death, from the cradle to the grave,) when we point out the universality of the causes of disease we do not do so with the thought or the desire of alarming any one, but with the intention, as we have said before, of familiarizing every one with the facts as we see them.

The Evils of Adulteration.

We are continually reading about the all-pervading presence of adulteration in articles of food and drink. The Legislatures of our States and the Congress of our nation have, almost continually, before them bills supposed to be capable of remedying this condition of affairs. It was recently stated before Congress that very many thousands of children and adults are annually killed by the consumption of adulterated food. This agitation for Legislative suppression of adulteration has been going on for several years, yet the practice of adulteration is more prevalent and the sale of adulterated articles is greater to-day than ever before, and is sadly on the increase. Therefore does it seem to us that it is almost a hopeless task to endeavor to suppress this evil by Legislative enactment. Rather would it seem to us is the remedy to be found in the education of the people to that point where they will demand and be willing to pay for the pure article. Looking for the reason why adulteration is so prevalent, we are forced to the conclusion that it is due to the fact that the people want cheap goods. They buy that which is supplied to them for the least money ; this necessarily brings about a competition among the manufacturers to offer cheap, and yet cheaper, their goods. The only way in which they can reduce the price of these articles is by substituting a cheaper article as a portion of that which, if pure, would bring a greater price. If the people would ask, first, for a pure article, and, secondly, for a cheap article, rather than asking first for a cheap one and secondly for purity, the question of adulteration would be more practically solved than by any amount of Legislative enactment, which, however stringent it may be, will always be successfully evaded by the manufacturers.

The Habit of Disputing.

The venerable Father Curley, who a few years ago died at the age of more than ninety, and who was one of the foremost, if not the leading, astronomer of the world, reads us a lesson on the necessity of keeping the heart in peace, and of the folly of being disturbed by passing events. He said once that when he was young he had fallen into the habit of disputing and always liked to carry his point; but, noticing that it disturbed his peace and led him into faults he had made a firm determination never to forget himself and never to dispute on any subject. He had adhered so strongly to this resolve that for thirty years he had never been a party to any dispute. There is a world of wisdom in this little bit of advice, for who can say that a dispute has ever been productive of any special good, and who can deny that it has often bred ill-temper, fretfulness, peevishness, anger and ill-will, all of which we can set down as strong enemies to good digestion and the health that is dependent upon it.

The Duke of Westminster's Hares.

We learn that the Duke of Westminster has decided to abandon his hare hunt this year, because of the disease among the hares threatening to make them scarce unless they are given a rest. We do not know whether the Duke of Westminster has any children or not, but if he has, we wonder whether he has ever thought of taking them away from school lest the unhygienic surroundings of such places might make them *scarce*. We remember reading once of a farmer who, when asked how many children he had, was obliged to stop and count them on his fingers, and even then forgot to enumerate the baby; but when this same man was asked how many sheep he had, he was able to answer " 83 " without a moment's thought, and a subsequent count proved that he had not forgotten a single one ; looking, to our way of thinking, as though the sheep were much more prominent in this farmer's mind than were his children, and we venture to say that when it came time for an increase in the sheep-fold this farmer was much more critical in his selection of a ram than he would ever think of being in the choice of a husband for his daughter. Which all goes to show that from the highest to the lowest, from England's great and noble duke down to the lowliest farmer, brute creation seems to hold a higher place in the estimation of humanity than do the offspring of their own bodies.

Bowing in Austria.

It would truly seem that there is really a silver lining to every cloud. Thus far, there would seem to have been but one aspect to the late epidemic of the " grippe," and that an aspect of grief, so to speak. We learn from Austria, however, that, owing to the prevalence of this epidemic, the ridiculous habit of removing the hat in salutation on the street has been abandoned. Going down the street on a cold winter day we have frequently thought, as we would see a man remove his hat and expose to the cold blast a bald head in a state of perspiration, that therein was probably to be found the cause of very much of the neuralgia that afflicts humanity. Owing to the influence of the "grippe," as we have stated, this practice has been abandoned throughout the empire of Austria, being replaced by the salutation " *a la militaire.*"

Clerical Wisdom.

In church the other day, when we saw the clergyman, coming in to prepare for service, remove from his shoulders, not a tight-fitting overcoat, but a large, loose, roomy, voluminous cloak, we felt that in this cloak we saw another evidence of the wisdom of the clergymen. How frequently will a man run out of his house or his office and go around the corner for a moment, neglecting to put on an overcoat, as it is too much trouble and he does not want to be bothered with it, whereas, if instead of an overcoat, he was in the habit of wearing a large cloak, that could be thrown over the shoulder while he was going down stairs and drawn closely around the body, covering not only the body itself, but enclosing the hands, thereby doing away with the necessity or the trouble of putting on gloves, he would be much less likely to venture out unprotected. From an æsthetic point of view, the cloak should be called an improvement on the overcoat, for what is more graceful than the flowing folds of such an ample garment. Certainly our distinguished brethren of ancient times, the artistic inhabitants of ancient Greece and the martial citizens of ancient Rome, seem to have thought that garments patterned somewhat the same as the cloaks to which we refer were much more graceful and much more ornamental to the human body than the great coats of our present day and generation.

The Hygiene of our Changing Climate.

It would really seem that in this section of the country we are undergoing an absolute change of climate. While it may be only temporary, yet the character of the past two winters has been such as to give some reason for believing that we are not going to have in this region any more such winters as we used to know. If such be the case we will, of course, while becoming accustomed to the change, be liable to suffer in our bodily health, but when this acclimatization, so to speak, has become accomplished, we see a far greater advantage in this likely change, because if we are always to have spring-like or summer weather, the growing tendency towards suburban life will be immensely fostered. As it is to-day, there are few people who do not prefer the country to the city during the summer days. It is only when the cold, snowy, icy, penetrating days of winter come upon us that they feel drawn towards the crowded city. If, therefore, we are to have perpetual summer, so also will we have a perpetual desire for country life, the only objection to which will be thereby removed.

A Christian Sanitarian.

There is a deal of truth in the answer made to a man by his wife, who, when looking over a house into which he had just moved, said "I wonder who lived here last;" when she replied, "I don't know; but the lady was a Christian." Being asked how she could tell, her characteristic reply was: "She left no rubbish in the cellar." Acting on the principle that we should do unto others that which we would have others do unto us, one of the first rules of the Christian should be, not only not to leave any rubbish in a house that she is about to vacate, but also never to tolerate any rubbish or dirt of any kind in the house she is occupying.

Celery and Typhoid Fever.

Where do you think, said an eminent chemist to us recently, a great deal of typhoid fever comes from? The Schuylkill River, we promptly and dutifully replied, having learned our lesson well. Yes, he said, with a smile, but do you know that a great deal of it comes from our vegetables from down the " Neck ?" It is a fact that our odorless excavating companies convey the contents of cesspools that they empty to these vegetable farms, where it is used as manure, and if it should so happen that the germs of typhoid fever have existed in one or more of the cesspools, the contents of which are so used, then we can readily understand how vegetables so nourished might themselves contain and convey to the consumer the germs of disease. This chemist tells us (and he is no less an authority than Dr. Charles M. Cresson) that he has found, more than once, the germs of typhoid fever in the juice that he has squeezed out of celery. Of course, this is no reason for us to abandon the use of celery, neither is it an argument for us to deprive ourselves of the immense value, as a fertilizer, of the contents of cesspools, but it is a strong reason why every' one should be instructed that it is absolutely essential that wherever a case of typhoid fever exists in a household, the evacuations should be treated with a solution of corrosive sublimate before being deposited in a cesspool.

Tenement-House Mortality in New York.

Dr. R. S. Tracy, the Registrar of Records of the Health Department, has submitted to the Board of Health a report on the tenement-house mortality of 1888, supplementary to a report made by him on the same subject in June, 1889, The doctor says that since the beginning of 1880 all tenement-houses have been constructed under the supervision of the Health Department, and the construction of rear-tenements has not been permitted. The records show these things: 1. The death-rate was lower during 1888 in houses standing singly on a lot than where there were both front and rear houses. 2. The death-rate in houses built since 1888 was lower than in houses built before that time. 3. The death-rate was remarkably lower in houses built since 1886, both for adults and children. 4. The highest death-rate in the district south of Fourteenth Street and west of Broadway was below Reade Street. 5. The highest child death-rate was in the Ninth Ward, and the next highest in the Fifteenth. 6. The highest death-rate of persons over five years of age was in the First and Third Wards, and the next highest in the Eighth.

Ventilation in Iceland.

The extreme cold of the winter in Iceland reduces the system of domestic ventilation in that country to very primitive principles. A traveler there was so choked one night by the close atmosphere of the air-tight little chamber in which' he slept, with all the male members of the family, as to be compelled to wake his host, who sprang out of bed at the call, pulled a cork from a knot-hole in the wall for a few minutes, and then, replacing the cork with a shiver, returned to bed.—*College and Clinical Record.*

The Barrenness of the Rich.

The *New York World* has been compiling a census of productiveness among the wealthy and the poorer classes of New York City, with the result that, during the past year, the poorer classes of the metropolis have been eighteen times as prolific as the more wealthy and more fashionable. The *World*, and many of its readers, deplore this state of affairs, but, to our way of thinking, it is really a wise dispensation. Of course, it is according to nature for married people to have children, and anything which obstructs the course of nature is to be deplored. But, viewing this question from a materialistic view, we are forced to the assertion that the offspring of rich parents are very rarely of any use to themselves or the world at large, so that we must not regard the limitation of the production of a useless commodity as an unmixed evil. It is the poorer classes that have given to the world all, or nearly all, of its truly great and useful men and women, and so-long as this class continues to produce we need have no fear for the welfare of society. While, therefore, we must feel an instinctive reverence for the mother of a large family, as must have felt the husband who placed on his wife's tombstone in a church-yard in Delaware County the following inscription :

> Some have children and some have none;
> Here lies the mother of twenty-one.

yet we must not consider it an unmixed evil that the rich and fashionaole—very many of whom are unfit for the responsibilities of maternity—should be limited in their productiveness.

The Strangers' Cold.

A writer in the *Pall Mall Gazette* gives the following account of a curious phenomenon which has been noticed and commented upon by several observers before : During a seven years' residence in Norfolk Island—the well-known settlement of the descendants of the Bounty mutineers—he writes, he had opportunities of verifying the popular local tradition that the arrival of a vessel was almost invariably accompanied by an epidemic of influenza among the inhabitants of the island. In spite of the apparent remoteness of cause and effect, the connection had so strongly impressed itself on the mind of the Norfolk Islanders that they were in the habit of distinguishing the successive outbreaks by the name of the vessel during whose visit it had occurred. But the phenomenon is not confined to Norfolk Island. Whatever may be its explanation, there are evidences of its appearance in widely sundered localities. In *Chambers's Journal* for July, 1888, an article headed "The Strangers' Cold," gives various instances of influenza appearing among remote populations simultaneously with the arrival of strange vessels on their coasts. The island of St. Kilda is quoted as having a fixed tradition to this effect, while in Wharekauri, an island about four hundred and thirty miles east of New Zealand, the circumstance is so well recognized that the mere appearance of the influenza is sufficient signal to the inhabitants of the interior that a strange vessel is in port.

The Salutary Effect of Small-Pox.

Commenting on the appearance of small-pox in Connecticut, Dr. C. A. Lindsley, the Secretary of the State Board of Health, says :

"Possibly an occasional outbreak of this dreaded malady is not an event altogether bad in its influences. There are several ways in which by the sacrifice of a few citizens, such public action has resulted, as has doubtless preserved many other lives. Thus, the indifference to the importance of vaccination in the public mind grows so rapidly when for a short period the public are exempt from small-pox, that the only thing which will induce a renewal of the practice is an occasional human victim of the disease.

"It may therefore be well that the intervals between these sacrifices for the public good should not be too long, lest the neglect of vaccination should make so large a part of the people unprotected that when the disease did come it would find victims in every household.

"Again, there is nothing known in the experience of this State that will animate a local board of health like a case of small-pox within its jurisdiction. Boards which have been in a state of profound hibernation through all seasons for many years, have been aroused into the most exalted activity, as if by an electric shock, when a small-pox case has been reported to them. And in some cases this recovery from general paralysis has been more or less permanent, with corresponding benefit to the communities they served. So that in the language of the bard of Avon we may say :

> "'Sweet are the uses of adversity ;
> Which, like the toad, ugly and venomous,
> Wears yet a precious jewel in his head ;
> And this our life   .   .   .
> Finds   .   .   .   .
> Sermons in stones, and good in everything.'"

A Ventilating Dado.

At a recent meeting of the Glasgow Philosophical Society the subject of house ventilation was brought up by Mr. D. J. Hoey, who said that he was a disciple of Sir Humphrey Davy, and that the method he had elaborated was founded on Davy's work. A dado of three to four feet in height was placed round the walls of the apartment, with a narrow space between the dado and the wall to form a reservoir for fresh air let in from without by inlets in the wall. On the top of the dado, wire gauze or perforated metal was placed, through which the air percolated into the room. The area of the exit from the top of the dado being much greater than that of the inlet, and the total space inclosed by the dado being much greater still, the fresh air passing through this extended space lost its initial velocity, and percolated gently into the room. The total area of the inlet was proportioned to that of the hot-air shaft for carrying out the impure air. The needful column of hot air, for carrying off the impure exhausted air, could best be supplied by a chimney of suitable capacity, with a close-throated fire-grate, having an opening in the room at a high level into the flue. When a suitable chimney was not available, the same results were produced by a tube of sufficient area and height erected above a sunlight in the roof of the hall.

The Journey Through Life of the Babies of 1890.

Take your pencil and follow us (says *The Scotsman*,) while we figure out what will happen to the 1,000,000 of babies that have been born in the last 1,000,000 seconds. We believe that is about the average—one every time the clock ticks. First December, 1890, if the statistics don't belie us, we shall have lost 150,000 of these "little prides of the household." A year later 53,000 more will be keeping company with those who have gone before.

At the end of the third year we find that 22,000 more have dropped by the wayside. The fourth year they have become rugged little darlings, not nearly so susceptible to infantile diseases, only 8,000 having succumbed to the rigors imposed. By the time they have arrived at the age of twelve years but a paltry few hundred leave the track each year.

After threescore years have come and gone we find less trouble in counting the army with which we started in January, 1890. Of the 1,000,000 with which we began count but 370,000 remain ; 630,000 have gone the way of all the world, and the remaining few have forgotten that they ever existed.

At the end of 80, or, taking our mode of reckoning, by the year 1970 A. D., there are still 97,000 gray-headed, shaky old grannies and grand-fathers, toothless, hairless and happy. In the year 1984 our 1,000,000 babies which we started with in 1890, will have dwindled into an insignificant 223 helpless old wrecks, "stranded on the shores of time."

In 1992 all but 17 will have left this mundane sphere forever, whilst the last remaining will probably, in seeming thoughtlessness, watch the sands filter through the hour-glass of time, and die in the year 1998, at the age of 108.

Thus, we see, that, as things are, after 80 years have passed by, more than nine-tenths of all our babies have disappeared. But things are not as they should be ; for, were we all sanitarians the very great majority of our 1,000,000 babies should reach the age of 80, and should then gradually die *natural* deaths.

Wash and Grow Fat.

Sir Edwin Chadwick, at the recent Health Congress and Exhibition at Hastings, England, spoke of what he considered a great sanitary factor—the power of washing cheaply with tepid water. The German army was the lowest death-rated of any in Europe, being only five in a thousand, while our army was eight, France ten, and Italy eleven. One means of this was the practice of washing with tepid water. That, he had shown in England, was the great means of reduction of the children's diseases in the district schools. In Germany half a million of soldiers were being washed with tepid water at a cost of about 6d per hundred, soap included. He expected that when the exhibition opened he would be able to display a power of washing children with tepid water at the rate of a working expense of not above 1d for a dozen, and they would accomplish at the rate of a little more than three minutes for each child. He had long shown elsewhere that pigs that were washed put on one-fifth more flesh than pigs that were unwashed, and more than this was the result with children.

Hay and Straw and Filth in Street Cars.

Every now and then when we pick up a paper we notice an agitation against the use of hay and straw in our street cars, it being claimed that such commodities furnish a convenient place for the propagation of disease germs. This is an indisputable fact, and we feel that no one competent to form an opinion would argue against it, but would, unhesitatingly, condemn such use of hay and straw. We feel like going further and in the most emphatic terms condemn the whole general filthy condition of the street cars of this city, since by centralization the stimulus of competition has been removed. To speak in plain words, we must say that of all dirty, stinking, pest holes, we feel that the street cars of this city take the lead. And it is because there is no just reason that this should be so, that we speak thus plainly. If the business was not a profitable one then we could find abundance of excuse for the disgusting conditions offered by the managers of these lines to their patrons, but since the street car traffic is possibly the most enormously profitable of any form of business, we can see no earthly reason why the patrons of our street cars should not be vouchsafed the same cleanliness, the same elements of comfort, the same safeguards against filth diseases as are offered to those who patronize the suburban traffic of the Pennsylvania Railroad.

Recent Saving of Life in Michigan.

In a carefully-prepared paper read before the Sanitary Convention at Vicksburg, the proceedings of which are just published, Dr. Baker gave official statistics and evidence which he summarized as follows : .

"The record of the great saving of human life and health in Michigan in recent years is one to which, it seems to me, the State and local boards of health in Michigan can justly 'point with pride.' It is a record of the saving of over one hundred lives per year from small-pox, four hundred lives per year saved from death by scarlet fever, and nearly six hundred lives per year saved from death by diphtheria —an aggregate of eleven hundred lives per year, or three lives per day saved from these three diseases ! This is a record which we ask to have examined, and which we are willing to have compared with that of the man who 'made two blades of grass grow where only one grew before.''

A Travesty on Justice.

Were it not likely to prove serious to the victim, we would incline to say that justice recently made a ridiculous aspect of herself in this city when she ordered the incarceration, in the county 'jail, for a period of ten days, of a little boy of eleven years of age, whose offense was that, with a tin-kettle as a drum, he, with some of his little companions, disturbed the pious meditations of a so-called Christian sect who claim to model after Him who said, "Suffer little children to come unto me, and forbid them not," etc. This period of imprisonment cannot help but have an injurious effect upon this little boy, and we feel very strongly that he who set the example that this little fellow's accusers are supposed to be following, would not approve of this demonstration of their Christianity.

The Pan-American Congress on Sanitation.

The Committee on Sanitary Regulations of the Pan-American Congress has made a unanimous report, in which it condems absolute isolation in preventing the spread of epidemics, and recommends in its stead the disinfection of all articles from infected localities before they are permitted to be imported into healthy places. The following propositions have been adopted by the Congress on recommendation of the committee:

" That, taking the existing state of the relations between the nations of America, it is as practicable as it is advisable for the promotion of these relations to establish perfect accord with respect to sanitary regulations.

" That the greater part of the ports of South America, on the Atlantic, are guided and governed by, the decisions of the International Sanitary Convention of Rio Janeiro of 1887.

" That although it does not appear that the plans of the Sanitary Congress of Lima of 1889 have passed into the category of international compacts, it is to be hoped that they will be accepted by the Governments that participated in the said Congress, because those plans were discussed and approved by medical men of acknowledged ability.

" That the Sanitary Convention of Rio Janeiro of 1887 and the draft of the Congress of Lima of 1889 agree in their essential provisions to such an extent that it may be said they constitute one set of rules and regulations.

" That if these were duly observed in all America they would prevent, under any circumstances, the conflict which usually arises between the obligation to care for the public health and the principle of freedom of communication between countries.

" That the nations of Central and North America were not represented, either in the Sanitary Convention of Rio Janeiro or the Congress of Lima, but that they might easily accept and apply to their respective ports on both oceans, the sanitary regulations before cited."

A draft of the provisions adopted by the Sanitary Conventions of Rio Janeiro and Lima, forms an appendix to the report.

Health and Wealth.

The Philadelphia *Press*, in a recent issue, tells us of an interesting interview with Russell Sage, of New York, who by his own energy has accumulated a fortune of $50,000,000. The purpose of this interview was to learn from Mr. Sage what were the requisites necessary for a man who desired to be wealthy. Of course, the old-time, trite injunctions of industry, economy, honesty, sobriety, and the like, were referred to, but we were instructively edified to hear this old millionaire say that a man's HEALTH has much to do with his success in life, because ill-health will deprive him of that energy which he must use to attain success. Therefore, says Mr. Sage, it behooves one to look well after his bodily condition. As we go on from year to year we become more firmly impressed with the indisputable truth of the assertion that we have so frequently made, that health is really the foundation stone of all material success in this world.

The Life-Giving Power of " Kind Words."

It has been said that a "kind word turneth away wrath," and we would now say that a "kind word" will add to the length of life and increase the happiness of both him who says and him who hears it. If a person would make it a rule never to say anything disagreeable, such a person would be a pleasure to himself and to those about him. Such, we fancy, must have been the practice of Lady Morgan, whom the Hon. Richard Vaux describes (in a recent issue of *The Times*) as having been, more than a half century ago, the most genial, accomplished and fascinating woman in all London. So, also, must it have been with Tom Moore, whom this same authority describes as a most delightful companion.

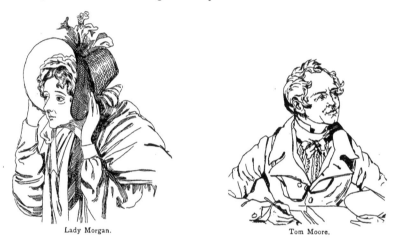

Lady Morgan.   Tom Moore.

In the same way do we believe that the life-long habit of saying *something nice* has had much to do with the popularity of the Hon. Richard Vaux himself, who, now at the age of probably seventy-five, is one of our most thoroughly respected and admired and *typically healthy* fellow-citizens. It is just as easy to say pleasant as unpleasant things, and we are absolutely sure that the former practice will give to us all much more of that mental contentment, so essential to our physical welfare, than will the latter.

A Royal Sanitarian.

It is related of Louis XVI of France, (whom his chroniclers record as one of the best of men,) that, when the infuriated, wild, unreasoning, French mob came to tear him and his family away from the palace at Versailles and consign him to a Parisian prison, his greatest source of grief was not the loss of his throne, but the thought that his children would be thus deprived of the health-giving country air, for above all selfish thoughts of kingly power was the beautiful *kingly* thought of care for the health of his offspring.

An Important Use for State Boards of Health.

The question is often asked, "Of what use are State Boards of Health?" The answer to this question is, that, if all their uses were enumerated, they would fill many pages. But we were recently struck with one very important mission that they have to perform when we read in the daily papers that Dr. Benjamin Lee, the Secretary of the Pennsylvania State Board of Health, had received information from the Secretary of the Connecticut State Board of Health that small-pox existed in certain towns in the latter State. It was recommended that persons who might be about visiting these infected regions should be vaccinated before leaving home. Before the organization of State Boards of Health and the custom which now holds among them to notify one and another of any contagious disease that may be prevalent in any of their respective States, persons visiting other localities were never warned of the dangers which they were about to encounter, but were allowed to rush headlong into the abyss, just as might have done a train, loaded with passengers, before the discovery of the telegraph had placed it in our power to give warning of the destruction of a bridge over a river. It is worth one's while to stop and reflect what an enormous advantage has come to us now that we have a system, through the intervention of the State Boards of Health, by which we may know of the presence or absence of contagious diseases in any particular locality that we may propose to visit.

Disease in Barber Shops.

It is not an imaginary danger when we state that barber shops, as at present carelessly conducted, may be the means of conveyance of disease of a more or less unpleasant, and even dangerous, nature, from one to another. In certain portions of Europe this danger has become so thoroughly recognized that barbers and hairdressers are required by law to disinfect their instruments each time they have been used. Such a custom need entail but little trouble and practically no expense. A disinfectant solution, into which might be placed the combs, brushes, razors and the like, would cost but little and would prove an absolute safeguard against the conveyance of disease as intimated. We would also strongly urge upon barbers to abandon the use of sponges for washing the face after shaving. We can hardly conceive of a more proper place for the breeding and multiplication of disease germs than a sponge, in place of which we would strongly urge that the face should be washed with a wet towel.

The Faith Cure.

Fortunately for suffering humanity (according to the Faith Cure Society of Brooklyn,) the Almighty has seen fit to open the eyes and change the hearts of those dangerous fanatics. Now that they have allowed several of their deluded dupes to die for want of proper care, and now that the Coroner and the District Attorney are getting ready to make them feel the power of the law that they have violated, they have been brought to reason. They now assure the authorities that they will in future employ doctors and use medicine in cases of sickness, for which wise conclusions they are promptly to be congratulated.

The Punishment of Children.

Of course we will not attempt to say that children should not be punished. This would be flying in the face not only of public sentiment, but of common sense. But we most heartily concur with the views recently expressed by Mr. Cadwallader Biddle, the Secretary of the State Board of Public Charities, when he says that he does not like the idea of depriving children of food as a punishment. A growing child requires an abundance of nutritious food, and he who would punish a child by depriving him of this food would be somewhat on a par with a man who would punish a refractory horse by starving him. So, also, must we most heartily condemn the incarceration of children in a room by themselves as a means of punishment. Such practices will have a very evil influence upon the child's nervous system that may possibly result in making him, practically, an unwell person for life. Moral suasion should be the mainstay of those who have the care of children. Of course there are exceptional cases wherein stronger measures may become necessary, but nothing that will interfere with the physical growth or will shock the nervous system of a growing child should be tolerated.

Impure Candy.

Dr. Chevalier Q. Jackson recently contributed an admirable article on the adulterations of candy to the *Pittsburgh Dispatch*, and since he suggests a very wise and practical remedy for the dangers of these adulterations, we quote him, as follows:

" Now the remedy for this state of things is not in letting candy alone. The writer has received many letters stating in effect that : ' If the advice given in the adulteration articles recently published in *The Dispatch* were followed, one's daily dietary would be narrowed down to air, and it is questionable if even that is pure.' No such advice has, however, been given in these columns; what has been urged is to pay reasonable prices for things, or do without them. This is doubly true of candy. If you want to get pure goods of this kind don't expect to get them for less than glucose is worth; if you do you will get pipe clay and worse. If your money is limited buy clear, uncolored goods such as rock candy. The good old-fashioned taffy is as wholesome as anything in the candy line; though commonly considered as very prone to ferment in the stomach, it is not so. Never buy cheap imitations of fine grades of confectionery, such as so-called French candies for they are pretty certain to contain pipe clay or similar substance. Highly flavored preparations should be avoided for the reason that they contain large quantities of essential oils or artificial essences, both of which are objectionable. The oils are irritating to the stomach, and the artificial essences are made in most instances from fusel oil, an acid, and oil of vitriol. Few, if any, of the 'pure fruit essences ' used for flavoring confectionery and various other things contain any fruit juice whatever; they are products of the chemical laboratory. For instance, the acid of rancid cream cheese, when mixed with methyl alcohol and oil of vitriol, yields on distillation a fragrant essence of pine-apple. So it is with the rest of the commercial 'pure fruit juices.' "

The Effect of Corsets on Monkeys.

If our fair readers will pardon the inferential comparison we would tell of some experiments that have recently been made as to the effect of tight-lacing on monkeys. Female monkeys were put into plaster of Paris jackets, to imitate stays, and a tight bandage was put around the waist to imitate a petticoat band. Several of the monkeys died very quickly and all showed signs of injuries resulting from the treatment. Of course, with a human being, generations of use have bred a tolerance so that while we do not find such immediately fatal results, those who are capable of forming an opinion yet know that the constriction of the vital organs of the body caused by tight lacing is continually working mischief within.

Safety in Railroad Traveling.

An association of some railroad employees are anxious to have Congress legislate so as to insure greater safety in the management and handling of trains. We are strongly in sympathy with all their recommendations, but especially must endorse that which calls for shorter hours of work so that lives and property will not be entrusted to men worn out with fatigue. Of course, there is not much use in arguing with railway corporations unless such arguments are backed by overwhelming popular sentiment, but we would assert, as an unquestionable fact, that any railroad forcing its trainmen to work more than ten hours out of the twenty-four is not only requiring from the employee that which they have no moral right to exact, but they are treating with unfairness their patrons, whose lives they are entrusting to men, who, because of overwork, are not capable of *properly* working. Again, there is a selfish reason why railways should not over-work their employees. The time has now come when we should recognize quality rather than quantity of work, and we must understand that he who works for ten hours and rests for fourteen hours, will, during these ten hours, produce much better and more productive work than he who labors for fourteen and rests for ten. Therefore, does it seem to us that for moral reasons, so far as the employee is concerned, and for selfish reasons, so far as the employer is concerned, the great public would be justified in appealing to our railroad companies not to overwork their employees.

The Need of One Day's Rest in Seven.

Some interesting experiments conducted at Munich show that a hard day's work diminishes the amount of oxygen in the system about one ounce. It has been found that the laborer does not recover during the night the oxygen he has thus overdrawn. But an occasional day of rest, coming at just the right time, will serve completely to restore the equilibrium and make him as good as new. It has been found that the amount of exhaustion of the oxygen of the system—in other words, of the life power—by six days of labor, is the amount that can be supplied by a day of complete rest.

Pea Soup as a Substitute for Beef Tea.

Dr. Ris, of Switzerland, emphatically recommends pea soup as an excellent substitute for beef tea for invalids, convalescents, and especially for patients suffering from cancer of the stomach or *diabetes mellitus.* Take peas, water, and a sufficient amount of some vegetable suitable for soup; add one per cent. of carbonate of soda, and boil the whole until the peas are completely disintegrated; then let the soup stand until sedimentation is complete, and decant the fairly clear thin fluid above the deposit. The product is said to resemble a good meat soup in its taste, to be at least equally digestible, and at the same time to surpass the very best meat soup in nutritive value. The latter statement will appear less surprising if we consider that peas contain a considerable portion of legumen, that, is a vegetable albumen, which is easily soluble in a faintly alkaline water, is not coagulated by heat, is easily absorbed, and equal to the albumen of eggs in its nutritiousness,

Peddlers as Disseminators of Disease.

In a recent issue we called attention to the fact that peddlers undoubtedly were the means of propagation of contagious diseases. Going from house to house, they would be just as likely to carry the germs of the disease from a house in which scarlet fever, measles, or the like existed to another house as they would be to carry the goods they were peddling; for the germs of disease are in reality just as much of an entity as the soap or the shoe-strings, or the combs or the suspenders, that the peddler carries in his basket. Again, some member of the peddler's own immediate family may be suffering with a contagious disease which he may be the direct means of bringing into your house. Therefore is it with great pleasure that we note that the Supreme Court of this State has rendered a decision by which it is unlawful for any person to peddle goods from house to house in any of the streets of this city. Unfortunately, however, this restriction applies only to this city, whereas it should, in reality, be made to hold good throughout the State.

Ripe Fruit the Best Remedy.

Neuralgia and diet are more intimately associated than most people are apt to imagine, says the *Anti-Adulteration Journal.* Romberg somewhat poetically says: " Neuralgia is the prayer of the nerve for healthy blood." Disease, generally, may be regarded as "prayer for healthy blood." Thus the great question for the invalid or sufferer should be how to make pure blood. The dead carcasses of our fellow creatures cannot form healthy blood, but ripe fruit most certainly will. Nothing can equal ripe fruit, be it for the invalid or the healthy and strong. It is an excellent rule to commence every meal with fresh, uncooked, ripe fruit. Should such a course destroy or diminish the appetite for savory, so much the better.

Common Soaps.

An intelligent writer expresses the opinion that diphtheria and typhoid fever, and some other diseases, are frequently caused by the soap we use. Soap fat is generally made up of diseased animal matter, taken from beasts which have died of putrescent maladies ; and where this is not the case the fat is generally in a putrid condition, no amount of perfumes used in the soap being able to act as an antidote to the poisons that penetrate the pores of the skin. Another writer, who has been investigating the subject called at a large soap manufacturing establishment, when the head of the firm acknowledged that the fat used in soap was in anything but a healthy condition. He said : "We get the article from the fat rendering establishments. They, of course, take all the carcasses of dead animals and boil them down together. They do not stop to examine as to what death the animal died. Their disease impregnates the fat, and will cause disease in the person using the soap if it is not properly prepared. I found that the only thing to counteract this putridity in fat is borax."—*Anti-Adulteration Journal.*

Moral : Don't buy COMMON SOAP.

The English Amazon.

England has been greatly agitated of late by the side-saddle question. Strong-minded members of the weaker sex have not hesitated to write to the *Field*, advocating a change from the present system, and some huntswomen are already seen in the field wearing a modification of the divided skirt. But two young ladies at Bournemouth have outstripped everybody else, and the cut, reproduced from the *Pall Mall Gazette*, shows the costume which they have been permitted by their families to adopt. While we heartily approve of the innovation, so far as the position on the horse is concerned, believing, as we do, that the ordinary female position on horseback has a tendency to distort the figure, yet we think that the costume that has been adopted by Miss Mabel Jenness, of New York, will be less objectionable and more likely to become popular than that depicted in our illustration, from

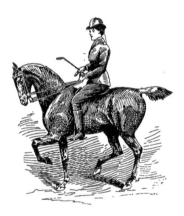

The Times. Miss Jenness dresses in a trim, close-fitting habit of green silk, with pleated waist and skirts. On the street no one would suppose the skirts were bifurcated, the edges of the two overlapping perfectly. Within each skirt is a well-fitting trouser leg, about which the loose pleated outer garments hang in graceful folds.

The young woman, taking the two sets of reins in her left hand, and the whip in her right hand, places both together on the pommel of the man's saddle, and springs into an upright position, resting her whole weight on her hands. The same second her right leg is thrown over the horse's back, the skirts separating, and she sits erect and sure of place.

Seen from either side she looks like an ordinary woman rider mounted on that side from which the view is had. It is only when she is coming towards one or going directly from one, that the unusual impression is given of there being two ladies mounted on opposite sides of the same horse, of which the head and body of but one is visible.

Lavatory Accommodations.

Mr. Horace J. Smith writes to *The Times :*

" In Europe abundant provision is made at frequent intervals along the streets for the necessities of human nature. The delicacy of the American people will not permit the public places for these necessities that are universal on the Continent; and yet we must find some method of meeting the wants of men, women and children, a method that will accord with the feelings and usages of our countrymen.

" From all around the city are daily coming large numbers of people who are ignorant of the places where they can find the thing that they need. Many physicians would give painful testimony as to the results of this lack of accommodation. Oftentimes in the places provided as a gratuity, the accommodations are unclean and unsuitable.

" The only way to secure cleanliness is that the person using these accommodations should pay as in Europe. We have a right to demand the value of what we pay. In this way only can the wants of the community be met.

" We already have conventional signs, such as the barber's pole, and so the notice referred to might be a conventional sign, but need not be anything near as large ; in fact, need only be a few inches in diameter, or it might be a simple card, as follows :

LAVATORY ACCOMMODATIONS

FOR

LADIES AND CHILDREN.

———

PRICE, FIVE CENTS.

" The modest lady passing along the streets, seeing the sign in a suitable store, goes in, pays her money for that which she and the children need. Having paid for the service, she can demand such cleanliness and such accommodations as she has in her own house.

" This is a subject which should be taken up by such associations as are formed among ladies, by the plumbers and sanitary organizations and by medical associations ; when once fairly demonstrated as the suitable method of solving this difficulty, it will spread itself over the whole of America. But no one need wait for anyone else. Any store-keeper or householder is entirely competent to carry out this idea at once and without conference with any organization, if, indeed, any organization is needed.

" There is no vulgarity in speaking of these matters so essential to the health and well-being of the community ; but vulgarity is the speaking of those things about which there is no necessity of talking."

———

IT is the misfortune of the electric light wire that when it gets in its deadly work, it does so under conditions of thrilling spectacular interest. The unobtrusive plumber's pipe, which has slain its thousands where electricity has killed tens, works so modestly, and effects its purpose so gradually, that it constantly gets extension of time and new opportunities for reform.—*Rochester Union.*

Tight Collars and Short Sight.

If, at a fire, one were to tightly constrict with a strong cord the fireman's hose, the stream of water passing through it would be so much reduced in calibre that its effect upon the flames would be much lessened. So it is identically the same with those who wear tight collars. Pressing upon the large blood vessels in the neck they interfere with the free and proper circulation of the blood therein, lessening the quantity and interfering with the regularity of the supply to the head and all contained therein. Hence, we may be prepared to understand the statement made by Dr. Forster, that in three hundred cases of short-sightedness that have come under his observation, the trouble has been due to the pressure of tight collars upon the blood vessels of the neck. It is a cardinal rule of life that no portion of the body should be pressed upon more than another; that the free circulation of the blood should in no place be interfered with. But when this pressure comes to be applied to so important a portion of the body as the neck—important, because through that portion passes the blood vessels supplying the brain, the eyes, the ears and all the more vital portions of the body—then is it that the evil effect of this pressure becomes doubly great.

Free Quinine.

We would probably be accused of exaggeration were we to assert that the popular use of quinine has been as injurious to health as has the popular use of whiskey; yet we do not fear that we would be very far from the truth in making such an assertion. We are called upon to make this remark by noting that certain manufacturers of this drug are urging upon Congress that a tariff shall be placed upon quinine and the revenue taken off alcohol. We should all understand that quinine is a drug, and a powerful one at that; potent for immense good when properly used, but equally potent for mischief if used when not indicated. The enormous fortunes that have been accumulated by those who have devoted themselves in a special manner to the manufacture of quinine clearly demonstrate how great has been the popular use of this drug. We fear not contradiction when we assert that, owing to its popular use, quinine has, on the whole, done more harm than good.

The Origin of Cigars.

The use of cigars by civilized people is much more recent than most people suppose, says a correspondent of the Pittsburgh *Times*. The real cigar, which is a pure roll of tobacco alone, probably originated in Cuba, where the very best cigars are still made. If not there it was undoutebdly in one of the West India Islands. Their origin with us, as in Europe, did not begin until early in the present century. It is said that of all the various cook-books published between 1800 and 1815, and books which treat of the pleasures and adjuncts of taste before the last named date, no one refers to the after-dinner cigar or to cigars at all. Cigars are now made all over the civilized world. They are produced very extensively in Bremen and Hamburg, and at Seville, in Spain. But at Manila, in the Philippine Islands, the largest factories are to be found, in some of which 10,000 girls are employed.

Activity a Factor in Longevity.

It is really a mistake to say, as some do, that over-work is prejudicial to health. Of course, if a man works twenty hours out of the twenty-four, his strength will give out, because he will not have provided sufficient time for rest and sleep. We would

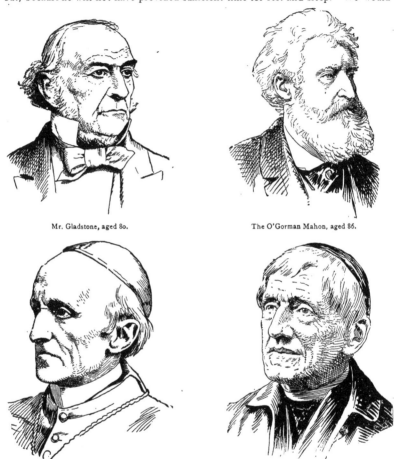

Mr. Gladstone, aged 80.

The O'Gorman Mahon, aged 86.

Cardinal Manning, aged 81.

Cardinal Newman, aged 88.

ask our readers to differentiate between active, prolonged work, and misdirected, unsystematic effort. Such a thing as over-work on the part of a business man is well-nigh impossible, since the hours alloted to business by custom would, of necessity, preclude this. A professional or literary man might be tempted to devote too much time to work; but if he be methodical and systematic, if he devote a portion of his day to exercise and recreation, and secures a sufficiency of sleep, it is very unlikely (save in extremely rare cases) that any amount of work will do injury to his health. It is not work but improper methods of life that do the harm that is so often attributed to over-work. An active life (other things being equal) will be much more conducive to health and longevity than will a passive one. Man was meant to be an active and not an indolent animal. Here are four of the most eminent octogenarians in the world of to-day.

The lives of each of these men have been of the most *active* kind. The O'Gorman Mahon, who was a contemporary of Daniel O'Connell, has, all his long life, been ardently fond of out-door *active* sports, and to-day, at 86 years of age, he is still an *active* member of the British Parliament. Cardinal Newman's *activity* has been displayed in the field of letters ; Cardinal Manning has been probably the most *active* religio-social leader of the century, while the politico-social *activity* of Mr. Gladstone's long life is too well known to need mention here. These four famous characters forcibly remind us that *activity*, health and longevity are closely allied. We have always urged against hurry and worry, but, equally forcibly, do we argue in favor of systematic, methodical, well-directed *activity*.

A Test for Water.

A test for the purity of drinking-water is given as follows by Prof. Angell of the Michigan University: "Dissolve about half a teaspoonful of the purest white sugar in a pint bottle completely full of water to be tested, tightly stopped ; expose it to daylight and a temperature up to 70 degrees Fahr. After a day or two examine, holding the bottle against something black, for floating specks, which will betray the presence of organic matter in considerable proportion."

Transportation of Corpses.

Only a short time ago a child died of diphtheria in Ravenwood, Ill. The body was removed to Zanesville, O., where, doubtless, sympathizing friends and others "viewed the remains." As a result an epidemic of diphtheria broke out, with five deaths of children at last accounts. In this case there is some question as to who is to bear the blame, it being alleged on one hand that the doctor gave a false certificate, and on the other that the certificate showed the cause of death to be diphtheria ; but the railroad company took the responsibility.

Salus Populi.

The real wealth of a people is not counted by its gold, silver, or broad acres. These are sources of material interest and physical greatness ; above these, as high as the heaven is above the earth, as a simpler question of value, is the health of the people. Here is the manhood, the real civilization, the source of its content, happiness, and its good will to men.—*Dr. J. W. Jones, in The North Carolina Bulletin.*

Mental Aberration in Paris.

Dr. Paul Garnier, in a report addressed to the Society of Medical Jurisprudence, has brought to notice the alarming increase of cases of mental aberration that occur in Paris. In the last fifteen years this increase has been more than thirty per cent. The principal causes of the increase of insanity are, according to the author, alcoholism and excessive intellectual work. Mental aberration is a little more common in men than in women. The proportion is fifty-six men and forty-four women out of one hundred lunatics, but this proportion tends to be equalized, as the progression of insanity is more rapid for the female sex than 'for the male.—*Paris Correspondent Boston Medical and Surgical Journal.*

A Brief History of the Small-pox in Connecticut.

D. C. A. Lindsley, the Secretary of the State Board of Health of Connecticut, thus writes:

"Small-pox which started, as it very commonly does, from a rag department of a paper mill, appeared in January in Windsor Locks. It appeared soon after in some of the adjoining towns; one case in Waterbury. These cases were immediately put under proper regulations and controlled; but in Meriden the disease has been allowed greater liberty. The first suspicious case was reported to the health authorities. Six doctors examined it, but as four asserted it was chicken-pox, and only two thought it varioloid, the majority of course ruled and no protective measures were taken. The laws of nature, however, are not subject to majorities, like the health authorities of Meriden. Meriden was also unfortunate in being a double-headed town, having two boards of health, a town board, and a city board. So that when a little after, other cases of "chicken-pox" ripened into the genuine small-pox, there was still no decisive and energetic action taken to control it and protect the public. On the contrary, with astonishing deliberation the two boards of health officials called a joint meeting for the *next day*. This meeting, which the Secretary of the State Board of Health was invited to attend, was not called to decide upon the best methods of guarding the public. Those questions did not seem to be interesting. The chief discussion was whether the town or the city was liable for what expense might be incurred. Upon this pitiful dispute, with small-pox in several places in the city, these two august bodies, the representatives of sanitary administration in the town and in the city of Meriden, wasted time wrangling about results, when every passing hour was precious to prevent the spread of the contagion. Is it remarkable that with such guardians of the public health there were a dozen cases of small-pox in Meriden before the end of the month?"

A BILIOUS MAN, hunting for something to get mad at, is generally successful in his search.

ALPHONSE DAUDET and Prince Bismarck have smoked more tobacco than any other two men in Europe.

AN hour's industry will do more to produce cheerfulness, suppress vile humors and retrieve your affairs, than a month's moaning.

A Model Russian Community.

We have been fond of advocating the Chinese plan of practice, by which a physician is employed by the year to keep his patients well, rather than the more general plan of endeavoring to cure them, when, perhaps, it is impossible to do so. Hence it is with gratification we read that in Tiflis, Russia, a club of one hundred and twenty-five families has made an arrangement with a physician, who agrees, for a definite sum, to visit the families regularly and give them advice as to how to keep healthy; to attend them if sick, and besides to give the club occasionally short lectures upon hygiene. The cost to each family for this service is only fifty cents per month.

To Practise Deep Breathing.

1. Stand erect, the feet separated, the right slightly in advance. 2. Shoulders and head in natural position. 3. Hands lying lightly on the abdomen, the fingers pointing to the umbilicus. Compliance with this rule enables the child to be sure she is using the abdominal as well as the pectoral muscles in respiration. 4. Empty the lungs of air, then close the mouth. 5. Inhale slowly through the nostrils, using abdominal as well as chest muscles. The lungs thus receive the utmost possible amount of pure oxygen and muscles have exercise. 6. Hold the breath as long as possible, and meanwhile use the ordinary calisthenic exercises. 7. Never exercise except with the chest well expanded with air. 8. Exhale slowly, enunciating the vowel sounds as the air passes the lips.

The Death of General Crook.

The recent sudden death of Major-General Crook, United States Army, in Chicago, teaches a valuable lesson. We were told by the newspapers that he was cognizant of some heart trouble, yet, when he gets out of bed, with his system weakened by a prolonged absence from food (as is always the case early in the morning before breakfast), he commences to exercise with chest weights and pulleys. His weakened heart is not equal to the strain placed upon it; he gasps for breath, falls upon the sofa and, in a few minutes, this noblest of hearts is still in death forever.

We do not believe in gymnasiums nor in apparatus as an aid to exercise for any one; believing that the efforts thus put forth are too violent; but, when a man, sixty-one years old, with a weak heart, undertakes to pull heavy weights, in the early morning, before his breakfast, we are forced to the conclusion that he has had more to do with his own death than most persons would, at the first blush, perceive.

An experiment in photographing the bottom of a well 1,700 feet deep was recently made, and a perfect picture obtained. The instrument was let down, and the moment it touched the bottom a bright flash lighted up the cavity, revealing, as the effect of the explosive shock, a very large hole.

Burial reform in England contemplates the prohibition of leaden and other solidly constructed coffins, the effect of which is thought to retard complete decomposition, and so prolong the period during which the dead are not only æsthetically objectionable, but are an indisputable source of danger to the living. It is proposed to use wicker-work or papier-maché receptacles.

BUREAU OF INFORMATION.

The Restriction of Diphtheria.

EDITOR ANNALS OF HYGIENE:

Diphtheria has broken out in two families in my district. Two have died and another cannot possibly live. What do you consider the best disinfectant and the best treatment to observe in regard to the corpse, so as to prevent, if possible, the spread of the epidemic.

LEWIS P. T.,

Hulmeville, Bucks Co., Pa.

We would refer our correspondent, as well as all who may be interested in this vital question, to THE ANNALS OF HYGIENE for October, 1889, page 490, where full instructions will be found.

The Danger to Health in Ready-Made Clothing Establishments.

EDITOR ANNALS OF HYGIENE:

In the February number of your useful and instructive issue, you show the great danger of peddlers and hawkers spreading infection from house to house. Does it not strike you that contagious diseases can as readily be conveyed by clothing? If so, what more ready agent can be found than the rapidly increasing number of all grades of the ready-made clothing establishments? A coat, a pair of trousers, etc., may be tried on by a dozen or more of individuals before the same is sold. Is there no danger in such a custom? ITCH.

We believe this to be a real danger, and thank our correspondent for calling the attention of our readers thereto.—[ED. A. OF H.]

SPECIAL REPORT.

Special Meeting of the State Board of Health of Pennsylvania.

A special meeting of the Board was held, on the call of the President, *pro tem.*, Dr. Groff, at the request of Dr. Edwards, Mr. Murphy and the Secretary, at the Executive Office, Saturday, February 22, 1890, at 3 P. M. Present: Drs. Groff, Davis, Dudley, Mr. Murphy and Drs. Edwards and Lee. The President, *pro tem*, Dr. Groff, presiding.

The Secretary stated the objects for which the meeting was called to be the auditing of accounts, the appointment of delegates to Sanitary Conventions, and the arranging for the State Sanitary Convention, to take place in May.

Vouchers No. 305 to 247 inclusive, amounting to seven hundred and sixty-three dollars and forty-two cents ($763.42), which had been passed upon favorably by the Executive Committee, were presented and approved.

A communication was read from Dr. C. O. Probst, Secretary of the State Board of Health of Ohio, and Secretary of the National Conference of State Boards of Health, announcing that the Executive Committee of the Conference had fixed on Louisville, Kentucky, as the next place of meeting and the early part of May (date not definitely decided) as the time.

On motion of Dr. Dudley, the Secretary was authorized to issue credentials to any members desiring to attend the Conference.

On motion of Mr. Murphy, it was *Resolved*, That, after the present time, the regular meetings of the Board shall be held on the second Thursdays of May, July, and November, instead of the second Wednesdays of those months as heretofore.

An invitation from Dr. George I. Garrison, Secretary of the Tri-State Sanitary Convention, to be held at Wheeling, West Virginia, February 27th and 28th, to the members of the Board to attend said Convention was presented.   On motion of Mr. Murphy, the Secretary was instructed to issue credentials to any member desiring to attend.

The Secretary then read a communication from the Secretary of the Board of Health·of Norristown, requesting that the next State Sanitary Convention might be held in that town.   On motion of Dr. Davis, the Secretary was instructed to accept the invitation with thanks.

Drs. Edwards, Lee and Dudley were appointed by the Chair a committee of arrangements with power to act.   The determination of the date for the Sanitary Convention was left to the discretion of the Committee after consultation with the Norristown Board.

The Secretary announced that he had in preparation a circular on the subject of Precautions against Consumption, and that on submitting it to the President *pro tem.*, he had suggested the inquiry " Whether inveterate smokers were ever known to die of consumption?" Mr. Murphy moved that the Secretary be authorized to prepare a circular letter to the medical profession in the State, asking for the results of their observation upon this subject.   It·was carried, and the Board then, on motion, adjourned.

(Signed)   BENJAMIN LEE,
Secretary.

State Board of Health and Vital Statistics of the Commonwealth of Pennsylvania.

PRESIDENT,
GEORGE G. GROFF, M. D., of Lewisburg.

SECRETARY,
BENJAMIN LEE, M. D., of Philadelphia.

MEMBERS,
PEMBERTON DUDLEY, M. D., of Philadelphia.

J. F. EDWARDS, M. D., of Philadelphia.	GEORGE G. GROFF, M. D., of Lewisburg.
J. H. McCLELLAND, M. D., of Pittsburgh.	S. T. DAVIS, M. D., of Lancaster.
HOWARD MURPHY, C. E. of Philadelphia.	BENJAMIN LEE, M. D., of Philadelphia.

PLACE OF MEETING,
Supreme Court Room, State Capitol, Harrisburg, unless otherwise ordered.

TIME OF MEETING,
Second Wednesday in May, July and November.

EXECUTIVE COMMITTEE,

PEMBERTON DUDLEY, M. D., Chairman.	JOSEPH F. EDWARDS, M. D.
HOWARD MURPHY, C. E.	BENJAMIN LEE, M. D., Secretary.

Place of Meeting (until otherwise ordered)—Executive Office, 1532 Pine Street, Philadelphia.

Time of Meeting—Third·Wednesday in January, April, July and October.

Secretary's Address—1532 Pine Street, Philadelphia.

Bureau of Registration and Vital Statistics—Department of Internal Affairs, State Capitol, Harrisburg.

State Superintendent of Registration of Vital Statistics—BENJAMIN LEE, M. D.

THE
ANNALS
OF
HUGIENE

VOLUME V.

Philadelphia, May 1, 1890

NUMBER 5.

COMMUNICATIONS

President Harrison; Vice-President Morton and "The Cabinet" on Hygiene.*

President Harrison is a sanitarian in every sense the word implies. He is so instinctively, without rule or method, but in such a manner as to insure him a natural life when he retires from the executive chair. It is because he obeys the warnings of nature that he is enabled to withstand the death breezes which float from the swampy lowlands just south of the White House, and fill every nook and cranny of that historical building with its life-destroying malaria. The Chief Magistrate is not averse to conversation bearing upon his daily modes of living, but they are so many and varied that it would require a larger book than this to give a complete description of them. The temperature of his bath does not worry him in the least, neither does the hour for taking a walk or drive. While he is careful what he eats he is not an abstainer to any great extent. "I attribute my present good health more to my own good sense than to anything else," he said. "Understand me, I don't say this egotistically. I merely contend that a man with a sound, healthy body must necessarily be possessed of clear mental faculties. Now, reverse this and you have my case. I know that when my brain feels tired from overwork or any kind of worry it needs a rest. Some people will hurry to their rooms and indulge in a nap as the best medicine. Do I do that?—not much. On these occasions I take a dose of nature's own physic. It costs nothing and is far more exhilarating than all the devices known to medical science. A most natural mistake made by many is that to tire out the body in order to induce sleep is the best method of recreating the mind. That is nonsense as far as I am concerned. I am very careful in my pedestrian exercise. I take particular care to fill my lungs with plenty of good oxygen and walk with as little effort as possible. In some of my rambles I have met with some peculiar experiences. When General Schenck was alive he was a great walker. One Sunday afternoon I met him up near Iowa circle and in the course of conversation he asked me how long my daily walks were prolonged. I told him that they varied from one to two hours and sometimes longer. Looking at me quizzically for a

---

* Being views expressed in the course of personal interviews—specially prepared for this journal by E. S. Conner.

moment the old General said, ' Do you know that if I were to be taken so ill that it would be impossible for me to take my daily walk, I think it would end me.' It was not long after that before General Schenck was taken sick, and, as he said, it was

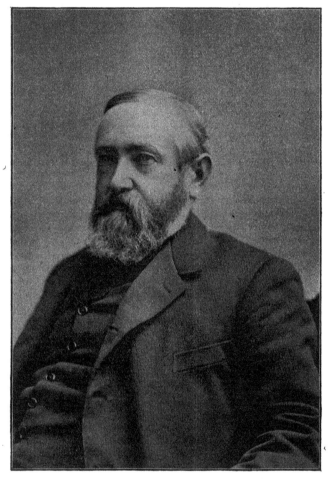

President Harrison.

impossible for him to get out doors, and he died. The cares of a Chief Magistrate are of such importance that he cannot always put his business in his desk and lock it up. This rule, however, I have made and adhered to, never to allow my mind to get the best of me to such an extent that any worriment or cares of the day shall interfere with my sleep.''

"Do you find your periodical fishing and gunning trips benefit you?"
"Indeed I do. The papers all speak of me as being fagged out when I start on one of these trips. Nothing of the kind. The 'fag' is just beginning, and

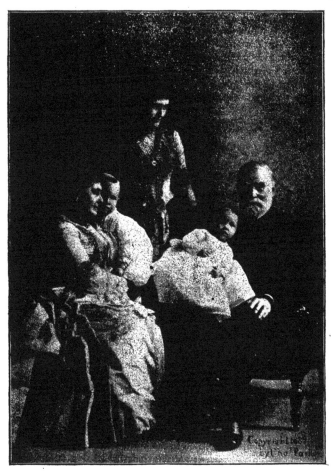

Mrs. Benj. Harrison.　Baby McKee.　Mrs. R. B. McKee.　Mary L. McKee.　Rev. Dr. Scott. (In his 90th year.)

FOUR GENERATIONS.

This picture was taken in the White House.

I know that were I to remain here after I have been warned that something is bound to be weakened about my physical machinery. Nature applies a smooth oil to the multiplex wheels of life on a two or three days' duck shoot. As a matter of course, the excitement of the day is somewhat tiring, but it is a diversion—a recreating diversion—I find, and when I reach my bed at night you may be sure that I fall into a sound, dreamless slumber. On returning from these trips I have received such a goodly supply of invigorator that it is really a pleasure to work. The secret of my present good health may be summed up in a few words,—keep clean, take plenty of exercise, and don't allow the body or mind to become tired.''

It would be hard to find a better example of the result of living a natural life than Vice-President Morton's. Though he has led a political life—one of the hardest of all lives—for many years, has been senator, diplomat, and Vice-President, Mr. Morton is a remarkably well-preserved man. When I spoke to him, he said :

"Hygiene? I don't believe that I know much about it in the sense that physicians use the word—if that be a scientific sense. But I think I am what is

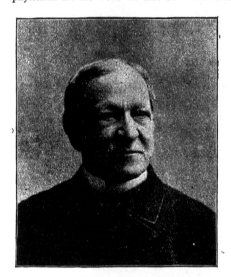

Hon. Levi P. Morton,
Vice-President of the United States.

called a man of regular habits and abstemious. A natural life? That is a good word to use in speaking of my case. Nature is my law. When she warns me to stop work I do it and unconsciously follow her guidance. The labor leaders say the day should be divided into three parts—eight hours for work, eight hours for play and eight hours for sleep. I get the eight hours' sleep, but work a good deal more than the eight hours that they want to make the limit. But I make it a rule to take recreation whenever I feel that it is necessary. I am sixty-five years of age and I flatter myself you wouldn't take me to be so old by five years. I have led a natural life to the best of my ability and have tried to follow the dictates of nature as much as possible, slowing speed or turning off steam when she whistles. To this I ascribe my present good health, and I believe that such a course of treatment is more beneficial than all the medicine, dieting and 'early to bed and early to rise' habits in the world. But nature used me pretty well in the first place, all my ancestors being long-lived. My father was a country clergyman, and, brought up in the fields, I have always had a fondness for out-door life. About six months of my time is spent at my country place on the Hudson, where I take a keen delight in looking after my farms. I am fond of hunting, but just now am too old to do much of it. That is about all I can tell you about myself as a sanitarian.''

Notwithstanding the unnatural pallor of Secretary James G. Blaine's face, he is a healthy man. His clear, shrewd mind, like that of President Harrison is free from debilitating influences and he is to-day one of the strongest and heartiest men in the Cabinet.

"To what do you ascribe your present state of health?" was asked of him the other day.

"I don't know," he replied, "unless it is that I have always taken good care of myself. I like plenty of ventilation, keep good hours and worry as little as possible."

"Have you ever taken your business to bed with you?" he was asked.

"Oh, yes; on several occasions, but not in the sense you imply. I found him a very pleasant bedfellow. It was when I was studying law and I recollect often placing my books beneath my pillow at night and repeating sentences, etc., until I feel asleep. Since I have grown older, however, I have stopped all that and now when bed-time comes I divest myself of my thoughts together with my garments. From long practice I have become the master and, unlike Banquo's ghost, he will "down at my bidding."

"Do you get plenty of fresh air?"

"Yes, considerable; but that is too thin a diet |to subsist upon. The goods that the gods provide I partake of, but not to excess. If I feel that I have eaten a little too heartily, a good brisk walk will relieve me of all feelings of uncomfortableness.

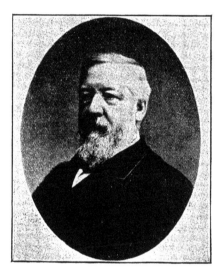

Hon. James G. Blaine,
Secretary of State.

The seashore is the best place to recoup the lost physical forces. There is a health-restoring atmosphere in such places that cannot do otherwise than build up. Had not James A. Garfield been taken to the seashore it is my opinion that he would not have lived nearly as long as he did. Take a clerk in a city store for example. He is pale, sickly and thoroughly worn out when the time comes for his vacation. He goes to the seashore for a couple of weeks and as a result, he is not the same person when he comes back. He is invigorated, has a healthy coat of tan on his face, a good appetite—in fact he is completely renovated. Does he live in the house, or breathe the atmosphere made fetid by hundreds of breaths, while he is there? Not by any means. He lives on the beach nearly all of his time. He fills his weakened lungs with good salt air and in consequence his debilitated constitution is so strengthened that he comes back to his work a new man. Look at that same individual three months afterwards, with the cares and worry that devolve upon his position. He has returned to his old habits, he breathes the close air of a city store, his appetite is gone, and all the good that was accomplished by nature has been undone. In my case it is almost the same, but only to a certain extent. I have my daily cares and toil—only when night comes I leave all that behind and in the summer months I hasten to the pure atmosphere of Bar Harbor and there set myself to work to regain what I have lost. It is an exceedingly pleasant occupation I assure you."

" Was your health just as good while you were a congressman ? "

" I hardly think it was. You see it was different there, especially when I was Speaker of the House. The heat and light were nearly always artificial. Many times have I sat in the Speaker's chair amid all the noise and confusion, when I felt that I should be in bed. Breathing the atmosphere of three hundred breaths is not conducive to good health, and no matter what arrangements are tried the Capitol cannot be ventilated as it should be. My office in the State Department is well lighted and ventilated and there is always a supply of fresh air in it. Living a temperate life in all things, taking plenty of exercise and getting nature's full quota of sleep will, in my opinion, counteract the bad influences of an unhealthy body.

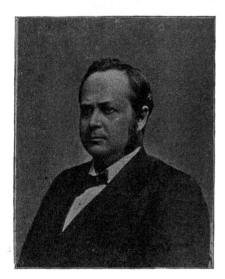

Hon. William Windom,
Secretary of the Treasury.

" I don't believe that I ever paid any particular attention to Hygiene," said William Windom, the Secretary of the Treasury, " but I had the stationary washstands taken out of my office in the Treasury building and the sewer pipe plugged up. I now use a wash-bowl and pitcher to wash my hands and face. This was because it was said that Secretary Manning's health was affected by the sewer-gas. That, I believe, is the sum total of my experience with sanitation. I go to bed early and get up early, sleeping about eight hours. One rule I make—that is, never to take my business to bed with me. I don't work after dark, and when I leave my office I leave my official duties behind me, too, and try my best to forget them. I generally walk two or three miles a day, or drive myself twice the distance. It is quite a nice little walk from my house to the Treasury building, and I take it every day unless it is raining, and then I think my health and dry feet more important than the exercise, and that the exposure would do more harm than the walking good. My vacations are spent in a different way than are those of most men. Last summer I went with my family to the hills of New Hampshire, and we went from town to town, stopping at the little inns along the roadside, breathing the fresh pure air and thoroughly enjoying ourselves. I can recommend that to anyone who is not too closely wedded to the luxuries of existence in a large city as a most delightful way of spending a vacation."

"Mr. Windom, how is it that, although you are the oldest man in the Cabinet, you are, in appearance, one of the youngest?"

"I have been in public life since 1859, when I came here to Congress from Minnesota, and yet I venture to say you speak the truth when you say I don't look my age. The only reason I can give for this is that I never allow myself to be angered without cause. Rage don't do anyone any good, or the person at whom it is aimed any harm, and it often does the person who is angered considerable harm. This I have learned, and I try to apply the knowledge in my every-day life. My habit of leaving my official duties and office at the same time, I think, also has something to do with my present good health."

"I have spent a great deal of my life in the country," said Secretary of War Proctor, "and I take a great deal of out-door exercise, though not as much as I ought to, or as much as I did formerly. I ride and walk a great deal, and find that the exercise is beneficial. Walking is a great medicine, so cheap as to be accessible to the humblest beggar and far-reaching in its benefits. I have found its effect on me very beneficial. It keeps up my health and physique. Yes, I reiterate that the power of pedestrianism is one of the greatest boons conferred upon mankind. Fishing is a recreation, and a medicine as well, with me. When the Rebellion was quelled, my health was shattered, and I have always told my friends that fishing cured me."

"Fishing?"

"Yes, fishing. I used to go to my private fishing reserve, near my

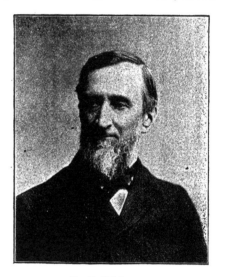

Hon. Redfield Proctor,
Secretary of War.

country place in Vermont, when I was so feeble that my wife had to support me and help me to the spot. The out-door exercise and the breathing of the fresh air, instead of remaining cooped up in the house, did me a wonderful amount of good, and I honestly believe that it was the prime cause of my restoration to health. If I hadn't been such an enthusiastic follower in the footsteps of Izaak Walton I might not be here now. Sleep is another medicine of mine that I always try to get a good dose of, and I always feel better when I get as much as I ought to have, which, in my opinion, is about seven hours. I have had to work pretty hard lately, but now that I have been given an assistant I am going to Vermont for a couple of weeks or so to take a rest and fish. I will then be far enough away from the seat of war to be able to throw aside the cares of business. I am hardly a sanitarian, you see, but I know enough to take good care of that great blessing with which God has endowed me—good health."

The awful calamity which fell upon the head of Secretary of the Navy Tracy and his family recently, has left him pale and haggard, but he bears up well beneath the strain. When questioned upon the subject of Hygiene, he said :

" I am not very well posted on the subject, though perhaps my health would be better if I had a more extensive acquaintance with the principles of sanitation. All my life I have been a great sufferer from dyspepsia and find that walking is almost a necessity. I am always glad to walk as much as I can, and invariably feel better for the mild exercise and am able to sleep more soundly. I sleep only about six hours, which I don't think is enough. I suppose doctors would be shocked to learn that I go to bed at any time from 8.30 P. M., to 2 A. M., and sometimes pass one or the other extreme. With me walking is a duty which I owe to myself, and I find that I suffer less from dyspepsia when I take a stroll of a mile or two. I have no regular distance mapped out to walk. I like to talk as I walk and the length of my walk is often in proportion to the length of my talk. If I have an interesting companion, it is long. Sometimes, when a friend calls to see me and have a little chat, I will put on my coat and go out-doors, talking as I walk, and keeping my legs going as long as the tongue of either myself or my friend is wagging. Whatever observance I may pay to the laws of Hygiene is not of my own volition. As an instance—I only smoke one or two cigars a day, although I am fond of tobacco. This is not because I don't want to smoke, but because the doctor told me that it would be the right thing for me to do to stop smoking or smoke as little as possible."

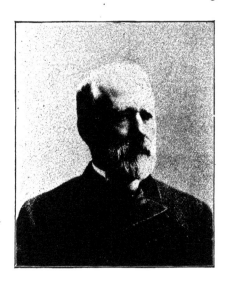

Hon. B. F. Tracy,
Secretary of the Navy.

" *Mens sana in corpore sano*," quoted Secretary of the Interior Noble, as he leaned back in an arm-chair, which seemed more luxurious than would have been tolerated by the sanitarians of the early schools, who believed that privation was essential to good health. " I believe in that motto thoroughly and in it may be summed up my views on the question of Hygiene. The two are inseparable, and the first cannot get along without the latter, and I don't know but one is as great a blessing as the other. For of what use would be a sound mind without a sound body to enjoy it. The brightest intellect would not be long undimmed unless due regard was paid to the laws of nature.

One of the best ways in which to secure the indispensable " *corpore sano* " without any very great exertion, is by walking, or driving, or some other outdoor exercise. This is a method of acquiring health which may be used by everyone. I don't walk five miles a day, but I suppose I ought to, and that it would do good to anybody on earth to cover that amount of ground regularly every day. I take frequent baths; this is another cheap, but effective medicine. When I bathe I rub my body briskly with a crash towel until I produce a bright glow. I am not an athlete, but I am particular about these two things which I regard as indispensable to good health—my walks and my bath. Anybody who will follow my example in these two respects will, I honestly believe, in that way prolong their lives by weeks, months or years. But then we are never able to find out how much this course of treatment, or that, adds or subtracts from the span of life, as we were never told how long it was allotted that we should live. I think horseback riding is beneficial. Public men lead a sedentary life and in that way are inclined to corpulency; now a good way in which this surplus of avoirdupois can be prevented, is by riding a horse for an hour or two every day. It is a very pleasant medicine to take, which is another advantage. I am also a believer in the efficacy of sleep. An untroubled sleep will do wonders, it is the only time when the brain is almost completely free from worry, and for that reason it is of great benefit to the health. Now I have given you my sanitary platform."

Where can a better illustration of healthy manhood be found than Postmaster-General Wanamaker? Yet when questioned upon the subject of Hygiene he was as ignorant as a school-boy. What he does know, however, is how to take care

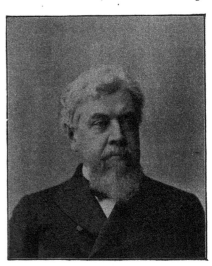

Hon. John W. Noble,
Secretary of the Interior.

of his body, and as a result he is blessed with a keen, shrewd mind, that has brought him up from the ranks to a lofty position in the circle of Presidential advisers. Mr. Wanamaker has not run his race yet, and that gigantic intellect of his is, sooner or later, going to see him far above his present position and in the right place to give his broad views the wide scope which they so richly deserve.

"Can you tell me the secret of your success?" was asked of the "General," as he is familiarly called in Washington.

"I might give you the history of my life as far back as I can remember," he answered, "and even then I doubt if you would be any wiser. In fine, it is simply this: Take advantage of your opportunities as they present themselves. Keep your body in good working order, and cultivate your mind assiduously. 'Be temperate in all things' is the text I have so often written in my youthful days, and it conveys more in its brevity than a whole bookful of scientific rules to govern the health." The healthy glow of Mr. Wanamaker's face is never paled by late hours or social dissipation or study. He applies his mind to business only during business hours, and when he returns to his home in the evening the cares and worries of a political position are either left to his private secretary or they are left at the Post Office Department. No close rooms for him. No burning of midnight oil to

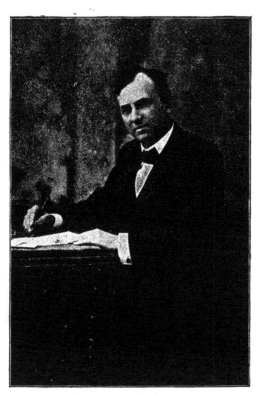

Hon. John Wanamaker, Postmaster General.

sap away his wonderful vitality. He is a man who is faithful to his work, but more faithful to his own health. He walks but little, but it is a noticeable fact that when he enters his unpretentious little coupé one or more of the windows are invariably lowered.

I saw him in the room with Samuel J. Randall on the night that illustrious statesman died. He felt the temperature of that sick room with the unerring instinct of a sanitarian. From time to time he would walk quietly to the front window, and either raise or lower the sash as the occasion required. After the death vigil had ceased, the Postmaster-General put on his hat and overcoat, and took a brisk walk of half an hour, returning to the afflicted household apparently as fresh as ever. On

Christmas Day of 1888 I saw Postmaster-General Wanamaker alight from a train at Jenkintown, on his return from the celebration at Bethany Sunday-School. He sniffed the bracing air gratefully, and placing his hands on my shoulders said, "What a glorious thing it is to be able to get in some quiet spot where one can fill one's lungs with God's own medicine." Mr. Wanamaker believes in the old text "Cleanliness is next to Godliness," and in this only does he live by rule. Not once—no matter how pressing his duties may be—does he neglect his daily bath and shave. In another important fact does Mr. Wanamaker demonstrate that life is too short to worry. He never loses his temper. Affairs may go wrong in every branch of his official business, but he always maintains his quiet, unobtrusive demeanor. Office-seekers may harangue him, Congressmen may badger him, but not for an

instant does he lose his courteous, gentlemanly demeanor. Fresh air he wants, and fresh air he gets, whether at his office or at home. Apollinaris water is his strongest tipple, and tobacco in any shape never touches his lips. Let him have a couple of days and a clear country stretch, and Mr. Wanamaker would not willingly exchange them for all the social enjoyments of modern times. In his everyday life he is humble and unassuming, but there is no man in the United States who enjoys better mental and physical health than he does.

"Miller as a Sanitarian," and the Attorney-General laughed incredulously. "Well, I am afraid you won't find that I am very much of a one, although I believe that it would be better for me if I

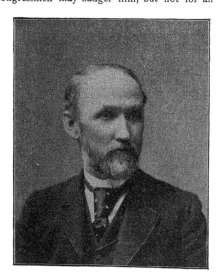

Hon. William H. H. Miller,
Attorney-General.

paid more attention to the subject. I always try to take a reasonable amount of exercise, but I should take more. I walk a great deal, and used to ride horseback, but I don't do as much of that as I used to. I find a slight period of relaxation after hard work of great importance. I believe that if I were to fail to observe nature's warnings when given I would not be here now, as I am not naturally a very strong man. I try to keep my family well, and so far as I am able, make them do those things which experience, observation and reading have taught me are conducive to health. What are these things? Well, I hardly know how to explain them to you. I have no stereotyped rules and regulations which are to be followed and observed like the laws of the Medes and Persians, but I make the law when the occasion arises. I always try to take a vacation of a couple of weeks, usually starting about February or March, and I have not neglected this sanitary precaution for many years. I have found this rest often a necessity, always useful, as I am generally worn out after a hard winter's work. These two weeks are usually spent as far from the scene of my work as convenient, in order that I may free my mind from its usual cares and forget business as much as possible. I generally make the Southwest my destination, New Orleans, Texas or Mexico. I try to get eight hours sleep, and always feel better for it, though I am not always able to get it. I think there are but few men in public life who do not heed nature's warnings. If they did not pay attention to her cries of distress they would hardly be able to attend to the affairs of state or nation. Yes, I think that nothing could be more beneficial than a natural life, and that is an excellent summing up of my views on the subject of Hygiene.''

"Uncle Jere" Rusk, as the Secretary of Agriculture is called by his friends, is one of the most picturesque figures of the present administration. He is a wonderful example of what out-door life will do for a man.

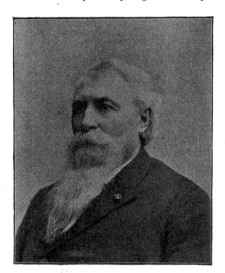

Hon. Jeremiah Rusk,
Secretary of Agriculture.

"I probably have more muscle than any other man in the Cabinet," said Mr. Rusk, as he held out his arm for me to feel. "That is because I have lived out-doors all my life. No bird is fonder of the green fields than I, and the sight of the seeds from which the plants are grown is all that keeps me from beating by wings against the iron bars of my cage. I got some of that muscle I just showed you from wielding a scythe, and I venture to say that I can mow grass with almost any man in public life in Washington. I can handle a rake or hoe and drive a plow or harrow as well. Walk and ride? Why, I have done it all my life, though I hardly call that exercise. It is very good, however, if you can't do anything better. There is nothing I enjoy more than a canter on the back of a lively nag, and I believe that horse-back riding will do anybody a world of good. As for walking, I have done a good deal of that ever since I was a little youngster 'so high,' and a day seldom passes without my taking a stroll of a few miles. But handling a hoe is the thing to get up your muscle. If any one who has a pale face and feels generally run down from over-work will go out into the country and do some light work on a farm, he will come back with an amount of muscle, a springy step and sunburned face that will be a surprise to himself and his friends. Yes, country life is the thing. We don't need to bother ourselves with such questions as sanitation or Hygiene where we live any more than with Chaldaic or some other dead language. We just live a plain, natural, every-day life, without any thought of scientific notions.''

The Ideal Disposition of the Dead.

By REV. CHARLES R. TREAT,

Of New York.

(Concluded from page 68.)

Within a few years it has become unquestioned that some of the deadliest diseases that attack mankind owe their origin and propagation to living organisms, and it may yet appear that the field of their operation is far wider than we now think. Not to attempt to tell all that has been ascertained, it will be sufficiently convincing to quote from Sir Henry Thompson's utterance in the *Nineteenth Century*, in 1880: "I state, as a fact of the highest importance, that, by burial in earth, we effectively provide—whatever sanitary precautions are taken by ventilation and drainage, whatever disinfection is applied after contagion has occurred—that the pestilential germs, which have destroyed the body in question, are thus so treasured and protected as to propagate and multiply, ready to reappear and work like ruin hereafter for others. . . . Beside anthrax, or splenic-fever, spores from which are notoriously brought to the surface from buried animals below and become fatal to the herds feeding there, it is now almost certain that malarious diseases, notably Roman-fever and even tetanus, are due to bacteria which flourish in the soil itself. The poisons of scarlet-fever, enteric-fever (typhoid), small-pox, diphtheria, and malignant cholera are undoubtedly transmissible through earth from the buried body." That the burial of a body which contains the seeds of zymotic disease, is simply storing them for future reproduction and destruction, is amply proven by the researches of Darwin and Pasteur; of whom the former has shown that the mould, or fertile upper layer of superficial soil, has largely acquired its character by its passage through the digestive tract of earth-worms, and the latter, that this mould, when brought by this agency to the surface from subjacent soil that has been used as a grave, contains the specific germ of the disease that has destroyed its tenant.

We may fitly close this portion of the discussion with the conclusion, so strongly stated by Dr. James M. Kellar, in his report to the session of the American Public Health Association, at St. Louis, in 1884, which is far from an overstatement of the truth: "We believe that the horrid practice of earth-burial does more to propagate the germs of disease and death, and to spread desolation and pestilence over the human race, than all man's ingenuity and ignorance in every other custom."

It may now be asked: "Granting that these evils are inseparable from the burial of the dead in the earth or in tombs, what is the remedy? What else can be done?"

To this question not many answers can be given, because the modes of disposing of the dead have always been and must always be few.

Plainly, no such novel mode as casting the dead into the sea will be generally adopted. Plainly, also, the mode of the Parsees, grounded as it is in ancient, if not original, use—to give the dead to beasts and birds—will not become universal. And, plainly also, cremation will not be welcome to the many, free as it is from objection on the score of public health, if a method equally sanitary, and at the same time satisfactory to a reverent and tender sentiment, can be devised.

The inquiry, then, has reached its limit. For, apart from the modes that have just been named, there are no others but earth-burial and entombment; and earth-burial, as we have seen, cannot be made sanitary under common conditions. Therefore, if the demands of affection and sanitation are both to be met, entombment is to do it, or it cannot be done.

Happily, better than any other method of disposing of the dead than has ever been devised, entombment has met the demand of affection. Never has any other

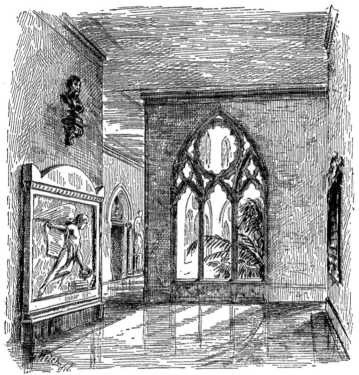

"Campo Santo," Angle of Cloister.

mode so commended itself to men as this. There may have been at times a general adoption of cremation, and there may have been a general prevalence of earth-burial, but the one has not long satisfied the sorrowing survivors, and the other has owed its beginning and continuance to the apparent absence of alternative. Wherever the living have been able, and the dead have been dearly loved or highly esteemed, the tendency to entomb and not to bury has been constantly manifested.

To call attention to this tendency is enough to prove it, so easily accessible is the evidence and so familiar is its operation in the human heart. The most natural reference will be, first, to the Mausoleum, the tomb of Mausolus, that was erected by his sorrowing Queen, Artemisia, at Halicarnassus, upon the Ægean's eastern shore; and that became at once one of the few great wonders of the ancient world. This was intended to do honor to the loved and illustrious dead; and this it did, as no grave or pyre could do. This was also intended to protect the lifeless form from ruthless robbery and reckless profanation; and it performed this task so well that, for near two thousand years, no human eye beheld the mortal part of Mausolus and no human hand disturbed its rest. At a far earlier time, Abraham, the Father of the Faithful, while he illustrated this tendency to entomb the dead, also offered an influential example to all who would do him reverence, as, in the hour of his great sorrow, he sought the seclusion and the security of Machpelah's cave for the last earthly resting-place of his beloved wife. There he buried Sarah; there he and his son and his son's son and their wives were all laid to rest, and the place of their repose hath not been violated even at this distant day. To this constant tendency constant testimony is borne by the massive and magnificent tombs in which India abounds, the tombs and pyramids that make marvelous the land of the Nile, the tombs that stood thick upon the Appian Way and that rose superb upon the Tiber's shore, the modern use to which the Pantheon is put, the Pantheon at Paris and the Crypt of the Invalides, the Abbey of Westminster matchless in memorials, the sepulchres within the hills that gird Jerusalem, and the sepulchre in which the Nazarene was gently laid when His agony was ended.

It remains to consider whether entombment can be made sanitary; if it can be, the problem is solved, for entombment has ever been the best that the living could do for their dead, and, with the added advantage of promoting, or ceasing to be prejudicial to, the public health, entombment will be the choice of all whom cost or caprice does not deter.

That entombment can be made sanitary is evident from the fact that, in countless instances, in many lands and through long periods of time, it has been made sanitary by the ingenuity of man or by unassisted nature; and it is also evident from the fact that decomposition and disease germs are the dangers to be guarded against, and that against these both ancient and modern science have been able to guard. Not to enumerate all the modes that have been chanced upon or that have been devised by men, there are two that have been notable and are available for modern use—embalming and desiccation.

It is a delusion to imagine that embalming is a lost art; that, like some other marvels of the ancient time, this is a secret process that perished with the people that employed it. Did we desire it, we could embalm our princes and our priests, and retain their shrunken similitudes for distant coming times to gaze and gape upon, as skillfully as they who practiced this art in Egypt's palmiest days. Nay, it is doubtless far within the truth to claim that, better than they did we could do; and we are actually apprized of better methods and results than they employed or could attain, and it is not unlikely that we shall hear of better methods still. But Egypt's method, or its modern counterpart, will hardly now be popular. It involves too much mutilation and too much transformation. When it has done its work little is left but bone and muscular tissue, and these are so transfused with foreign substances, that a form moulded from plastic matter or sculptured from stone could almost as truly be considered that of the lamented dead as this. Moreover, indefinite preservation of the dead is not desirable, and is not desired. The uses to which the Egyptian Pharaohs and their humbler subjects have been put in these days of indelicacy and unscrupulousness in the pursuit of science or sordid gain, are not such as to make many eager to be preserved for a similar disposition, when the present shall have become a similarly distant past.

Desiccation, in striking contrast with embalming, is the process of nature rather than of art; and involves no mutilation and no substitution of foreign substances for human flesh; and does not by unnatural means preserve the semblance of the human form so long that a susceptible sentiment is shocked and a due return of material humanity to the elements that gave it birth prevented. Desiccation is so far a natural process that it seems not to have been thought of, until nature had done the work and shown the product; and through many centuries, and upon an extensive scale, nature had employed the process before it occurred to man to copy her, and adopt her method for the disposition of his dead.

Wherever the air that enwrapped the lifeless form of man or beast was dry, desiccation anticipated and prevented decomposition. In deserts, upon elevated plains, upon the slopes of lofty mountain ranges, to which the winds that passed their summits bore no moisture, the dead have not decayed, but have dried undecomposed. In the morgue attached to the Hospice of St. Bernard, the dead, lifted too late from their shroud of snow and borne thither to await the recognition of the friends, dry and do not decay. In the "Catacombs" of the monastery of the Capuchins at Palermo, and in the "Bleikeller" at Bremen, the same phenomenon has appeared. Even Egypt is a confirmation of these statements, for it is probable that, had much less care been taken to preserve the dead, they would not there have yielded to decay as in other lands; and that moisture is so far absent from the atmosphere that the dead would have been preserved from decay by desiccation had not embalming been resorted to. Upon the elevated western plains of this continent, the bodies of beasts and men, by thousands, have been preserved from decomposition by desiccation. To take one instance out of many that might be cited: A cave was not long ago discovered high up among the Sierra Madre Mountains within which were found, where they had rested undisturbed for many years, the lifeless figures of a little aboriginal household, dried and undecayed. Father, mother, son and daughter, one by one, as death had overtaken them, had been brought thither, bound so as to keep in death the attitude that had marked them when at their rest in life, and there they bore their silent but impressive witness to the beneficent action of the unmoist air that had stayed decay and kept them innocuous to the living that survived them. In Peru, instances of this simple, wholesome process abound on almost every side; upon the elevated plains and heights, as also beside the sea, the dead of Inca lineage, with the lowliest of their subjects, are found in uncounted numbers, testifying that in their death they did not injure the living, because desiccation saved them from decomposition; and a recent traveler has vividly described the scene that a battle-field of the late war presents, and that illustrates the same process, where, though years have passed since the last harsh sound of strife was heard, the fierce and bitter combatants still seem eager to rush to conflict or to sink reluctant into the embrace of death. And all these instances furnish conclusive proof that decomposition can be controlled, and that its loathsome and unwholesome transformations can be prevented, if only the simple conditions are secured that have already so extensively effected this result. That these conditions can be secured no one can doubt; for, every day, in almost every clime, by processes familiar and available to man, the atmosphere has moisture added to it or taken from it; and the extraction of the moisture from a portion of the atmosphere is all that is required to introduce the process of Peruvian desiccation into the sepulchres of Chicago or New York.

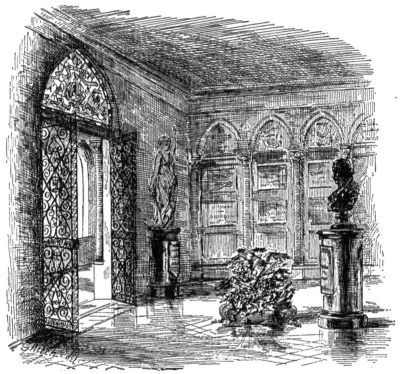

"Campo Santo," Family Compartment.

It will naturally be further asked, " Is this all that has been done to demonstrate the efficiency and availability of desiccation for the dead ?'' To this the answer would be sufficient that the evidence that has been adduced is ample; and that, at once, in perfect confidence as to the result, mausoleums might be erected, with provision for the withdrawal of the moisture from the atmosphere and for the passage of the desiccated air through the sepulchres in which the dead should rest. So little is involved, and so much has been accomplished without the application of any human skill, that it seems inevitable that, as soon as the resources of modern architecture and sanitary science are drawn upon, the desired result will be at once attained. But, to make assurance doubly sure, several carefully-conducted experiments have been made, under the supervision of the directors of the New Mausoleum movement, that prove that the conditions of desiccation can be controlled, and that decomposition can be prevented, that where it has begun it can be stayed, and that prolonged preservation, with a fair approximation to the appearance in life, can be made sure, for the recognition of absent friends, for transportation, or for the furtherance of the ends of justice.

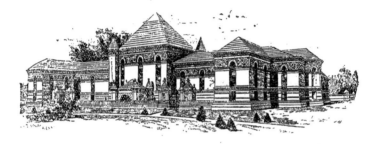

When, now, it is added, that desiccation has been ascertained to be an efficient agent in the destruction of disease germs, as proved by the experiments of Dr. Sternberg, of the Hoagland Laboratory, and by the investigations of other experts, enough seems to have been said to establish the truth of the assertion, that entombment can be made sanitary, and that, therefore, entombment offers the satisfactory solution of the problem how to dispose of the dead so as to do no violence to a reverent and tender sentiment, and at the same time not to imperil the public health.

The proposition, then, soon to be submitted for public approval is this: to erect in the suburbs of our large towns and cities, perhaps in their most thickly-populated parts, extensive and handsome edifices that will provide sanitary sepulchres for the dead. To be comparatively inexpensive, they will have to be comparatively plain; and it seems not too much to hope that our cities will soon adopt this mode of disposing of the dead that depend upon the public care for burial, and that the horrors of a "Potter's Field," of which it cannot be divested even in a fair and sea-girt isle, may be forevermore unknown of men.

All these structures, however, will not need to be inexpensive and plain. Many of them, as the rich shall lavish their wealth upon them, will be spacious and splendid, as no tombs of earlier time have ever been. These will naturally differ in design and plan, and while one will incline to one order of architecture another will incline to another; one will incline to the light and graceful style of the Greeks, another to the substantial and enduring Roman type, another to the still more firmly-built and time-defying type of the Egyptians, another to the rich and exquisitely decorative Byzantine style, and another to the Gothic type, with its suggestions of spiritual aspiration and heaven-sent consolation and heaven-born peace. It should certainly be the architect's study to avoid, as either of these styles is adopted, the appearance of edifices with familiar and established secular or sacred uses. These must, if possible, be so designed as to speak of repose and loving care and undying recollection, and should appear to be homes for the dead, and yet temporary habitations in which they only rest until the resurrection.

Perhaps the most favored style will be that of the " Campo Santo," like that at Pisa, where the Holy Field lies light upon the dead, and where the softened sunshine and the tempered wind and the hushed notes of happy birds and the sweet seclusion

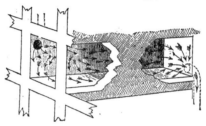

of the spacious and graceful Gothic cloister, with its memorials of many who have been loved and lamented, and its rare pictorial teaching of the life to come, all speak soothingly of hope and peace and comfort. Such a "Campo Santo," modified to meet the demands of modern life and art, might well be one of the crowning monuments even of this wondrously achieving age. To what a grand and noble consummation would it seem to lead the race in their efforts for a fitting disposition of their dead! And what honor would it reflect upon the men who should erect it and place it at the command of their fellows, in due regard for what both health and heart require!

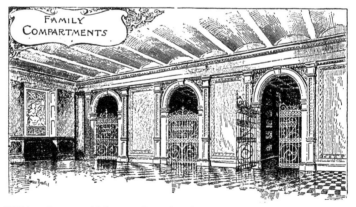

Within, there would be, as the unit of construction, each sepulchre so constructed that anhydrous air could enter, or would be made to enter, and withdraw, laden with moisture and morbific matter, which it would convey to a separate structure, where a furnace would complete the sanitary work that the anhydrous air had begun, and return to the external atmosphere nothing that would be noxious. Each sepulchre, in itself and its surroundings, would appear to provide a place of repose, and would have electrical appliances attached to it for the instant indication of the return of consciousness to any who had been prematurely entombed; and would promise and provide the most perfect and permanent protection against intrusion or theft that can be found on earth. In arrangement these sepulchres would have to conform to the price paid and the taste of the purchaser. Many would be like the single graves that thickly ridge portions of our cemeteries; many more would be grouped together after the semblance of a family-tomb, as in the

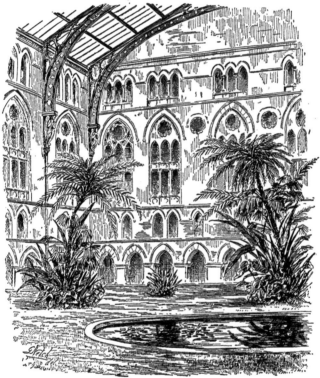

" Campo Santo, " Inner Court.

illustration; but in the general impression, in the surroundings and suggestions, the resemblance to the provisions of a cemetery would go no farther. For here, there could be no burning sun, no chilling cold, no inclement storm; for the living, as they should pay the last sad honor to the dead, or in any subsequent tribute of affection, there could be no exposure, and for the dead, there would be only the constant semblance of the comfort and the quiet of the best-ordered and most tranquil home. Thus, in providing the utmost that exacting affection and sanitary science can require, and in taxing to the utmost the resources of art, in architecture, in sculpture and in the use of subdued and according hues and forms for appropriate decoration, these " Campo Santos," or " Mausoleums," or " Mansions of the Dead," will seem to have realized the ideal disposition of the mortal remains of those who depart this life.

In conclusion, it is evident that the present modes of disposing of the dead are unscientific, unwholesome, repulsive, and, in a word, unworthy of this enlightened age.

On the other hand, it is apparent that the New Mausoleum method of disposing of the dead affords relief from all these obnoxious features, inasmuch as it provides for the perpetual care of the dead ; protects from premature interment ; protects the dead from theft ,. protects the living from exposure, while paying the last duty to the dead ; meets the demand of the most reverent and tender sentiment ; meets the urgent sanitary demand that the dead shall not endanger the living ; meets the medico-legal demand that the evidence of crime shall not be destroyed ; and costs less, in view of its manifold advantages.

Bad Air as a Disease Producer.*

By J. A. De ARMOND, M. D.
Leclaire, Iowa.

An item in the daily press states that Professor Brown-Séquard has lately informed the French Academy of Science that he had, by condensing the watery vapor coming from human lungs, obtained a poisonous liquid capable of producing almost instant death. The unreliability that would naturally cling to any statement touching a technical subject as found in a newspaper would be more than counterbalanced by the reasonableness of the fact stated. To those practitioners who have, by force of circumstances, been forced to extract teeth as a side issue to the general practice, the discovery of Dr. Brown-Séquard will not appear unreasonable. Nor, indeed, will the extreme virulence be attributed to the presence of carbonic acid, whose presence in expired air has long been recognized. When this fact, if fact it be, becomes a matter of certain knowledge, it may be the forerunner to important discoveries concerning the origin and spread of infectious and contagious diseases. It is, at least, most reasonable, and when the relation which we know exists between respirable and irrespirable air is called to mind, the body is admitted to be an important battle-ground.

In the very laudable desire to discover, if possible, the causes that underlie the origin and aid in the spread of infectious and contagious diseases, sewers and water supply surely have had a monopoly of attention. Not that they do not merit all the care and supervision they receive, but may it not be possible that in noting the large evils we overlook smaller and apparently insignificant ones, which future investigation may find worthy of supervision and correction ? Of the so-called filth diseases there can be no question but that any violation of the atmosphere, whereby it is rendered unfit for respiration, must be regarded as a cause of the disease. Bad sewers and bad

*From the *Medical Bulletin*.

drainage simply mean that the air is contaminated by being loaded with odors and gases arising from decaying vegetable and animal matter. Admitted, then, that these causes acting, can and do produce the diseases alluded to, and also aid in the spread of the diseases by lowering vitality, and thereby not only producing a disease but furnishing suitable soil for its full development, let us see what similar causes might do in more restricted quarters.

In investigating and attempting to track an epidemic of diphtheria, a few decaying potatoes in a damp cellar has satisfied many a board of health that the monster had been run to cover.

Did you ever hear of a board of health having a word to say about the old, filthy pipe that finds resting-place in so many houses? How common it is for the head of the family to sit down by the fireside of an evening and smoke an old pipe until the air of the room, and of all the rooms, in fact, is so dense that you could almost hang your hat in mid-air. Especially is this state of domestic affairs likely to be found in the small houses of the working people. When at the most three small rooms comprise the living and sleeping rooms of these families, it will be seen that it will not take one vile pipe and a vigorous smoker long to so pollute the air as to render it unfit for a brute, and still less for a human being. In the winter season economy in fuel prevents almost all attempt at ventilation. Crowd three to six or more people into a couple of small rooms, shut off all outside air, supply and then fill the house with rank tobacco-smoke, and the system has an uphill contract on hand to get enough oxygen, and what a lot of chaff must be taken in to get the little wheat needed ! Add to this vile atmosphere the smoke and odors of the cooking, and you have a state of affairs that is at once appalling. In time the inmates become yellow and smoke-cured. The children especially suffer, and when an epidemic is abroad what better place for it to anchor !

Then there is a state of domestic poisoning that is even worse than this. If added to this, as it often is, it is beyond computation, while if it is alone it is awful to contemplate. I refer now to the breath that so many people possess. Bad breath depends upon a very few causes. Bad teeth, abused stomach, and neglected mouth comprise the causes that are easily remediable. That growing class who have catarrh in various stages of development may not be able to secure such treatment as their needs demand ; but the man or woman who cannot afford to eat at meal-times and at regular stated periods, and also devote five minutes after each meal to the care of the teeth, must indeed be overworked. The price of a good, clean breath is eternal vigilance and a tooth-brush. When the truth of Dr. Brown-Séquard's discovery becomes generally known, maybe a slight impetus to keep the mouth in a healthy condition will be given.

What makes bad breath, dismissing for the time those cases of catarrh which render the possessor a sort of moral skunk ? The expired air as it leaves the healthy lungs can not and does not have the odor it is laden with when it passes out of the mouth. In a very large percentage of these cases the mouth and teeth are to blame. A filthy mouth, if it contaminates the expired air must also contaminate the inspired air, and it then follows that the foul-mouthed man not only breathes out bad air, but he also breathes it in, and in this fact there is some consolation ; but the trouble is he is not forced to smell it, and while he is poisoning himself he does not know what a nuisance he is to those around him. A man who will not clean his teeth, on the ground that it is only necessary for dudes and beaux to do that, would not wash his face if he did not have to show it to the public. Think of the man who marries a nice, clean girl, and after the honeymoon is over adopts an old pipe and neglects his teeth ! How soon his breath smells like a school-boy's slate ! The children even avoid him, and the boys are mamma's boys, and the girls are mamma's girls, and he, after twenty years' devotion to the old pipe and as long neglect of the tooth-brush, has a breath that is a terror in its way, and those who know him sit on the windward side of him when he finds consolation in reminiscent pastimes.

A custom that is yet far from extinction is largely observed by women, and relates to the insane desire of a large majority of women to kiss little children, whose inability to resist makes them powerless victims. What there is about innocent childhood that suggests to the average female mind that the child should be kissed has not yet been reported to the academy of science. A woman who has a breath like a jackal has no more right to kiss a little child than she has to slap it for walking pigeon-toed. One of these days some legislative body will embalm itself in immortal memory by making it a penal offense for an old or a young woman to kiss a baby simply because of its alleged sweetness. Like the boy in the school-fight, let them take one of their size ! Without a doubt many diseases are spread and many children rendered far from well by this kissing habit, which is very fine when properly observed, but very wrong when abused.

Sleeping-rooms are, as a rule, the poorest ventilated rooms in the average house. The havoc one inmate can work on several other occupants of a small room, with outside air closely excluded, is very great. Especially is this state of affairs liable to be found among the poor, who are forced to economize in fuel, and in the end do economize in health. When medical men fully appreciate what a powerful factor in the causation of ill health impure air is, and when the source of impure air is looked for in the house and not around it, I feel very sure an important step will be taken in locating the cause of so many ailments that have heretofore escaped detection, or been ascribed to unreliable and uncertain causes.

Cooking.

From experiments made by Jansen in the laboratory of the University of Tübingen, it appears that raw meat is much sooner digested than cooked meat. Cooking, as far as animal food is concerned, has the effect of making it more pleasing to the taste, but is unnecessary ; whereas, with certain vegetables, especially those composed principally of starch, as grain and potatoes, it is required to fit them for use. The proper preparation of food is a question that has not received the attention it demands. A badly cooked meal is more apt to disorganize the system than to prove nutritious and beneficial. The general teaching of cooking in our schools, both public and private, to girls, would undoubtedly result in much improvement in this regard.—*Science, February 7, 1890.*

The Pine Belt of New Jersey.

By BENJAMIN LEE, A. M., M. D.,

Secretary of the State Board of Health of Pennsylvania.

The establishment of a new health resort in the immediate neighborhood of a large city is always a matter of interest to the physician and the sanitarian. Not less so is the revival and rehabilitation of an old resort. For well on to a century it has been known to a limited number of the citizens of Philadelphia that there was a highly favored spot in the Pine Belt of New Jersey where the breezes of the Atlantic were drained of their dampness, without being deprived of their ozone, by passing over twenty miles of warm sand—where pine forests stretching in every direction filled the air with balsamic fragrance ; where a picturesque lake and a swiftly flowing stream tempered the fierce heats of summer, affording opportunities for aquatic sports and tempting the gentle angler, and where the surface of the country was sufficiently undulating to give zest to the scenery—just the spot which the convalescent would desire for recuperation ; the jaded and overworked, whether by the demands of business or of society, for rest ; the invalid for refuge from the noise, the dampness, the confinement and the foul air of the miles of brick and mortar and cobble-stones and sewers, which constitute an American city. This spot was known, appreciated and resorted to, we say, by a few, to whom it was known as Brown's Mills. But it had its drawbacks—it was difficult of access. The accommodations for guests were limited in extent and defective in character. The drainage was conspicuous for its absence. Now, however, all this is changed. The Pennsylvania Railroad conveys Philadelphians in its well-equipped trains, directly to the door in about an hour from Camden. A superb hotel, complete in all its appointments, has sprung up on the site formerly occupied by the old hostelry. The noteworthy features of this house, called the "Forest Springs Hotel," are the dryness of its location, the perfection of its sanitary arrangements, the spaciousness of its corridors, the profusion of open fire-places, the comfortable character of its furniture, and the soft, pleasing tone of its decorations—a matter of considerable importance to an invalid. While the temperature of the halls and sitting-rooms is made equable by steam radiators, the objectionable character of this form of heat is entirely obviated and perfect ventilation secured by roaring wood fires. Although within twenty-five miles of the ocean, its altitude is 102 feet above sea level. The drainage system of the hotel and of the laundry, which is several hundred yards distant, are entirely distinct, and neither is likely to be a source of ill-health, or even of annoyance, being carried into the current of the Rancocas. The water supply is brought from the same stream higher up, and is pure and palatable. A hydraulic elevator takes the guests to all the upper stories, and the waste water from this, which is in itself a small river, constantly flushes the drain pipes. The fall of the stream is also utilized in the production of electric light, which, as well as gas, is distributed profusely all over the house. In addition to this unfailing supply of pure drinking water, the curious anomaly is presented of the existence of two mineral springs upon the property, one sulphurous, the other chalybeate. The following are the analyses of the springs :

ANALYSIS OF SULPHUR SPRING AT BROWN'S MILLS-IN-THE-PINES.

One gallon contains

Magnesium Carbonate	0.802
Calcium Carbonate	0.897
Sodium Sulphate	0.884
Calcium Sulphate	0.269
Silica	0.249
Sulphureted Hydrogen	
Carbonic Acid	
	3.101

ANALYSIS OF IRON SPRING AT BROWN'S MILLS-IN-THE-PINES.

One gallon contains

Calcium Carbonate	3.02
Sodium Carbonate	0.12
Ferrous Carbonate	3.40
Magnesium Carbonate	1.02
Magnesium Sulphate	4.03
Calcium Sulphate	1.02
Magnesium Chloride	0.02
Alumina	.10
Silica	.13
	12.86

The kitchen forms a wing by itself, one lofty story in height, with ventilators running the entire length of the ridge pole. No odors of cooking can, therefore, offend the sensitive stomach.

Under its present liberal management the house cannot fail to soon become as popular with Philadelphians as Lake Wood is with New Yorkers. Its natural advantages are certainly greater. The capabilities of this entire tract, just at our doors, as a winter sanitarium, especially for persons with pulmonary affections, are only just beginning to be understood. The next few years will undoubtedly witness many enterprises for the sake of utilizing them.

Deaths following the use of a Soothing Syrup.

Dr. A. G. Belleau has called the attention of the Quebec Board of Health to six fatal cases among children following the use of a so-called soothing syrup, which upon examination showed the presence of opium in large proportion. It is supposed that a mistake was made in the compounding of the syrup and four or five times the amount of opium required by the formula was introduced by the mixer. In the case of five of the children, the medicine produced convulsions in which they died ; so that their deaths were certified as due to that disorder. But when the sixth child fell ill and had a coma, and not a convulsion, this irregularity led to the discovery that this intensely soothing syrup had been used, and an inquest by the coroner was ordered. The ordinary soothing syrups of the shops contain more or less opium or morphia, and are essentially so dangerous that their sale should be forbidden by law, except under the same conditions as the other preparations of known strength which must be sold and labeled as poisons, if indeed their sale cannot be interdicted altogether.—*Jour. Am. Med. Ass.*

THE ANNALS
   OF HYGIENE,
THE OFFICIAL ORGAN OF THE
State Board of Health of Pennsylvania.

The State Board of Health is not responsible for
anything appearing in this Journal except that
which bears the official attestation of the Board.

❋ ❋   PUBLISHED
        MONTHLY.

Subscription, two dollars ($2.00)
a year, in advance.

Address all communications to

The Hygienic Publishing Company,
224 SOUTH SIXTEENTH STREET,
PHILADELPHIA, PA.

EDITORIAL.

Please Remit.

On the first of April we sent bills, by mail, to all of our subscribers whose subscriptions were then due. We have heard from a few of them, but quite a number seem to have overlooked the matter. We would, therefore, take this opportunity of saying to our friends and subscribers that a remittance of the amount called for by the bill would be duly appreciated and received by us with thanks.

Proposed Wholesale Suicide in Erie.

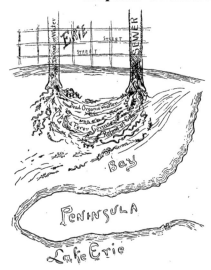

It has come to our knowledge that the authorities of the city of Erie, in this State, have recently authorized a measure which we can only characterize as "AN ORDINANCE TO RUIN THE WATER SUPPLY AND DESTROY THE HEALTH OF THE PEOPLE OF ERIE." We imagine that the city council would have been surprised, to say the least, had an ordinance, with this title, been presented to them, yet the ordinance which they have passed and which has been signed by the Mayor, should be properly designated as we have stated.

What this ordinance contemplates, or rather what it will accomplish, will be made clear by a study of our sketch. This ordinance provides for the construction of a sewer, which is liable, in time, to receive the drainage of 15,000 persons, and which will empty into the Bay, less than 2,000 feet from the intake of the water-works. Extended comment is unnecessary, for our sketch plainly shows how the people of Erie will, in reality, be taking back again in their water, that which they have voided into their sewer, if this proposition becomes a reality. We are forced to the conclusion that the full danger of this proposed measure was not realized when the ordinance was passed. The water supply of Erie is good, as we demonstrated in our January issue, and we cannot think it possible that the people will endorse its ruination and the destruction of their own health when they clearly realize the danger that is before them.

The Disposal of Refuse.

The longer we live and the more deeply we, inductively, penetrate into the nature of the causes of disease and the means for its prevention, the more thoroughly do we become impressed with the fact that the improper removal, or, we should rather say the improper *conversion*, of refuse material is at the bottom of most disease, and that one of the greatest safeguards to health is to be found in bettering the methods of disposal or conversion.

That we may have a clear understanding of what we mean by "refuse," we would remind our readers that there is no more matter in the world to-day than there was a thousand years ago and that there will not be any more a thousand years hence. Every particle of matter has its use, its own duty to perform, its own ends to accomplish, and just as we find these duties properly performed, do we find an approach to the perfection of natural laws.

Dealing, principally, with man, we can say that all particles which have been part of him, or which have been deprived of life that they might become part of him, or that are intended by nature to become part of any living thing by giving nourishment thereto, that all such particles, once deprived of life, either within or without the body of man, become refuse matter. That which has had its own life destroyed in the act of giving life to others will become capable of giving death to that life which it has helped to sustain, unless, after having performed its mission, it be handed over to NATURE to be renovated, as it were, to be treated in nature's laboratory. Just as the sweetest cider will change into the sourest vinegar, so the very elements of human life, having once been deprived of their own life will become the agents of destruction.

Therefore all *dead* organic matter, as such, is poisonous to human beings and will continue so until it has been, by nature, infused with new life. This dead organic matter will be just as fatal as will be the breathing of an atmosphere charged with illuminating gas and just as we will surely avoid the latter, so also should we shun the former. But, it would be very inconvenient, to say the least, for us to get away from the vicinity of all dead organic matter, hence does it become imperative that we should get this matter away from us. But how; in the way that nature intends. Organic matter is loaned to us by nature, that we may use it for the perpetuation of our lives; but, she wants the loan repaid; she knows that we have, by our use of it, vitiated the matter that she has loaned, but she is willing to receive it back in its damaged condition, because she is able to make the necessary repairs. Believing, as we said in the beginning, that the presence of dead organic matter is at the basis of most of the ill-health afflicting humanity, we are constrained to ask why we do not more effectually and more *naturally* combat this condition, and the answer forces itself upon us that it is, so to speak, because of our ignorance. Ignorance, first, of the prime importance of removing this matter and, secondly, of the *natural* way in which to do it. We are forced to conclude that the methods now generally in use are not satisfactory. This, we have felt for a long time, but we hesitated about saying so, because we remembered the old saying that "Any fool can find fault, but that it takes a wise man to find a remedy." We were averse to finding fault until we had a remedy to suggest. This we now have and in our next issue we will demonstrate by word and by illustration what we really believe to be an ideal, natural, perfect method of disposing of organic refuse.

NOTES AND COMMENTS.

To Keep Closets Dry.

A small box filled with lime and placed on a shelf in the pantry, or closet, will absorb dampness and keep the air in the closet dry and sweet.

Cairo Sanitation.

A Sanitary Engineer, who has been commissioned to report on measures to improve the sanitation of Cairo, recommends a sewer system of two hundred and forty miles in extent, costing $2,500,000.

Catholics and Cremation.

The Archbishop of Paris has informed the *curés* of his diocese that the Pope has forbidden Catholics to cremate their dead, or to belong to cremation societies. Catholic priests are therefore directed to refuse the usual rites when bodies are burnt.

Death from Fright.

An extraordinary case of death from fright is reported from Rangoon. It appears that a young Eurasean lad was crossing the road, when the rumbling of the wheels of a mail car frightened him, and he dropped down lifeless, the cause of death being heart failure.

Hospital for Infectious Diseases in Chicago.

Several ladies of means have undertaken to supply a "long-felt want" in Chicago—a hospital for infectious diseases, particularly diphtheria and scarlet fever. Such cases are turned away from all existing hospitals. The amount of subscription already received indicates success.

A Sanitary Court.

It was a wise Court, and a far-seeing Court, and a Court to be congratulated (up in Canada), that recently decided that a potato that was not thoroughly cooked was, in reality, a deadly weapon. Its fatal power may not be as obvious as that of the revolver, nor as rapid as that of strychnia, but it is there, all the same.

Turpentine Oil Baths.

Turpentine baths for the treatment of rheumatism, etc., may be quickly prepared by shaking up 90 to 120 grams of oil of turpentine with a very strong solution of green soap, and mixing this emulsion thoroughly with warm water when the latter is poured into the bathing-vessel.

Sweat-Bands in Hats.

Sweat-bands of hats may contain even twenty-eight per cent. of fatty acids, which in summer may penetrate into the forehead and cause inflammation, and corrode deeply into the skin. Rub with burnt magnesia every little while, so as to leave a small film on the band; wipe it off with a cloth before applying again.

A Natural Turkish Bath.

A natural Turkish bath has been discovered near Salida, Col. In digging a well not far from the Wellsville Hot Springs a cave was struck with apartments similar to the rooms of a house, the heat being so intense as to cause a veritable sweat-bath. The largest room was twenty feet long, ten feet wide and ten feet high, and the walls and ceiling perfectly smooth.

Hygiene and Hurry.

There are many simple rules of health violated because it is considered inconvenient to obey them, but it is the violation of these same simple rules that burdens life with that greater inconvenience—ill health. The busy man will find that it takes far less time to comply with hygienic laws than it does to suffer the sickness resulting from their violation.—*Sanitary News.*

A Fortune from Antipyrin.

Dr. Knorr, the discoverer of antipyrin has found a mine of wealth in the late epidemic of influenza, having taken in, by means of his royalties, considerably more than a million of dollars. He gets sixty cents on every ounce produced, and the drug sells at $1.40 per ounce. This, if true, would indicate a consumption of not less than forty tons of the article by the victims of *la grippe.*

To Stop Palpitation of the Heart.

Distressing or excessive palpitation of the heart can always be arrested by bending double, the head down and the hands hanging, so as to produce a temporary congestion of the upper portion of the body. In nearly every instance of nervous palpitation the heart immediately resumes its natural function. If the movements of respiration are arrested during this action, the effect is still more rapid.

The Hygiene of Infants.

The Paris Academy of Medicine has just opened to competition a prize of the value of 1,000 francs for the best work on the hygiene of infants. The following is the question proposed : To determine what are, in the artificial feeding of infants, the value and the effects of raw milk, warmed or boiled milk respectively. The papers, which should be written in French, the other academical rules being observed, are to be forwarded to the Academy before March 1, 1891.

Intemperance and Insanity.

Dr. Kraft-Ebing, of the University of Vienna, recognized in Europe as an authority, thinks that no proper legal measure should be neglected that may combat intemperance, and that the formation of societies to counteract it should be urged. He declares that in 20 per cent. of all cases intemperance is found to be the sole or chief cause, and in 30 per cent. more one of the causes of mental disease.

To Prevent Tuberculosis.

It is proposed to appoint veterinary inspectors in Pittsburgh, who shall be empowered to condemn all tuberculous meat, a reasonable compensation being paid to the owners of animals found in that condition; and who shall visit all milk dairies and condemn every cow found suffering from tuberculosis, particularly those with mammitis. It is also proposed to make it illegal to breed from tuberculous animals.

Perils of Foot-ball.

A recent number of the London *Lancet* had a list of seven casualties reported to it during the previous week from various parts of England. One of these was attended by a fatal result, and one of the correspondents remarked inquiringly if it would not be expedient to revive the enactment of the Scottish King James, who in 1524 decreed fifty shillings fine against any person who should be caught playing foot-ball.

Breathe Through the Nose.

Do not breathe through the mouth unless it is impossible to breathe through the nose. The nose was made for breathing, and air, passing through the long, moist, nasal passage, is purified, and leaves behind dust, disease germs and various impurities, while the air is warmed and tempered for the lungs. But when the mouth is left open, dust, dirt and disease rush down into the lungs, and fastening there, develop and destroy the whole system.—*Good Housekeeping.*

Separation of Oxygen from the Atmosphere.

A novel industry is the separating and storing of oxygen from the atmosphere. This interesting process has a unique application in the maturing of spirits and in improving the quality of beer. It is claimed that the oxygen, in its contact with spirits, actually accomplishes in a few days what, if left to the natural process, required a period of from three to five years. The oxygen gets rid of the fusil oil quickly, and when used on beer produces a rapidly maturing effect.

Sickly Children at Two Dollars.

When Stanley's expedition reached Usambiro, the station of Missionary Mackay on the south shore of the Victoria Nyanza, the sick-list was so heavy that a halt for rest was imperative. Mr. Mackay soon found that the feeble and sick children were being bought up by the natives, for two goats apiece; so that he was led to purchase about twenty-five weak children, "On Mission account," to save them from slavery. To use his own words: "The amount I have paid is two dollars per head."

Selling at Cost.

In Paris, whenever a local shopkeeper advertises to sell "at cost," a government official, detailed for the purpose, swoops down upon him, and makes a careful inspection in order to satisfy himself that the merchant carries out what he advertises. If the latter is detected in fraud an adequate punishment is at once meted out to him. They don't deny a man's right to sell his goods at less than cost if he chooses, but he must not publish any lying advertisement.—*Canadian Journal of Fabrics.*

Labor Better than Luck.

It is not luck but labor that makes the man. Luck is ever waiting for something to turn up. Labor, with keen eyes and strong will, always turns up something. Luck lies in bed and wishes the postman to bring him news of a legacy. Labor turns out at six, and with busy pen or ringing hammer, lays the foundation for a competence. Luck whines; labor whistles; luck relies on chance, labor on character; luck slips downward to self-indulgence; labor strives upward and aspires to independence.

Shaking Senators.

The report of the Secretary of the United States Senate shows that during the year ending June 30, 1889, 1,700 two-grain and 1,600 three-grain quinine pills were purchased by the Government for the use of Senators. This may seem to some persons a small kind of pickings for United States Senators to be after, but may it not also be that these dignified gentlemen having heard so much about the Potomac malaria, and believing quinine to be a good preventive, are determined to be prepared for emergencies.

Grace.

Miss Mabel Jenness, in a lecture on Grace to New York ladies, said: " Correct sitting does not mean sitting stiffly upright, tiresome to yourself and to your friends as well, and demoralizing to social approachableness; neither does it mean sliding to the front of the chair to rest on your backbone, with your shoulder bent against the chair and your abdomen in prominence. Spinal columns weren't made to sit on, but to hold the body erect. In sitting, relax every muscle except the chest muscles; they must always be doing duty. "

A Food for Infants.

In the summer diarrhœal troubles of infants, where milk in any form disagrees and vomiting is easily provoked, Jacobi says that a mixture which has rendered him valuable services is about as follows: Five ounces of barley-water, the white of one egg, from one to two teaspoonfuls of brandy or whisky, some salt and sugar; a teaspoonful every five, ten or fifteen minutes, according to circumstances. Mutton-broth may be added to the above mixture, or may be given by itself, with the white of an egg and some salt.—*Archives of Pædiatrics.*

How to Rest.

The genial president of the New York Central Railroad, Chauncey M. Depew, lets it be plainly seen that he knows "how to rest," when he tells us that during his recent trip to Florida he was not there to "study the race problem, nor the necessity for a Federal election law, nor the industrial development of the new South, nor any other novel or brain-straining question, but only to chase alligators, smell magnolias, suck fresh-picked oranges, get outside of juicy steaks and honest milk, and take in ozone."

To Clear Waste Pipes.

At night, pour into the clogged pipe enough Banner lye to fill the trap or bent part of the pipe. Be sure that no water runs in it until the next morning. During the night the lye will convert all the offal into soft-soap, and the first current of water in the morning will wash it away and clear the pipe clean as new. One thing is very important to remember, namely, that the lye is a most powerful caustic and very dangerous if used carelessly. It should never be left where children could possibly get at it.

Harvard's "Sabbatical Year."

A little paragraph recently caught our eye wherein it was stated that a certain professor of Harvard University will have leave of absence next year; it being his "Sabbatical Year"—the one in seven when he has twelve months' vacation on full salary. What a wisely glorious rule this is. A man thus periodically refreshed will do infinitely better work than he who is forever and eternally *driven* to his duty. We doubt not that this wise regulation has had much to do with the great reputation as a seat of learning that is enjoyed by Harvard.

Royal Fees for Royal Work.

The doctors who attended the late King of Portugal during the last few weeks of his illness, presented bills for their services amounting to nearly $100,000. One of them demanded $14,000 for ten visits, another demanded $17,000 for fifteen, while a third thought that $30,000 was not too much to ask for his attendance at eighteen consultations. Eventually, the new king succeeded in effecting a settlement of their claims by means of a lump sum of $60,000. The present infant king has a staff of nine physicians to look after his health.

Cosmetics.

Dr. Albert E. Ebert, in a paper on "Cosmetics," shows that the public is flagrantly swindled by manufacturers of cosmetics. He gave as an instance the case of a little pot of "cream," which has a wonderful reputation on the strength of its secret formula. It is sold for $1.50, and costs 10 cents, being composed of common zinc oxide, ground in equal parts of water and glycerin, and perfumed with rose. Another well-known wash, which retailed at $18 a dozen, was shown to consist of water and calomel, which cost 66 cents per dozen to manufacture.

Aristocratic Drainage into Philadelphia's Water-Supply.

Marshall P. Wilder, of New York, recently interviewed a colored hotel waiter on the subject of Schuylkill water:

"Sam, I hear the water you give guests to drink soaks through a graveyard. Is that so?"

"That's right, boss, that's right, shu' enough; but de people buried in dat yer graveyard am mighty high-toned people, sah: mighty so."

A Double Monster.

There is now on exhibition in England a double monster, known as the Tocci Brothers. The children are thirteen years of age, and were born of an Italian woman living in humble circumstances. The body as far as the shoulders is single, but is double above. The stomach is common to the two children, and if one eats heartily the other has no desire for food, yet it is said that the two are very unlike in their appetites and tastes, one being fond of sweets, while the other cares only for substantials. The genital organs are male, but the face of one of the children is very feminine in its appearance.

Cremating the Garbage of New York.

A New York company has offered to enter into a five years' contract with the city, under good and sufficient bonds, to take charge of and dispose of all the garbage, ashes, and street refuse of every kind at a sum not to exceed the present outlay for the disposal of garbage, which is about $250,000 a year. The company has a capital of $1,000,000 and purposes, if its offer it accepted, to erect crematories at each dumping station—fifteen in all, with extra ones for emergencies, making a total of eighteen—and to have the first of them in operation within three months, and all within a year.

"The End Crowns the Work."

Henry M. Stanley, emerging from the "Dark Continent," writes to a friend, beginning with the words of our caption and referring to those whom he had rescued, saying:

"'The end crowns the work,' did I say December 10, 1886? I say it again this date of 1890. I have brought exiles back to their homes. I have re-united parted families. I have rescued those who were in sore straits. I have borne the young and aged and placed them in their loved land of Egypt. I have brought the beleagued Governor out of his threatened bondage; wherefore as these were the aims of the work and they have been accomplished, I say: 'The end crowns the work.' True, I am blanched and white, but what matters it? I have naught to regret, and if any mission of like nature presented itself I should still wish to do it. For whatever here or there life stays not, but rushes on apace, and men must work and strive; but let us do it bravely and fitly with all our strength.'"

And the whole civilized world is ringing with the praises of Stanley. That which this intrepid explorer has done for a handful of his fellow-creatures, the sanitarian is doing for the whole of humanity. He is exploring the hitherto "Dark Continent" of disease, that he may rescue afflicted humanity from its slough of despondency and bring it out of its threatened bondage, into the glorious happiness of a sanitary enlightenment.

A Newly Reported European Epidemic.

According to cablegrams from the Continent a new plague has sprung up, called Nouna or Noma, in Russia, Austria and Italy. It bears no resemblance to any malady of recent times. The marked feature of the attack is a stupor or prolonged sleep, of twenty-four to forty-eight hours duration. This may come on suddenly in the midst of apparent good health or may be preceded by two or three days of insomnia, headache and malaise. Fatal cases have occurred, the patient never awakening; or the stupor passes off and recovery follows. Whether the disease is contagious, or otherwise, is not yet known.—*Jour. Am. Med. Ass.*

Healing Salve.

The following salve will be found a useful application for chapped lips and slight abrasions:

℞ Boric acid . . . . 2 parts.
Vaselin . . . . 30 "
Glycerin . . . . 3 "
M.

The above may be perfumed by the addition of a few drops of attar of roses, if intended for a lip salve.

Chapped Hands.

The following is a pleasant and efficacious application for chapped hands:

℞ Quince seed, ... ½ oz.
Water, ... q. s.
Glycerin, ... 1 oz.
Alcohol, ... 4 oz.

Macerate the quince seed with a pint of water for twenty-four hours, stirring frequently, strain with gentle pressure through muslin, and make the volume up to one pint with water; then add the glycerine and finally the alcohol containing the perfume and stir briskly.

Polluted Rivers.

At the meeting of the Public Health Association, held recently in Brooklyn, Dr. L. S. Kilvington, of Minneapolis, then presented a paper on "Statistics of River Pollution," with some observations relating to the destruction of garbage and refuse matter, and said that the majority of health officials in this country favor the cremation system. He also stated that in the Mississippi River, during the past year, eight cities alone deposited 152,675 tons of garbage and offal, 108,250 tons of night-soil, and 3,765 dead animals. In the Ohio River, five cities, in the same period, dumped 46,700 tons of garbage, 21,157 tons of night-soil, and 5,100 dead animals. In the Missouri River, four cities cast 36,000 tons of garbage, 22,400 tons of night-soil, and 31,600 dead animals. No theory of self-purification of running water will dwarf the magnitude of this sanitary crime.—*Medical and Surgical Reporter.*

Aids to Digestion.

1. Proper selection of food.
2. Best treatment of food as regards cooking, flavoring and serving.
3. Proper variety of food, with occasional change of diet.
4. Moderate exercise; warmth and a genial state of mind.
5. Sufficiency of sleep.
6. Pleasant social surroundings at the table.
7. Thorough mastication.
8. Regularity in eating, and proper intervals between meals.—*Anti-Adulteration Journal.*

Waxy Concretions in the Ear.

The following formula is proposed in *La Clinique* for a preparation to aid in removing accumulations of wax in the ear :

Boric acid	1 dram.
Glycerin	1½ fl. ozs.
Distilled water	1½ fl. ozs.

This should be warmed and instilled into the ear, leaving it there for a quarter of an hour, repeating the process daily for several days. The result is to soften the plugs and make their removal comparatively easy by means of the syringe.—*Druggists' Circular, February, 1890.*

Eau Dentifrice.

The following is indistinguishable from the well-known *Eau Dentifrice de Dr. Pierre*:

℞ English oil of peppermint	♏ lx.
Oil of aniseed	♏ xc.
Oil of cloves	♏ xc.
Oil of cinnamon	♏ xv.
Rectified spirit	f ℥ xx.
Saffron	gr. x.
Macerate a week, and filter.	

National Druggist, January, 1890.

What Man is made of.

Dr. Lancaster, a London physician and surgeon, recently analyzed a man and gave the results to his class in chemistry. The body operated upon weighed 154.4 pounds, The lecturer exhibited upon the platform 23.1 pounds of carbon, 2.2 pounds of lime, 22.3 ounces of phosphorus and about one ounce each of sodium, iron, potassium, magnesium and silicon. Beside this solid residue Dr. Lancaster estimated that there were 5,595 cubic feet of oxygen, weighing 121 pounds; 105,900 cubic feet of hydrogen, weighing 15.4 pounds, and 52 cubic feet of nitrogen in the man's body. All of these elements combined in the following: One hundred and twenty-one pounds of water, 16.5 pounds gelatine, 1.32 pounds fat, 8.8 pounds fibrin and albumen and 7.7 pounds of phosphate of lime and other minerals.

An Athletic Lady.

An English paper asserts that there is a titled lady whose chief pleasure is found in exhibiting her muscular powers in her own drawing-room to a circle of admiring and astonished friends. Attired in a long and clinging gown, she lies down at full length upon the floor, with arms held closely to her sides. A friend is then requested to fasten her skirts securely around her feet and place her handkerchief upon them. This done the handkerchief is conveyed by her feet to her mouth. She then resumes her first position, and, without moving her arms, gradually raises herself until she stands upon her feet, without a hair out of place or the tiniest bead of moisture on her brow.

Indian Corn.

Says an exchange: When Dr. Johnson, in preparing his dictionary, defined oat-meal as something on which the English fed their horses and the Scotch their men, Boswell remarked: "Yes; but what men and what horses!" An enterprising American now wants to show the Scottish people the advantages of Indian corn as a wholesome and strengthening food, and proposes to make an exhibit of it at the Edinburgh International Exhibition, which is to open on May 1st next. Corn-meal has an advantage over oat-meal in the varied methods of preparing it for the table, and in the fact that it can be used not only as food, but as an addition to the dessert. There will be an economic value in such an exhibit.

Important in Fumigation.

Dr. Squibb, of Brooklyn (*Medical News*), in a recent address on sulphur fumigation in the prevention of infectious disease, directed attention to the important fact that, in the absence of moisture, the penetrating power of sulphurous acid gas is only slight, and for this reason there should be an abundance of aqueous vapor in the apartment in which the sulphur is burnt. Boards of Health neglect to emphasize this fact, which is not known to the laity. The *Medical News* recommends that water be kept boiling in the room in which gas is being generated. Dr. Squibb also called attention to the relative uselessness of chlorine gas as a disinfectant in the absence of aqueous vapor.—*The Pacific Record.*

Hereditary Transmission of Peculiarities.

A singular instance of the transmission of hereditary peculiarities has been brought to the notice of the German Anthropological Society. The correspondent tells of his meeting a farmer by the name of Loewendorf, who had a peculiar habit of writing "Austug" for "August," his Christian name. Some years later he was inspecting a school, and heard a little girl read "leneb" for "leben," "naled" for "nadel," and so on. Upon inquiring, he found that her name was Loewendorf, and that she was the daughter of his former friend, the farmer, now dead. This defect was noticeable in the speech and writing of both father and daughter. It appeared in the father as the result of a fall that occurred some time before the birth of his daughter.

Gum-Chewers' Teeth.

The chewing-gum habit is looked upon favorably by some dentists (says a writer in *Epoch*) and by all dealers in dental supplies; by the latter because chewing-gum is being sold as a tooth-cleansing agent. Chewing-gum is supposed to aid digestion, for the increase in saliva is usually retained in the system in contradistinction to tobacco-chewing, in which case it is expectorated. It has also been claimed that the constant use of chewing-gum prevents sea-sickness, and some think that it benefits sufferers from lung troubles, although by such the pure spruce gum only should be selected. Gum-chewing is liable to enlarge the muscles which control the movements of the lower jaw, thereby changing, possibly for the better, both the contour and the expression of the face. If the gum be pure, I see nothing in the habit to condemn except its vulgarity, as it has no effect upon the teeth beyond that already stated.

Perspiring Feet.

Not long ago the relative values of various remedies for the treatment of perspiring feet were being tested by military surgeons abroad. A weak chromic acid solution seemed to yield the best results, and was adopted for the German army. Still, the acid solution is not entirely satisfactory, since it must be used most cautiously and, when applied to sore feet, not unfrequently gives rise to severe inflammation.

A simple and perfectly harmless preparation is the following:

℞ Talc . . . . 10 parts.
  Alum . . . . 2 parts.
  Mix, and dust freely and frequently on the feet.

This preparation has proved most efficacious, and is largely used in the Swiss army.—*Medical and Surgical Reporter.*

Mouth Washes.

Hygiene of the teeth is as important as that of other parts of the body; and prophylaxis in this direction will prevent decay as well as keep the teeth clean and the breath sweet. Monte, in the *Deutsche med. Wochenschrift*, October 31, 1889, gives the two following formulas for prophylactic mouth washes:

℞ Acidi borici . . . . gr. xxxviij
  Aquæ destillatæ . . . . f ℥ vij
  Tincturæ Myrrhæ . . . . ℳ xxxxviij
  M.
℞ Sodii salicyl . . . . gr. xxxxiij
  Aquæ destillatæ . . . . f ℥ vij
  Tincturæ Myrrhæ . . . . . . ℳ xxxxviij
  M.
Sig. Wash out the mouth several times daily with either of the above formulæ.

PLAYS affect the sexes differently. At a recent performance there was hardly a woman in the house whose eyes were dry, but to gauge by the men going out between the acts the dryness must have left the women's eyes to get in their throats.

Treating Infectious Diseases.

M. Letulle proposes that the following regulations should be adopted in hospitals, and by doctors treating infectious diseases. Every patient brought to the hospital suffering from a contagious affection should be immediately placed in an isolated ward, so that all contact between infectious cases and surgical cases should be avoided. The clothing of each patient should be disinfected on his arrival at the hospital. A hot bath and subsequent cleansing with a solution of corrosive sublimate at 1 in 1,000 should be practiced. The hospital furniture should be made of iron and easily taken to pieces, so that it may be disinfected at the departure of each patient. The different rooms should be thoroughly aired and disinfected, and all cases of contagious disease isolated. In his hospital practice the physician should avoid importing or carrying away any morbid germ. He should therefore wear a blouse in the wards and disinfect his clothes daily. The same rules apply to his private |practice when he has cases of contagious affections to attend.—*Paris Correspondence British Medical Journal.*

Wash Your Hands.

Surgeons understand how readily disease may be carried by the hands, and, under favorable circumstances, communicated to others, particularly certain specific diseases. In referring to the subject of unclean hands, the *Sanitary Era* says that cases of infection, that could be accounted for in no other way, have been explained by the fingers as a vehicle. In handling money, especially of paper, door knobs, banisters, car straps, and a hundred things that every one must frequently touch, there are chances innumerable of picking up germs of typhoid, scarlatina, diphtheria, small-pox, etc. Yet some persons actually put such things in their mouths, if not too large! Before eating, or touching that which is to be eaten, the hands should be immediately and scrupulously washed. We hear much about general cleanliness as "next to godliness." It may be added that here, in particular, it is also ahead of health and safety. The Jews made no mistake in that "except they washed they ate not." It was a sanitary ordinance as well as an ordinance of decency.— *Sanitary Volunteer.*

Artificial Ice.

We are glad to learn that a company has been recently formed in Germantown for the manufacture of "artificial ice"—glad, because therein we see the possibility to secure absolutely pure ice. We must know that impure ice is as dangerous to health as impure water or foul milk, and oftentimes we know but little of the source of the ice delivered at our doors. It will be an easy matter for this company to make its ice from pure water; and if they start out with this resolve and adhere firmly to it, they ought to find a ready sale for all the ice they can make.

PROF. GEORGE H. ROHE has been appointed to the honorable and responsible position of Commissioner of Health for the City of Baltimore. He will bring to the accomplishment of his work experience, culture, and rare executive power. The city is to be congratulated for this selection.

Precautions Against Cholera in Caucasian Russia.

According to the Voljsky Vestnik, 1890, February 21, the Caucasian governor-in-chief has issued an order of the day (prikaz) in which, while pointing out that cholera still prevails in Mesopotamia and Persia, and that it is very possible that the disease may spread to the Caucasian military district, he lays down a series of precautionary measures to be immediately adopted all over the district. The chief measures are as follows: Strict sanitary supervision of barracks, hospitals, and lazarettes; the formation of military sanitary commissions; arrangements for opening cholera wards and infirmaries; special courses for army surgeons and medical assistants (feldshers) in connection with the first aid to cholera patients, and so on.

Disinfection of Rooms by Ozone.

Make a mixture of equal parts of manganese dioxide, potassium permanganate and oxalic acid. This mixture, moistened with water, evolves ozone instantaneously. For a room of ordinary size two spoonfuls of this powder are placed on a plate and moistened from time to time; ozone is given off, and the atmosphere is disinfected without exciting coughing. Care should be taken to remove all metallic articles from the room (save silver and gold) since ozone oxidizes them more or less. The disengagement of ozone can in part be substituted in close apartments for a changing of the air; the organic matters derived from respiration which pollute the atmosphere are gradually destroyed by the ozone and the air purified.—Rhode Island Board of Health.

The Art of Prolonging Life.

Somewhat different advice must be given with regard to bodily exercises in their reference to longevity. Exercise is essential to the preservation of health; inactivity is a potent cause of wasting and degeneration. The vigor and equality of the circulation, the functions of the skin, and the aëration of the blood are all promoted by muscular activity, which thus keeps up a proper balance and relation between the important organs of the body. In youth the vigor of the system is often so great that if one organ be sluggish another part will make amends for the deficiency by acting vicariously, and without any consequent damage to itself. In old age the tasks cannot be thus shifted from one organ to another; the work allotted to each sufficiently taxes its strength, and vicarious action cannot be performed without mischief. Hence, the importance of maintaining, as far as possible, the equable action of all the bodily organs, so that [the share of the vital processes assigned to each shall be properly accomplished. For this reason exercise is an important part of the conduct of life in old age, but discretion is absolutely necessary. An old man should discover by experience how much exercise he can take without exhausting his powers, and should be careful never to exceed the limit. Old persons are apt to forget that their staying powers are much less than they once were, and that, while a walk of two or three miles may prove easy and pleasurable, the addition of a return journey of similar length will seriously overtax the strength.—Dr. Robson Roose, in Popular Science Monthly for October.

Antiseptic Property of Coffee.

It has been lately shown by Lüderitz, from a series of experiments conducted by him in the Berlin Institute of Hygiene, that coffee as a drink (infusion) possesses very decided antiseptic properties. Several different forms of bacteria were experimented on, and their growth was found in all cases to be interfered with by the addition of a small quantity of coffee infusion to nutrient gelatine. In pure infusion the bacteria were rapidly destroyed. The question as to what constituents exercise the antiseptic action cannot yet be answered. The caffein is certainly only active to a slight degree, the tannic acid to a greater extent, but probably of greatest importance are substances which are formed during roasting. It is interesting to note that a cup of coffee left lying in a room remains almost free from microörganisms for a week or more.—*Berlin Klin. Woch.*

Vaccination and Small-Pox.

We are reminded again by *Gesundheit* that while the German Empire and some other countries, as the result of their wise and salutary compulsory vaccination laws, are seeing small-pox almost wholly excluded from their borders, those neighboring lands in which vaccination is optional are still suffering from the old-time pestilence. The following table shows the number of deaths from small-pox in each million of inhabitants, in each country named:

		1887.	1888.
Austria-Hungary,	} Vaccination optional,	583.7	540.4
Russia,		535.9	231.5
France,		167.0	191.9
German Empire,	} Vaccination compulsory	1.8	0.8
Denmark,		0.0	0.0
Sweden and Norway,		0.0	0.0

—*Sanitary Inspector.*

The Clothing of Babies.

Although I own that children are now more sensibly clothed than was the case thirty years ago, it is still common to see an infant, who can take no exercise to warm himself, wearing a low-necked, short-sleeved, short-coated dress in the coldest weather. The two parts of the body—viz., the upper portion of the chest and the lower portion of the abdomen—which it is most important to keep from variations of temperature, are exposed, and the child is rendered liable to colds, coughs, and lung diseases on the one hand, and bowel complaint on the other. What little there is of the dress is chiefly composed of open work and embroidery, so that there is about as much warmth in it as in a wire sieve, and the socks accompanying such a dress are of cold, white cotton, exposing a cruel length of blue and red leg. I can not see the beauty of a pair of livid-blue legs, and would much rather behold them comfortably clad in a pair of stockings. If the beauty lie in the shape of the leg, that shape will be displayed to as much advantage in a pair of stockings; if it lie in the coloring of the flesh, beautiful coloring will not be obtained by leaving the leg bare ; and, from the artistic point of view, a blue *or* red stocking is infinitely preferable to a blue *and* red leg.—From " Mental and Physical Training of Children," by Jessie O. Waller, in the *Popular Science Monthly for December.*

The Profit of Amusement.

The daily *Telegraph* (of this city) commenting on the fact that twenty-five thousand residents of Boston, recently, dropping all business, turned out to witness two games of base-ball and, noting that the same story comes from all our great cities, says that "It might be supposed that the world had turned backwards several thousand years and we were living in an age when the highest purpose of human existence was to find some sort of amusement." Would to goodness, that this thought may be realized. Innocent amusement should be the first thought of humanity and the business necessary to furnish it should be a secondary consideration. Let us encourage this growing tendency towards harmless recreation by every means in our power, for it means good health and all the happiness that is necessarily attendant upon it.

Clearing-Houses of Disease.

The "Dime Savings Banks," that are so rapidly springing into existence throughout the country, may be, not inaptly styled "Clearing-Houses for Disease," because to them will be brought dimes and nickels, greasy and decorated, in many cases, with the germs of disease. We do not make this observation as a reproach, but that we may make a suggestion whereby these banks may become great blessings to humanity. If the authorities will arrange (which they can do at but little cost), to submit all the metal money brought to them to the beneficent action of steam. they will thus destroy all germs of disease thereon, and will thus become not only a boon to the poor by the facilities they offer for saving, but they will be in reality benefactors of humanity, as they will become the agents for the centralization and destruction of very many germs of disease.

The Dwellings of the Poor.

Prof. Ely very truly says, in *The Century*, that it is a sad commentary on our Christian civilization that when there is more than one man in New York city claiming to be a Christian who, alone and unaided, could reconstruct the entire tenement-house district or districts of the city, the unspeakable wretchedness and squalor of its slums continue almost unabated. But, if the Christians do not, the Jews do see the appropriateness of this work, for we are informed that Baron Hirsch, the great European banker, has concluded to send to this country $10,000 monthly to be used in supplying better classes of habitations to the poorer classes of Jews. So, also, we learn that Sir Edward Guinness has selected several sites in London for the erection of dwellings for the working classes, which are to differ from the famous Peabody houses in that they will be let only to the poorest class of laborers and that the rent will be almost nominal .These are moves in the right direction. The filthy tenement houses of a large city are veritable breeding places for disease germs, from which they go forth to slay without mercy or fear the occupants of the more fashionable and richer palaces of the city. Self preservation, to say nothing of philanthropy, should prompt us to improve (and that thoroughly) the habitations of the poorer classes.

Meat Inspection and Pure Food.

The United States Senate recently passed a bill providing for the inspection of meats for exportation and forbidding the imposition of adulterated food or drink. The bill provides for an inspection, under the direction of the Secretary of Agriculture, of salted pork and bacon, to be exported, whenever the laws of any foreign country to which the pork or bacon is to be shipped require inspection upon its importation into such country.

The bill also forbids the importation of adulterated or unwholesome food, or adulterated wines or liquors, and provides suitable penalties. It authorizes the President to suspend the importation of animals by proclamation when such a step is necessary to prevent infectious or contagious diseases.

The Health of London in 1889.

Remarkable as has been the continual decline of the death-rate in England and Wales in recent years, the decrease of the rate of mortality in London, with its aggregate population of more than four millions, with constantly increasing density, is still more remarkable. The Registrar-General, in his last annual summary, reported that the death-rate in registration London in 1888 was 18.5 per 1,000, being "far the lowest death-rate as yet recorded in London," the next lowest being 19.8, 19.9, and 19.6 in the three immediately preceding years 1885–86–87, previously to which the London death-rate had never fallen below 20 per 1,000. The death-rate in 1889, moreover, again fell, and was considerably below the low rate in 1888. The Registrar-General's return for the fifty-second week of 1889, just issued, affords the means of calculating that the mean annual death-rate in London in the fifty-two weeks of last year did not exceed 17.5 per 1,000, was 1 per 1,000 below the rate in 1888.—*Lancet, January 4, 1890.*

Emotion as a Power.

If there was not so much "common sense" about hygiene, we fancy it would be even more popular than it is. It is has been repeatedly and truthfully said that the rarest of all senses, is "common sense," and since it requires "common sense" to make one appreciate the "common sense" value of hygiene, it may be that, in the comparative rarity of this commodity, we will find the reason why so few, comparatively, seem to take a lively interest in the subject. That which appeals to the more illy defined attributes of humanity, such as the emotions or the superstitions, seems to take a much stronger hold than that which is directed towards the "common sense." We recently read that the "Salvation Army," (appealing to the emotions) now numbers more than two million souls. So also, we see men grow rich from the sale of a drug, which they claim will kill microbes, but, when the sanitarian tells us of a "common sense" way, in which we can destroy these microbes he is, at once, regarded as a "harmless lunatic." There are no charms, mysteries, incantations, amulets, moon-stones or trade-marks about hygiene; there is nothing emotional about it; it is merely the results of experience viewed from the standpoint of "common sense;" hence its votaries are, comparatively, limited. But, do let us all cultivate a little more *common sense.*

Prolongation of Life.

Why should men, women and children die of disease at all? (asks Dr. Alfred Carpenter). There is no provision for death in early life except by accident, ignorance of the laws of health, and neglect of duty towards our neighbor on the part of somebody. * * * Why do some die, and some recover? Why should disease be fatal at all? Fatality is connected to some extent with the surroundings in which the patient has lived before he became affected, and is living at the time at which the disease commences in a given district. If there has been a large number of fatal cases of inflammation of the lungs, you may be certain that the air of that district is not so pure as it ought to be, and the habits of the inhabitants are not so prudent as they might be. No man dies of inflammation of the lungs in middle life, or indeed of any acute disease, be it what it may, if he has lived healthily both as to habits and character of surroundings. If a district has a death rate of 24 in the 1,000, it is double what it ought to be. The half of the deaths which takes place might have been prevented if the people would obey the laws of health, keep their houses and their persons clean, dispose of their excreta in a proper way, and be temperate in their habits of living, and at the same time do their duty to their neighbor by avoiding the sophistication of articles of diet, or the mischief of adulteration.—*The Monthly Bulletin.*

Danger in Preserved Food. '

Dr. Charles M. Cresson, Chemist of the Philadelphia Board of Health, reported to that body recently, that for several months past he has been engaged in making an examination of vegetables packed in glass jars in some preserving fluid covered with a loose plate of glass, which is held in place by a metallic cap. Over the whole cap is placed one of the ordinary stamped metallic caps.

"The evident intention is to use a metal cap," says the report, "which is not affected by the prevailing fluid or by the juices of the vegetables, and tin has been selected by the packer for the purpose. If pure tin had been selected, it is probable that but little action would have taken place upon the metal; but unfortunately the tin employed in the jars which I examined contained the metal lead, and this metal has been dissolved to a greater or less degree by the preserving fluid. The asparagus and peas were notably contaminated with lead and to a degree which I consider unwholesome. In addition to lead, the sprouts contained copper, which was probably introduced either by boiling the vegetables in copper vessels, or by the use of copper salt for improving the color of the goods.

"It should not be forgotten that the action of nearly all the metals, when introduced into the human system, is cumulative, that is to say that the dose of one day is added to that of the day following, so that, however small and comparatively harmless, the quantity of the metal introduced at a meal may be, the time at length arrives when the system becomes so impregnated as to occasion injurious and even poisonous results. This view of the matter demontrates the necessity of insisting upon the absolute freedom of all articles consumed as food from even the minutest amount of avoidable metallic contamination."

Philanthropy and Hygiene.

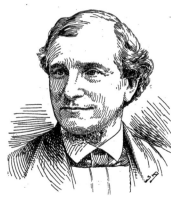

George H. Stuart.

As we have taken occasion, elsewhere, to assert that avarice and hygiene are incompatible, so now we would formulate the close relationship that exists between philanthropy and hygiene. The true philanthropist, he who like the late George H. Stuart, (so universally known as the efficient head of "The Christian Commission" during our late war,) really loves his fellow creatures so truly that the best efforts of his life are devoted to bettering not only their spiritual but their temporal conditions, such a man is a sanitarian in the highest sense of the word. That serene, inner self-contentment, the ever-present result of an effort to think well of humanity and to practically aid our fellow creatures, must, of necessity vouchsafe to its possessor an integrity of function, both mental and physical, that will not only prolong his life, as it did in the case of Mr. Stuart (he was seventy-five years of age when he died), but that will make life worth living while we live.

Boxing the Ears and its Results

We would fain hope that, in deference to repeated warnings from various quarters, the injurious practice of boxing the ears, once common in schools, is fast and surely becoming obsolete. It is too much to say that this desirable end has yet been realized. Certainly the recent observations of Mr. W. H. R. Stewart do not give color to any such view. In a pamphlet on "Boxing the Ears and its Results," lately published, and referred to in the *Lancet*, December 21, 1889, he briefly summarizes his own experience in the matter. Notwithstanding the toughness of the aural drum-head, its tense expanse will rupture only too readily under the sudden impact of air driven inward along the meatus, as it is in the act of cuffing; and Mr. Stewart shows that in one instance at least this injury resulted from a very slight though sudden blow. Given early and skilled attention, the wound may heal very kindly, but if the beginning of mischief be overlooked, as it often has been, further signs of inflammation soon follow, and a deaf and suppurating tympanum is the usual result. There is practical wisdom in the statement that this consequence most readily follows in the case of the poorly developed and underfed children who abound in every Board school. In them, an earache would probably receive no very strict attention, and disease might for a time work havoc unimpeded. Where chronic suppuration exists already, and it is only too common, a random knock on the ear may, and has resulted, in fatal brain complications. The close connection between ear and brain should never be forgotten, and the reflection that injury to the former organ most easily terminates in total deafness, and in suppuration which may any day take a fatal course, should assist in the preservation of a sometimes difficult patience.
—*Lancet.*

The Wearing of Veils.

No doubt a young and pretty girl decked out as our illustration depicts, is a pleasant sight to the beholder, and is calculated to produce a sense of pleasure, regarded as a specimen of nature's handiwork, that will tend towards a more happy and inspiriting view of life. But such a young lady is not doing justice to herself, howsoever much she may gratify the æsthetic sense of others. The bad practice of wearing veils must prove injurious to the sight, however gratifying they may be to human vanity. Particularly is this so of the dotted veils, for the presence of one of these little dots close up to the eye will not help to keep the eyes in good condition. As far as possible we believe in sailing with fashion, but we can have no word of commendation for the fashion of veil-wearing, it will certainly not do the eyes any good and it is more than likely that it will do them a deal of harm.

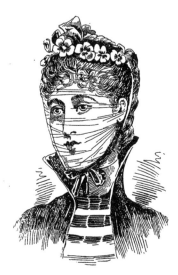

The Transmission of Typhoid Fever by the Air.

It is generally admitted that the transmission of typhoid fever takes place principally through the water supply. Experience, indeed, has proved this to be the case ; but—as the *Medical Press* of February 5, 1890, says—it must not be overlooked that other ways may exist, and speaks of introduction of typhoid bacilli by the breathing of air contaminated with the spores. Some observations by Dr. Chour, of an epidemic of typhoid fever among soldiers, commented upon in the *Revue Scientifique*, serve to show the importance of not concentrating one's attention too exclusively upon any one vehicle in the endeavor to prevent the spread of the disease. Two regiments stationed at Jitomir, and supplied with drinking water from the same source, suffered in a very different degree from the disease. The soldiers belonging to the regiment which suffered most severely were quartered in various barracks, and it was remarked that at one particular locality the men were attacked in a far larger proportion than their fellows, who were located elsewhere. In December, 1886, the buildings were evacuated and thoroughly cleansed and disinfected, whereupon the mortality fell to 1.7 per thousand in 1887, and to 0 in 1888. In the other barracks, which had not been thus dealt with, the mortality rose to 22 per 1,000 in 1887, and to 33 per 1,000 in 1888. It occurred to Dr. Chour to institute an examination of the dust from the infected barracks, and he found in it an average of fourteen million microbes per gramme, among which the typhoid bacillus was easily detected. The evacuation of the rooms and their thorough disinfection promptly put an end to the epidemic.—*Medical and Surgical Reporter.*

The Emperor William.

A recent despatch tells us that the Emperor William of Germany has been at Wartburg, "the place where Luther threw his inkstand at the Devil," and we are tempted to suggest to the Emperor that he should throw his inkstand, loaded with dynamite, at the heads of the "leading medical authorities of England and Germany," for this same despatch tells us that these wiseacres have assured him that he has before him not more than ten years of life, or, at least, of sanity. This, they claim, because of the reappearance of a hitherto dormant scrofulous trouble. Such advice would directly tend to kill or drive mad anyone to whom it is given. We are glad to learn that these wise gentlemen have *ceased to administer drugs, recommending instead exercise and change of scene*, which, if persisted in, with a suitable regard for other hygienic rules, will vouchsafe to the Emperor many times ten years of both life and sanity.

The Lesson of Randall's Life.

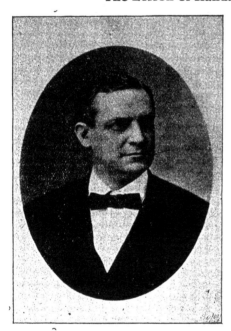

Hon. Samuel J. Randall, late Congressman from Pennsylvania.

If we accept the statements from all sources, opponents, politically, as well as friends, the late Congressman Samuel J. Randall was a man who, preeminently, wished to be right in all that he did. Just, to an unusual degree, toward the people whom he served, he was unjust to himself, in so far as the thought of self-preservation was never within him. Thoroughly versed in the law of the land, he was, we must presume, woefully ignorant of the natural laws of his own humanity. Ignorant, we presume, because, being so thoroughly imbued with the desire to do right, it would have been impossible for Mr. Randall to have ignored the laws of nature, or of hygiene, had they been familiar to him.

In the death of this great man, cut down before his time, we strongly read the need for all, and particularly for those whose services can be illy spared, to familiarize themselves with the laws of nature, to master the art of self-government, to learn how to live.

There are so few such men as Mr. Randall was that we cannot afford to lose them, particularly, when we know that it is within the pale of possibility to keep them with us for a time longer.

Bicycling for Young People.

. Dr. B. W. Richardson discusses this subject in a recent issue of the *Æsclepiad.* He admits that since he first warned the public of the dangers of immoderate cycling, changes have taken place in the construction, both of bicycles and tricycles, which materially modify the old drawbacks. He is still, however, of opinion that cycling should never be practiced by boys and girls, since it differs from other exercises in the fact that it moulds the bodily framework, as it were, to its own mode of motion; and riders in course of time almost invariably acquire what he calls "the cyclist's figure," which is not graceful, and is not indicative of the possession of perfectly balanced powers. Of two things at least he is satisfied: they are that the temptation of competition is, to an earnest and practiced cyclist, a "demon of danger," and that the systematic pursuit of cycling should never be fully commenced before the age of twenty-one.

Kissing the Bible.

Judge Arnold, of the Common Pleas Court of this city, deserves the sincere thanks of all sanitarians for having officially decided that it is not necessary for one to kiss a dirty and, perhaps, disease-germ bedecked bible, when taking an oath in his Court. When a witness in his Court declined to kiss the bible, she was sustained by Judge Arnold, in the following emphatic and unmistakable language :

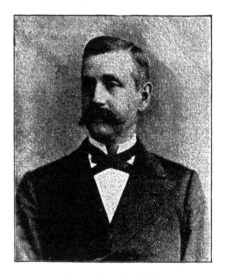

Judge Arnold, of Philadelphia.

"I am not surprised that this witness did not kiss the book. I would not do it either, a dirty book like that. This custom is a relic of idolatry, and the sooner it is abolished the better it will be. I don't think this witness objected to kissing the book because she intended to lie, but because it is a dirty book. I respect her regard for her person and her health."

After the trial Judge Arnold was asked what he meant by kissing the bible being a relic of idolatry that ought to be abolished. He replied:

"I mean that it was established by the Church to show the humiliation of the people before the first judges, who were clerics. It has been abolished in England; judicial declarations subject to penalties being substituted.

"I mean that it is a relic of a superstitious age and superstitious people. It is a relic of that age in which trial by fire took the place of trial by jury; when a man's guilt or innocence depended on his physical capacity to resist pain and torture; but its worst feature is the dirt and disease which is imparted to the book by the constant handling it receives from dirty witnesses, and I not only would not kiss such a book myself, but have a respect for those who have enough respect for themselves to refuse to do so."

The Dangers of Kissing.

The daily papers are strongly condemning, rather ridiculing, the efforts of a society recently formed for the suppression of the "kissing habit," one paper saying :

"Forswear your war on kissing, unhappy beings, lest you be forsworn by every soul whose veins run blood, not ice water. There are some forms of caprice so fantastical that the human race—patient and long suffering as it is—openly revolts against them.

"The kiss is inviolable. No vandal need hope to profane it by hurling medical sophistries at it. Joyous the thought that kisses will be given in boldness and taken with blushes thousinds of years after the feeble voice of these protesters has been stilled by the icy kiss that no man can shun."

Now, then, this paper is wrong, because it does not properly comprehend the question. It is promiscuous, indiscriminate kissing that is to be condemned ; the prevalent habit of every one kissing children that is to be deprecated. There is no harm in the kissing of relatives, of intimate friends, of those who know all about each other, but, sentiment and newspapers to the contrary notwithstanding, there is a real danger in promiscuous kissing and it is not at all to be questioned that much disease is transmitted thereby.

Arsenical Wall-Paper.

The danger of using hangings or wall-paper which contains arsenic was very forcibly illustrated in Berlin not long since by the famous chemist and expert, Dr. Paul Jeserich, the head of the renowned Sunshine Laboratory.

A woman and her little child were taken suddenly and dangerously ill without any apparent cause and the family physician was summoned in haste. After a careful examination he decided that his patients had all the symptoms of arsenical poisoning. He did everything in his power to help them and finally they were removed into another room to see if any change would prove beneficial and they very soon recovered. Upon going back to their former sleeping place they were again prostrated and once more removed.

Dr. Jeserich was summoned, and he at once attacked the wall-paper. He found that the walls carried three layers of paper, having been repapered twice. A most careful examination revealed no trace of arsenic whatever in the two outer papers, but the inner or original covering contained an enormous quantity of the poison. To a surface of twelve square metres, which is about the area covered by wall-paper in a room of moderate size, the paper contained twenty grammes of arsenic acid.

The incident affords striking evidence of the danger of selecting wall-papers without knowing the acids which are used in their coloring.

However, we need not worry much about this danger in this country to-day, as there are very few arsenical wall-papers to be found in our better class of stores, because the shades of green that are now fashionable are not made with arsenic.

Leprosy in China.

Leprosy is viewed by the Chinese as infectious, contagious and hereditary, but it is prone, they think, to exhaust itself in four generations. As many as eight varieties of leprosy are recognized. In the interior of China there are leper villages, to which all suffering from this disease must be sent.

Avarice and Hygiene.

As with water and oil, so with avarice and hygiene, they will not mix. He, who like Tamagno, the famous tenor, who has been lately receiving $2,000 of our good money for one evening's singing, is so avaricious that he will resort to every subterfuge to save his pennies, cannot have good digestion, an active liver, nor healthy and refreshing sleep. We do not, of course; favor extravagance, but we hold that he who can command $2,000 for two hours' services, yet washes his own handkerchiefs, as a measure of economy, is a mean, miserly fellow, to whom serenity of mind, so essential to health, happiness and longevity, must be a stranger.

The Health of Hebrews.

One of the Jewish pastors of Montreal, the Rev. Mr. De Sola, has been lecturing upon a very interesting subject, that of the Jewish dietary laws, which account in such great measure for the healthfulness of the race.

The Mosaic law, he pointed out, permitted for use as food only the flesh of such animals as divide the hoof and chew the cud. In the killing of these animals the strictest examination had to be made to prevent the communication of disease to man. Mr. De Sola said that, so far as his own congregation was concerned, lambs and calves usually passed examination, but 50 per cent. of sheep and 50 per cent. of cows slaughtered in Montreal were rejected. Yet the rest of the population eats this contentedly enough. As to fish, the Jews only eat those with both fins and scales, and oysters, in Mr. De Sola's opinion, are simply "the scavengers of the sea." Lobsters, crabs, and other crustacea are likewise tabooed. The result of the great care taken by the Jews as to their diet is famous everywhere in the extraordinary low death rate of this people and their immunity from epidemics which decimate other sections of the population.

How to Keep Down Fat.

The fact that so many *anti-fat* suggestions are made is pretty good evidence that the course that will be successful in one case will not do for another. Hence, whenever we hear of any method that has been successful, we reproduce it for the benefit of our readers, so that if one fails another may be tried, thus hoping to bring comfort to our adipose friends who wish to reduce their incumbrance. Here follows the course that has been successfully persevered in for two years by the Duchess of Marlborough :

"Not a morsel of bread, cakes, rolls or pastry. No tea, coffee, chocolate or sweet wine. No potatoes, peas, rice, carrots, turnips, macaroni, cheese, butter, cream, custard, jellies or sweets. Not a drop of ice-water. No warm baths. No flannel and only enough clothing to keep from taking cold. No bed-room heat. Not a drop of any liquid food at meals In place of bread she had fruit. Her diet was limited to two meals a day, breakfast at 10 and dinner at 7, with the following bill of fare to select from : Rare, lean meats, game and poultry, soft-boiled eggs, sea foods, toast, lettuce, spinach, celery, cresses, fruits.

"She had half a gallon of hot water to drink every day, with lemon juice in it to take away the flat taste. Cold water was denied her, and ales, frappes, champagne and claret strictly forbidden. She was even forced to forego the luxury of bathing in water, in place of which she had sponge and vapor baths. Every few days she took a fast, allowing the system to consume the adipose tissue. While no limit was put upon the pleasure of driving or riding, she was asked to select the roughest, rockiest roads, and to walk from five to ten miles a day in the open air."

Powdered Milk.

The *American Analyst*, March 6, 1890, quotes from the *American Dairyman* the following in regard to a proposed substitute for milk :

The idea of reducing cows' milk to a dry powder, and shipping it in this condition all over the world, seems to have originated with Dr. Krueger, a Swiss savant, and under his management a company was organized to make milk powder in Switzerland. It is claimed that milk in this form is much better than canned or condensed milk ; for one reason, it has no sugar in it. It is well known that condensed milk cannot be used in many departments of cooking on account of the sugar, and this also makes it objectionable for use with very young children, not that the sugar itself is injurious to the babies, for it is always put into their milk, we, believe, but it is better that this sugar be put in fresh at the time of preparing milk for the child. How far this powdered milk will answer these objections remains to be seen. One thing is certain, the powder will be much better for transportation and more handy to have in the house than either plain or condensed milk, provided it is a success. It looks somewhat dubious as a complete substitute for plain milk, not only on account of necessary expenses, but we do not find any kind of food capable of being thoroughly dried and afterward made over with water so as to closely resemble the original article, and we never expect to see it done with cows' milk. Nature has a way of mingling these things that thus far man has not been able to closely imitate.—*Medical and Surgical Reporter.*

Blood Poisoning from a Glove.

A somewhat sensational paragraph has appeared in a London lay paper relating to the death of a lady which is said to have been due to blood poisoning derived from a glove. The facts, as stated, are as follows : A young Jewess from Kieff was visiting her friends in the Polish capital, who, in honor of her visit, gave a large ball. The young lady, well known for her beauty and other attractions, purchased for the occasion a pair of long Danish gloves. While in the middle of a dance she suddenly felt a severe pain in her left wrist, which rapidly became inflamed and swollen. Upon reflection she remembered to have slightly pricked the wrist with a pin while making her toilet. Subsequently medical examination showed that the young lady was suffering from carbuncle and blood poisoning, contracted from the glove. The medical men in attendance expressed their conviction that the glove had been made from the skin of an animal suffering from anthrax. Within forty-eight hours their unfortunate patient was dead. The rapidity of the development of the symptoms is not the least remarkable feature in this case ; we do not question the theory which has been advanced to account for the attack ; it is a quite possible one, though without corroborative evidence it sounds just a little transcendental. In view of the process through which "skins" have to pass before being cut up into gloves, a perfectly disinterested person can only feel some admiration for the robustness of the individual microbes whose tenacity of life and purpose enabled them at the proper moment to give expression to their malignity.—*Med. Press and Circular, January 8, 1890.*

What Produces Death.

Some one says few men die of age. Almost all persons die of disappointment, personal, mental, or bodily toil, or accident. The passions kill men, sometimes even suddenly. The common expression, "choked with passion" has little exaggeration in it, for even though not suddenly fatal, strong passions shorten life. Strong-bodied men often die young; weak men live longer than the strong, for the strong use their strength, and the weak have none to use. The latter take care of themselves, the former do not. As it is with the body, so it is with the mind and temper. The strong are apt to break, or, like the candle, run; the weak burn out. The inferior animals, which live temperate lives, have generally their prescribed term of years. The horse lives twenty-five years, the ox fifteen or twenty, the lion about twenty, the hog ten or twelve, the rabbit eight, the guinea-pig six or seven. The numbers of all bear proportion to the time the animal takes to grow its full size. But man, of all animals, is one that seldom comes up to the average. He ought to live a hundred years, according to the physiological law, for five times twenty are one hundred; but, instead of that, he scarcely reaches an average of four times the growing period. The reason is obvious: man is not only the most irregular and most intemperate, but the most laborious and hard-working of all animals. He is always the most irritable of all animals, and there is reason to believe, though we cannot tell what an animal secretly feels, that, more than any other animal, man cherishes wrath to keep it warm, and consumes himself with the fire of his own reflections.—*Scientific American, November 9, 1889.*

Antiseptic Vapor.

A recently devised method of supplying buildings with antiseptic vapor has met with considerable success, the plan consisting, briefly, in forcing fresh air from the purest available source outside into the building, by means of a rotary fan or air-blower; this fan can be driven by the waste steam from an engine on the premises, and the atmosphere at the same time heated by the steam. The temperature thus given to the air is regulated by the simple device of mixing cold air with it in the proportions required; flues or pipes convey the warmed air to the various parts of the building where it is desired, and the outflow from the pipes is controlled by simple regulators—both the temperature and supply being thus under the complete control of the persons in the building.

The advantages of forcing the fresh air into the building under a slight pressure are that cold draughts are excluded and the vitiated air is forced outwards by every available opening. In a building supplied with electric-lighting apparatus, the waste steam of the dynamo engine is used to warm and ventilate it at the same time. By inserting in the flue trays of porous materials such as cotton waste, soaked in essence of eucalyptus, pinol, or any other antiseptic and aromatic extract of a volatile nature, the air in its passage to the various rooms of the building, or it may be to any one particular room, is impregnated with antiseptic vapor. For hospitals, this system is regarded as well-adapted, and for private individuals suffering from diseases of the breathing organs it is said to be almost equally applicable, whether in the office or the home.

Artesian Water at Memphis.

The *Bulletin* of the Tennessee State Board of Health, February 20, 1890, contains a very interesting account of the system of water-supply at Memphis, which is now as fine as any city could have. This account would interest any one who cares to know the principles and methods of artesian water-supply, and would prove instructive to any who are not familiar with the subject.

So far as Memphis is concerned, it is gratifying to learn that the supply of artesian water at Memphis is practically inexhaustible. Such is the capacity of the water-bearing sand, and so enormous its area for gathering its store, that it is thought that Memphis, in using profusely all she may need for years to come, cannot make an impression on the sea of supply below. It is assured that there is no possibility of an admixture of the river or surface waters about Memphis, or of sewage fluids, with the waters of the artesian wells. The upward pressure from the wells, to a point even above high water of the Mississippi, gives this assurance.

The quality of the water for all city purposes has proved highly satisfactory. Its source is from a region boasting of its water, and from that it percolates through miles of sand, coming out transparent and sparkling, unaffected by washing rains or turbid streams. Its introduction was an epoch and a blessing to all concerned. Finally, the system for gathering and controlling the self-flowing water, and for sending it through the iron arteries of the city, is not only unique, but admirable in conception and execution.

While congratulating the inhabitants of Memphis upon securing so magnificent a supply of water for drinking and domestic uses, it is pleasant to know that artesian well-water is within easy reach of many other cities in our country, especially in the great Valley of the Mississippi.—*Medical and Surgical Reporter.*

Early History of Water Supply.

During the first century of our era the water supply of ancient Rome was so abundant "that whole rivers of water flowed through the streets." It has been estimated at 375,000,000 gallons per day, or 375 gallons for each inhabitant, and was conducted through nine costly conduits of masonry, in whose construction wonderful engineering skill was shown. Their aggregate length was 249 miles. The principal aqueducts were the Aqua Martia, erected 431 B. C., 38 miles in length, and partly composed of 7,000 arches; the Aqua Claudia, a subterranean channel for 36¼ miles, for 10¾ miles a surface conduit, 3 miles a vaulted tunnel, and 7 miles on lofty arcades, with a capacity of 96,000,000 gallons daily; and the Nova Anio, which was 43 miles in length. Some of these aqueducts rose in three distinct arches, which conveyed water from sources of different elevations. In Constantinople, the capital of the Eastern Empire, the Romans left numerous subterraneous reservoirs covered with stone arcades resting on pillars. In France, also, the famous Pont du Gard aqueduct, which supplied the town of Nismes, is still an object of interest. It consists of three tiers of arches, the lowest of six, supporting eleven of equal span in the central tier, surmounted by thirty-five of smaller size. Its height is 180 feet, with a channel 5 feet high by 10 feet wide. The capacity was estimated at 14,000,000 gallons per day.

India is noted for numerous ancient impounding reservoirs of vast dimensions. The Poniary reservoir has an area of 50,000 acres, and banks 50 miles in extent. In Mexico and Peru the aboriginies left water channels of wonderful length. The great aqueduct of Peru, built by the Incas, was 360 miles long.

The works of the Romans left nothing to be improved upon in the method of transporting water from a distance until recent times ; but in the early part of this century it was found that by sinking artesian wells a supply could be obtained more economically.—*Maverick's National Bank's Manual, Boston, Mass.*

Treatment of Obesity.

In an article on the Physiological Treatment of Obesity in the *N. Y. Medical Record*, February 15, 1890, Dr. Walter Mendelson gives the following diet list made up as an average of two by Oertel and somewhat modified for American habits. Such a list is only to serve as a *general guide* to the patient to whom it is to be given. No absolutely hard-and-fast rules can be laid down, and patients under treatment should be seen—and weighed—from time to time ; increasing one kind of food and diminishing another as occasion demands.

Breakfast : 1 cup (6 ozs) tea or coffee, with milk and sugar. Bread, 2½ ozs. (2 or 3 slices). Butter, ½ oz. 1 egg or 1½ oz. meat.

Dinner : Meat or fish, 7 oz. Green vegetables, 2 ozs. (spinach, cabbage, string beans, asparagus, tomatoes; beet tops, etc.) Farinaceous dishes, 3½ ozs. (potatoes, rice, hominy, macaroni, etc.), or these may be omitted and a corresponding amount of green vegetables substituted. Salad, with plain dressing, 1 oz. Fruit, 3½ ozs. Water, sparingly.

Supper or Lunch : 2 eggs, or lean meat, 5 ozs. Salad (radishes, pickles, etc.), ¾ oz. Bread, ¾ oz. (1 slice). Fruit, 3½ ozs. Or fruit may be omitted and bread, 2 ozs., substituted. Fluids (tea, coffee, etc.), 8 ozs. No beer, ale, cider, champagne, sweet wines and spirits. Claret and hock in great moderation. Milk, except as an addition to tea or coffee, only occasionally. Eat no rich gravies, and nothing fried. Patients should always feel *better*—never worse—under treatment. Lassitude and fatigue are signs that the muscular tissue, as well as the fat, is being reduced, and that more non-nitrogenous food must then be allowed.

Dr. Mendelson says : Never yield to the wishes of the patient to grow thin *quickly*. All reforms, to be lasting and beneficial, must be slow in action, they must be the result of education, they must be a growth from within, not an impress from without. And the cells of the body, in their infinite diversity of occupation resembling the citizens of a state, can by slow degrees be habituated to better things, to change their vicious mode of action to one harmonious with the welfare of the commonwealth. And when this education has once been established, continuance becomes a mere habit.

Professional Athletes.

" Show me a professional athlete 40 years old," said an eminent physician, "and I will show you a man old beyond his time, with bones out of shape, muscles injured, and joints stiffened, and no one would promise him five years more of life."

National Conference of the State Boards of Health.

The sixth annual meeting of the Conference of State Boards of Health will be held at the Maxwell House, Nashville, on Monday, May 19th, preceding the annual meeting of the American Medical Association. The meeting will be called to order at 9 A. M.

The following questions for the consideration of the Conference have been received by the Secretary :

Proposed by State Board of Michigan. The editing and printing of annual reports of State Boards of Health, and other methods of disseminating public health knowledge.

Discussion opened by Dr. Henry B. Baker and Dr. C. A. Lindsley.

Proposed by State Board of Rhode Island. By what means can a proper comprehension of the principles and practices of hygiene be most effectually promoted.

Discussion opened by Dr. C. H. Fisher and Dr. Ezra M. Hunt.

Proposed by State Board of Kentucky. Resolved, That upon the outbreak of yellow fever or other epidemic disease, rendering the establishment of quarantine necessary, this Conference urges such co-operation in administration on the part of threatened States as will confine the disease to the point of initial attack, in place of the expensive, unscientific and unsatisfactory so-called quarantines at distant State lines.

Resolved, That this Conference urges upon the health authorities of each State the importance of such an administration of any quarantine they may establish as will furnish proper protection to, and show due regard for the rights of States lying beyond them.

Discussion opened by Dr. Pinkney Thompson and Dr. J. D. Plunket.

Proposed by State Board of Pennsylvania. What steps should the United States Government take to prevent the introduction of leprosy into this country ?

Discussion opened by Dr. L. F. Salomon and Dr. Granville P. Conn.

Proposed by State Board of Michigan. To what extent is it necessary to moisten the air of rooms at the time sulphur is burned for the purpose of disinfection, after the occurrence of diphtheria, scarlet fever, and small-pox ?

Discussion opened by Dr. Victor C. Vaughan and Dr. C. W. Chancellor.

Proposed by State Board of Kansas. Is it not both important and very desirable for all State Boards of Health to have a uniform system of blanks for the reports of vital statistics ?

Discussion opened by Dr. J. F. Kennedy and Dr. S. W. Abbott.

Proposed by State Board of California. How to prevent contamination of potable waters ?

Discussion opened by Dr. C. A. Ruggles and Dr. J. T. Reeye.

Proposed by State Board of Ohio. Should State Boards of Health have executive powers ?

Discussion opened by Dr. Henry B. Baker and Dr. Benjamin Lee.

Fourth State Sanitary Convention of Pennsylvania.

A Sanitary Convention, to which the public is invited, will be held at Norristown, Pa., on Friday and Saturday, May 9 and 10, 1890, under the auspices of the State Board of Health, acting in conjunction with the Board of Health of Norristown. There will be three sessions on the first day, and two on the second.

OFFICERS.—President, Hon. Henry K. Boyer, State Treasurer elect ; Vice-Presidents, Hon. Thomas J. Stewart, Secretary of Internal Affairs ; Surgeon-General

L. W. Read, M. D.; Hon. A. S. Swarts, Prest. Judge; Hon. H. K. Weand, Additional 'Law Judge; Hon. Charles Hunsicker, Rev. Isaac Gibson, Rev. Charles Fulton, Rev. Thomas Beeber, Hiram Corson, M. D., Hon. H. R. Brown, State Senator; Hon. I. Newton Evans, Hon. Austin P. Taggart, Member House of Representatives; Hon. Alan Wood, Mr. Charles Heber Clark, Mr. S. Powell Childs, Mr. Samuel Anders, |J. K. 'Reid, M. D., Hon. Charles Moore, Member House of Representatives; Mr. Morgan R. Wills, Editor *Norristown Herald;* Mr. William Rennyson, Editor *Norristown Times;* Secretary, William B. Atkinson, M. D., Hon. Professor of Sanitary Science, Med. Chi. College; Assistant Secretary, H. H. Whitcomb, M. D.

It is intended that the essays and discussion shall be entirely of a practical 'and popular character. The object of the convention will not be scientific research, but the unfolding of the results of such research with such clearness and simplicity that " he who runneth may read." It is especially desired that ladies, on whom so much of the hygiene of the home depends, shall attend. The occasion will be one of especial interest and profit to Health Officers and Municipal Authorities, who, it is trusted, will avail themselves of the opportunity.

The Annual Address will be delivered on Friday evening, by Mr. A. Arnold Clark, Member of the State Board of Health of Michigan.

Among the eminent gentlemen from whom papers are expected are the:

Hon. H. K. Weand, of Norristown, on " The Necessity for Sanitary Organization of the State under Legislative Sanction."

Dr. C. W. Chancellor, Secretary of the State Board of Health of Maryland, on " The Purification of Drinking Water."

Gen. D. H. Hastings, on " Some of the Sanitary Lessons of Johnstown."

Prof. Pemberton Dudley, of Philadelphia, Member of the State Board of Health, on " The Importance of the Early Diagnosis of Cummunicable Diseases and their Immediate Report to the Health Authorities."

Rev. Mr. Bridenbaugh, Pastor of the Church of the Ascension, Norristown, on " The Dangers Arising from Public Funerals in the Case of Contagious Diseases."

Prof. Henry Leffmann, of Philadelphia, on " The Employment of Salicylic Acid as a Food Preservative."

Dr. S. D. Risley, of the University of Pennsylvania, on " The Eyes of our Public School Children."

Subjects connected with the Sanitary Necessities of Norristown will be treated by the members of the medical profession resident in the borough. It is desirable that the length of papers should not exceed twenty minutes, as free discussion is solicited, and ten minutes will be allowed to each participant. The papers are expected to be original contributions, and will be left with the Secretary of the State Board of Health.

Arrangements for reduced transportation have been made with the Railroad Companies.

Committee of the State Board of Health: Dr. Joseph F. Edwards, Dr. Pemberton Dudley, Dr. Benjamin Lee. Committee of Norristown Board of Health : Dr. P. Y. Eisenberg, Joseph K. Weaver, M. D., Mr. Samuel E. Nyce.

For further information, address   Dr. P. Y. EISENBERG, *Chairman,*

Norristown, Pa.

Second-Hand Coffins.

Somewhat of an agitation has recently been created in this city in reference to the subsequent use of coffins in which bodies have been carried to the crematory. As a similar question may arise at any time in any place, it might be as well to have a clear understanding on the subject. We do not think it wise policy to make an observance of the laws of hygiene an unnecessary hardship, and since the repeated use of the same coffin tends to lessen the cost of a funeral, we do not see why it should be forbidden unless there is real danger in such a practice, and we do not think that there is. Of course, if death has been due to a contagious disease then the coffin and everything that has been about the body should be destroyed; but, if this element of danger has not been present, then we see no reason why the destruction of the coffin should be deemed necessary, due regard for proper cleanliness being, we think, all-sufficient. This question coming up, causes us to suggest to funeral directors that the "ice-box," in which a corpse, dead of contagious disease, has been preserved, may prove a menace to the health of some household into which it is subsequently introduced, and to urge upon them the importance of thorough disinfection (with corrosive sublimate) in all such cases.

State Board of Health and Vital Statistics of the Commonwealth of Pennsylvania.

PRESIDENT,
GEORGE G. GROFF, M. D., of Lewisburg.

SECRETARY,
BENJAMIN LEE, M. D., of Philadelphia.

MEMBERS,
PEMBERTON DUDLEY, M. D., of Philadelphia.

J. F. EDWARDS, M. D., of Philadelphia.	GEORGE G. GROFF, M. D., of Lewisburg.
J. H. McCLELLAND, M. D., of Pittsburgh.	S. T. DAVIS, M. D., of Lancaster.
HOWARD MURPHY, C. E., of Philadelphia.	BENJAMIN LEE, M. D., of Philadelphia.

PLACE OF MEETING,
Supreme Court Room, State Capitol, Harrisburg, unless otherwise ordered.

TIME OF MEETING,
Second Wednesday in May, July and November.

EXECUTIVE COMMITTEE,

PEMBERTON DUDLEY, M. D., Chairman.	JOSEPH F. EDWARDS, M. D.
HOWARD MURPHY, C. E.	BENJAMIN LEE, M. D., Secretary.

Place of Meeting (until otherwise ordered)—Executive Office, 1532 Pine Street, Philadelphia.

Time of Meeting—Third Wednesday in January, April, July and October.

Secretary's Address—1532 Pine Street, Philadelphia.

Bureau of Registration and Vital Statistics—Department of Internal Affairs, State Capitol, Harrisburg.

State Superintendent of Registration of Vital Statistics—BENJAMIN LEE, M. D.

THE
ANNALS
OF
HYGIENE

VOLUME V.

Philadelphia, June 1, 1890

NUMBER 6.

COMMUNICATIONS

The Necessity for Sanitary Organization of the State under Legislative Sanction.*

BY HON. H. K. WEAND,
Of Norristown, Pa.

The increasing interest shown in all matters relating to the public health, and the adoption of sanitary laws, and the beneficial results arising from investigation into the hidden causes of diseases and the best means of preventing them, is a subject for congratulation not only by the medical profession and sanitarians, but by all who believe that, to a certain extent, contagious diseases at least can be met and fought in a practical manner in our everyday life.

When the subject of our health thus becomes a practical one, and when it can be brought home to the knowledge of thinking men that by studying the cause and origin of disease it will be found that much of it can be prevented by simple rules, and that we ourselves, by ignorance or indifference, are indirectly, if not directly, the cause of much suffering and distress, which could be easily avoided, and thus add to our daily comfort and prolong our lives, the matter will appeal to us as one of such general importance as to deserve for it the same consideration which we give to the protection of our persons and property.

If we can by the study of disease, the elements which cause it, how and where it is propagated and how best it can be defeated, become insurers of our health, the plainest dictates of common sense and humanity require us to adopt such methods as will procure these results.

I feel safe in assuming that this body, at least, recognizes the necessity and advantage of some general system of sanitary regulation throughout the State, which shall at the same time be the most practical, thorough and effective in its purpose to ascertain the cause of and to prevent, as well as to arrest, disease arising from any source which may create it, either by polluting the air or

---

*Read before the State Sanitary Convention at Norristown, Pa., May 9th and 10th, 1890.

water ; by insufficient drainage ; the maintenance of cesspools or the disposal of garbage, and which shall, by the proper enforcement of laws adapted for the purpose, preserve the public health from these and other agencies, and also to disseminate useful and practical knowledge upon this all-important subject.

That combined effort in this regard is more likely to accomplish the end desired than individual action is self-evident, but the question still remains, ought it to be done by legislative sanction, as a measure in which the State is or can be interested ?

I therefore propose to treat the subject with reference to the duty of the Commonwealth in relation to health laws, and the advantage and necessity of general sanitary regulations capable of enforcement.

The paramount object of all organization is to protect and benefit those who enter into it. To most effectually accomplish this purpose, power must be lodged in some person or body to enforce obedience, and to counsel and advise by proper rules and laws, else if each is allowed to act upon his individual opinion the object of the organization fails. For where all are left to do as they please, there are none to be governed, and hence no necessity for government.

The primary object of State government is, therefore, the protection of the people in their lives and property ; so that each may pursue that course which is best conducive to the enjoyment and defending life and liberty ; of acquiring, possessing and protecting property and reputation, and of pursuing their own happiness. In the pursuit of these objects there must necessarily be some rule of conduct laid down by the superior power, to which all must yield obedience. To state that every individual in the community ought freely and voluntarily to do that which will produce these results is but to recognize the dictates of reason. Self-preservation is the first law of nature, and men will return blow for blow in defence of their persons ; shoot the midnight thief to protect their property, although this may be replaced or restored. How much more, therefore, ought they to endeavor to prevent the loss of health, which when once lost may never be restored or regained, and which in every condition of the social scale is more important than mere worldly wealth. But even though the individual should, after being robbed, condone the offence or consent to injuries which may render him unable to pursue his ordinary occupation, or may so far forget his duty to himself, his family or society, as to attempt his own destruction, the State will not consent that these acts shall go unpunished. At common law to attempt suicide is a crime ; to render oneself habitually drunk is punishable, and so of many acts committed by individuals in a manner only directly affecting themselves, yet indirectly affecting the community by impairing their usefulness. All this proceeds upon the theory that in an organized political body, such as a State, city, or other municipality, each individual in return for the protection afforded, owes a duty to the whole community, and that the power to enforce this duty must be lodged in the organization as an entire body.

Manifestly, it is to the interest of the State that its citizens should be honest, that each may enjoy his own ; that they should be intelligent, diligent and frugal, for this produces prosperity ; that they should be temperate and moral, for this prevents crime ; and that they should be healthy, for without this the other good results are less likely to follow or may be of no benefit. People of intelligence recognize the fact that sickness means pain and distress leading to premature death ; that health means pleasure and contentment or the means of acquiring it, and prolonged life through natural causes. Besides our natural instincts teach us that cleanliness is more desirable than filth ; and what is fair and pleasing to the eye and taste is more desirable than the reverse. But as unfortunately all do not think alike or agree as to what constitutes cleanliness or what is proper in a given case, and as there always have been and always will be those who set themselves in opposition to all laws human and divine, natural or political, who imagine that the only true rule of life and government is that every one should so live as to violate no written and positive law, and who only obey these from fear of the punishment following the violation, it becomes absolutely necessary for the State, as a guardian of the public interests, to interfere for the general good. For while many will eagerly resent an attempt of an individual or set of individuals to correct an abuse or to reform an evil, they will consent to such action when it appears to be sanctioned by positive law ; and if not willing to yield obedience, they must be forced to do so. In our everyday life we constantly do that which our conscience may question, but which we sanction merely because it is the law. To say to a man, " You ought not to do so, because the act is morally wrong," provokes the reply, " Who made you the judge ?" But to say to him, " The law forbids it," generally disarms him and insures obedience.

If, therefore, as an eminent prime minister of England once said, " The health of the people is the first duty of the statesman," it would appear that the Legislature of our State could have no more important subject brought to their attention than that which relates to the protection of the public health, and if this can be better accomplished by a general sanitary system under the protection of the law, and having for its main purpose the enforcement of rules and regulations which will tend to prevent disease, remove and abate nuisances which affect the health, and by the collection of vital statistics enable us to study and comprehend more effectually the origin and nature of our everyday ailments, they will simply be doing that which in this age of advancement and progress becomes a duty and its neglect a crime.

That the members of the State Board of Health recognize the necessity for some general and systematic action must be apparent ; for to them now, with their limited organization, powers and means, is entrusted the subject of all those matters involving the causes of disease, with the duty resting upon them to disseminate information upon the subject which shall be best calculated to prepare us for such action as will make the appearance of contagious diseases, especially, less likely to happen, as well as to instruct us how we shall in everyday life so act as to protect our health.

To the credit of the medical profession it may be said that much of the indifference shown with reference to the enforcement of sanitary laws arises from the faith which we have in their power to do the proper thing at the proper time, and hence the general indifference on the part of laymen. As a result, nearly every effort looking to good results in these matters comes from the medical profession ; and yet, with all their efforts, the result is not entirely satisfactory.

It is reasonable to assume that much of this indifference arises from our ignorance, and not because we do not value or truly estimate the benefits shown to follow. Until danger appears, few think of it. We are apt to speak of cranks and theorists, and to the average mind to guard now against an epidemic not immediately apparent is a waste of time ; and to pass laws even against ordinary nuisances is regarded as nothing more than an attempt to be better than your neighbor.

Thus, indifference leads to delay and neglect, until contagious disease appears ; and then in our frantic efforts to ward off its effects and arrest its spread, we blame the doctors and the law, without reflecting that we ourselves are responsible for the result.

As in all movements of the kind, the first thing to do is to interest every intelligent thinking man, woman and child in the subject by teaching the danger of non-attention to health laws ; to show how disease is created and how to avoid it ; and by pointing out the danger resulting from a violation of those sanitary laws which modern science and learning have demonstrated to be the sure cause of contagious diseases, arouse public sentiment by an appeal to reason.

When a community becomes thus alive to the importance of the subject, it will be found that public sentiment will induce that which otherwise it might be difficult to accomplish.

For when a community is taught that acts manifestly for their own good and advantage are prompted not by selfish, arbitrary, vain or personal motives, they make the cause their own and unite in enforcing obedience. But if good is thus to be accomplished it ought to be systematic, general and uniform, and not confined to a few localities ; for, whilst in a certain sense this would be a gain to the localities immediately affected, it does not meet the trouble.

Contagious diseases cannot be arrested in their progress by geographical lines, and a community in which the strictest rules of health are enforced is still liable to be affected by a communicable disease brought to it from other places.

If, therefore, the individual owes it as a duty to the State to give it his best efforts, and if such efforts can best be obtained by healthy bodies, so far as individuals can ordinarily produce such results ; if his duty to himself, his family and his neighbors require him to be an active worker for his, their and the general good, he should be in favor of such measures as will best produce that result.

On the other hand, if the State as the guardian of the citizen owes him the duty of education and protection in health as well as in life and property, the necessity for some general system regulating the observance and enforcement of health laws must be apparent.

If it is wise to enact a law prohibiting the sale of unwholesome food, because of the evil effects likely to follow, why not equally wise to forbid the pollution of water, or rendering the air which we breathe impure, if they also affect the health ? These remarks, of course, can only apply to those acts which naturally and inevitably tend to create disease, and which, from their public character, are likely to seriously affect the community, and which are based upon hygienic laws, which experience has shown cannot be violated without producing evil results.

This subject has already received the attention of many of the States, including Pennsylvania ; but it has only been done in such a qualified manner as not to meet the requirements of the subject, and further legislation would be justified if for no other reason than as an educational measure. If to be forewarned is to be forearmed, then to be forearmed is half the battle. The good which results from knowing what to do in a given emergency and how to do it well, especially in case of sickness, cannot be overestimated.

Thus, local organizations, by acquiring a knowledge of the laws of health, especially with reference to those diseases contagious in their nature, the treatment of epidemic and other diseases, the proper application of sanitary principles to practical life, and then being able to act intelligently and advise others how to do so in matters requiring speedy action on questions of public health, must be of inestimable benefit to a community. We all know how we dread the approach of contagious diseases, how easily a community is alarmed and almost thrown into a panic by the sudden appearance of cholera, smallpox or kindred diseases in our midst, and what a feeling of comfort follows when we know that there are those at hand who, by previous study and preparation, with authority to act and with knowledge what to do, and a willingness and desire to afford relief. In many cases speedy and judicious action has saved a community a loss of life and property which otherwise might have been disastrous.

To be armed with knowledge adapted to the situation, wisdom and courage to properly apply this knowledge, and authority to enforce obedience to all needful rules and regulations is at once to be master of the situation. The benefits of such local organizations, even limited in their sphere, is shown by our own local board of health, who have already done so much good by their efforts to prevent nuisances, and to direct the attention of our people to those thoughtless acts which experience has shown produce disease and death. Would it not therefore be wise if in each locality organizations could be formed, composed of energetic, public-spirited citizens and physicians, who would act in concert with a State board, and thus make that general which is now confined to but few localities ?

But to make this good the more effectual, local boards should, if possible, be compulsory, and be under the sanction of law, armed with proper authority, without which they lose much of their value. Generally, under their police powers, municipalities have authority to protect the public health, but such authority is usually exerted, if at all, when too late, and rather as a cure than prevention. Boards of health should be compulsory, and not as now left to the option of cities, boroughs or townships.

It has been found from experience that local authorities are slow to act in these matters except in cases of emergency, and then find themselves unprepared. Besides, when optional, it will be found that when such organization is effected. in many cases it becomes useless by reason of influences brought to bear upon its members.

Too often politics enter into these matters, and thus a few influential citizens can prevent any action whatever. Neighborly kindness and a desire not to wound the feelings of others often restrain us from doing that which we know to be a duty, and which we would not hesitate in doing if the law commands us to act. It may also be doubted whether, under existing laws, there is sufficient power vested in municipalities, except in the large cities, which would warrant certain summary proceedings at times made necessary. But even if there is, the threats of law-suits and the doubt as to the right to proceed makes us hesitate to act when the effect of such action may cause loss and damage to others even though it be for the public good.

The rights and duties of health officers should be clearly defined by law so that well-meaning officials may not be made to suffer when acting for the public for mere errors of judgment. Every lawyer is aware that when an officer of the State Board of Health is called into the community to investigate and report upon an alleged nuisance, or to report upon a matter affecting the public health, that there is at once created a prejudice against him as an intruder, and if a suit is the result, the party accused most generally has the sympathy of the locality with him, and the officer considers himself fortunate if he escapes without payment of costs. This would not be the case if a local board acted in the matter. It would be felt at once that they could not be actuated by any other than proper motives and a desire to benefit the community. Another most important advantage to be gained is through the information communicated by the local to the State board, in the shape of reports as to particular cases not 'of frequent occurrence. Such cases invite discussion, research and investigation leading to good results. To a great extent, of course, this end is obtained through local medical societies, but this depends upon the disposition and will of the physicians having the case in hand.

Given a case involving symptoms of contagion, it must be of inestimable benefit to the physician to have the opinion of a competent body, such as we assume a State board would be, upon the subject, rather than to rely solely upon his own judgment, or his particular county society, no matter how competent its members may be. The benefits of discovery, the interchange of thought, combined action and the result of careful consideration upon such subjects cannot but be of advantage.

It is as wise to enforce and enact laws to protect health as property, when it can be done without infringing upon the rights of individuals ; and it is no more wrong to treat that which affects our health as an enemy to be punished, than it is to punish the thief or the common scold. How this shall be done can safely be left to those who have made these matters their special study. Details are at present unimportant ; the necessity now arises for some expression of opinion that will result in bringing the matter before the law makers.

The Legislature of Pennsylvania has to some extent seen the wisdom and necessity of State action in this matter, and the result has been the Act of June 3d, 1885, establishing a State Board of Health ; but this was a feeble beginning, and although the results have been highly beneficial it is not entirely satisfactory, owing to the limited appropriations for its support. It consists of six physicians whose duties extend all over the State. It is required to make sanitary inquiries respecting the causes of disease and especially of epidemic diseases, including those of domestic animals ; the sources of mortality and the effect of employments, conditions, habits, foods, beverages, and medicine upon the health of the people ; and it shall disseminate information upon these and similar subjects.

The organization of local boards in cities, boroughs, or other districts is entirely optional with those localities. It is also authorized from time to time to engage suitable persons to render sanitary service, or to make or supervise practical and scientific investigation and examinations requiring expert skill, and to prepare plans and reports relative thereto ; and the total expenditure of the board for one year shall not exceed $5,000.

The present law is defective in not supplying the proper machinery to enforce the proper sanitary regulations, and in not requiring the formation of local boards to aid the State Board. In some localities this has been done, and with good results, but it should be general throughout the State, aided and assisted by the necessary power to enforce obedience.

When it is remembered that the duties of the State Board extend over the whole State, that they are charged with the duty of abating nuisances wherever found, and of bringing offenders to justice, that they must make careful inquiry into all complaints, and make accurate reports of their investigations—and this unaided, except by volunteers—it will be seen that the necessity for the enactment of more stringent sanitary laws and a general system for their enforcement is absolutely necessary. Borough and city councils, school boards or township officials should be constituted local boards of health, to aid the State Board ; and to them should be added an advisory committee of physicians and citizens.

There always will be found in every locality medical and scientific men, and public-spirited citizens, who are willing thus to act in conjunction with local boards, whose advice and co-operation would lighten their duties and add to their efficiency ; and thus would be provided all over the State competent bodies whose investigations and conclusions upon sanitary measures would banish much of the ignorance now existing upon the subject, and by their valuable suggestions as to preventive measures and the enforcement of the laws bring about results beneficial to the general good. The State should treat this as a practical matter deserving of immediate attention, and thus fulfil one of its primary and most important objects.

DISCUSSION OF ABOVE PAPER BY GEORGE W. ROGERS, ESQ.,

OF NORRISTOWN, PA.

Mr. President, Ladies and Gentlemen:

In looking over the programme for this convention I see the names of gentlemen representing all the professions interested in a work which contributes not so much to their own profit as to the good of others.

The medical gentlemen to care for the health, the clergyman to care for the spiritual welfare and the lawyers to guard the morals and give tone to the body. The anomaly of my position is somewhat embarrassing. The paper just read by the gentleman who occupies the bench of our county with so much grace and ability is for discussion. But I have not been so educated. We are taught that when an opinion is delivered by a member of the judiciary, discussion is at an end and criticism is out of taste, and though we sometimes think and often know they are wrong, they are not convinced of their error until a gentle suggestion in the form of a peremptory order comes from that august body who may be found during business hours at the new city hall in Philadelphia. If Judge Weand had concluded with the usual order, *that the Board of Health conduct its labors in accordance with the principles of the opinion,* then judgment of approval would at once have been entered and the case ended.

But the subject of sanitation is of momentous importance not only to those who are advising its enforcement, but reaches the health, happiness, comfort and prosperity of every man, woman and child, whether in town or country. Life and death, health and disease have been waging a conflict since men had existence, and in the early ages, long before civilization had advanced until comfort, convenience and style had led to a disregard of the more important considerations of health, happiness and prosperity, the subject of hygiene was of individual and national consideration. The scrupulous attention to cleanliness ; the extreme care in the preparation of food ; the isolation of the sick and the frequent and thorough ablutions and perfect ventilation enjoined by the old Mosaic code, attest the necessity for a strict observance of sanitary laws and the singular immunity from disease that was enjoyed by the ancient Jewish nations, has long since passed into history. But within the last century a new interest has started, and scientific men with a philanthropy that has rivalled the ancient philosophers, have pushed their researches into every domain of nature. And now the valuable discoveries that have been made are no longer confined to the laboratory of the chemist or the consulting room of the physician. But the press is carrying into every household the results of their researches, and the lecture platform is calling around it the people, and eminent scientists are instructing them as to the dangers that exist in their own homes and around their own firesides, and the best known remedies for their extinction. In fact, a new science has been evolved called the Science of Prevention. Food and drink, water and air, are being analyzed, and every enemy of life and health is being exposed and attacked, and, if possible, destroyed. From our youth we were taught that the mystical Pandora box contained all the diseases, and when they escaped to prey upon the race hope was left behind. But upon a scientific analysis of the contents of that wonderful box it was found filled with microbes and bacteria, and when they departed the Board of Health remained behind. Now, it is to them that we turn for suggestions whereby health may be preserved and disease and death prevented.

The proper ventilation of sleeping and other apartments, the preservation and preparation of food, the purity of water for drinking and culinary purposes, the arrangement of sewers and other drains, the disposing of garbage and the abatement of all stagnant pools and miasmatic marshes, and the necessity for thorough cleanliness, are subjects that no longer are treated as the whim or interest of men may suggest, but must be subject to the revolution made by the retort and the microscope. Infection and contagion are no longer mysterious terms belonging to some mystical science, but are the names of subjects entering into and affecting the health and life of every member of the human family. The prevention of disease from whatever source is of more importance than its cure. Health continued and unimpaired is of more value than doctor's fees, and life enjoyed as intended by its Great Author a boon whose preservation calls forth every effort that reason and science can suggest. The overcrowding of our towns and cities ; illy-ventilated school-rooms, where our children must breathe an atmosphere laden with poison ; the reckless disregard of human life manifested in the dilapidated tenement houses, where the poor are compelled to seek a home ; the penurious neglect with which alleys, streets and gutters are allowed to be the hotbed of disease ; the inadequate remedy for the removal of noxious bodies, and an occasional outbreak of an epidemic, call for notes of alarm and warning to be sounded everywhere. The people must be instructed so that not only the officers in charge, but the subjects to be affected, must understand that danger and death are lurking on every side ready to strike the fatal blow at the most unexpected moment. Now, I endorse all that Judge Weand has said, and the people of the State should rise up and insist that our lawmakers use the power they have to not only furnish the State Board with the means to do their work thoroughly, but so they can organize local boards, that every infectious spot, no matter how secluded or hidden, shall be sought out and removed. When science, with a disinterestedness that characterizes this age, has done so much, give her all the aid she wishes, so that a high degree of health and long life may be the heritage of the people of our beloved Commonwealth.

The Sanitation of Rural Homes.*

BY SAMUEL WOLFE, M.D.,
Of Skippack, Pa.

In one way or another the idea has rooted itself that the residents of the country districts are the healthy, the robust, the strong, and the long lived ; that city life tends to weakness, disease and early decrepitude ; that as to matters of health, the country with its pure air, its fresh, green vegetation, its crystal springs of cool water, its rivers, lakes and mountains, will take abundant care of itself; that the city with its crowded populace, its polluted water, and its impure atmosphere, demands the closest scientific, sanitary supervision ; that to be bodily vigorous, and mentally callous, it is only necessary to live in the country ; while to live in the city means affliction with physical delicacy, but endowment with intellectual astuteness.

Indeed, so firmly fixed are these notions that physicians do not even generally recognize that some patients in the country should be sent to the city, while the merest tyro of a city practitioner is ever ready to recommend change of scene and air ; ever ready to send his patients into the country.

These opinions embody much that is true, but also some that are mistaken. There is no doubt whatever that the children born in the slums of a large city, or even in the poorer quarters of a smaller town, exposed as they are to all the dangers there occurring, incident to season, overcrowding, and moral degradation, have less chance of survival of the period of infancy than is usually the case in the extremest poverty or parsimony of the country. There is no doubt that the country, during at least a certain portion of the year, offers even to

* Read before the State Sanitary Convention at Norristown, Pa., May 9th and 10th, 1890.

adults in the best stations conditions more favorable to the maintenance or recovery of health than does the city.

Indeed, I am ready to admit that the country people should be the healthiest, but I regret that, to be true to my convictions, I am constrained to deny that they are.

And here let me say, by way of parenthesis, that those living in the suburban districts, very many of them in the open country, but who have their employment, their association, their interests altogether in the city or in what pertains to it, cannot be justly regarded as country people. These have all the privileges and perquisites of both city and country, without the disadvantages or drawbacks of either, and are the typically healthy if such a class at all exists. Indeed, no one so well knows how to utilize the sanitary benefits of the country as the denizen of the town.

What then are the problems that present themselves for solution? Are they such as concern our sanitary authorities?

I take it that State Boards of Health or, more correctly speaking, Sanitary Conventions, are in some way concerned with every factor of disease or physical incompetency, as well as with every method applicable to their removal or control, whether educational or legislative. Some subjects may be remonstrated with; some may be legislated against; and still others may be wiped out by the execution of already existing laws; by the infliction of ready provided penalties.

To the administration of health laws, it seems to me the country presents many obstacles that are not met with in the town. The people are widely scattered; there is no machinery for surveillance and execution such as exists in the police force of every municipality; they would strenuously resist, and openly rebel against inquisitorial procedures such as town people from habit readily submit to.

The main problem lies perhaps beyond the reach of a health board, and is largely a moral question. Though connected with rural homes, it deals more especially with the condition of rural character, of rural sentiment. There is a loss of rustic individuality in the attempt to introduce urban customs. There is the "little knowledge" which is a "dangerous thing." There is the occasional contact, the frequent yet not constant intercourse with the city and its people, brought about by the facilities of interchange, by railroads, telegraphs, telephones, freight and express lines. There is the sacrifice of that distinction, that consecration to sectional influence that nature intends, art desires and policy demands.

These are some of the circumstances which have engendered a race of rural malcontents, with slight frames, uneasy manners, and anxious faces; with weakened bodies, perturbed hearts, and worried minds.

A race which cannot give to our great Eastern cities the brawn and brain which in the past generation has so largely figured in the perpetuation and success of their great commercial concerns, their political institutions, and their educational forces; which cannot put the heads into their largest mercantile houses, the scientists into their colleges, and the judges on the bench ; which cannot take up the line of succession, as the boys who have been acted on by the degenerative influences of high metropolitan life for a few generations drop out and back into obscurity. The Bucks and Montgomery County mothers of this generation had better look well to their laurels, if for the next, Philadelphia is to depend on them for a fresh supply of Jameses, Rothermels, Leidys and Paxsons. These fathers will hardly send sons with rugged but strong and powerful characters to their commercial apprenticeship or to their classical curriculum, but will more likely send out pale, rickety clerks or dudish sycophants, to vie with the man about town in his listless, useless, corrupting life.

Why needs the rustic to be ashamed of his station ? He is quite as good as his city brother, and his wife and daughters are the peers of their polished relatives, except in so far as they attempt to be like them ; except in so far as they overtax all their energies of body and mind with exhausting shopping tours, full of strained, anxious observation of the furniture and the embellishments of city houses, and of the attire and manners of city pedestrians ; full of painful worry how to fill their expensive longings from meagre purses, ending in remorseful regret at the final selection of what the invited criticism of their city friends will stamp as shabby or out of taste ; except in so far as they degenerate from what they should be—the leaders and promulgators of rustic sentiment into cold exclusiveness ; in so far as they fall from the high place of rural commanders to the obscurity of urban privates ; except in so far as they drop their genuine qualifications, yield their graces, resign their possessions in order to assume the borrowed plumes which they fancy brighter and more becoming.

Let our farmers, our country artisans and all classes come back to themselves ; let them once more deserve the title of sturdy yeomanry, and tempt the poet again to consecrate their lives in the immortality of the pastoral, the lyric and the ballad.

What ! you cry ; do you wish to relegate the rustic to his primitive condition ; to push him back into the darkness of barbarity ; into the superstition of the mediæval ages ? I would say, yes ; rather than let him remain what he now is—the unsuccessful imitator of the citizen. The standards of country life will not permit success after this fashion. The bankruptcy that stares the honest agricultural people of Eastern Pennsylvania in the face ; yea, that has already almost engulfed them, and plunged them into disastrous ruin and distressful despondency, owes one-half of its cause to this very thing.

But to make the picture not too black ; out of all this chaos may come beautiful order; out of this wholesale panic there may come blessed tranquillity. This is a formative period, and the country people need not balk their true advancement ; need not retire to primitive ignorance ; need not relapse into the rudeness of frontier life. They have only to recognize the helpful influences that would act on them ; only to appreciate that refinement and culture and health are conditions that though having certain external essentials are not dependent in one station upon the type or stage of such essentials existing in another. I say, let the country people educate heads, hearts and hands to the maintenance of a clear-cut rural individuality ; of a high-toned, but distinctly rural character. Let them stamp their life with a rank as specific and respectable as that of the city. Let them realize that servile imitation is the mark of the sluggard and weakling, and the begetter of misery and disquiet, while healthy, heroic independence not only springs from power, but creates and commands it, along with respect and success, and what is above all, peace and happiness.

But by this time all of you who have been sufficiently indulgent and self-sacrificing to follow me, are ready to exclaim, "What has all this to do with the sanitation of rural homes?" Too little, I fear, on which to make a clear case for acquittal from the charge of vagary.

But if you, ladies and gentlemen, through either personal or official influence, can bring about such a condition as that obscurely pictured, as a desirable one for rural sections, you will have overcome the abject despondency, the forced submission to circumstances, the abnormal longing for changes which can never come, or which, if they do come, will meet with no graceful acceptance. You will have aroused in the breasts of the rural inhabitants such a spirit of interest in their humble homes that they will accept with most hearty gratitude any plans for making them salubrious. Such a people will not permit the supervisors of their public roads to leave in front of their houses stagnant pools, reeking with organic putrescent matter, teeming with malarial germs, or possibly still more virulent poisons, awaiting the first drouth to resurrect them from their watery graves, and the first gentle evening zephyr on which to float silently and unseen into bedrooms on their mission of destruction and death. Such will not permit cupidity to embargo the head spring of every rivulet, only to liberate it from the greasy portals of a creamery, laden with a vile, malodorous scum, to steal stealthily out over meadow and lawn, from which to rise on the misty air of night to taint the very life blood of the unconscious sleeper whose last thought had been a thanksgiving to a Gracious Providence for having cast his lot in pleasant places. Such will create a sentiment of respect for the few remaining patches of woodland that still remain to grace the rich agricultural bottoms, as well as for the already sadly devastated mountain forests on whose aspect there is written a pitiful prayer for protection. Such people, I say, will create, maintain and enforce a policy that will stay the hands of the defiler more effectively than any mere abstract agitation of the forestry question. Such will not deliberately pollute their own surroundings by horrible quagmires of filth and acridity, fed daily by a torrent of offensive offal, pouring like an intermittent deluge from the kitchen door or window.

Such will not drink water from a well that owes its sparkling brilliancy, which is supposed a guarantee of its purity, to the quantum of organic impurities it has borrowed from the barnyard, the pigsty or, horror of horrors ! the cesspool on the banks beyond. Nor will they offend the transient guest, whom a cruel fate has thrown for a night on their hospitality, by the stale, sickening must of the whited sepulchre, which within is full of rottenness and death,

·although without a too hard-earned pittance has furnished an exuberance of tinselry, embroidery and tapestry that seeks to allure the eye ; but, alas ! the nose detects the spare room. Nor will the viands that now grace the table, arrayed with all the fashionable daintiness of the city epicure, have but lately parted company with a cellar whose atmosphere is a mixture of noxious gases ·emanating from mud floors and decaying vegetables.

Nor will they, when no "company" is present, dine in swine-like haste in hot kitchens swarming with flies, and even in midsummer off fat pork, when the city artisan or mechanic takes his meal of fruit and vegetables leisurely in his dining-room, sharing it with his best company, his family. Such, in short, will throng the sessions of our sanitary conventions, and give ready application ·to the general principles of sanitary science, falling thus within easy reach of the laudable efforts of that self-sacrificing, public-spirited, earnest body of men which constitutes that important arm of the administration, the State Board of Health.

The Mission of Sanitation.[*]

By HON. SAMUEL T. DAVIS, M.D.,
Of Lancaster, Pa.
Member State Board of Health of Pennsylvania.

Mr. President, Ladies and Gentlemen :

It has fallen to my lot to respond, on the part of the State Board of Health, to your kind invitation to hold the annual State Sanitary Convention in your beautiful town. We not only feel gratified for the invitation, but commend your local board for the manifest interest which prompted them to extend it.

Now that we are here, your words of welcome and encouragement place us under still more obligations, and cheer us on in our earnest endeavors to ferret out from all the abnormal conditions of air, water and food the causes of their contamination and consequent common carriers of disease and death to ·our fellow-citizens.

The prevention of disease from clearly defined specific causes is a subject worthy the investigation of a lifetime, and a moral and political duty which man owes to his fellow man. To those who cure diseased conditions we would vote a crown of earthly glory and sufficient of this world's goods to enable him or her to enjoy all of this world's enjoyments.

To those who prevent disease, we grant everlasting honor and peace as benefactors of the race of man, and entitled to all the honors of the former, ·and in addition the extolation of Divine preferment beyond this short struggle with things temporal.

· Born June 3d, 1885, your Board of Health of the State of Pennsylvania is as yet but a small boy in kilts, but it has gotten into line, made its mark, and

-----

*Being the reply to the address of welcome delivered at the State Sanitary Convention at Norristown, Pa., May 9th and 10th, 1890.

its influence has been felt throughout the length and breadth of this great Commonwealth. Our circulars, containing sanitary instructions and wholesome advice to the people, find their way to every hamlet in the State, and are sought for by sanitarians in every State in the Union.

A limited and barely sufficient appropriation for current expenses and the want of proper legislative enactments for the enforcement of sanitation in the rural districts have, to a great extent, retarded the work of the Board ; but, on the other hand, the efficiency of the Secretary, whose ability as a sanitarian is second to none in the country, has, as far as it was possible, made up in part for the lack of State aid.

In the cities of Philadelphia, Pittsburgh, Allegheny, Erie and the larger population centres self-preservation has long since necessitated the establishment of well-organized and efficient health departments. But I am sorry to say, in the rural districts and small towns of the Commonwealth the prevention of disease in man and domestic animals is sadly neglected, and responsible for results of the most disastrous character. The necessity for small town and township boards of health is as urgent as that the rootlets of the growing tree should have nourishment.

A well-organized board of health, with proper authority, willingness to exercise it, and always on the alert, would have prevented over one thousand persons from being affected with typhoid fever, saved over one hundred lives and thousands of dollars to the plague-stricken inhabitants of Plymouth, Pennsylvania. The history of that memorable epidemic and the possibility of its prevention beyond the shadow of a doubt, are no longer debatable subjects.

Without well-organized, intelligent local boards of health over the whole State, the same calamity is liable to occur just as often as the necessary circumstances and conditions are brought together. As true as that water seeks its level ; that certain substances always crystallize in the same form ; that nature's laws are inevitable, so will the germs of contagion cause disease. While I am not an alchemist, nor in search of the philosopher's stone or the fountain of eternal youth, the fact that the microscope has, within the last few years, developed so much of the heretofore unknown, I am inclined to think sometimes that all diseases are preventable, and that the only disorder which the human form divine should be afflicted with is old age and a useful physical condition for more than threescore years and ten. Who can tell, or even imagine, what the result of another century of scientific investigation as to the cause and prevention of disease will develop ? Many years ago Dr. Franklin caught from the clouds and bottled the electric spark, and won the applause of the scientific world. The latent force remained in its lethargic condition until but a few years ago. May we not be in our daily walks of life stumbling over small and apparently worthless or insignificant substances, which will some day, when properly applied, counteract the spread of disease in man and beast ? Three scientists of Paris but lately assert that essence of cinnamon, when sprinkled in the room of a typhoid fever patient, kills bacteria within twelve hours and prevents the disease from spreading. Whether this be true or otherwise, time will prove, and if the discovery is freighted with the same good results as vac-.cination in the prevention of that loathsome disease, smallpox, the civilized, educated part of the world will rise and call Drs. Chamberland, Mermier and Cadiac blessed benefactors.

The objects of holding sanitary conventions throughout the State are manifold, and suggest themselves to anyone interested without the formality of an introduction. The special object of this convention is to awaken an interest in the minds of the citizens of Norristown in such matters as pertain to the public health and prevention of disease in the borough, the discussion of local measures of reform needed as regards drainage and sewerage, the disposal of garbage, the registration of births and deaths, and last, though not least, the condition of the water supply.

When Isaac Norris purchased from William Penn the site upon which this ancient town stands its sanitary condition was, no doubt, first-class. The sparkling waters of the picturesque Schuylkill were pure, healthful and unde-filed, and the air, ladened with ozone and perfumed with the odors of the virgin forests, sweet and invigorating. The tide of civilization reached Swede's Ford, and in 1812 the borough of Norristown was incorporated. From the little hamlet on the North bank of the river blast furnaces, rolling mills, woolen and cotton mills, a glass factory and oil refinery have sprung up, and with them a population nearing 20,000 souls. The forests along the stream have given way to the husbandman's axe, and the soil in which they grew to the plow; and where once rustled the leaves of the majestic oak now waves the growing grain. Towns, cities, farmhouses and factories nestle on both its banks and tributaries, and the once pure and healthful water of the Schuylkill has become a common sewer on its way to the ocean. It may be true, as someone who had more faith than facts has said, that impure water becomes pure when it has run over three rocks, but sanitarians nowadays don't believe it. One instance alone will refute the silly assertion. The village of Laussane, near Basle, Switzerland, is situated at the foot of a mountain out of which flows a beautiful spring, and from which the inhabitants, save six families, were supplied with water. On the opposite side of the mountain was an isolated farmhouse, near a small brook. In this house was an imported case of typhoid fever. The brook received the dejections and the linen was washed in it. After the water had been thus polluted it was used for irrigating some of the meadow land close by, and the effluent water filtered through the intervening mountain to the spring in the village, and every inhabitant, except those in the six families, who used the water from private wells, was stricken down with typhoid fever. The passage of water from the irrigated meadows to the spring at Laussane was proven by dissolving in it at the meadows eighteen hundred weight of common salt, and then observing the rapid increase of chlorine in the spring water. But the most important and interesting experiment consisted in mixing uniformly with the water fifty hundred weight of flour, not a trace of which made its way to the spring, thus showing conclusively that the water was filtered through the intervening earth and did not pass by an underground channel.

Two years ago, when the State Sanitary Convention was held at Lewisburg, my better half, after considerable persuasion, accompanied me. At that interesting session, Dr. Edwards, during a lecture on home sanitation, exhibited, by the aid of a stereoscope, a number of photographic views thrown upon a screen, entitled the "Mistakes of the Plumber"—the architect, the fouling wells, animalculæ and other inhabitants of the microscopic landscape. The good lady became so much interested in the whole subject that she can scarcely wait for the monthly visits of the Annals of Hygiene. The water in the old well, which had quenched the thirst of thousands for half a century, was looked upon with increased suspicion, and to-day it is used only for washing cuspidors and the surface drain.

Soon the cistern had to be remodeled, and since its completion its pure, sparkling water, filtered through eight inches of hard-burnt bricks and six inches of charcoal, is used entirely for drinking and culinary purposes. Several additional traps in waste pipes were also necessary, as well as some changes in ventilation. The home is the unit of sanitary reform, and successful sanitation must begin there. The prevention of disease is one of the subjects of which the school of experience teaches much, and aided by sad illustrations, but to which the pupils pay but little heed. Our good housewives, the queens of our homes, are in the most favorable position to first discover when anything is wrong, and while they may be active and useful members of missionary societies, temperance organizations, ladies' aid associations, and blessed with health, education and intelligence, if they are not familiar with the action of foul gases, contagious poisons and the causes of disease, both sickness and death, which might be averted, may steal upon them through an almost imperceptible crevice in the wall.

Much has been said and written upon the subject of home hygiene, but the importance of interesting the ladies particularly in the great work has been neglected or overlooked. Our home rules for what and how to do when the dread monster diphtheria or scarlet fever has fastened its talons on one of the little flock of home-lambs should be studied, understood and cherished by every lady who is or ever expects to be a mother. What a grand field for woman's work! Thousands of dollars are collected yearly by penny and nickel contributions in Pennsylvania, and find their way to foreign lands, to be used in the enlightenment of the heathen. I say "Amen," but self-preservation should be the first law of nature. Our duty should be to look first to our vital interests at home, and as long as there is a leaking sewer or a pile of decayed vegetables in the back yard or cellar, see that it is attended to first.

Before closing these remarks I earnestly take the liberty of making a suggestion to the ladies of Montgomery County, and sincerely trust my words may not fall unheeded ; that is, to ask you to form a Montgomery County Ladies' Sanitary Society. Hold regular monthly meetings. The Norristown Board of Health will hail your new departure with delight and render you all the assistance in their power. Request Dr. Alice Bennett, president of the Montgomery County Medical Society, to help you organize and give you a plain talk occasionally. Ask Dr. Benjamin Lee, secretary of the State Board of Health, for literature, and I guarantee it will be forthcoming. Open up the subject of prevention of disease and the prolongation of human life, and follow it from the cradle to the grave ; and don't stop there, for the dead are often the greatest enemies of the living. Send representatives to our sanitary conventions, and we will be proud to receive your delegates.

The Use of Salicylic Acid as a Preservative.*

BY HENRY LEFFMANN, M.D.,

Of Philadelphia.

Food Inspector for the Pennsylvania State Board of Agriculture.

The question of the use of salicylic acid as a preservative is a hackneyed theme. Attention has repeatedly been called to it in sanitary journals, and the restriction of its use has been discussed by many sanitary conventions, especially in Europe. The evil is not, however, abating in this country, and it seems therefore to be appropriate to say a few words again on the topic. Concerning the general effects of this body I need only refer to a paper previously contributed among others, to an account of experiments made by my assistant, Mr. William Beam, and myself, published in the *Polyclinic*.

The facts now at hand show that this acid interferes with important digestive processes so that, independent of any unwholesomeness in itself, it is an objectionable ingredient. Furthermore, since it is now made on a very large scale, less care is used in its preparation, and it is more likely to be impure. The usual method of manufacture is from carbolic acid. Several observers have recorded the danger of small amounts of carbolic acid being present. When such impure acid is used in food, a greater degree of objection of course arises. The employment of this body is resorted to to prevent decompositions and fermentations to which organic infusions and mixtures are liable. It is not commonly employed in those preserved foods which—canned fruits, for instance—are easily sterilized by heating, but in beers, malt extracts, catsups and similar perishable articles it is now used without stint. Briefly summarizing the knowledge as to the effect of salicylic acid, I may say that it has the power to suspend the action of the pancreatic secretions as far as regards the digestion of starch, and also to interfere with the action of diastase. Administered, therefore, in ordinary food it will when reaching the intestine prevent an important function from being fully operative ; administered in a malt extract or beer it will stop any beneficial effect that such materials might have as far as regards the malt present. The above remarks apply to the pure salicylic

*Read before the State Sanitary Convention at Norristown, Pa., May 9th and 10th, 1890.

acid ; more serious results would follow the use of that not containing any appreciable amount of carbolic acid.

Concerning the effects of salicylic acid, a paper has recently appeared in the *British Medical Journal*, detailing experiments made by Drs. Charteris and Maclennan, of Glasgow. These show that the artificial salicylic acid, by which is meant that obtained from carbolic acid, is decidedly more poisonous than that obtained from either salicin or oil of wintergreen, which are the so-called natural sources. The symptoms produced in animals were first paralysis of flexor muscles, and then death by convulsions. The artificial acid will, of course, be used in trade on account of its price. The experimenters are of the opinion that the greater danger of the artificial is due to impurities, but they have so far been unsuccessful in identifying the particular ingredient. It is worth noting that not only will the artificial acid be used in foods, but that when prescribed in the ordinary course of medical practice the same form will also be used. Data are not at hand of sufficient extent to show precisely what effects on the general health are produced by the continued use of salicylic acid. But there can be but little doubt that it must be objectionable. Several of the governments of Europe have investigated this question through commissions including some of the most distinguished medical authorities, and as a result of reports made by these have prohibited the employment of this body. An incidental objection to its indiscriminate use is often overlooked. It is in some cases, at least, a cover for carelessness or imperfection in manufacture. It is easy to rely upon it for the preservation of any article, and thus to neglect other and less objectionable methods, or to take less care as to cleanliness in preparation. Liberal doses of the preservative will make amends for all errors or imperfections. Thus, by the want of restriction and the competition between dealers the condition grows continually worse. At the present time a number of prepared preservatives are upon the market intended for a variety of uses; and many of these are composed largely of salicylic acid.

The question, of course, arises what practical method is there of reaching this abuse. The system of government under which we live does not permit such summary measures as have been resorted to in the same emergency in Europe. We can not secure an imperial decree, nor an order of council. There is, however, a preliminary method of approaching this evil which I think is entirely practical and as fair as any one could expect. That is, to insist that all persons who employ salicylic acid in the preservation of any article of food or drink should be compelled to place in a conspicuous place on the label of each package a statement of the amount used. Farther, the amount used should not be permitted to exceed a certain proportion. As investigation pro-gresses, it will be found possible to dispense more and more with the use of the acid, and the limits should gradually be drawn in. Thus it is known that malt extracts can be preserved without its use, for good extracts are now on the market that do not contain it ; therefore it would be perfectly permissible to for-bid its use in these. Its employment in beer is also not necessary, and conse-quently should be forbidden. Concerning the label indicating its presence, it may be said that since any attempt to prescribe in writing the form of such label is generally circumvented by dealers, the proper plan would be for the sanitary authorities to reserve the right to design, and approve the form of label, and to place severe penalties upon any attempt to employ the article without the label or to conceal or render it invisible when attached.

The Disposal of Garbage in Norristown.*

BY J. K. WEAVER, M. D.,
Of Norristown, Pa.

To gather and dispose of the waste matter under the different forms in which it exists in domestic life and as a result of business activities of our larger towns and cities, without offending the senses or polluting the air we breathe or the water we drink, is one of the questions which is agitating the sanitary world to-day, and to the solution of which the best efforts of sanitarians in this and the old world are directed.

There was a time when this question did not press so hard for an answer. When what are now cities were villages sparsely populated, and waste matter limited, and its disposal could well be left to take care of itself or to those secret forces of nature's laboratory in which its organic contents would be decomposed and rendered harmless.

But with the increase of population, the rapid growth of cities, the closely-crowded dwellings, and their still more closely-compacted inhabitants, nature's forces were found inadequate, and the ingenuity of man was called upon to devise a method by which the refuse of human life could be disposed of in a manner at once sanitary and give immunity from nuisance.

Happily for us, although we are still in the period of experimentation, rapid strides have been made in this direction in the last few years, and its complete settlement would seem to be almost within our reach.

These are the principal difficulties in the way, as in all matters pertaining to health : Ignorance on the part of the people, and indifference, often born of the same parent, on the part of the officials.

The education of the masses in the essentials of health, and the relation of filth and dirt to disease, is one, if not the principal duty of local and State boards of health.

It is no less the duty of borough and municipal authorities to provide such measures as will promote the health and prevent diseases among the inhabitants, than it is to give them good government or well-paved streets.

I doubt not that the State Board of Health in our borough at this time, and the presence of some of the leading sanitarians of this and other States,

---

* Read before the State Sanitary Convention at Norristown, Pa., May 9th and 10th, 1890.

as well as the active participation in these proceedings of the clergy and legal profession, will give a great stimulus to and quicken an interest in matters pertaining to the sanitary betterment of Norristown—may we not hope the whole Schuylkill Valley ?

The subject of the disposal of garbage in Norristown is the one upon which I am requested to make some suggestions.

Under the generic name of garbage I will, for my purpose, include all refuse and offal from the households, business places, markets, hotels, street sweepings, etc.

The question of the disposal of human excreta, or night soil, will not be included, as its consideration would consume more time than is at my disposal.

This waste or refuse may be divided into liquids and solids. Under liquids we have the discharges from the kitchen, principally dish water, bath room, washstands, etc. In a town like ours, where sewer connection is the exception, the disposition of these wastes is more important than at first sight would appear, both from the quantity discharged (constituting nine-tenths of the offensive residue of our homes) and the composition of the effluent.

From the basins and baths we have the feathery masses of dead epithelium, or outer skin of the body. From the laundry we have the organic scourings of soiled clothing, which are often specifically infected, and, therefore, a fertile medium for the development and growth of disease germs.

From the kitchen are discharged the dish and other general waters which have been very appropriately termed weak organic broths, readily responding to inoculation, and, in fact, all the waters which are used in the household are so charged with organic waste as to make its retention in or about homes imprudent, if not dangerous.

If there is sewer connection the best disposition that can be made is into a well trapped and thoroughly ventilated sewer, its convenience all the year round being a strong argument in its favor.

In the absence of this method of disposal, the waste pipes from the bath or wash stands are usually attached to or run into the rain pipes of the house and the contents find their way into the street or alley, where, together with the liquid waste from the kitchen, they find their way slowly for a square or two, or even three squares, giving off offensive odors, creating here and there stagnant pools of greasy and foul looking nastiness, until they finally discharge themselves into the nearest sewer, which they have had so long a way to go to find, or, what in many places is more likely, to throw the dish water in the immediate vicinity of the kitchen door, forming artificial swamps, and possibly finding its way to the foundation walls, rendering damp and offensive the soil and making all attempts at neatness and cleanliness impossible.

In cases where there is no infectiousness there can be no serious objection to thus disposing of liquids from bath and wash stands, especially if it is followed by copious flushings of clean water; but to make this disposition of kitchen or laundry water is, to say the least, questionable, and should, if possible, be avoided.

What then can be done with it ? It is possible and practicable in a property where there is a small plot of grass or garden to conveniently and economically dispose of these fluids by distributing them over the grass or around the roots of trees or shrubbery ; and it is not a little surprising to find the large amounts of fluids that are thus absorbed and how much they add to the fertility of the soil and the luxuriousness of the growth.

It has been found by experience that a space twenty feet by twenty-five feet would be ample to utilize all the slops of an ordinary household. An equally effective but more expensive method is by subsoil drainage, by which the fluids are conducted through loosely joined drain pipes at proper depths to different parts of the ground. The only drawback to this method is the danger of obstruction in the pipes when not properly laid and necessitating some means of periodic flushings.

Another method is to conduct them into a cistern, or other water-tight receptacle, and at intervals pumping out and distributing them as fertilizers.

If your premises are too limited to employ any of these methods, a very practicable and economical way, suggested to me a day or two since by a practical housekeeper, is to put all the refuse of the house, liquids and solids, into a barrel or box, mixing with them the ashes from stove or range, thus absorbing the excessive moisture, and have it all removed as often as necessary. The simplicity, convenience and economy of this plan will make it worthy of trial, the ashes serving the dual purpose of absorbing and disinfecting the mass.

The disposal of the grosser refuse matter of a borough like Norristown is a task of graver importance, and difficult of successful accomplishment. The welfare of the people, in all that pertains to their health, their prosperity and happiness, demands a plan which shall be economical, thorough in its execution, and without offense.

The methods among housekeepers are various. In small families, where the amount of waste is meagre, a very common way is to throw the offal into the chicken yard or over the back fence into the alley where the chickens, dogs, and cats become the scavengers. The most popular resort is to the slop barrel, or swill pail, near the window or door, or, among more tidy housekeepers, at some distant corner of the yard, and, when full, taken away by the scavenger and fed to pigs, or possibly to milk cows.

A very small proportion of housekeepers have adopted the most cleanly, economical, and rational method—incineration in the stove or range.

There are few, if any, houses where the ordinary kitchen range or house furnace will not be found a rapid and complete consumer. That it can be done has been demonstrated in our own home where, for years, all animal and vegetable matter is consumed in the ordinary kitchen range, the liquid waste is disposed of in the way above mentioned, and the slop barrel and the swill tub are things of the past. A little time and patience and judgment are all that is necessary to be successful.

Put the refuse inside the range near the fireplace, first removing excessive moisture, and in a few minutes the mass can be put on to the fire, and you will be surprised to find in what a short time it will be consumed, the material itself becoming a very fair fuel. If this method were adopted in households of ordinary size it would do away with much if not all the accumulation around the house, and the question of the disposal of garbage would be largely solved. The growing importance of this question is being appreciated by our housekeepers, and an organization is in existence in New York City, and one is now forming in Brooklyn, to look into the matter and make this method still more efficient.

There has been devised, and it is now in process of perfection, "a family garbage burner," that can be attached to the ordinary kitchen range into which the refuse is placed and rapidly destroyed or consumed, and without odor or inconvenience. The price being within reach of all it ought to become popular, and is especially adapted to small hotels or restaurants or large families.

There is a device called the Fire Closet, which is used for the same purpose, intended for use in large hotels, public institutions, colleges and seminaries, and which is said to accomplish the purpose of its construction with small cost and without offense.

There is a borough ordinance which prohibits the throwing into the streets or alleys of any animal or vegetable matter, which, up to the time of the formation of the Board of Health, was entirely unheeded, and any convenient lot or hollow or low place was regarded as all-sufficient for the purpose. But the offal from grocery stores, markets and manufactories is now deposited upon dumping grounds selected by the Board of Health and adopted by the borough authorities.

Under the supervision of the street supervisor the offal from the market and scrapings from streets, are frequently and systematically collected in the carts of the borough and deposited in the same place and carefully covered.

We want it understood, however, that this dumping ground is not to be used as prospective building sites for the "gradual murder of future tenants," but is the location upon which, as the progress of our rapidly growing borough, (soon we hope to be a city) demands, a street is to pass.

This spot being a deep hollow of considerable area, the deposits will be deeply buried out of sight, and at such distance from any future dwelling as to preclude the possibility of the air, any cellar or house being contaminated, or the pollution of the stream of the Stony Creek, which is not far removed.

Conscious of the imperfection of the present method of disposing of the garbage in our town, and the need, nay, the necessity, for a cleanly, speedy and economic one—the Board of Health a few weeks ago recommended to the borough authorities to take into consideration the advisability, so soon as the finances would warrant, of the construction of a furnace at some convenient location for the destruction by fire of the refuse accumulation of our town.

The advantages of this method are enhanced by the important fact that they are equally adapted to the destruction of dead bodies of domestic animals of all sizes and in whatever conditions, also the waste products of the abattoir and slaughter houses, and likewise the contents of the cesspools, and all human excreta.

These furnaces or crematories are in successful operation in several large cities in this country, and still more extensively in foreign countries, especially England, where more than three hundred are in use ; and so rapid is the growth of sentiment in favor of this method that it is likely that it will soon become the recognized means in all English cities.

That the same sentiment exists in this country, which is also on the increase, is attested by the fact that they are successfully used in New York City, Coney Island, Governor's Island, Minneapolis, Des Moines, St. Louis and other large cities of the West. As an indication of the general character of the awakening on this subject I see that it is proposed at the International Medical Congress, which meets in Berlin in August, to take steps looking to the more general adoption of fire as the great destroyer of all human waste. And it is likely that steps will also be taken to make cremation of the human body legal in the different countries of the world.

A New York company has offered to enter into a five years' contract with the city, under good and sufficient bonds, to take charge of and dispose of all the garbage, ashes, and street refuse of every kind, at a sum not to exceed the present outlay for the disposal of garbage, which is about $250,000 a year. The company has a capital of $1,000,000 and purposes, if its offer is accepted, to erect crematories at each dumping station—fifteen in all, with extra ones for emergencies, making a total of eighteen—and to have the first of them in operation within three months, and all within a year.

So complete in construction, so thorough in their execution, are the crematories in their work, that several tons of the most promiscuous collection are consumed in a few hours, and that, too, without odor, or the giving off of noxious gases ; are economical in the use of fuel, demand a small outlay of labor to conduct them, and that the cost of construction and of maintenance is within the easy reach of any town of the size and population of Norristown.

It is further claimed that the ashes of products resulting from the combustion are of such a value as a fertilizer as to make up a considerable share of the expense of maintenance. It is also claimed that when once the fire in these furnaces is fully under way, that the contents themselves become valuable fuel for their own destruction.

And so, while our provision for the disposal of the refuse of our town is somewhat crude and imperfect, it is the best we can do for the present. But we are alive to the importance of the subject, and our authorities and people are becoming interested, and we are looking forward to a time, which we hope is in the very near future, when Norris City will be noted not only for beautiful location, comfortable homes, and well-laid streets, but shall have made such advancement in all matters pertaining to the health of the citizens as to entitle her to stand among the foremost of sanitary municipalities.

The Funeral Director as a Sanitarian.*

BY R. R. BRINGHURST,

Of Philadelphia.

President of the International Funeral Directors' Association.

Mr. Chairman, Ladies and Gentlemen :

Those of my calling certainly feel highly honored in the knowledge that for the first time we are permitted to be heard on your platform in a public meeting of your organization ; but that honor is somewhat abated when we remember we are here by sufferance, not on earnest and oft-repeated invitation. Only last Tuesday evening was I informed of the meeting here yesterday and to-day, and having attended a similar gathering in Philadelphia a few years ago, I was anxious again to be present.

I received word that ten minutes would be set apart in which we could be heard and I will have to be brief; but some, or in fact all, may ask why do you wish to be heard at all ? or what on earth can the funeral directors have to say of interest to us ? As my authority for this exhibition of assurance on our part I will refer to An Act

" *To establish a State Board of Health for the better protection of life and health, and to prevent the spread of contagious and infectious diseases in this Commonwealth ;*" the authority under which our State Board " lives and moves and has its being."

Section 5 of that act reads thus :—

The State Board of Health and Vital Statistics shall have the general supervision of the interest of the health and lives of the citizens of the Commonwealth, and shall especially study its vital statistics. It shall make sanitary investigations and inquiries respecting the causes of disease and especially of epidemic diseases, including those of domestic animals, the sources of mortality, and the effects of localities, employments, conditions, habits, food, beverages and medicine on the health of the people. It shall also disseminate information upon these and similar subjects among the people. It shall, when required by the Governor or the Legislature, and at such other times as it deems it important, institute sanitary inspections of public institutions or places throughout the State. It shall codify and suggest amendments to the sanitary laws of the Commonwealth, and shall have power to enforce such regulations as will tend to limit the progress of epidemic diseases.

If, as stated in the first part of this act, you have general supervision of the interest of the health and lives of the citizens of the Commonwealth, why not call to your aid a calling that can, and under your direction, should be compelled to, render all assistance in their power ; and if the members of that or any other calling are not sufficiently imbued with a desire or the ability to render that assistance, then take advantage of your prerogative as laid down in the latter part of the section quoted—" It shall codify and suggest amendments to the sanitary laws of the Commonwealth, and shall have power to enforce such regulations as will tend to limit the progress of epidemic diseases." Now to you as medical men and women and as sanitarians, I put the question, who stand

---

*Read before the State Sanitary Convention at Norristown, May 9th and 10th, 1890.

⸻more in need of enlightenment on sanitary subjects, or can, when properly edu-cated, render you greater assistance in stamping out epidemics, or, better still, aid you in preventing contagion from becoming epidemic, than the undertakers of our State? I say when properly educated : for I here repeat a statement I made in Toronto at our last International Association, and I made it without any desire or intention of belittling those of our calling, but rather to arouse them to the true condition of affairs and the application of a remedy. There is a greater amount of ignorance among the undertakers of our country than in any other semi-professional class. This should not be, nor would it if the people of our State were thoroughly cognizant of the fact. Why are we brought face to face with such a deplorable state of affairs? Simply because the proper amount of importance is not attached to our calling by just such people as are gathered together here. You throw around our citizenship, in the shape of legislative enactments, the strong arm of protection against the unqualified physician, druggist and lawyer ; even the baseball player has rights in the eye of the law that unscrupulous managers are bound to respect ; but the under-taker is allowed to go his way and ignorantly and blunderingly shamble with his patient from the death-bed to the grave.

I will not treat discourteously a privilege, nor do I wish to be understood as under-rating the ability of the followers of an honored profession, or cast dis-credit upon our institutions of learning, but I will give voice to an honest con-viction, born of sights I have witnessed and discussions I have heard, in that I believe your work as sanitarians would be greatly benefited if the standard for graduation in our colleges was considerably raised. When the college door closes upon the graduate, and he faces the world of active practice, he has but the rudiments of that education which must be built upon and added to by practice and application, practice in that he honestly and conscientiously applies that which he has already learned, and application in that he not only sub-scribes for but gleans from the periodicals and literature of the day the advanced ideas of giant minds of his profession. If this be so in your case, why not in ours? Give the undertaker a chance. We have local and state organ-izations in twenty-three states, and an international organization. Our last international convention was held in Toronto, Canada ; our next is at Omaha, in October. At our State conventions we have lectures on scientific subjects. Dr. Joseph F. Edwards, of your State Board, has addressed us on several occasions, as has also Dr. John B. Deaver. But, you may ask, how can the undertaker become a sanitarian? In what can he become in any way a help to us in the truly great work we have in hand?

Allow me to suggest he may and should become a great help to you and the public in general by being able to decide the oft-raised question, "has death really taken place ?" by being able to take up the work of disinfection where the doctor often leaves off at the death-bed of the patient, to render non-infectious the dead body, the clothing, the furniture, the very atmosphere of the house, and as equally important his own person and clothing, so as to avoid even the resemblance of a possibility of carrying contagion from the house of

death to his own or any other family. He should be able, and at all times prepared, to so prepare a body dying of a non-contagious disease that its shipment to
any portion of the globe might be made without any risk of inconvenience or
unpleasant odors to railroad employés or patrons. He should be so educated to
the importance and responsibilities of his office as not to go direct from a case
of contagion to street car or other public conveyance, or his own family. He
should exercise the same care as to the safety of the public after attending a
case of diphtheria or scarlet fever, as he should after that of small-pox or spotted
fever ; and yet how many undertakers are there who attach but very little
importance to the two former diseases ? It is not necessary, nor will time allow,
to enter into details ; but all sanitarians should go hand in hand, be he doctor,
lawyer, merchant or undertaker, and I beg to indulge the belief that if all physicians would but give your pet theme due consideration ; were all funeral
directors thoroughly alive to their responsibility, and our citizenship in general
properly educated upon this subject of sanitation, your educational gatherings
such as this would be attended by the leading minds in medicine, surgery, law,
and mercantile pursuits, and the largest building in the State would not accommodate the attendance.

The physician when called to a case requiring prompt and heroic treatment, understands the cause and can apply the remedy, but does not have time to
explain details to family or friends. So it is with our appearance here to-day.
We come to call your attention to a place in your sanitary fence where the bars
are down ; to say to you here is a line of business that should, as far as contagion
is concerned, be a company mustered in the grand army of the Red Cross, to
offer our assistance in your noble work and ask your aid in placing ourselves in
proper position. In making this offer we modestly ask our experience be considered and we be allowed some small voice in shaping the necessary rules and
regulations that may be made so as best to control our actions and bring out the
largest results.

It would be considered the veriest presumption and display of ignorance
on the part of an undertaker to suggest to the doctor or family the quality or
size of a dose to be given a patient, or, in other words, to interfere with the
family physician ; and yet how often is it the case where the physician continues to exercise authority and give directions after the undertaker has been
called in ? This is explained by the fact that we are not credited with any knowledge or given much of a sphere in which to cut a caper. That we have not a
collegiate education is true, and only within the last few years we have had the
benefit of the experience of others, and yet we claim our knowledge, based on
experience, fits us to aid the legally constituted authorities of the State to mark
out a line of action that will, with the efforts of other sanitarians, bring the
desired results. What we ask is a law compelling every present or prospective
funeral director to prove to your State Board of Health, or some other efficient
and trustworthy board, his or her fitness to follow their calling.

We ask that this matter be not dropped. Some time ago warnings from
the Conemaugh Valley were given, oft-repeated, yet unheeded, and the terrible

calamity of Johnstown plunged a nation in sorrow ; a grand jury condemned the shortsightedness and the action that left green fields for grass and truck and reared a six-story building in which to confine the feeble-minded ; that warning was born away on the wind and we with all nations stand aghast at a calamity that penned up and incinerated a large number of the most afflicted of God's creatures. Our history is made up of successes and failures, and until the law-making power of the land is influenced by the thinkers of our country, the failures will be well up with the successes.

The time has passed when embryo editors, the minstrel and humorist, point the finger of scorn or ridicule at any one, and figure the doctor or under-taker with a broad smile when they contemplate cash profit from a visitation of contagion. We are willing, yea, anxious, to go hand in hand in this grand and glorious work. Allow us to aid you, or, in other words, demand and invoke the law to compel a compliance with your demand that all branches of professions and business may do their share to bring about cleanliness, carefulness and sanitary education, so that in the near future the bright sun-light of intelligence, application of preventives and remedial agencies may drive contagion and epidemics from our shores, and all as sanitarians may say of our effort as explorer Stanley says of his, '' The end crowns the work.''

Women and Their Wants.*

BY SHIRLEY DARE.

Here, on the page from which I have just risen, in a prose poem exquisitely carried out in Hawthorne's vein, are these words: ''And what of all things that monuments are built in memory of, is most loved and soonest forgotten ? Is it not a beautiful woman ? Who loves her for the beauty she once possessed ? Is there in all history a figure so lonely and despised as that of the woman who, once the most beautiful in the world, crept back into her native land a withered being.'' It is true. Yet against this decree of age and ugliness should not women set themselves with all the skill their fertile brains furnish ? The hand has been put back nearly twenty years on the dial of human life, which lasts till the sixties, where at the beginning of the century it was doomed to fail at forty. Men have forced back death, should not women outwit age and decay ? These are questions to be repeated and pressed upon the consideration.

Women look less beautiful than usual this Spring. Many of them have had a sore struggle with the Winter epidemic, whose after-effects on those of sensitive physique are as tedious as the sequelæ of scarlet fever or typhoid, from which a patient cannot call himself recovered under a year. It will take many days' basking in the warm sunshine, many days' breathing the deep free winds which stir the blood, and many nights of sound sleep to restore the tone to unstrung nerves. If the work is half done, as it usually is, the penalty will

---

* From the *Philadelphia Press.*

be visible in sallow faces, lack-lustre eyes and drooping forms. Women must, perforce, learn wisdom.

Not a few will find themselves forced to simplify their social work and drop much of the routine, useless duty which has absorbed them. The woman who is a member of eleven clubs, political, literary and charitable, will be obliged to ignore them so long as it is possible she may find existence more endurable without than with them. The mere routine of these time-stealing woman's clubs makes an enormous waste of time. So many letters of invitation and notification, so many explanatory notes and circulars are indispensable, and so much polite figuring must be done to make the meetings interesting, that no one with real aims in art or study but finds herself obliged to choose between her proper work and this formalizing and posturing mainly for the sake of giving Mrs. Manœuverer credit for being president over a large society. That is the most any of these women's clubs amounts to. It is the end and origin of their being, and keen-witted men awake to the fact. One of the most effective officers in a prominent association in a large city said lately in my hearing : "The ladies' auxiliaries want us to fly around and do the work for them while they eat cake and ice cream, send us on errands, and then take all the credit. When they come to our aid, it takes our available forces to wait on them, and a day to clear up after them ;" which confession could be echoed by many hard-working officers of benevolent societies. As to the glittering generality of literary clubs, their usefulness is summed up by a bright young member who speaks of them as "gossip served on trays with Shakespeare or Browning to float on the teacups." So if you mourn that your privileges are cut off, dear madam, by want of strength, rest consoled that the loss is not irreparable, either to the club or to you.

The only work worth mentioning in the world, the only kind that lasts and tells is individual work, whether of brain or hand. One can't object to gossip on any reasonable ground—indeed, has not Dr. Deems lately christened it with much insight " the humanities of conversation ?" That is when it is human and not fiendish, for there is a human interest in other people's affairs, and an inhuman one. But gossip weakens literature past toleration. Perhaps this is the reason why the most prominent woman's club in the country makes the melancholy confession in its yearly report that it has to depend for interest on the effort of six of its members, the rest being content with taking no part at all in its discussions. Now a man's club which depended on half a dozen members would turn up its toes and die, out of sheer decency. If you want an excuse for having a good time, christen your gathering gossip-club or the scandalmongery, and try to live up to it.

Every woman who values her health this chilly, stormy Spring, true breeder of typhoid pneumonia, should go into silk underwear, vests, chemiserie, skirts and nightgowns, if she has to economize on her dresses to provide them. Neuralgia and rheumatism are flying round, fell brood of the Winter scourge, and no cost can be reckoned dear which wards them off. Flannel has not the same warmth or electric action on the skin. A featherweight of a silk garment has more warmth than a thick wool one, with the advantage of lightness. The knickerbockers of black silk in fashion are commendable when Spring winds are abroad. At a sudden reel of wind at a street corner a glimpse of trim black silk stocking and rose-embroidered black silk ruffles has far less the effect of an exposé than a fleeting show of white garments. And the pink and blue slumber robes of India silk do so kindly keep off the pains in the shoulder next the crevice of the bedclothes when the tail of a cyclone is showing how full of drafts a $4000-a-year house can be.

Silk underwear doesn't mean combination suits in this instance, nor those nondescript attachments called "leglettes" by women with one lobe to their brain. Kate Field tells a witty and wicked story about an old woman up in Vermont whose only amusement was the village lecture course every season, which led off with Colonel Ingersoll one week and Mrs. Jenness Miller the next, when the old lady came home thunderstruck. "No hell and no chemise ! What was the world coming to ? For her part, if *both* were to be done away with, she didn't want to live in it any longer," and that's the way most nice women feel about their inner draperies. They are just as pretty in pale blue, rose or white India silk ruffled with feathery, firm thread lace, as the white cambric in which every woman ought to look like an angel that has laid off its wings.

If you love life and your families, don't stint fires this Spring, if you have to keep them mornings till the middle of June. An invention was shown in New York city last Spring which meets the wants of households better than any other warming apparatus. Perhaps its excellence is the very reason why it was hustled out of the way so that its present address cannot be found. It would not be the first invention so useful it had to be killed for fear of its superseding everything else of its kind. A sheet-iron tank, holding several gallons of kerosene, was fixed on the wall, with a quarter-inch pipe leading to a fire-box of porous clay or stone, through which the oil filtered, filled the box with flame. Any more complete economy of fuel is not to be found, and the ease with which it was regulated was a great recommendation. The room once warm with a quick fire the oil could be turned off to the merest dribble, sufficient, with slight flame, to keep the house at even warmth all day or night without attention. It was said to be so safe that the insurance companies charged no extra risk for it, and one gallon of oil was enough to keep a fifteen-foot room warm for twenty-four hours. I want to know what has become of this invention.

People must take to eating food which has the fullest nourishment. The new process has nearly ground and bolted the life out of flour, so that bread, the staff of life, is slighter than a wheat straw. A new company in Philadelphia has started the business of making perfectly nutritious bread without the yeast or powders, which is a surprise to everyone who eats it, two of their muffins with a cup of coffee making more of a working breakfast than a whole meal besides. The company furnishes a dozen forms of these cakes, made from whole wheat meal mixed with water and salt, and baked by steam, the application of quick heat raising them perfectly. The brown sweet little "breads" are gaining in favor with all brain workers who try them. One physician, well known in New York, has five dozen sent by express each Monday for his supply, an excellence of the new process being that the bread is as good for a week as the day it is baked. It feeds the nerves, it satisfies the appetite, the eyes grow brighter for using it, the complexion clearer, the color richer. Wheat entirely supplies a nearly complete food, or the foundation for it, with a small amount of the best meats and fruits and vegetables in variety.

Sedentary women, as a rule, eat far too much meat. It should be taken hot and well served at one meal, with fish broth, salad or croquettes at another, but certainly omitted at the third meal. Less work for the digestion means more vigor for the brain. Where even the steam-baked cakes are a tax on the system, a lighter food is the stale muffins dried in the great oven and pounded into a coarse meal, very nourishing, crisp and nice to take. Two or three tablespoonfuls of this, with a cup of broth or grape juice, furnishes a repast on which one can do more brainwork than on an ordinary dinner.

So, if the grip has left you feeling only half yourself, the first thing is to build up the ruins by supplying good nutrition, suited to weakened powers. Then the black lines under the eyes will disappear, and the pallid blueness, or the flush which alternates ; smooth, fresh cheeks will replace gaunt, sallow outlines, while mental improvement keeps place with the outward.

Lastly; keep in the sun and pure air, and if you cannot go out for it, let sun and air come to you. Choose the sunny window for your work, and keep the room ventilated, opening windows every hour for a few minutes. Rest with the lounge or bed drawn into the sunshine, an hour of which is better than many grains of quinine for giving strength. Not an hour of the priceless sun should be wasted between this and July by those who would undo the ravages of disease.

The Laughing Plant.

Palgrave, in his work on Central and Eastern Arabia, mentions a plant whose seeds produce effects analogous to those of laughing gas. The plant is a native of Arabia. A dwarf variety is found at Kasum, and another variety at Oman, which attains a height of from three to four feet, with woody stems, wide-spreading branches and light green foliage. The flowers are produced in clusters and are yellow in color. The seed pods contain two or three black seeds of the size and shape of a French bean. Their flavor is a little like that of opium, the taste is sweet, and the odor from them produces a sickening sensation and is slightly offensive. These seeds, when pulverized and taken in small doses, operate upon a person in a very peculiar manner. He begins to laugh loudly and boisterously, and then sings, dances and cuts up all kinds of fantastic capers. The effect continues about an hour, and the patient is extremely comical. When the excitement ceases, the exhausted individual falls into a deep sleep, which continues for an hour or more, and, when he awakens. he is utterly unconscious that any such demonstrations have been made by him.

THE ANNALS of HYGIENE,

✧ ✧

THE OFFICIAL ORGAN OF THE

State Board of Health of Pennsylvania.

The State Board of Health is not responsible for anything appearing in this Journal except that which bears the official attestation of the Board.

PUBLISHED MONTHLY.

Subscription, two dollars ($2.00) a year, in advance.

Address all communications to

The Hygienic Publishing Company,

224 SOUTH SIXTEENTH STREET,
PHILADELPHIA, PA.

EDITORIAL.

The Natural Disposal of Refuse.

To follow out the idea suggested in our last issue, we will repeat the assertion that all matter in reality belongs to nature ; that by her it is loaned to us that we may, by its use, perpetuate our existence, but, having so used this matter, it is imperatively necessary that we should return it to nature, failing to do which will surely bring upon us the punishment of nature which we are wont to call disease.

All the animal kingdom, in a state of nature, do faithfully and conscientiously return this loan ; man, alone, of all nature's creation, man, in what he is pleased to style the height of civilization, man alone fails to render unto nature that which is nature's own.

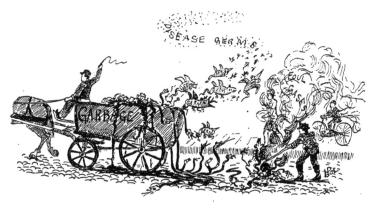

Nature's beautiful law provides that the matter which she has loaned to animal life, shall, having performed its mission therein, be passed on to do a like work in the vegetable kingdom. That which would prove detrimental to human health is the very matter that is greedily devoured by the vegetable world.

Let us clearly understand that by refuse matter we mean not only the solid and liquid waste from man, but what is commonly called garbage, waste bath water, dish water, soapy water of all kinds, everything, in a word, that contains organic matter.

How then does civilized man, living in a modern city, return this loan of nature. Let the dripping, reeking slop-cart, traversing the streets, depositing a goodly portion of its contents on the paving, there to putrefy and poison the atmosphere in the immediate vicinity of man, let this pestiferous sight answer the question.

Open up to view the miles upon miles of sewers underlying the streets of our cities, wherein the ingenuity of man has imprisoned tons upon tons of refuse, hidden away from nature's influence for good, yet subject to her inevitable law that dead organic matter *must decompose ;* witness herein not *natural decomposition*, but foul putrefaction, a resolving of this matter into its original elements, but an inability for these elements to do what nature wishes ; no chance for

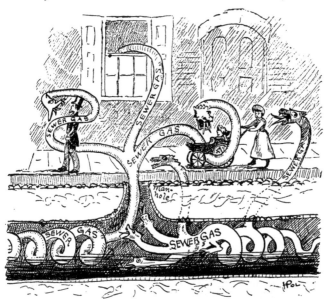

them to nourish vegetable life, but ample opportunity for them to poison humanity ; look here for our answer.

Let us follow this organic matter, leaking through the crevices of brick sewers and the broken joints and shattered sections of terra-cotta drains, percolating and saturating the ground, until we can truly speak of the subsoil of our large cities as a huge cesspool.

Let us remember that there is such a thing as " ground air," and let us watch this air, laden with putrefaction, rising from the soil and finding man's lungs, not six feet above the surface, ready to inhale it ; let us remember that he is thus taking back, practically unaltered, that which he but a short time previously has voided as unwholesome and injurious and in this picture let us read our answer.

Let us remember that it is the nature of gases to *ascend*, and let us realize that the very fact that man has invented all sorts of contrivances to prevent

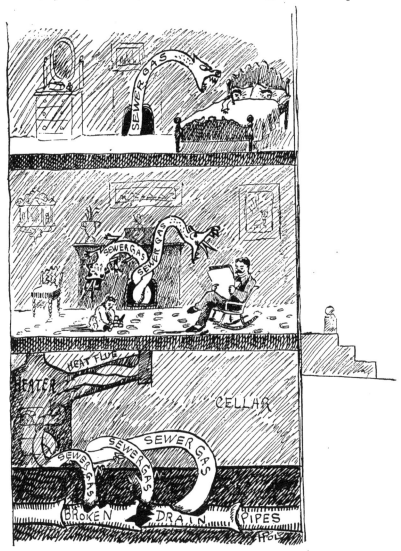

the return of sewer gases to our houses, is evidence of the natural tendency of these gases to so invade our homes, and as we see them doing so, let us have reason enough to admit that whenever *art* tries to overcome *nature*, that, while, sometimes apparently successful, nature is usually the victor in the end, and in this fact let us again read our answer.

In a word, let us critically inspect all the devices designed by man for the removal of organic refuse, and we will find them all eminently unsatisfactory, for the simple little reason that they are artificial and do not meet the laws and the requirements of nature.

Just as the contemplation of nature by a mind of keen penetrative powers has suggested to the world the wonderful powers of electricity as we see them to-day, just as the swinging lamp in the dear old cathedral at Pisa suggested the whole theory of the pendulum to the grasping mind of Galileo, just as the simmering teapot was pregnant with the possibilities of steam, and just as all these suggestive agencies lay unnoted for years, just so did a natural method for the disposal of organic refuse remain unthought of, though being continually suggested to us by nature, until the investigating mind of a man (who was returning from the funeral of two children who had fallen victims to disease, the result of our unnatural refuse disposal), determined to devise some means by which organic refuse could be disposed of in accordance with, rather than in antagonism to, nature.

Many years of deliberation and experimentation have enabled this mind to present to the world a *natural* system, with the theory and practical working of which we have thoroughly familiarized ourselves, and which, as a consequence of our investigation, we feel to be so *natural* as to constitute *perfection*. By this system all dead organic matter is deposited in a vault on an elevated surface, so that a current of air is passed over it and under, traversing the vault at the rate of fifteen or twenty miles an hour, gathering up from this decomposing mass all the gases of decomposition, carrying them up a tall flue, and casting them out into the atmosphere to be wafted away to feed vegetable life, as nature intends. Let us place our noses over a closet from which human deposits have been made into this vault, and is our sense of smell offended by the odors that arise? Far from it; for all such are being carried from us and up the flue at the rate of twenty miles per hour. Do we see a *putrefying* mass, such as our sewers would disclose? Such is impossible, for it is *natural* decomposition that is going on therein. Are the results of organic disorganization imprisoned from nature until they are forced back into our homes to poison and to slay us? On the contrary, they are, as fast as generated, hurried away to nature at the rate of twenty miles per hour. Is the atmosphere poisoned by the discharge into it of these gases of decomposition? Not any more so than would be the water of the Delaware River at Philadelphia were one to place in it, forty miles above, *one drop* of prussic acid, the poisonous agency, in each instance, being so infinitesimally small in comparison to the enormous proportion of the diluent, that its specific power for harm would be destroyed, in addition to which, in the case under consideration, these gases are wafted away by the winds toward the vegetable life to which nature intends that they shall give nourishment.

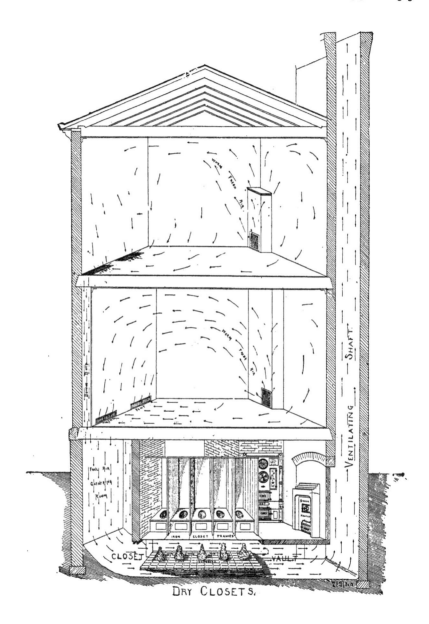

DRY CLOSETS.

Let us look into one of these vaults, in a public school, we will say, twenty-four hours after it has been used by, perhaps, 500 children. Will we be sickened by the odor and disgusted by the sight of a reeking mass of moist filth, such as would present itself to view did we penetrate the mysteries of a sewer? On the contrary, we will find a mass of thoroughly dry, odorless, *mummified* organic matter, similar to the cow manure of the field that has been subjected to the forces of nature; we will find a mass of matter that we can handle, if we choose, with impunity, over which we can pour some coal oil, touch a match thereto, and in an hour or two that which has been the refuse of 500 children will present to us but a small mass of ashes that one could swallow, if he so willed, without fear of injury. Can the mind of man conjure up a more natural or a more beautiful picture? We plead guilty to having fallen a complete and unqualified captive to this system. We started out to briefly describe the features of this system, but our enthusiasm has run away with our pen until we fear that we have run away with the patience of our readers. It is not our wish or intention to make this editorial an advertisement for any man's business, hence we have purposely refrained from saying anything that would unfold the identity of this system to any of our readers save those who may be already familiar with it. But, in conclusion we would say that if our pen picture presents a scene of nature to any of our readers that, as it was with ourselves, they can have no conception of the perfection of the system until they have seen it working. It is the system, and not its inventor, that we are advocating, and while, therefore, we fail to reveal its identity in our pages, we will be only too glad to personally say to any of our readers where they may see it in operation, hoping, as we believe, that anyone who once sees the system in operation will become as ardent an admirer thereof as we ourselves now are.

A Just Retribution.

It is related of a doctor "down East" that although several eminent physicians, as well as the health authorities, had pronounced a disease that was prevalent in the town to be scarlet fever, he persisted in denying this fact and even went so far as to tear down the flags of warning that had been displayed upon infected houses by the authorities. For this latter act he was arrested and will probably be a wiser and sadder man before he gets through with his trouble. But for the retribution; denying the nature of the disease and, consequently, neglecting to observe the simplest precautions, he carries the disease into his own home and infects his own children. The moral of this true story is that whenever there is a doubt as to whether a given disease is contagious or infectious or not, the benefit should be given to the side of contagion. The precautions to prevent spreading that will then be in order cannot do any harm under any circumstances, while if the disease is contagious, their neglect may prove fearfully and fatally retributive.

NOTES AND COMMENTS.

Onions for Insomnia.

A writer in a daily paper recommends eating raw onions before bedtime as a remedy for insomnia. Evidently he sleeps alone (says the *Medical Record*) and by an open window.

The Absent-Minded Doctor.

An absent-minded doctor recently took unto himself a wife. During the marriage ceremony when she held out her hand for the ring, he felt her pulse and requested to see her tongue.

A Small Baby.

Dr. C. G. Hubburd, of Hornellsville, N. Y., reports in the *New York Medical Journal* the birth of a living child which weighed one pound and two ounces and measured ten inches in length. It lived eight hours.

To Remove Fruit Stains.

Pour boiling water on chloride of lime, in the proportion of 1 gallon to ¼ pound ; bottle it, cork it well, and in using be careful not to stir it. Lay the stain in this for a moment, then apply white vinegar and boil the table linen.

Fish as an Invalid Diet.

It is remarked by a contributor to the *London Lancet*, that many medical men may be unaware of the fact, simple as it is, that boiled fish, fried fish, and almost any other kind of cooked fish, are all inferior in digestibility to steamed fish.

Ozone for Bedrooms.

A simple plan for obtaining ozone in small quantities is to mix very gradually three parts of strong sulphuric acid with two parts of permanganate of potash in a jam-pot, and place the vessel under the bed. Ozone will be given off from the mixture for some weeks.—*N. Y. Medical Times.*

How to Bathe the Eyes.

To bathe the eyes properly take a large basin of cold water, bend the head close over it, and with both hands throw the water with some force on the gently closed lids. This has something of the same effect as a shower bath, and has a toning-up influence which water applied in any other way has not.

A Cure for Snoring.

It has been recommended that when a person can breathe readily through the nose, if they will tie a band or handkerchief over the mouth it will cure the habit of snoring. We have had no experience with this procedure, hence cannot endorse it ; but, as it is simple and harmless, it is worthy of trial.

An Album for Pasteur.

The *Semaine Médicale* reports that a committee, composed of British and American notabilities, has been formed to offer an album to M. Pasteur. The first page of this album bears, in French, under the signature of the Princess of Wales, the following inscription : "To the Great Monsieur Pasteur; the Benefactor of the human race."

Use of the Kola-Nut in Armies.

During the manœuvres of the German Army last Autumn, numerous experiments were made to determine the practical utility of the kola-nut in enabling men to endure severe and prolonged physical labor. So satisfactory were the results obtained that the authorities are said to have ordered thirty tons of the drug for use of the army.

Liniment for Neuralgia.

R Camphorated alcohol,   90 parts.
   Ether,   30   "
   Tincture of opium,   6   "
   Chloroform,   20   '   M.

To be applied on flannel.—*Courier Médicale.*

Bound to Kill Them Somehow.

Mary—said the sick man, feebly—those yowling cats annoy me terribly. Can't they be reached by a shot-gun or something of that kind ?

No—replied his wife—they are on the flat roof of the adjoining house.

Mary—exclaimed the invalid again, after a pause, and his face grew hard and pitiless—throw some of these medicines up on the roof.

Gelatine as a Food.

We are glad to find Dr. F. P. Henry, of this city, calling attention to the fact that the merits of gelatine, as a food, are not sufficiently recognized. Jelly is a favorite dish for the invalid, but the man in health seldom thinks to eat it. We are satisfied that gelatine is a most nutritious and healthy food, and we would bespeak for it a larger degree of popular favor than it now enjoys.

Persistent Headache.

It will be well for those of our readers who may suffer from persistent headache for which they cannot assign satisfactory cause, to know that such a condition is, not infrequently, due to some eye trouble. If, therefore, any one is troubled in this way, often thinking it to be neuralgia, it will be wise to consult a *good* oculist and see if relief cannot be procured by attention to the eyes.

Keep on Your Hat at the Grave.

A society of clergymen of Topeka, Kan., has passed resolutions opposing the custom, on the part of pall bearers and friends, of uncovering the head at the commitment of bodies to the grave, and has requested the local medical society for their opinion on the matter. The society has unanimously endorsed the ministers' views, and so do we also ; most emphatically.

For Indigestion.

For indigestion, the external application of something warm to the stomach, a piece of flannel, or anything to keep the stomach warm and promote a supply of blood, is sometimes of great benefit. In taking hot water internally, it is best to sip it by spoonfuls, waiting a moment after each for an eructation of the gas disengaged by the hot water from the fermenting contents of the stomach.

Connecticut Tobacco.

An item, in the paper, recently caught our eye, to the effect that the value of Connecticut tobacco has depreciated fully 50 per cent. because the proper kind of manure is not supplied to the growing plant. If, we thought, improper food (for manure is the food of vegetable life) will depreciate the value of a vegetable growth 50 per cent., is it unreasonable to claim that improper food will depreciate the value of a human being equally as much?

No Time for Health.

People are too hurried to think of health—are under too much pressure to pause for physiology. They bolt their meals, race for the train, jump for the boat. Those who live fast do not live well. The steady, moderate, methodical man does more work and better than one who tries to do in a day the work of a week. The racer gives out sooner than the plodding draught horse. Yet there is nothing that shortens life like laziness.—*Monthly Bulletin.*

The Eiffel Tower as a Mother's Mark.

The Paris correspondent of the *Medical Press* is responsible for the story that a woman from St. Quentin visited (being at the time about four months' pregnant) the late Paris Exhibition. One of the sights which seemed to strike her the most and to have an extraordinary influence on her nervous system was the celebrated Eiffel tower. Small blame to the poor woman! Recently she was confined, and the child bears on its chest a well-defined reproduction of the monument.

The Abolition of Capital Punishment.

There has perambulated down the ages a legend to the effect that "the doctor takes life easily," and it might be inferred that he would regard the taking of life by society without any sentimental protest at least. We believe it is true that the physician looks at the question of capital punishment very objectively, and passes judgment upon it mainly as he would upon a question of therapeutics—for this is what it is. If society can better preserve and protect itself against criminals by their strangulation or electrothanatosis, why, then, these measures should be employed. No question of first principles or inherent rights or sentiment is involved. The public mind is being exercised upon this matter just now, and we hope with fruitful results. It appears as if the death penalty were a necessity in the early stages of social organization, but that as civilization advances it becomes useless and unwise.—*Medical Record.*

Glass Water and Sewer Pipes.

We have always felt that if glass could be used for water and sewer pipes, it would be a great step forward. Not only would lead contamination of water be then impossible ; not only would corrosion by sewage and occlusion of the pipe be unheard of, but if placed in view (as all pipes always should be), it would be always possible for us to see and know just what was going on inside of our pipes. Hence do we record with extreme gratification that a glass pipe for water service has been placed upon the market by a firm in Dresden.

Married at 90.

It must have been a pleasant sight to one who admires longevity to have witnessed the marriage ceremony that recently took place in West Virginia, wherein the groom was 90 years of age. This old man walked twenty miles to greet his bride, then six miles more to get a license, and was then married. There is no earthly reason why in time, by a process of physical regeneration, the result of a *universal* observance of the teachings of hygiene, all of us might not, at 90 years of age, be as vigorous and as interested in the affairs of this world as was this ardent and athletic lover.

Bismarck's Retirement Not an Unmixed Evil.

One result of Prince Bismarck's retirement will, says the *British Medical Journal*, perhaps, be a notable improvement in the eyesight of his countrymen. German oculists almost unanimously attribute the extraordinary prevalence of myopia and other defects of vision in the Fatherland to the use of the national black-letter type in school-books. Prince Bismarck has always resolutely stood upon the ancient ways in this matter, and has opposed the substitution of the Roman for the Gothic character in German books. The party of typographical reform is now hopeful of succeeding in its object.

How Smallpox Epidemics Originate.

The following account of the origin of a recent epidemic of smallpox in Meriden, Conn., as furnished by Dr. C. A. Lindsley, the secretary of the Connecticut State Board of Health, is very instructive, in so far as it clearly shows how one *suppressed* case was the cause of communicating the disease to twenty-six persons and causing the sacrifice of ten lives :

A man boarding with a saloon-keeper in Meriden visited Windsor Locks during the prevalence of the disease in that place. After his return he was ill and had an eruption, which was thought so suspicious that he was kept out of view in his rooms until it had disappeared, and advised to say nothing about it. In due time the little daughter of the saloon-keeper was also taken sick and had an eruption ; and her physician reported it to the City Health Committee as varioloid. A consultation with other physicians was held upon the case, and the majority being of the opinion that it was chicken-pox and not varioloid, the Health Committee took no precautions about it. The case was not even kept under observation for the brief time necessary to settle the doubt concerning it.

The experience of Meriden will afford a notable illustration of the importance of immediate notification of every infectious disease, and of the danger of neglecting any cases about which there is reasonable uncertainty of the diagnosis.

Spitting in Street Cars.

An evidence of the way in which sanitary teaching is taking possession of the popular mind is to be found in an order recently issued by the Traction Company, of this city. The company controls the majority of our street car lines, and within a few days placards have been conspicuously placed in all of their cars to the effect that "spitting in the cars is positively forbidden." This rule has resulted from the publication to the public of the fact that the expectoration of consumptives contains the seeds of the disease and that promiscuous expectoration is a ready means for diffusing this fearfully prevalent malady.

Dont's.

Don't read in omnibuses or other jolting vehicles. Don't pick the teeth with pins or any other hard substance. Don't neglect any opportunity to ensure a variety of food. Don't eat and drink hot and cold things immediately in succession. Don't pamper the appetite with such variety of food as may lead to excess. Don't read, write, or do any delicate work unless receiving the light from the left side. Don't keep the parlor dark unless you value your carpet more than your children's health and your own. Don't endeavor to rest the mind by absolute inactivity ; let it seek its rest in other channels, and thus rest the tired part of the brain.

A Swiss Cure for a Fresh Cold.

Camphor, says the *Lancet*, has often been recommended for colds in the head, although Dr. George Johnson and others have long since indicated the dangers from concentrated alcoholic solutions. A Swiss pharmaceutical journal gives the following method : Into a jug half filled with boiling water put one drachm of powdered camphor ; over it place a funnel-shaped paper from which the apex has been torn off so as to admit the nose. The camphorated steam may thus be drawn in through the nose for ten or fifteen minutes. Any cold in the head, it is maintained, however severe, will yield to three such applications. —*New York Medical Journal.*

The Hygienic Aspect of Life Insurance.

There are but few arguments left unpresented to would-be victims by life insurance agents, but there is one that we have not yet seen written about. Serenity of mind, contentment, is, we must all admit, a most potent factor in the preservation of health and the promotion of longevity ; while worry and anxiety will do much to produce ill-health and shorten life. To the man who loves his family what thought can possibly be more wearing or harassing than the fear that should he be taken away they will be left unprovided for. On the other hand what refreshing sleep will come to the man who places his head on the pillow conscious of the fact that should he die before morning his life insurance policy will provide for the loved ones he has left behind. Thus then, will the insuring of our lives not only protect those who are dear to us, but it will actually tend to lengthen our own lives by the peace of mind it will vouchsafe to us.

Swelled Heads.

The man who, as a result of material success, allows his head to swell, is a man whose liver will be very apt also to swell, and he will become so generally swollen that he will prove a nuisance to himself and to all about him. Edison, the great inventor, when it was recently remarked to him that since his great success he must have forgotten his old associates, replied that he would "rather have the smallpox than a swelled head." A man with a "swelled head" is an abnormal man, and an abnormal man cannot be a healthy or a happy man, so, for goodness sake, let us avoid "swelled heads," not only in ourselves, but in others.

A Grasping Lot.

The story is told in the newspapers that a certain M. Heriot, the owner of a big store called the Louvre, in Paris, was sent to the insane asylum by his relations because he insisted upon giving $1,000,000, which he could readily afford to lose, to founding an orphanage for soldiers' children. The local authorities finally ordered that he should be removed from a private asylum and placed in a public one, and it was quickly found that he was not insane at all. For thirteen months' treatment the private asylum doctors demand $22,500, the local doctors want $20,000, three medical students who helped find him crazy, $13,500, and the keepers, $5,000.

Cleaning the Teeth.

Strange as it may seem to say so, yet we imagine but few persons really use a tooth brush as they should. We recall, many years ago, when a student of medicine, the advice given in this connection by the famous Dr. Leidy, who called attention to the fact that it is not enough to brush the teeth alone, but that the whole inside of the mouth should be scrubbed as well. Many of those annoying cases of "bad breath" are due to neglect of this simple practice. The dead tissue in the mouth should be brushed loose and rinsed away, otherwise it will decompose and prove very unpleasant and offensive to both the individual and any one who may be in close proximity to him.

Living by Rule.

A lady recently said to one of our agents, who was soliciting her subscription to "The Annals," that she did not care to read about hygiene, because she did not believe in "living by rule." If there is one point that we instruct our agents to impress upon those whom they visit more strongly than another, if there is one strong vein running through our journal, it is that "living by rule" is not hygienic. He who would so live must by so doing concentrate so much thought upon self, must become so self-conscious, so introspective, as it were, that his life would be an artificial one, and since a natural life only can be hygienic, we do not see how it is possible for one who "lives by rule" to lead a hygienic life.

Quarantine Against Epidemic Influenza in Saranac Village.

Dr. E. L. Trudeau wrote recently to the *Medical News* that he had been enabled to carry out, with apparent success, a policy of protective non-intercourse against "la grippe" at his Cottage Sanitarium in the Adirondacks. Fearing that an incursion of influenza would prove disastrous to the invalids under his care at that institution, he undertook the experiment of a quarantining of the place as soon as the disease appeared in that neighborhood. Since that time a considerable portion of the population of the surrounding country have been attacked, but no case has occurred among those connected with the sanitarium itself. That establishment is not more than a mile distant from the village, where had been a number of cases of the epidemic disease.

The Light of Publicity upon Contagion.

We are heartily in accord with the efforts of Dr. P. D. Keyser, who would like to have the casket containing the body of a person dead of a contagious disease marked with a sign of warning. This is an effort in the right direction. If we make evident to the people the spot where contagion exists, they will avoid it. If a man places an obstruction on our streets he is obliged to mark it by a red light when the shades of night have hidden it from view; neglecting which, he is liable for any damages that may occur. So should it be with contagion. Let us recognize contagion as an entity and treat it as such; let us mark the place where it exists, just as we would indicate the pile of building material or the cave-in of a street.

The Shortcomings of Soap.

There are probably few people who do not find the joy of living made less keen by having to read each day the advertisements of popular soaps. Their good qualities are so superlatively good, their effect on the complexion, the health and longevity so unfailing, their chemical composition in each case so remarkably in accord with all that exact science and dermatological art could produce, that it discourages the medical man, who finds so much in his own measures that are imperfect and incomplete.

We read, therefore, with a certain sense of relief the results of an investigation made by Dr. B. H. Paul, in the *British Journal of Dermatology*, on the composition of these highly lauded toilet soaps. Dr. Paul states that for bodily ablution soaps should not contain an excess of alkali but should be neutral or nearly so. He found, however, that among the toilet soaps, as usually met with, a perfectly neutral soap is the exception, and that a trustworthy soap of that kind is still a desideratum. Three of five soaps of the higher grade were described as "super-fatted" soaps, one of them being alleged to have been prepared according to Una's formula. But in fact they all were found to contain the full proportion of alkali required for the saponification of the fat, besides some additional potash, which in one of them was considerable. It seems, therefore, that the perfect soap is yet to be made.—*Medical Record.*

Lead Poisoning.

There are but few complaints that will present symptoms so obscure, so misleading, so little directly pointing to the cause, as will be the case with comparatively mild chronic lead poisoning due to the continual ingestion of small quantities of lead in the water that we drink, this same being derived from the leaden pipes through which the water is conveyed:

Competent and observing authorities are now agreed that lead poisoning from this cause is infinitely more common than we generally suppose, and it is sufficiently prevalent and its consequences sufficiently alarming to warrant the assertion that leaden pipes for the conveyance of water ought to be abandoned. In another part of this issue we tell of the introduction of glass for this purpose, or we could, if we so wished, use iron pipes. Of course the expense would be somewhat greater, but if we would do that which we should do, we will abandon leaden pipes for the conveyance of drinking water.

A True Story of Boarding-School and Measles.

We relate the following because it has just transpired in a family very near to us and we can vouch for its absolute accuracy. This family consisted of father, mother, daughter, aged 12, boy, aged 8, and little boy, aged 3½. Though opposed to boarding-schools, it was, for certain reasons, deemed expedient to have the daughter spend the past Winter at a convent. On the sixth day of last month this girl came home to spend a couple of days. She was somewhat droopy and not just "like herself" upon arrival. On the 8th she was in bed with well-marked measles. At the time of writing all three children are sick together, with measles, in one room. Some of our old-fashioned readers who still hold to the idea that it is necessary for children to have measles, scarlet fever and all the so-called "children's diseases," will see a wise dispensation in this order of things, whereby the inevitable is received in one instead of in divided doses. But to such we would propound this query: "Is it possible for corn to grow in a field wherein the seed has not been deposited?" Of course there can be but one answer, and this same reply applies with equal force to all these contagious diseases. *It is not necessary for children to suffer from these diseases, and they will not so suffer unless the seed be deposited in their bodies.* It is perfectly possible to keep such disease away from the house, but when it has been once brought therein it is next to impossible to prevent its being spread from one to another of the children. Just as the morning-glory will not grow without first planting the seed, neither will disease ; but every one knows how profusely this vine will grow until it invades every possible place and becomes a nuisance. So will the germ of disease, once brought into the house, spread and multiply until it will invade every susceptible resident thereof. We can, however, keep this seed away from the home, and there is no more favorable place for the propagation, multiplication and dissemination of disease germs than large schools wherein a large number of children, of whose home conditions we cannot be sure, are congregated in the closest of communion.

The Suppression of Street Music.

We cannot sympathize with the movement now in course of agitation in this city for the suppression of street musicians. Music, even though it may be bad music, will prove a pleasure to the healthy and a most valuable remedial agent to many who are not well. The strains of music may disturb the serenity of some, whose lives and whose stomachs are out of gear, but we cannot see any valid reason why this honest means of gaining a living should be denied to those who would select it, and we do see many reasons, from a hygienic point of view, why the streets of our city and the homes of our citizens should be made cheerful and pleasant by the strains of music (good, bad or indifferent) floating therein. Let the bands play, or at least, before suppressing them, let us get at public sentiment on the question and learn whether the great mass of *natural* persons who desire them would not far outweigh the handful of bilious, dyspeptic, nervously deranged, *artificial* persons who would suppress them.

Dangers of Tight Clothing.

Now that rational ideas as to dress have acquired a definite place in public esteem, it may be imagined that the practice of tight lacing and customs of a like nature, if known at all, are not what they used to be. A case of sudden death lately reported proves that it is still too early to indulge in such illusory ideas. The deceased, a servant girl of excitable temperament, died suddenly in an epileptoid fit, and the evidence given before the coroner respecting her death attributed the fatal issue to asphyxia, due in a great measure to the fact that both neck and waist were unnaturally constricted by her clothing, the former by a tight collar, the latter by a belt worn under the stays. We have here certainly those very conditions which would lead us to expect the worst possible consequences from a convulsive seizure. There is no organ of the body whose free movement is at such times more important than the heart. Yet here we find, on the one hand, its movement hampered by a tight girdle so placed that it could with difficulty be undone at a critical moment; on the other, a contrivance admirably adapted to allow the passage of blood to the brain, while impeding its return. This is no isolated case as regards its essential character, though, happily, somewhat singular in its termination. Minor degrees of asphyxiation, we fear, are still submitted to by a good many self-torturing children of vanity. The tight corset and the high heel still work mischief on the bodies of their devoted wearers. Taste and reason, indeed, combine to deprecate their injurious and vulgar bondage, and by no means unsuccessfully. Still the evil maintains itself. Cases like that above mentioned ought to, if they do not, open the eyes of some self-worshippers of the gentler sex who heedlessly strive by such means to excel in a sickly grace. We would strongly impress on all of this class the fact that beauty is impossible without health, and would advise them, in the name of taste as well as comfort, to avoid those methods of contortion, one and all, by which elegance is only caricatured, and health may be painfully and permanently injured.—*The Analyst.*

Quarantine Your Nurses.

How many cases of measles or scarlet fever or diphtheria, for which the family is unable to account, have been brought into the house by the "new nurse" but few imagine, and it would be absolutely impossible to accurately determine; but that many such cases do occur we have no doubt. A nurse comes into the household; she has a slight sore throat, of which she may or may not speak; in a few days one of the children has diphtheria and we wonder where the disease came from. The relation between the "new nurse's" *sore throat* and the child's diphtheria does not occur to us. Just as we require references of honesty and capacity, so should we also inquire into the health not only of the prospective nurse, but of the household wherein she has been lately temporarily or permanently residing. Even after this, even should she be able to present a clean "bill of health," we should not think of allowing baby to sleep with nurse until the latter has been under observation for at least two weeks.

An Octogenarian Athlete.

When we read that which we reproduce below, the thought suggested itself to us that it must give to a man who has reached the age of 80 years a feeling of gratification, a sense of superiority, a self-contentment, a consciousness of a well-spent life, to find himself in the physical condition in which the hero of this episode is. Then came the reflection that this condition, which in this particular case is probably rather accidental than intentional, could be by design the happy boon of each and all of us did we so order our lives. Here comes the story :

A queer looking little specimen of humanity with an armful of newspapers stood outside of the Grand Central Depot, New York, the other afternoon, crying his wares. His hair was long and unkempt, his trousers were frayed at the edges, there were patches of poverty on his little jacket, but his eye was clear and his flattened nose showed that he was the hero of many a gutter battle. A pompous-looking individual, with his great coat thrown open, a heavy cane in his hand and dressed in the height of fashion, came swinging himself down the street in gorgeous style. The boy pulled one of his papers out, offered it to the swell, and was rewarded for his efforts by a thump on the back with the heavy cane. The little fellow howled with pain. The cabmen who were at the gate at the depot smiled and the other boys laughed in derision. The swell had proceeded about three steps on his way, when a firm hand grasped him by the collar, shook him vigorously, and an old man six foot two, as straight as a grenadier and holding a heavy malacca stick threateningly over him, asked : "How dare you hit a boy?" The swell tried to shake himself loose, but it was no use. The old man's hand was firm. The crowd was growing larger and the boy was howling as though his heart would break.

"You, sir," went on the old man, as the blood mounted to his face, "are a disgrace to humanity. Old as I am I can thrash you for that cowardly act. And if I ever know you to again lift your hand to a boy I will take the law into my own hands."

The swell's head dropped a little and his face was pale. The old man looked him firmly in the eye, shook him again as a cat would a mouse, and walked on. As he did so, the little boy, wiping the tears from his cheeks, followed after and thanked him. The old man patted him affectionately on the head and disappeared in the crowd. There was no comment except by the small boy, who exclaimed : "Ain't he a daisy?" He brushed the tears from his eyes, and in a moment was as busy as ever selling his papers.

The old man was a daisy. It was none other than David Dudley Field, the greatest constitutional lawyer in the world, brother of Cyrus W. and Stephen J. Field. He is nearly eighty-three years of age, but as vigorous as a man of fifty. In his young days he was a famous boxer and athlete, and the way he tackled the howling swell showed that his good right hand had not forgot its cunning.

How Drunkards are Treated in Norway.

The London correspondent of the *American Practitioner and News* says that a well-known medical man, who has recently been in Norway, gives a glowing description of their manner of treating dipsomaniacs. An habitual drunkard in Sweden and Norway is treated as a criminal in this sense, that his inordinate love of strong drink renders him liable to imprisonment, and while in confinement it appears he is cured of his bad propensities on a plan which, though simple enough, is said to produce marvelous effects. From the day the confirmed drunkard is incarcerated no nourishment is served to him or her but bread and wine. The bread, however, it should be said, cannot be eaten apart from the wine, but is steeped in a bowl of it, and left thus to soak an hour or more before the meal is served to the delinquent. The first day the habitual toper takes his food in this shape without the slightest repugnance ; the second day he finds it less agreeable to his palate, and very quickly he evinces a positive aversion to it. Generally, the doctor states, eight or ten days of this regimen is more than sufficient to make a man loathe the very sight of wine, and even refuse the prison dish set before him. This manner of curing drunken habits is said to succeed almost without exception, and men or women who have undergone the treatment not only rarely return to their evil ways, but from sheer disgust they frequently become total abstainers afterward.—*Northwestern Lancet.*

A Wise Employer.

John B. Stetson, of this city, is the largest hat manufacturer in this country, yet we doubt if, with all his facilities, he could make a hat large enough to cover the wisdom within his head. Mr. Stetson is a pioneer in that class of employers who have wisdom enough to know that a healthy employé will do healthy work, and *vice versâ*, and he is large-hearted enough to regard his employés rather as those over whom he should exercise a fatherly care than as mere machines to be forced to do all the work of which they are physically capable. These remarks were called forth by reading recently of the opening ceremonies of a gymnasium which Mr. Stetson has provided for the use of his employés. Adjoining the office of the manufactory Mr. Stetson has founded an institution where the mental, moral and physical condition of his employés may be improved. On the first floor is a dispensary presided over by six physicians. There is a clinic from 12.30 to 1.30 P. M. daily. Last year upward of 7000 patients were treated. Adjoining is a well-stocked library, which also contains newspapers and magazines. It is always open, and many persons avail themselves of the privileges. There is a Sunday school on the second floor. The average attendance is 1600. The primary class and kindergarten are located on the floor above. The fourth floor contains the headquarters of the Guard cf Honor, a semi-military temperance association. There are four companies of 150 to 200 men each.

There is also the John B. Stetson Union, which is similar to the Young Men's Christian Association. Its membership is large.

The Spare Bed.

A friend recently gave us the following eulogy, clipped from we know not where, with the request that we help to extend its circulation. We comply, not without a strong feeling of the uselessness of such effort. It requires more than ridicule to convert the average housekeeper from her blind devotion to the traditions of her foremothers concerning the "spare room."

"Who first called them 'spare beds?' Why didn't he name them 'man-killers' instead? I never see a spare bed without wanting to tack the following card on the headboard:

NOTICE!

THIS BED WARRANTED TO PRODUCE NEURALGIA, RHEUMATISM, STIFF JOINTS, BACKACHE, DOCTORS' BILLS AND DEATH!

"When I go out into the country to visit my relatives, the spare bed rises up before my imagination days before I start, and I shiver as I remember how cold and gravelike the sheets are. I put off the visit as long as possible, solely on account of that spare bed. I don't like to tell them that I would rather sleep on a picket fence than to enter that spare room and creep into that spare bed, and so they know nothing of my sufferings.

"The spare bed is always as near a mile and a half from the rest of the beds as it can be located. It's either upstairs at the head of the hall, or off the parlor. The parlor curtains haven't been raised for weeks; everything is as prim as an old maid's bonnet, and the bed is as square and true as if it had been made up to a carpenter's rule. No matter whether it is Summer or Winter, the bed is like ice, and it sinks down in a way to make one shiver. The sheets are slippery clean, the pillow slips rustle like shrouds, and one dare not stretch his leg down for fear of kicking against a tombstone.

"Ugh! shake me down on the kitchen floor, let me sleep on the haymow, on a lounge, stand up in a corner, anywhere but in the spare bed! One sinks down until he is lost in the hollow, and foot by foot the prim bedposts vanish from sight. He is worn out and sleepy, but he knows that the rest of the family are so far away that no one could hear him if he should shout for an hour, and this makes him nervous. He wonders if anyone ever died in that room, and straightway he sees faces of dead persons, hears strange noises, and presently feels a chill galloping up and down his back."—*Sanitary Volunteer.*

The Hygienic Treatment of Constipation.

The instructions which Sir A. Clark asks his pupils to give to their patients for the management of simple constipation are as follows: 1. On first waking in the morning, and also on going to bed at night, sip slowly from a quarter to a half pint of water, cold or hot. 2. On rising, take a cold or tepid sponge bath, followed by a brisk general toweling. 3. Clothe warmly and loosely; see that there is no constriction about the waist. 4. Take three simple but liberal meals daily, and, if desired, and it does not disagree, take also a slice of bread and butter in the afternoon. When tea is used, it should not be hot or strong, or infused over five minutes. Avoid pickles, spices, curries, salted or otherwise preserved provisions, pies, pastries, cheese, jams, dried fruits, nuts, all coarse, hard and indigestible foods taken with a view of moving the bowels, strong tea and much hot liquid of any kinds, with meals. 5. Walk at least half an hour twice daily. 6. Avoid sitting and working long in such a position as will compress or constrict the bowels. 7. Solicit the action of the bowels every day after breakfast, and be patient in soliciting. If you fail in procuring relief in one day, wait until the following day, when you will renew the solicitation at the appointed time. And if you fail the second day, you may, continuing the daily solicitation, wait until the fourth day, when assistance should be taken. The simplest and best will be a small enema of equal parts of olive oil and water. The action of this injection will be greatly helped by taking it with the hips raised, and by previously anointing the anus and the lower part of the rectum with vaseline or with oil. 8. If by the use of all these means you fail in establishing the habit of daily or alternate daily action of the bowels, you may try, on waking in the morning, massage of the abdomen, practiced from right to left along the course of the colon ; and you may take at the two greater meals of the day a dessert spoonful or more of the best lucca oil. It is rather a pleasant addition to potatoes or to green vegetables.

Treated upon physiological considerations, Sir Andrew believes that in the vast majority of cases simple constipation may be successfully overcome without recourse to medicine.—*New York Medical Times.*

The So-Called Sewers of Philadelphia.

This city has recently created a loan of several millions of dollars, a liberal slice of which has been appropriated for the construction of sewers. In his inaugural address, referring to the use of this borrowed money, President Smith, of Common Council, made the assertion that there never had been a time when our citizens were more willing to submit to reasonable and necessary charges, but that they would insist upon the wise and honest expenditure of their money. This we believe, but we are constrained to say that while the money devoted to sewers has been honestly appropriated, we cannot feel that it will be wisely expended. The fact is that none of our large cities have any real system of sewers ; they have accumulated in patchwork style, as occasion demanded, but there is no system, properly speaking, about them. Hence do we feel that money expended to extend and enlarge this unscientific network of sewers is not money wisely expended. We must begin at the beginning and go all over the work again in a proper and scientific way and the sooner we begin the better and cheaper will it be. Let our small and growing cities profit by the predicament of their elder brethren and start their sewerage on a scientific basis, sufficiently comprehensive to meet all possibilities of future growth.

The Sleep of Death.

How few, we imagine, have ever moralized over this familiar saying, yet how much suggestiveness there is about it. Look at one in deep sleep, when the movements of respiration are but feeble: is the resemblance to death not great? Is not a dreamless sleep as thoroughly full of oblivion to the sleeper as death can possibly be? So that, to both the sleeper and the beholder, is there not a close resemblance between sleep and death, the one a temporary slumber, the other an everlasting sleep. Dr. Oliver Wendell Holmes has truly said that "Death to the aged man wears as pleasing a face as sleep does to one who is tired," and we would add that death to the young and ambitious man is as repellant in aspect as the most horrible of nightmares. The old man who has rounded out his measure of life regards death as the *natural* termination of his existence, and he quietly and willingly falls asleep ; while the young man, who is by disease cut down before his time, can only regard the sleep that is thus forced upon him as an *unnatural* nightmare, a termination of that of which he feels, instinctively, he has not had a surfeit. Is it not wise, therefore, for all to so strive that death shall come to them as a welcome, expected slumber rather than to be regarded as a horror too horrible to quietly contemplate?

An Element of Health in Suburban Life.

It has been frequently noted, and many efforts have been made to furnish a scientific explanation therefor, that railroad engineers and conductors are usually stout, healthy-looking men.

It would seem to us that the explanation might possibly be found in the passive exercise to which they are almost continually subjected by the jarring and the jolting of the trains. We all know that motion, which is but another word for exercise, is essential to healthy life, and we should know that passive exercise, that is to say, motion of the tissues of the body produced without the expenditure of the will power of the individual, is a most admirable form of exercise. The manipulator, who is called in to aid the physician restore his patient to health, works on this hypothesis. He works and kneads and moves the different parts of the body, thus giving them motion, while the will of the patient remains passive : he, himself, has nothing to do with the production of this motion. Is not the situation somewhat identical with the motion received from the jarring and jolting of a railroad train. If so, if our ideas be correct, then the daily ride to and from the city, enjoyed by the suburban resident, will procure for him the passive exercise so beneficial to his health.

The Abnormal View of Hygiene.

The person who said that he would rather be ignorant of hygiene, because it made him nervous to think so much about himself; to be told that he could not eat this or that, and that he must do so and so, was a man who could not be convinced of the fact that the preconceived, ascetic notions of hygiene which he entertained were erroneous. Such a person ought to be present at a gathering of sanitarians and see whether they deprive themselves of any of the good things of the table. Far from it ; we believe that each man should be a law unto himself, but we hold that he should take a little trouble to familiarize himself with the special laws that may govern his special humanity. In this manner of eating, we believe that a person should eat just exactly what he pleases, with the single, simple proviso that he should avoid that which his experience teaches him will disagree with his special organism. Do not let us unnecessarily surround the practice of hygienic teachings with an austere and disagreeable enclosure that does not belong to it.

Nutritive Value of Certain Foods..

Speaking roughly, a quart of oysters contains, on the average, about the same quantity of active nutritive substance as a quart of milk, or a pound of very lean beef, or a pound and a-half of fresh codfish, or two-thirds of a pound of bread. But while the weight of actual nutriment in the different quantities of food material named is very nearly the same, the quality is widely different. That of very lean meat or codfish consists mostly of what are called in chemical language, protein compounds or "flesh formers"—the substance which makes blood, muscle, tendon, bone, brain, and other nitrogenous tissues. That of bread contains but little of these, and consists chiefly of starch, with a little fat and other compounds, which serve the body as fuel, and supply it with heat and muscular power. The nutritive substance of oysters contains considerable of both the flesh-forming and the more especially heat and force-giving ingredients. Oysters come nearer to milk than almost any other common food, their values for supplying the body with material to build up its parts, repair its wastes and furnish it with heat and energy would be pretty nearly the same.— *The Century.*

Country Life.

There are two points to which we would like to invite especial attention in the admirable paper by Dr. Samuel Wolfe, which we publish elsewhere in this issue ; first the statement that he who lives in the country, doing business in the city and going to and fro leads an ideal life. We have always thought that variety was not only a sauce that gives spice and piquancy to life, but that it is a great factor in the promotion of health and longevity, hence we have always held that one should make his home in the country, visiting the city, daily, if business requires, or, at intervals, for pleasure, recreation and variety, such as the country does not afford. Secondly, we would emphasize Dr. Wolfe's condemnation of the loss of their identity by country people. To our way of thinking, this erroneous idea is one of the greatest arguments in favor of the artificiality that now rules humanity. The oldest, most respectable, and most independent pursuit in the world is that of farming, yet by a strange perversity the farmer seems to consider himself inferior to the city man, because the latter wears better clothes. Dr. Wolfe's paper is a thoughtful presentation of a most important subject and is well worthy of careful perusal.

Building a City Underground.

How the Model Paris System Compares with the Philadelphia—A Practical Illustration of the Reason of Our Bad Highway System.

As early as 1853 Paris inaugurated the present system of intercepting sewers which to-day accommodates the water mains, telephone, telegraph and electric light wires, as illustrated in the cut. With variations in shape and size the city continues the construction on the broad and comprehensive plan of the

HOW PARIS IS BUILT UNDERGROUND.

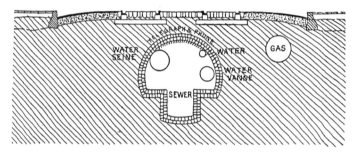

originator, Belgrand, which for years to come will furnish ample room, without disturbing the roadbed of the streets, for the several plants requiring sub-surface location. With the exception of gas mains one excavation suffices for all.

Under the present system of municipal government, the engineer reports

HOW PHILADELPHIA IS BUILT UNDERGROUND.

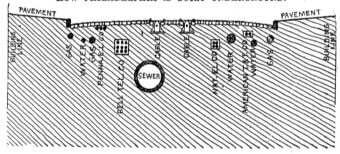

[Cross Section of Market Street, East of Eighth.]

his projects to the prefect. If he approves the work, he applies to the Municipal Council for the necessary appropriations. If it is a matter in which the State is also concerned, he represents the city in convention with ministers of all the State departments interested, before whom men recognized for high scientific standing are requested to give opinions, unbiased by a retainer from either side, as the government pays for the service, regardless of which side of the question their testimony supports. And on the report of this convention the government acts.

In contrast, observe the entire absence of systematic work in the sectional view of a Philadelphia street. Individuals, corporations and several city deparments trench the streets one after another for their varied interests, and often two and three times at short intervals the streets are opened either to increase the plant or to repair shoddy work. Under these conditions, the end of which is not yet in sight, it is obviously impossible to maintain good pavement, even if originally suitable and well laid. No matter how industrious or wisely directed the paving department may be, it is bound to suffer and finally be overthrown by unfavorable criticism, which it is powerless to disarm. Absence of uniform grade and uneven pavement defeat the best efforts of the street department, which in turn suffers for what it cannot prevent. Mud and water accumulate beyond reasonable possibility of removal, and the health department is held up for reprobation by the public, which can only judge by results of the capacity of the management.

The only distinction a man can gain under Philadelphia's present methods of conducting public work is in the degree of failure he is sure to make. Economy can only be secured by the co-operation of all interests under concentrated management.

Antique Meat.

The river Viloui, in North Siberia, is frozen a greater part of the year. In the cold season the natives follow its course to the South, and as Spring comes on they return. It was during one of these migrations that an entire rhinoceros was discovered. The river, swollen by the melting snow and ice, had overflowed its banks and undermined the frozen ground, until finally, with a crash, a huge mass of mingled earth and ice broke away and came thundering down. Some of the more daring natives ventured near, and were rewarded by a sight wonderful in the extreme. A broad section of icy earth had been exposed, and hanging from a layer of ice and gravel was a creature so weird that at first they would not approach it. It hung partly free, and had evidently been uncovered by the landslide. From the head extended a long horn, as tall as some of the children, while behind it was another smaller one. But the strangest feature of this curious monster was that it was covered with hair.

At first the astounded discoverers thought the creature was alive, and that it had pushed aside the earth, and was coming out. But the great rhinoceros was dead, and had probably been entombed thousands of years. The body was frozen as hard as stone, and the hair-covered hide seemed like frozen leather, and did not hang in folds, as does the skin of living species. Several months passed before the animal was entirely uncovered, and so perfectly had nature preserved it that it was then cut up and the flesh given to the dogs.

Buried Alive.

The belief that people are ever nowadays buried alive, or ever have been, except for criminal or judicial purposes, is one that is widespread, but also one that has very little foundation in actual fact. We venture to say that there are not in history any authentic records of cases of burial alive, where the deceased has been carefully examined by physicians, or even by intelligent friends. Of recent evidence of burial alive, there is certainly nothing of value. The *Medical Press and Circular*, of May 13th, 1874, reported the premature burial of a woman six hours after supposed death. But no evidence that the woman was not dead is given. The *British Medical Journal* of January 21st, 1871, cites the case of an infant that was *nearly* buried alive, but was heard to cry in its coffin. Here, too, the evidence as to the validity of the facts is wanting, while in effect the child was not buried alive. Another recent case occurred at Naples, in 1871. A woman in a state of trance is said to have been buried alive. The court sentenced both the doctor who signed the certificate, and the mayor who permitted the interment, to three months' imprisonment for "involuntary manslaughter." If these and other cases are analyzed, it will be found either that there was no proof of the premature burial, or else there was gross carelessness and criminal haste on the part of attendants. The belief in burial alive should disappear with the belief in ghosts and other bugaboos. It is, of course, possible that persons may be buried alive through some criminal conspiracy, or through some manifestation of monumental incapacity on the part of friends; but such contingencies can be easily avoided in modern life.—*Medical Record.*

Unhappy Childhood.

Sir John Lubbock, in "The Pleasures of Life" gives expression to the thought that the common phrase "Happy Childhood" is an erroneous one. Reflecting upon his assertion and his reasoning thereon, we are inclined to agree with him that it is a mistake to suppose that childhood is necessarily the happiest period of human existence. As it is to-day, a child is not a reasoning animal; he is guided solely by impulse; hence anything that would oppose his impulses is to him a real and grievous unhappiness, while to the thinking, reasoning adult, such would not be the case unless his reasoning would convince him that there was really cause for unhappiness. The point that we would make is that the reasoning powers of children should be much more cultivated than is now the case. He who is governed by impulse (whether he be man or child) is one who is either abnormally happy or despondingly miserable; there is no happy medium in the impulsive person, one extreme or the other always prevails. Let one however cultivate his reason or will power so that his impulses are subject thereto, and such a person will be a happy and healthy individual. If this education of the reason can be brought about at twenty, why can it not at ten years of age. Let us try, and when we have taught our children to reason with their impulses, then can we truly speak of happy childhood.

Cleaning-up Time.

It would seem that it was almost needless to suggest that the months of May and June are the time when preparation should be made to meet or avert the dangers to health which are incidental to the decomposition of organic and putrescible filth during the hot Summer days. It "goes without saying" that all intelligent persons have a knowledge of that fact. Nevertheless, there are few who are not benefited by being reminded from time to time of those duties which so largely conserve their best interests, and especially is this true of those duties which so largely concern the preservation and promotion of health. Very few individuals do as well as they know how. The good housekeeper, during the Spring months, makes a point of going through the inside of the house with a thorough turning out and overhauling the contents of every nook and corner, giving everything an airing, a dusting and a brushing, and all wood-work and floors a thorough washing and cleansing. No less is it necessary to have the outdoor premises cleaned up and put in order.

All heaps and piles, large or small, of decomposable material in or around the door-yard or premises near the house or work-rooms should be cleaned up and carried away to be spread upon the grass plots, if not too coarse and dry, or added to other fertilizers in the gardens and fields, where they may add to the luxuriance of forthcoming crops. Or if such disposal be quite inconvenient or not at all available, then let them be destroyed by the action of fire.

But to return to the indoor premises, it should not be forgotten that the cellar is often a source of unexplainable disease. When vegetables are allowed to decay and bits of animal substances, butter, cheese or lard, etc., are allowed to follow the same course, gases of decomposition will be set free and, carried with currents of the air or rising by their own lightness, will find their way into the living rooms above to poison slowly and insensibly the unsuspecting occupants. Closet shelves and corners, sink cupboards and cubby holes may furnish equally deleterious material if allowed to remain too long without a turning over and a turning out and a thorough cleansing. Clean up often and clean up thoroughly.—*Monthly Bulletin.*

What is Liquor!

A most estimable old gentleman, 86 years of age, some time before his death, said, in a letter to the editor of this journal that he had never tasted alcohol in his life. But a few days subsequently, dining at this gentleman's house, we were informed by him that a little bottle standing on the table was a tonic ordered by his physician because of the failing powers of his stomach, due to age. Upon inquiry we found that the tonic was the "compound tincture of cinchona." Feeling at liberty to do so, we propounded the query "What is the difference between your tonic and whiskey," and answered it by telling our venerable friend that while the latter was an *alcoholic* extract of rye or corn, the former was an *alcoholic* extract of cinchona. Now then, this good man had been really drinking a certain portion of alcohol daily, yet thought that he knew not the taste of alcohol because he had never consumed any whiskey, brandy, wine or beer. Our readers should understand that all tinctures are liquors, whether it be of ginger, of gentian, of quassia or of rye. Cologne is a liquor, anything containing alcohol is a liquor, and one can get just as drunk on sweet-smelling cologne as he can on foul-smelling beer or whiskey.

State Board of Health and Vital Statistics of the Commonwealth of Pennsylvania.

PRESIDENT,

GEORGE G. GROFF, M.D., of Lewisburg.

SECRETARY,

BENJAMIN LEE, M.D., of Philadelphia.

MEMBERS,

PEMBERTON DUDLEY, M.D., of Philadelphia.

J. F. EDWARDS, M.D., of Philadelphia.　　GEORGE G. GROFF, M.D., of Lewisburg.

J. H. McCLELLAND, M.D., of Pittsburg.　　S. T. DAVIS, M.D., of Lancaster.

HOWARD MURPHY, C. E., of Philadelphia.　　BENJAMIN LEE, M.D., of Philadelphia.

PLACE OF MEETING,

Supreme Court Room, State Capitol, Harrisburg, unless otherwise ordered.

TIME OF MEETING,

Second Wednesday in May, July and November.

EXECUTIVE COMMITTEE,

PEMBERTON DUDLEY, M.D., Chairman.　　JOSEPH F. EDWARDS, M.D.

HOWARD MURPHY, C. E.　　BENJAMIN LEE, M.D., Secretary.

Place of Meeting (until otherwise ordered)—Executive Office, 1532 Pine Street, Philadelphia.

Time of Meeting—Third Wednesday in January, April, July and October.

Secretary's Address—1532 Pine Street, Philadelphia.

Bureau of Registration and Vital Statistics—Department of Internal Affairs, State Capitol, Harrisburg.

State Superintendent of Registration of Vital Statistics—BENJAMIN LEE, M.D.

THE
ANNALS
OF
HYGIENE

VOLUME V.

Philadelphia, July 1, 1890

NUMBER 6.

COMMUNICATIONS

Annual Address before the Pennsylvania State Board of Health.*

BY PROF. A. ARNOLD CLARK, A. M.,

Of Lansing, Mich.

COMING, as I do, over many miles of territory and from a different State to be with you to-night, I am reminded how, one year ago, when your State Sanitary Convention was in session, word flashed across the wire from State to State telling of one of the greatest calamities in history—telling how the people of Johnstown had been buried beneath the great ocean of water which for years had threatened them, and nearly 4000 lives had been lost. For days the newspapers of Michigan were filled with the sad, the sickening details of this Conemaugh Valley flood. It was the one topic of conversation in drawing room and on the streets. Ministers preached about it, declaring that it could be compared only to the great flood where the waters of the great deep were broken.

Then as the waters subsided and the State Board of Health came to the rescue of the survivors—removing the débris and disinfecting to destroy the germs of disease—it was frequently remarked in other States that your State Board of Health was performing a noble work, and even grumblers admitted that in times of such catastrophies there was some reason for having a State Board of Health. But

EVERY YEAR MORE LIVES ARE LOST IN PENNSYLVANIA

from diseases which we well know how to prevent than in the great Conemaugh Valley flood—diseases which deprive us of our loved ones in the innocence of childhood, the joy of motherhood and the vigor of manhood, and it is to prevent such diseases that Pennsylvania has established a State Board of Health.

If I were asked to state the most important work of a State Board of Health I might quote from the law requiring your State Board to gather information

---

* Read before the State Sanitary Convention at Norristown.

concerning the causation and prevention of disease and to disseminate such information among the people. I would not underestimate the importance of those other questions with which hygiene was concerned fifty years ago. It is important that we have proper clothing, that we have pure food and pure air. You know Voltaire said that the massacre of St. Bartholomew was all because the king could not digest his food, and I do not doubt that bad food has made a great many bad tempers, and bad air, in close, unventilated schoolhouses, has made a great many dull brains ; but not one of these questions is so important as the saving of a human life. So it is important that nuisances should be abated, and very wisely your State Board is placed in charge of all sanitary interests. Our lives should not be made uncomfortable by unwholesome gases and odors, but as the most uncomfortable thing which can happen to a man is to die.

THE MOST IMPORTANT WORK OF A STATE BOARD OF HEALTH

is the stamping out of disease, the saving of human life.

How can this be done ? Let me illustrate :

From what part of the world comes the silk which you ladies wear to-night? Probably from Southern France. The people in Southern France practically do nothing but cultivate silk worms. When they meet in the street, they say not " How do you do?" but " How are the worms?" These worms are to be found in kitchen and parlor. In 1853 the raw silk produced by the worms of Southern France was worth $35,000,000.

But suddenly a great plague broke out among them, and in 1865 the silk produced was worth only one-fifth what it was twelve years before. The worms were found to be covered with little black spots—looked as though they had been *peppered*, and so the disease was called *pébrine*. When these spots appeared the worms became sluggish, stopped growing and died.

That great Frenchman, Pasteur, studying one of these little worms with a microscope, saw that its silk glands—the glands containing the fluid which it would spin into silk—literally swarmed with little microscopic germs, and though the worm itself was only one-half inch in length, so much smaller were the germs that he could see thousands of them swimming in the rivers of its body.

Rubbing up this worm in water, he spread the mixture over mulberry leaves, and

FED THE LEAVES TO THIRTY HEALTHY WORMS,

and in twelve days after they ate this infected meal every one of these worms was peppered with the characteristic spots of the disease, while the silk glands were literally charged with the germs.

Pasteur also found these germs on the claws of the worms, and saw that they communicated the disease by scratching one another with their claws. He also put a healthy worm in the same room with a diseased one, and it contracted the disease, showing that the germs of the disease might be carried through the air. He next discovered that moths contracting the disease invariably laid eggs which gave birth to worms which sickened and died without spinning silk.

Little faith was put in Pasteur's experiments until he took a number of eggs—every one of which the cultivators thought was healthy—and after examining the moths which laid the eggs, predicted, in a sealed letter, that twelve of these eggs would turn out diseased worms. At the close of the year the sealed letter was opened and read, and just those worms were found to be diseased which Pasteur had predicted, and those which he had pronounced sound yielded a healthy crop of silk.

Finally, by infinite painstaking, each of these little moths was placed, like a prisoner, in a numbered cell ; the eggs were laid in numbered cells, each moth laying about 500 eggs. Those eggs which were healthy were hatched in numbered cells, the diseased ones were destroyed, and thus, by this infinite painstaking, Pasteur saved the worms and restored this crippled industry to France.

Now, as the germ of pébrine passing from worm to worm will cause a great plague among them, so there are other germs which will cause disease in man—germs which, passing from person to person, from town to town, have been known to take whole cities by storm, stagnate industry, paralyze trade and even depopulate nations. And as Pasteur, by isolating the sick worms from the well, was able to save the life and labor of the worms, so the State Board of Health of Pennsylvania, by exactly the same methods, can

SAVE EACH YEAR THE LIVES OF THOUSANDS OF CITIZENS,

and if France could afford to spend thousands of dollars to save its worms, and if the life of the man who reels the silk is worth as much to the State as the worm that spins it, then we may well afford to spend a few thousand dollars to maintain State and local boards of health to protect us against these invisible germs swarming in the air we breathe.

The law establishing your State Board of Health requires this board to make scientific investigations concerning the causation of diseases, especially epidemic diseases, and as all work for the prevention of disease depends upon a knowledge of its causation, it seems perfectly proper to devote a few minutes to the consideration of the question just what part these germs play in the causation of diseases.

Nearly everyone in these days understands something about germs, and as it takes a microscope to see them, it is generally understood that they are "enormously small." Yet perhaps some of you are hardly prepared for the statement, that if an ordinary match were magnified as much as some of these germs pictured here it would stretch into the sky as far as the Washington monument—would even look as tall as the famous Eiffel tower.

Swarming in a drop of water, swimming like a fish, spinning around like a top, going together in pairs or forming beautiful chains, these little vegetable organisms at times seem almost possessed with consciousness and to be really having a good time. Dr. R. C. Kedzie, describing a drop of water filled with germs, said that it looked like an "animated skating rink." These germs reproduce by dividing, and so rapidly that, as someone has said, if their reproduction went on unhindered the descendants of a single germ would in three days fill all the oceans on the earth. Thus it is, that though only a few germs may gain an entrance to the body, they multiply so rapidly that in a few days the strongest man succumbs as Gulliver was bound by the little Lilliputians whom he carried in his pocket.

These germs assume as many shapes as those short-hand symbols which so bothered the brain of David Copperfield, and indeed the arbitrary characters of which he complained were not so arbitrary, despotic and disastrous as these germs. In general, a germ which is round like a dot is called a micrococcus, one which is shaped like a match is called a bacillus, while those shaped like corkscrews are called spirilla. Each of these germs has an official title of its own. Thus this germ is known among its neighbors as the *saccharomyces cerevisiæ*. Popularly it is known as the yeast plant.*

This leads me to say that not all germs produce disease. It is a germ which turns our milk sour, a germ which turns it blue, it is a germ which turns sweet meat into carrion, a germ which makes our fruit ferment, a germ which turns grape juice into alcohol. Indeed the process by which a man becomes sick and the process by which one becomes drunk are practically the same. When

THE GERMS OF FERMENTATION

gain an entrance to the grape juice they commence to grow and multiply, and in their growth possess the power of breaking up the grape juice into two substances entirely different—a gas, which escapes in bubbles, and alcohol, which remains. So the germs of disease, gaining an entrance to our bodies, break up our body compounds into a poison or ptomaïne, as it is called—each germ producing its own peculiar ptomaïne and each ptomaïne producing the symptoms of the disease just as the germs' of fermentation make the alcohol and the alcohol produces the symptoms of drunkenness—the bleared eye, the unsteady step, the nausea and headache. So similar are the two processes that some time ago those diseases caused by a germ were called "zymotic," because that word means a ferment. The difference between alcoholic intoxication and ptomaïne intoxication is that while the germs of fermentation make the alcohol outside of our bodies, the germs of disease make the ptomaïne inside of our bodies, so that a man sick with typhoid fever is not only being poisoned by a ptomaïne produced in the same manner that alcohol is produced, but he is himself the keg in whom the germs are working.

These germs of disease may be made to grow outside of the body like the germs of fermentation—in blood serum at the proper temperature, in gelatine or in beef broth. And you may go to-night to some biological laboratory and you will find there long rows of test tubes or bottles in which these germs, these

---

*see diagram on page 352.

little vegetable seeds, have been m•.de to grow in gelatine, and you will find among the labels on the bottles the words consumption, Asiatic cholera, glanders, malignant pustule, and just as Pasteur made thirty healthy worms sick by one infected meal, so if you wanted to commit suicide you could choose the disease from which you wanted to die and be sure of getting it. Or, as has frequently been done, you might arrange a dozen different animals in a row, inoculate each animal from a different bottle and produce a dozen different diseases, just as surely as a farmer may sow his farm with a dozen different kinds of seeds and produce a dozen different crops. And as the seeds of thistles always produce thistles and not corn, so

THE SEEDS OF SCARLET FEVER ALWAYS PRODUCE SCARLET FEVER

and nothing else. Or, as Florence Nightingale used to say : " Scarlet fever can no more generate measles than a race of dogs can produce a race of cats."

So these germs can no more arise out of the air out of nothing than can dogs and cats. You know it was formerly thought that animals might be generated spontaneously. Von Helmont once gave a formula for the spontaneous production of mice. Said he : " Take a dirty shirt, put into it some wheat, subject the whole to heat, and after a time you will witness a transmutation of wheat into mice." Now these germs are not easily generated, just because they are small. When you can your fruit you boil it to destroy the germs of fermentation in the can, then you seal it up tight to keep out the germs in the air, and when you do this the fruit does not ferment ; the germs do not develop spontaneously in the can. So you can no more spontaneously generate hog cholera than you can the hog that has it. If all the germs of scarlet fever could be destroyed to-night scarlet fever would be known only in history.

Before you there hangs a diagram* showing the deaths in Pennsylvania in 1880 from those diseases which your State Board of Health is endeavoring to prevent, showing in the relative order of their danger, consumption, diphtheria, scarlet fever, typhoid fever, smallpox, and every one of these diseases is caused by a living germ.

Some people do not know that

CONSUMPTION IS A COMMUNICABLE DISEASE,

but if you were to go to this biological laboratory, as I suggested, you would find among these test tubes one containing cultures of this rod-shaped germ pictured here,† and if you asked where the original germs were obtained you would be told that they came from the sputa of some consumptive patient. These germs have been found repeatedly in the sputa ; they have even been found on the walls of rooms inhabited by consumptives where the sputa had dried upon the floor and the sweepings had carried the germs into the air and to the walls of the room. These germs have even been found in the dried flyspecks on the windows of rooms inhabited by consumptives where the flies had

---

* See diagram on page 354.
† See diagram on page 352.

fed upon the sputa. These sputa have been pulverized, sprayed into the air, and dogs placed in an inhaling room and compelled to breathe this sputum dust, have contracted the disease and died. When Tappeiner was performing these experiments, a robust servant of forty laughed at the idea that consumption could be communicated in this way, and in spite of all warning he went into the inhaling room, breathed the sputum dust, caught the disease and died in fourteen weeks of consumption.

Now, thousands of citizens of Pennsylvania do every day in the week, unconsciously, just what this man did, consciously and wilfully, and when we think of the tens of thousands of citizens of Pennsylvania who, every day in the week, are expectorating on the floors of our public buildings, our post-offices and hotels ; when we think how these germs are being picked up and carried into the air at every sweeping ; when we think of the miscellaneous crowds sleeping in hotel bedrooms ; when we think of the close, unventilated sleeping car, with hangings so well calculated to catch the germs, and where, as some-one has said, the air is often as bad as in those boxes where dogs are placed for purposes of experiment, and then when we remember that man's lungs are a regular hothouse for the growth and multiplication of these germs, is it any wonder that ten thousand citizens of Pennsylvania every year yield up their lives to this great white plague ?

Now, my friends, the object of my remarks is not to make you afraid to breathe. It is quite likely that what I have said may sound like King Richard's cheerful request, " Let's talk of worms, of graves and epitaphs." I suppose there is such a thing as dwelling on the dangers that surround us until we become morbid, like the Irishman who used to stand each day before a mirror and shut his eyes to see how he would look when he was dead. It made him melancholy. You know Mr. Talmage says that a great many people kill themselves worrying about sickness and about dying. He says they bother about their digestion until the stomach finally gets tired of being suspected so much, and says : "Hereafter make way with your own lobsters," and the mistrusted lungs resign their office, saying : " Hereafter blow your own bellows."

But if we talk about these invisible enemies in the air we breathe, it is because we now know their military tactics and how to destroy them, and why should we cry " Peace ! peace ! when there is no peace ?" If this is an average Pennsylvania audience, one person in every seven here to-night will die from this disease, and this is true, with slight variation, over the civilized world. There are less deaths from consumption in Montgomery County than in other parts of your State, but forty citizens of Norristown will die each year from this disease. Yes ; during the hour that I will stand upon this platform some citizen of Pennsylvania—some seventeen men and women in the United States, men and women filled with happy, hopeful dreams—men and women to whom life is joy, will surrender their lives to this great white plague. And yet, if

THE RECOMMENDATIONS OF YOUR STATE BOARD OF HEALTH

were universally carried out, not one of those cases need occur.

What are those recommendations ? Is it necessary to shut up the consumptive—keep him from his family and friends? No; because the germs of the disease are not found in the breath. Bolinger caused a consumptive to breathe on a surface covered with glycerine and he caught no germs. Grancher caused a consumptive to breathe two hours a day for many days in an air-tight rubber bag filled with guinea pigs, and the guinea pigs did not contract the disease. The main danger is in the dried sputa from the consumptive.

Now, your State Board of Health has recently issued a circular—would that it had the money to place that circular in the hands of every citizen of this State—telling how to destroy the sputa. I have not time to-night to give those rules; but suffice it to say that your State Board recommends that in every instance the sputa from the consumptive should be disinfected or burned, and if that simple precaution were universally carried out, you might prevent consumption in Pennsylvania just as easily as you can stop your fruit fermenting by destroying the germs of fermentation in the can.

These other rod-shaped germs* which cause

TYPHOID FEVER

are found not in the sputa, but in the dejections from the typhoid patient. Thus finding their way from a vault to some well, as described this afternoon, some neighbor drinks the sparkling water and with it the germs of disease and death. If you are drinking water from a well situated thirty or forty feet, or fifty or sixty feet from a neighbor's vault, you may be tolerably sure what you are drinking. You know Artemus Ward used to say that when he went to a hotel he always ordered hash—then he knew what he was getting. Still, you say you have been drinking bad water all your life, and you never yet died of typhoid fever. This may be true. You may drink water from a well located only a few feet or rods from a neighbor's vault, and every time you drink from the well you may drain the vault, and you may keep this up for fifty years if you enjoy that sort of thing, and never get typhoid fever because the specific germ has never found its way into that vault, but the magazine is ready for the spark. Some day the germs of typhoid fever may find their way into that vault, and then you will drink not only filthy water, but the germs of typhoid fever as well.

These germs have been found in the water used by typhoid patients, and injected in dogs have caused the symptoms of typhoid in those animals.

Your State Board of Health has issued a circular telling how to disinfect the discharges, and if your Legislature would give your State Board the machinery for which it is pleading, if there were in every city, borough and township in the State a local health officer who had taken a solemn oath to carry out these recommendations of your State Board, typhoid fever might be, like smallpox, practically a disease of the past.

Not yet having the machinery, your State Board places a practical remedy in the hands of every man—that is, it recommends the boiling of drinking

* See diagram on page 352.

water, because boiling the water will destroy the germs of typhoid fever just as boiling your fruit will destroy the germs of fermentation. Let me emphasize this recommendation of your State Board to the people of Norristown. Boil the water you drink at the time of year when typhoid fever is expected ; boil it if you have any doubt about the purity of the water you drink ; indeed, if you drink Schuylkill water you might boil it all the time. It is perfectly practicable to have always on hand a supply of cold boiled water ; then, too, it is more civilized.

Civilized man cooks his food. ' The Australian puts a stick down into an ant hill, puts his mouth over the hole, lets the ants crawl up into his mouth and makes a very good dinner, but civilized man cooks his food. Still, civilized as we are, we insist on taking our water as Mr. Quilp took his whiskey—raw.

In this respect we are even behind the people of China—China where dog meat costs more than mutton and rats sell for ten cents a dozen ! Yet in China, though they have a filthy water supply, though they live in boats along rivers from which they derive their water supply and into which they empty their sewage, yet they do not have those diseases spread by contaminated water supply because they always boil the water they drink and would no more take it uncooked than they would eat uncooked potatoes.

The other two diseases which your State Board is making active efforts to prevent are

DIPHTHERIA AND SCARLET FEVER.

You will notice that no germs are pictured here as the cause of these diseases, because it is not yet known just what germs cause them, but there is no doubt that they are caused by some living germ. Indeed, during the past year there has been new evidence going to show that the so-called Löffler bacillus is the true cause of diphtheria. Six years ago Dr. Löffler found in the false membrane of those sick with diphtheria a bacillus which, cultivated and injected in rabbits, produced diphtheria in those animals, the germs being found on post-mortem examination. Three years ago, in ten recently examined cases, he again found this germ. Two years ago Roux and Yersin made similar successful inoculation experiments ; one year ago Kolisko and Paltauf found the bacillus of Löffler in a large number of cases of diphtheria and croup, from which they inferred, what many physicians have long believed, that there is a relation between the two diseases, and that croup may give rise to diphtheria. Only recently three different observers have made a bacteriological study of some cases of diphtheria in the Netherlands in which they found the Löffler bacillus which in cultures was fatal to rabbits in five or six days. And yet so cautious are sanitarians that they are not yet quite ready to accept the Löffler bacillus as the cause of this disease.

There is no doubt, however, that diphtheria is caused by some living germ. Three or four months ago word flashed across the wire telling of forty-nine cases of diphtheria and sixteen deaths in the little town of Zanesville, Ohio, and then the story was told how a little girl had died of diphtheria in Chicago, her body had been carried home, friends had gathered at the house to sympathize with the parents, the coffin was opened that the little children might take a last view of their little playmate, and in a week the brother and sister of the little girl followed her to the grave. In a family living only a block away four children were taken sick the same day ; two days later two of them died and the other two soon followed. The broken-hearted mother contracted the disease and followed her children to the grave ; the father returned from the Legislature and now sleeps in the same vault with his wife and children.

So it is not definitely known just what germ causes scarlet fever, and yet every day in the week cases occur in your State where the germs have been carried in the hair or clothing, where they have lingered in the carpet on the floor or the paper on the wall, where they have been carried a long distance by letter or have found a hiding place in the rubbish of the garret, as vigorous and vicious to-day as when they first emanated from the body of the infected person.

WHAT IS YOUR STATE BOARD DOING TO PREVENT THESE DISEASES?

As Pasteur, by isolating the sick worms from the well, was able to save the worms, so your State Board proposes to isolate every person in the State sick with diphtheria or scarlet fever, and then after death or recovery to thoroughly disinfect to destroy the germs of disease lingering in the room.

Just how many lives have been saved in Pennsylvania by those health officers who have followed these recommendations of your State Board I am unable to say, but I am better acquainted with the work in Michigan, where the facts have been collected, and as the recommendations there are similar to those in this State the facts apply here as well as there. There every health officer is required by law to report at once every case of a dangerous communicable disease, and they have learned that all doubtful cases must be reported, because, as we have seen, croup may turn out to be diphtheria, typho-malarial fever may turn out typhoid, scarlet fever may have been called German measles, and it is better to run on a false alarm than to miss a fire.

On the receipt of this information the State Board at once confers with the local health officer, telling him what to do and requiring regular weekly reports and then a final report after the outbreak is over. In this final report the health officer is required to state whether or not he isolated those sick with the disease and disinfected with the fumes of burning sulphur, as the State Board requires. He is also obliged to state just how much sulphur he used.

I am aware that some sanitarians put little faith in sulphur disinfection, basing their opinion on laboratory experiments by Koch with the anthrax bacilli containing spores which are very difficult to destroy, but it seems to me that the statistics which I am about to present prove beyond question that the fumes of sulphur will destroy the germs of scarlet fever and diphtheria.

Statistics ! Possibly you sometimes hear it said that State Boards of Health are simply bureaus for gathering statistics, and some people see no use in statistics. When Faraday was asked ''What is the use of statistics ?'' he answered, "What is the use of babies?" Within them are all the possibilities of future blessings. Now when a health officer reports to the State Board of Health that he did not isolate patients sick with diphtheria, that he did not disinfect premises, and that he had fifteen cases of the disease and three deaths, that is a statistic (if I may use that word); when another health officer reports that he did disinfect, and that he did isolate patients, and that he had only two cases and no deaths, that is a statistic. But when thousands of health officers make similar reports, they are statistics, but they are still all rubbish until some use is made of them—all in the dark—all in the clouds. But when these facts are placed side by side as in the diagram before you*, and when it is seen that universally where these precautions were not taken there were five times as many cases and five times as many deaths as in those outbreaks where these precautions were carried out to the letter, that is the compilation of statistics; that is where the lightning flashes from the clouds. These facts have been collected for both diphtheria and scarlet fever and for three years running, and, though only one year is represented in the diagram which I present*, facts covering three years, over five hundred outbreaks of diphtheria, over forty-three hundred cases and over nine hundred deaths show a similar result.

Now, just so surely as Pasteur could predict that those worms which ate the infected meal would sicken and die while the others would not, so

WE CAN PREDICT THAT WHERE HEALTH OFFICERS NEGLECT THESE
PRECAUTIONS

there will be five times as many cases and five times as many deaths as where they obey the instructions of the State Board*, and in this way we are able to prove that thousands of lives have been saved by those health officers of Michigan and Pennsylvania who have isolated patients sick with these two diseases, and after death or recovery have disinfected with the fumes of burning sulphur to destroy the germs. Sulphur has long been a good orthodox disinfectant for the next world; we now know that it kills the little devils in this.

You know it was an old idea that disease was caused by the possession of devils, and that the way to cure disease was to cast these evil spirits out. Our forefathers used to prick the affected part in the hopes of thus letting the evil spirit out, in much the same way that the Indian medicine men now gather about a patient, one playing the tom-tom to scare the devil out, one pronouncing an incantation to charm the devil out, another jumping on the patient's stomach to stamp the devil out. If the devil doesn't kill the patient the doctor usually does. Now, communicable diseases are caused by the possession of evil spirits, these germs; but these little devils, strange as it may sound, cannot live where sulphur is burning.

The one thing which hinders your State Board of Health in the restriction of these diseases is the failure of the Legislature to give it sufficient machinery.

* See diagram on page 353.

WHAT MACHINERY DO YOU NEED?

You have a local township school system, why should you not have a township health system? At least fourteen different states have such a system; there is such a system in the state where I live. There the common council of every city, the common council of every village, the board of supervisors of every township is the board of health by law, and as such is required to constantly have a well-educated doctor as health officer, and to report his name to the State Board of Health. Last year nine-tenths of the fifteen hundred localities in the State complied with this law.

More than that—every physician is required by law to report at once to the local health officer every case of a dangerous communicable disease in his practice, and he is fined if he fails. Every householder is required to report at once to the health officer every case of a dangerous communicable disease in his house, and he is fined if he fails. If he fails to pay the fine he is liable to imprisonment in the county jail.

The health officer is required to report at once to the State Board of Health, to isolate every case, to placard houses, to personally disinfect after death or recovery, and if he fails in any of these things he is liable to fine and imprisonment in the county jail.

More than this, any person who tears down the placard or in any way violates the orders of the health officer is liable to fine and imprisonment in the county jail.

Now, there may seem to be a good deal of "county jail" about this, but the time has come for people to understand that it is a misdemeanor—aye, a crime, for a man sick with communicable disease to expose a neighbor and kill him. We very properly boast in this country of our Saxon independence, and cry out against so-called sumptuary laws which needlessly interfere with personal liberty. The time was when nearly everything was regulated by law. In the old Massachusetts Colony a law was passed requiring the sleeves of all dresses to reach to the wrist and prohibiting anyone worth less than two hundred pounds wearing lace which cost more than two shillings a yard. Men who wore long hair were liable to imprisonment. I saw not long ago in the *Central Law Journal* a copy of a law still on the statute books of New Jersey, passed when that State was a British Colony, which reads: "All women of whatever age, rank, profession or degree, whether maids or widows, who shall, after this Act, impose upon, seduce and betray into matrimony any of the King's subjects by virtue of scents, cosmetics, washes, paints, artificial teeth, false hair, or high-heeled shoes, shall incur the penalty of the law now in force against witch-craft and like misdemeanors."

All of this is sumptuary law—a needless interference with individual liberty. Government has no right to interfere with the liberty of one man except where that man interferes with another's rights, but if

ALL MEN HAVE AN EQUAL AND INALIENABLE RIGHT TO LIFE AND LIBERTY,
it is the business of the State to maintain that right, and no man has any more right to go upon the street and infect you with the germs of disease so that you

sicken and die than he has some dark night to knock you on the head, and the government which punishes the one offense should punish the other.

The law makes it the duty of your State Board at such times as this to suggest to the Legislature certain necessary amendments. It seems to me that the one necessity in Pennsylvania—a necessity which overtowers all others—a necessity on which depends the lives of thousands of citizens, is the compulsory establishment of a local board of health and local health officer in every city, borough and township in the State. It is absurd to expect that your State Board can restrict every outbreak of a dangerous disease in your State without this

NETWORK OF LOCAL BOARDS.

You need a general at headquarters to keep track of the enemy, but you need in every locality a soldier. You have such a general in your able and tireless secretary, Dr. Benjamin Lee, but he cannot placard every house in the State where there is a dangerous disease. This is properly the work of the local board. Your State Board can furnish the inspiration—the steam—but you must have the machinery. The cities of Pennsylvania *may* establish a local board of health, *may* appoint a health officer, *may* make all needful regulations to preserve the public health, but your Legislature should make

A UNIFORM SYSTEM COMPULSORY

and should make it apply to the boroughs and townships. Your State Board has sent all over the State circulars urging the importance of these boards, but it needs a cracker on its whip, that it may say, not you can, but you must. If there were in every locality in this State a health officer who had taken a solemn oath that he would carry out the instructions of your State Board, that he would isolate patients sick with scarlet fever, that he would thoroughly disinfect, you might stamp out scarlet fever and diphtheria in Pennsylvania just as easily as Pasteur stamped out the silk-worm plague in France.

Now, can it be that anyone will still inquire, in spite of all these facts,

DOES HEALTH WORK PAY?

If France could afford to spend thousands of dollars to save its worms, as I said at the start, it is simply a question whether men are worth as much to the State as worms. If your State Board could save these lives and prevent this sickness, how much money would it save the State? I know it is almost absurd even to ask the question, for even savages admit that every life has a money value to the community. Two or three years ago a ranchman in San Juan County, New Mexico, killed an Indian, and the Indians at once demanded ten head of horses, or $200 in money as the value of the dead buck. They sent their squaws back into the interior and threatened to kill every white settler on the San Juan River if the money was not paid to the widow of the dead Indian. There was a squaw who would not lose her husband for a cent less than $200.

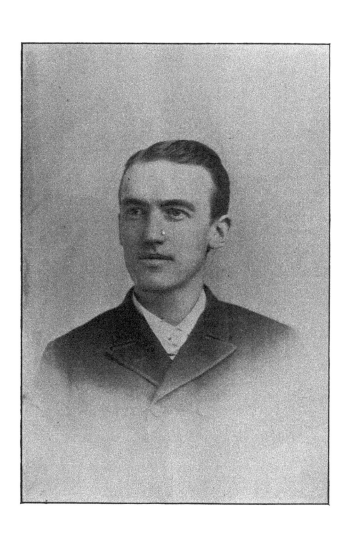

Our Teutonic fathers introduced a similar custom into England. They hardly regarded murder as a crime, but they did realize that every life had a money value to the community, and so everyone who took another's life was fined. The fine was paid in part to the widow and in part to the tribe, and this fine was intended to represent the value of the dead man to the community. Thus it cost little to murder a slave, more to murder an artisan, while taking the life of an English baron came very expensive.

So to-day there is on the statute books of most States a law providing damages for the wrongful taking of a human life whether by negligence or feloniously. The maximum is fixed in most States at $5000, and the minimum at $1000. Now, I know this sounds almost like sacrilege; it sounds almost like sacrilege to put the pound of sacred flesh in the same balance with the three thousand ducats. But it is a fact whether we consider man as the law considers him; whether we sit down as did William Farr with a life table in our hands and calculate the future annual earnings of a man at a given age, subtract his future cost of living and take the capitalized remainder as the value of the man; whether we say, as some have said, that every man is worth to the community what it will cost to train up from infancy another just like him, or whether we remember in a common sense sort of a way that in the slave markets of the South a man sold for a thousand dollars—the fact remains that every man who is not sick or a vagrant will give the world more than he will take from it. No man ever yet lived and labored but the world was richer because he lived and labored, and every death tends to bankrupt the nation.

More than that, every time one dies a dozen are sick, and

SICKNESS IN A COMMUNITY IS A FINANCIAL PANIC.

Do you doubt it? Reflect that when you are sick you spend at least fifty cents a day for medical attendance; that you spend at least as much for nurses; that when you are sick you lose your wages. Now, we have learned to-night that over one-third of all the deaths which occur in Pennsylvania each year might be prevented. Ten thousand deaths each year from consumption! 6000 from diphtheria! 3000 or 4000 from scarlet fever! 2000 or 3000 from typhoid fever. Over 20,000 preventable deaths! Over 200,000 cases of preventable sickness! Then calculate for yourself what a panic it is to have these diseases in your midst!

The amount of money which sickness costs your State is too great to be grasped even by the imagination. If you doubt it reflect that there are 8000 doctors in Pennsylvania. I suppose that they make on an average $1000 each. That is $8,000,000 which you pay to cure you after you get sick. Now, we would hardly agree with Dr. Holmes when he said that humanity would be infinitely better off if all the medicine were thrown into the sea, but it would be awful for the fish. And Lowell exaggerated some when he said that among doctors there were hydropaths, homœopaths and allopaths who agree in nothing except that the other fellow's path leads to the grave. No matter how much we may abuse the doctors, we are always ready to go to them when we get sick, and I do believe that nowhere is there to be found greater devotion to humanity than in the medical profession. They are ready to go at all hours of the day and night; they know that doctors die younger.than those in any other profession, because of the great exposure to communicable diseases, and yet they are willing to face not only personal discomfort but danger as well to allay pain. But my point is this : How much better it would be to salary these doctors to keep us well and then dock them their pay when we get sick—give them a money interest in keeping us well rather than sick.

How do you do that in Norristown ? You have here about thirty physicians—that is, you pay $30,000 to cure you after you get sick—and yet you pay your health officer only $200 (I believe) to prevent your getting sick. Now, prevention is better than cure. It is all right to pay these doctors to battle with these germs of disease after they enter our bodies, but you should pay one man at least $1000 a year to spend his entire time destroying these germs before they begin to destroy us. You have heard of the Irishman who swallowed a potato bug, and then swallowed Paris green to kill it. It is better to kill these germs before they enter our bodies—it is healthier and it is cheaper ; and yet we, who pay so much to cure disease, would probably grumble at a tax of five cents apiece to prevent disease. Some people seem to think that because they always have lived, all money spent to prevent disease and dying is money wasted. You have heard of the man who dropped his life insurance because he had kept the thing up twenty years, and never derived any benefit from it yet. That seems too often to be the policy of the city, the State, the nation.

While every second-rate power in Europe has its national board of health, ours has none. In 1887

CONGRESS APPROPRIATED $500,000

for the investigation of tuberculosis in cattle and of hog cholera—more, I believe, than it has ever appropriated for the prevention of diseases in man. New York State appropriated $105,000 more, Virginia $75,000 ; and yet, from the mere financial standpoint, all the cattle and hogs in the United States are not worth so much as the lives sacrificed each year in Pennsylvania to diseases which we might prevent.

Four years ago Edwin Chadwick, commenting on an appropriation of the Spanish Legislature for equipping war vessels, showed that the same amount of money expended in sanitary improvements would, in ten years, save over two hundred thousand lives and prevent two million cases of sickness. Such an appropriation would be laughed at, and yet Spain lost more lives during the last cholera epidemic than during the great Peninsular war. In the Crimean war 20,000 French soldiers died in battle, 75,000 died of disease. During our own late war disease carried off many times more than the fields of battle and the wounds of battle. And yet a nation which pays thousands of dollars to maintain a large standing army to protect us against foreign foes, with whom we ought to be at peace—a nation that spends thousands of dollars to study the diseases of peaches and pears, thousands of dollars to protect its fish and the young seals of Alaska, has done practically nothing for the prevention of diseases in man.

I have not time to continue this subject further, but no more important question was ever presented to any civilized audience in any civilized age. There is hardly a person here to-night who has not stood by the grave of some loved one whose death might have been prevented—one to whom death came, as the poet said,

"Like some untimely frost upon the sweetest flower in all the field."

If there are five hundred here to-night at the average age of forty-five years,

WE REPRESENT FIVE HUNDRED OTHERS,

who, forty-five years ago, started out with us on life's highway, and who have since joined the "Great Majority." One hundred and fifty dropped by the wayside during the first year of life ; at the close of five years three hundred were gone. We strewed the path with flowers and journeyed on. At 45 only one-half of the original band are here, and at 95 years of age only two of the original thousand are left to stagger to the grave. And yet if we prevented those diseases which we now know how to prevent, the average life of man would be 100 years.

Two of the original thousand will die from smallpox, 30 from typhoid fever, 35 from scarlet fever, 85 from diphtheria, 130 from consumption—over 300 * from diseases which we now know how to prevent.†

Do you remember Joseph Addison's "Vision of Mirza," where he tells how he was summoned to the mountain top, and there listened to the wonderful music of the "Genius of the Rocks?"

Cast thine eyes eastward, said the Genius, when he had finished playing, and tell me what thou seest.

I see, he answered, a prodigious valley, and through that valley a great tide flowing.

The tide thou seest, O Mirza, is part of the great tide of eternity ; but look again, and tell me what thou seest now.

And Mirza answered :

I see an immense bridge, which "from a cloud emerges and on shadow rests."

The bridge, thou seest, O Mirza, is human life.

And on this "narrow bridge 'twixt gleam and gloom" they watched the long procession of humanity hastening onward.

Come closer, said the Genius of the Rocks, and, following where he beckoned, Mirza saw that the bridge was composed of three score and ten arches—

---

* Including measles, whooping cough, etc.
† See diagram on page 353.

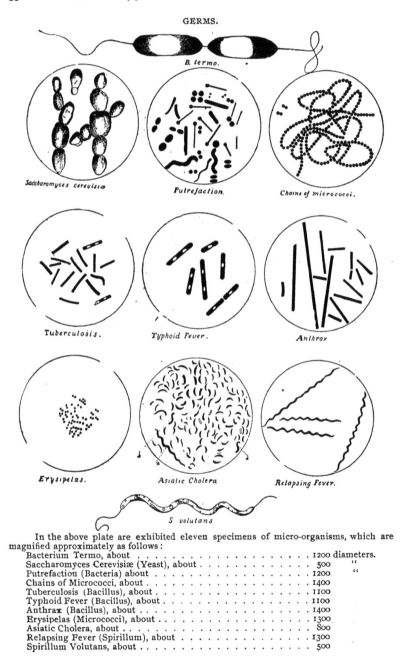

GERMS.

B. termo.

Saccharomyces cerevisiæ.

Putrefaction.

Chains of micrococci.

Tuberculosis.

Typhoid Fever.

Anthrax

Erysipelas.

Asiatic Cholera

Relapsing Fever.

S. volutans

In the above plate are exhibited eleven specimens of micro-organisms, which are magnified approximately as follows:

Bacterium Termo, about . . . . 1200 diameters.
Saccharomyces Cerevisiæ (Yeast), about . . . . 500 "
Putrefaction (Bacteria) about . . . . 1200 "
Chains of Micrococci, about 1400
Tuberculosis (Bacillus), about 1100
Typhoid Fever (Bacillus), about 1100
Anthrax (Bacillus), about 1400
Erysipelas (Micrococci), about 1300
Asiatic Cholera, about 800
Relapsing Fever (Spirillum), about 1300
Spirillum Volutans, about 500

ISOLATION AND DISINFECTION RESTRICT DIPHTHERIA.

Diphtheria in _Michigan_ in _1888_:- Exhibiting the aver-age numbers of cases and deaths _per outbreak_:- in those outbreaks in which Isolation and Disinfection were both _Neglected_; and in those outbreaks in which both were _Enforced_. (Compiled in the office of the Secretary of the State Board of Health, from reports made by local health officers.)

Scale for Cases and Deaths	Isolation and Disinfection neglected. Average.			Isolation and Disinfection enforced. Average.	
	Cases.	Deaths.		cases.	Deaths.
15	15.50				
14					
13					
12					
11					
10					
9					
8					
7					
6					
5					
4					
3					
2		2.38		1.74	
1					.53
0					

DEATHS, PENNSYLVANIA.
1880

CONSUMPTION.

DIPHTHERIA.

SCARLET FEVER.

TYPHOID FEVER.

SMALL-POX.

some broken, some complete. He ·looked again, and saw that in the bridge there were innumerable trap-doors, through which the passengers, long before they reached the last arch, dropped into the great tide beneath—"the dark and unknown sea which rolls round all the world." Some, while pursuing "glittering bubbles," others "with eyes toward heaven in thoughtful posture," slipped and fell, while it was very few indeed who survived the long and painful journey and hobbled at last under the last arch.

For the pitfalls and the trap-doors in life we are responsible. Prevent these diseases, and the natural span of life will be one hundred arches, not three score and ten ! Prevent these diseases, and the way will be not a "bridge of sighs," not a rack of pain, but a golden span, on which we journey safely to the unknown shore.

The Dangers Arising from Public Funerals in the Case of Contagious Diseases.*

BY REV. S. BRIDENBAUGH,
Of Norristown, Pa.

DEEPLY interesting to the living must ever be the disposal of the bodies of those whom they have loved and lost. The manner or method of treating the bodies of the dead is, in large measure, indicative of the condition and character of a people. Hence we find that funeral customs have always varied according to time and place, and that they have associated themselves with a variety of sentiments the expression of which has been attended, not infrequently, with actual cruelty toward the living.

Under the influence of the Christian religion some marked changes were made in funeral rites and observances, so that they became the direct antitheses to the customs of the Pagans. While the latter generally cremated their dead, the Christians always *buried* them. The Pagans buried by night ; the Christians by day. The Pagans carried the funeral cypress ; the Christians substituted palm and olive branches, symbols of victory and peace.

But while the general tendency of mankind regarding funeral customs has been one of advance, it must be clearly evident to any thoughtful person that further reform is needed in certain particulars, the importance of which will be seen and acknowledged by most people so soon as their attention has been directed thereto. Of these customs none call more vociferously for reform than that of *conducting public funerals in the case of contagious diseases.*

Before a convention such as this, it is unnecessary to cite authorities to convince you that contagious diseases, such as diphtheria, scarlet fever, smallpox, yellow fever, may be communicated by exhalations from the bodies of the dead as well as by contact with living persons afflicted therewith. This we

---

*Read before the State Sanitary Convention at Norristown.

assume on the strength of the almost universal testimony of the medical profession. We are assured by physicians that wherever bodies of those having died from contagious disease are exposed the germs of such disease are present, and that it is possible for these to find lodgment in the furniture of rooms, the walls of dwellings and in the clothing of those in attendance. This being so, what a probability there is that any one present, susceptible to the particular malady of which the person has died, may fall a victim to the disease and perhaps aid innocently in carrying it to others.

Such occurrences have, indeed, been very frequent in communities where public funerals have been permitted in the case of those dying from contagious diseases.

About twelve years ago, while pastor in a town of Western Pennsylvania, malignant diphtheria became epidemic. A child died of this disease in a house opposite the public school building. Burial did not take place until the third day after the occurrence of death. During a considerable portion of that time the remains were exposed to public gaze. More than a hundred pupils of the school availed themselves of the opportunity to linger around the corpse and take a last look at the remains of their departed schoolmate. The disease spread. In the town and surrounding country at least one hundred and fifty persons were infected with it. About forty died. This will not be surprising when I assure you that all the funerals were public. Whether held in the house or in the church in most instances crowds thronged to view the remains and aid in spreading the disease. There was no board of health, and a majority of the people were doubtless unaware of the danger to the living in their efforts to show respect for the dead.

Not very long ago a child died of diphtheria in Ravenwood, Ill. The body was removed to a town in Ohio, where sympathizing friends and others "viewed the remains." As a result an epidemic of diphtheria broke out and many deaths occurred in consequence thereof. On the 22d of last month a well-authenticated report from St. Paul, Minnesota, said: "Malignant diphtheria is epidemic in the village of Vining, in Otter Tail County. The village has a population of about one hundred and fifty persons, nine-tenths of whom are afflicted with the disease. There have been twenty deaths since April 1st, and thirty altogether. Instead of adopting measures to check the contagion the people, mostly Scandinavians, are seemingly doing everything possible to spread it. The funerals of all the victims have been public and largely attended."

In "THE ANNALS OF HYGIENE" for November, 1888, I find recorded this incident. "An adult person died of diphtheria. The corpse was taken a few miles distant to the home of a relative. The coffin was opened, and the body exposed to the view of relatives and friends. In a few days there was a severe outbreak of the same disease among the inmates of that home. There had been previously no case of diphtheria in that village."

Before the thirteenth annual meeting of the American Public Health Association, Dr. Stewart, health commissioner of the city of Baltimore, said: "I know that in an epidemic of smallpox that occurred in Baltimore two or three years ago, the great start the disease obtained was from a public funeral which took place in a church. Five or six hundred people were present. In that locality within two or three weeks the disease was dotted around in four or five houses, and hundreds of cases came from that one cause.''

We could multiply instances of like infection and fatal results arising from public funerals in the case of contagious diseases. But let these suffice.

Knowing the fact that infection does occur by persons coming within reach of the germs exhaled from the bodies of those having died of diseases such as we have mentioned, what is our duty with reference to the obsequies in connection with the burial of these departed ones? Clearly, it would seem, to discourage in every feasible way the holding of public services over the bodies either in the home or the church.

In instances of this kind three persons are invested with a special responsibility—the physician, clergyman and the undertaker. To evade this responsibility, and neglect to dissuade, if possible, sorrowing friends from having public funeral rites is to manifest a lack of proper regard for the welfare of the living. I know the difficulty that will confront us. There is, it would seem, planted deep in the human breast a desire to honor the dead. And, unfortunately, there are those who think that honor can best be shown by a public funeral pageant. Whatever is said to bereaved relatives at such a time, therefore, must be spoken with the utmost gentleness. But they should be instructed as to the duty of subordinating their wish to honor the dead to the important matter of preserving the health of the living. Let surviving friends be assured that whilst we esteem the sentiment which prompts them to testify their respect to the memory of the departed by public funeral services, we do not regard the omission of such services, when required by the public good, as resulting in any detriment to the dead, either in the way of dishonor to the body or injury to the spirit.

Whenever the public health requires it let the burial be private ; yea, if the safety of the living can be the better assured thereby, let the night season be chosen wherein gently to lay away in the bosom of the earth the body of the departed.

This need not, in any sense, prevent the living from showing all respect and honor to the memory of the dead ; for, if desired, at some later time, when there is no longer risk or danger of contagion, relatives and friends can meet together in the home or sanctuary and there engage in fitting services.

Certainly it must be considered very thoughtless, if not selfish, for the members of one household to insist that persons from many other homes shall be subjected to the danger of infection and consequently of being lost to those near and dear to them in order that a public funeral service may be held over the unconscious remains of one who can neither be benefited by it, nor injured by the omission of it. And most persons, we believe, will readily yield in this matter if properly advised. But, if any are unreasonable and insist upon public funeral rites with an apparent disregard of the health of others, and the fearful sacrifice of human life that may result, it becomes the duty of the proper authorities to call to their aid the strong arm of the law. If rendered necessary, the police power should be invoked to teach such persons that it is a high moral duty to forego their personal preference and to sacrifice their individual liberty that the welfare of the community may be conserved. In instances of this kind the Board of Health should take possession of the house when death occurs; direct when and how the burial shall take place; destroy clothing and other articles that have been in contact with the patient; disinfect the house and the corpse and take every necessary precaution for preventing further infection.

Fortunately, in this Commonwealth, legislation has been such as to endow councils of cities and boroughs with all the powers needed for the protection of the health of their respective localities. But, as we all know, such laws depend, in great measure, for their enforcement upon public opinion and the sentiment of the particular community. Hence the great importance of such education as this State Board of Health is seeking to give. These efforts of your Board should be supplemented by proper teaching on the part of the Church, to which the affair of funerals has been almost entirely delegated. Ministers can do much in the way of explaining to people how it is possible to manifest proper respect for the dead without disregard of the living.

The following words of John Ruskin, the celebrated English writer and critic, contain a truth that is worth pondering : " Our respect for the dead, when they are *just* dead, is something wonderful, and the way we show it more wonderful still. We show it with black feathers and black horses ; we show it with black dresses and black heraldries ; we show it with costly obelisks and sculptured sorrow. . . . This feeling is common to the poor as well as the rich ; and we all know how many a poor family will nearly ruin themselves to testify their respect for some member of it in his coffin, whom they never much cared for when he was out of it ; and how often it happens that a poor old woman will starve herself to death in order that she may be respectably buried."

To the members of my own profession I would say that, as a rule, brevity should characterize funeral services. The customary funeral discourse we have come to regard as of doubtful benefit. After reading that sublime discourse of St. Paul contained in the Fifteenth Chapter of I Corinthians, it is hardly possible for the minister to say much more of importance upon the hope of immortality.

And it would be well for all if we could "quit our habit of thinking that what we say of the dead is of more weight than what we say of the living. The dead either know nothing, or know enough to despise both us and our insults or adulation."

Sanitary Defects in Manufacturing Establishments.*

BY H. A. ARNOLD, M.D.,

Of Ardmore, Pa.

THE especial object of this paper is the consideration of those questions of heating, ventilating and disposing of the dust which so greatly concern the health of operatives in manufactories where cotton, jute, wool, camel's hair and shoddy form the basis of materials used.

Much time and thought have been given to the evolution of the best methods of heating and ventilating public halls, school buildings and churches. Truly a laudable work, and with the steady advances wrought out by painstaking and intelligent research in this particular much good has been done. But when we consider that neither church, hall nor school building are often occupied for more than three or four hours consecutively, and but rarely for six days out of the seven, we can readily understand that the temporary occupants of such places cannot long be exposed to noxious gases or injurious temperatures.

Seeing, then, the provision made for a maintenance of health during hours of study, recreation and devotion, it does not require any great stretch of the imagination to elicit the inquiry, What provision is being made for hours of labor of those who are compelled to occupy the same apartments for days and hours continuously.

The laws of acoustics demand high ceilings for public halls and church edifices, thereby furnishing a larger volume of air, and the almost constant ingress and egress assist in furnishing a change of air. Neither of these measures is available for the relief of the factory operative, who spends on an average ten hours each day in a close, confining atmosphere.

The relative healthfulness of different occupations has been a matter of consideration and conjecture—especially conjecture—and tables giving the longevity of individuals following the different pursuits of life are so frequently published in the various health journals, magazines and newspapers that it will not be necessary for me to try your patience or consume your time by rehearsing them. We will consider, rather, those defects of management and construction readily apparent to the casual visitor ; defects that are as remediable as they are apparent.

A visit to the ordinary factory reveals a rectangular room, with low ceilings and so cluttered up with machinery that, as you pick your way through the whirling maze, the danger of the situation, added to the discomfort arising from the air, superheated and surcharged with atoms of dust, begets a longing for the more salubrious atmosphere outside the buildings.

These defects are more noticeable in old mills using the machinery of a generation ago, and in small establishments, such as shirt and stocking factories, where, from limited capital, small, overcrowded quarters are considered a

---

* Read before the State Sanitary Convention at Norristown.

necessity and sanitary considerations luxuries unthought of and unattainable. The principal defects presenting themselves to me in the course of a self-imposed inspection of a number of manufacturing establishments in this and the adjacent counties of Philadelphia and Delaware were imperfect methods of heating, ventilating, disposing of dust, and failure to provide satisfactory water closet arrangements.

We will consider these defects in the order named.

HEATING.

The system of heating almost universally used at present consists of a number of coils of pipes running along the side walls between the windows and the floor. Through these pipes live steam, or what is more generally the case, exhaust steam from the engine is made to pass. As an abundant supply of steam is obtainable, the principal danger lies in overheating. Indeed, so essential is it in certain processes (such as spinning) that a high temperature should be maintained, that a complete check is thus placed upon any marked lowering of temperature. This is not operative, however, in the prevention of overheating, and the temperature may climb up away above the requisite degree, and the feeling of discomfort be scarcely noticed by the busy worker. In many mills storm sashes are made use of as an additional protection against cold. That they are effectual is evidenced by the fact that they are still excluding the cold air from some mills at the time of the writing of this article (May 7th). The only instances of a cold atmosphere menacing the health of employés that have come under my notice, have been at the starting hour in the morning, when, from tardiness or other reasons, the engineer has not been able to spare the steam necessary to properly heat the mill. This defect, which seldom lasts more than a half hour, is worthy of consideration where the employés have a long distance to travel through inclement weather.

VENTILATION.

The question of ventilating is one that has such an intimate relationship to that of heating, that as far as my observation extended, with but few exceptions, the only reason for ventilating was the sense of bodily discomfort arising from overheating. It was not that they loved fresh air more, but hot air less.

An article recently published in one of the Philadelphia papers, in the course of a glowing description of the work rendered by the inspectors appointed under the State law of May 20th, 1889, gives as a result of 720 inspections since January 1st, 1890, a grand total of improvements suggested as follows :

Elevator safeguards	50
Fire escapes	19
Closet changes	19
Belts boxed	24
Hours shortened	7
Better ventilation	1
Total	120

Had I known that the duties of the inspectors extended further than to matters relating to the employment of minors and providing fire escapes, I should have taken up the consideration of this subject very reluctantly.

And had I seen their statement of the uniformly excellent system of ventilating in existence in the various manufacturing establishments thoughout this Commonwealth, I am sure I would have considered it a work of supererogation to have commenced this paper. I do not stand here to criticise the results of laborers in so good a cause, but I do say that the results of my self-imposed task have led to far different conclusions.

What is designated in each instance in this quasi-official report, as "perfect ventilation," or "first-class ventilation," has, so far as I have gone, proven to be nothing more than the imperfect system of ventilating by raising or lowering a window sash.

In those rooms where the raw materials receive their first attention, the change of air in the room is augmented by the exhausting fans attached to the machinery, the primary object of which is the removal of all dust without its being disseminated throughout the apartment. Even in these rooms the outside air must needs find its way in through open windows or doors. The rooms which give the most flagrant evidence of imperfect ventilation are those where the spinning is done. This is especially the case in cotton mills, where it is necessary to maintain a temperature of 80° to 104° F., according to the degrees of fineness of the thread manufactured. In quite a number of these rooms I found not only every window tightly closed, but also heavy fire doors assisting to hermetically seal the apartment. In one such mill, of three stories, with forty-five windows on the South side, on a warm sunshiny day, four only were opened by partially raising the lower sash.

In maintaining the requisite temperature the thermometer is not referred to, indeed, it is conspicuous by its absence, the sense of bodily comfort, and the facility with which the labor goes on, furnishing the uncertain guide which is blindly followed both as to heating and ventilating.

This system of window ventilation at its best is very imperfect, and being under the control of no one reliable person very seldom receives proper attention. The overheated employé, during a respite from labor, throws up the lower sash, that being the handiest, and a very few minutes suffice to check the perspiration, and chill the superheated body. An exceptionally large number of cases of pleurisy have come under my observation, some of which have been directly referable to this cause.

One instance was met with where the top sashes in a factory of recent construction are stationary, and the only ventilation obtainable is through raising the lower sash and opening the doors at the end of the room.

DUST.

Passing one of our shoddy mills a few evenings since, just at the hour of stopping work for the day, I found it a difficult matter, at a short distance, to determine whether a certain number of the hands were not negroes ; and just as I decided that they were all white I saw a genuine negro among them.

This extreme change of appearance, giving evidence of the very considerable exposure to the dust and grease by certain laborers in shoddy mills, is well calculated to awaken the inquiry as to its effect upon the health of persons so exposed.

After eight years of observation and experience among these workers, I feel compelled to answer the question negatively.

Theorizing suggested a train of troubles leading from rhinitis, pharyngitis, laryngitis, bronchitis and pneumonia up to degenerative changes and phthisis itself. But theory and practice have not accorded, and I am compelled to state that I have noticed less indication of irritation and inflammation, either acute or chronic, of the respiratory mucous tract among such persons than is commonly present where the only possible irritant inhaled is the dust from city street or country road.

The only ill effect from this class of work that I have observed is a tendency to erythema and furuncles in certain individuals, who, attributing the trouble to the oil used, designate them "oil boils."

Cotton operatives do not enjoy this same immunity. Throat troubles have been more plentiful, dyspnœa frequently met with and emaciation common. Several cases of commencing phthisis pulmonalis were directly traceable to the constant inhalation of irritant dust and cotton filaments. And yet I am not prepared to agree with an accepted authority (Peterson, of Buffalo, quoted in Report of New Jersey Board of Health, 1886, p. 159) when he says of cotton workers : "They all suffer more or less from bronchitis, dyspnœa, etc ; " for a tour of inspection will reveal the fact that it is possible for cotton to go through all its processes of manufacture without the air becoming contaminated or the health of the operative endangered.

In explanation, I would state that different samples of raw cotton vary greatly in the strength of fibre and amount of dirt contained, and that, as a rule, the poorer the cotton, the more antiquated the machinery used for its manufacture. This statement seems to apply more especially to small establishments and very old mills, where the machinery is so far behind the times that they can no longer enter into competition in the manufacture of the finer yarns. It is true the picker house machinery in these mills has fan attachments, but through long use, the amount of work superimposed by reason of the character of the material used, and other reasons, they do their work but imperfectly, and become a menace to the health of the employés.

The lower grades of cotton continue to charge the air with dust and dirt through all the processes of their manufacture. This fact is very forcibly brought to one's notice where the different floors of one large building are used by several firms working different grades of materials. On the first floor of one such building, visited by me, there was a general air of tidiness and carefulness. The cotton was of good quality and contained but little dust ; the machinery was modern and in good order, and the exhausting fans attached to willow and picker were run at a high rate of speed and did their work so thoroughly that there was an entire absence of dust.

Ascending a flight of stairs, you find yourself facing a sanitary problem in reality. Entering the picker room, a cloud of dust is seen issuing from the broken front of a machine, which, by reason of this defect, has almost reversed the action of the fan from an exhaust to a blower. In the spinning room the loosely-twisted threads, as they are rapidly twirled, cause all incoherent particles to be forcibly thrown off and received by the air, where they are retained by the revolving machinery until they finally find lodgment. This being a stocking mill, nearly all the yarn is dyed, thus adding an additional element of danger to the unfortunates compelled to breathe it in. Upon leaving this mill particles of dyed cotton could be seen floating in the air for some distance after making their escape from the windows raised for ventilating purposes.

In such mills as these you see pale, thin, anæmic boys and girls, who evidently began this work too early in life, and in whom the struggle for an existence precludes the choice of either hygienic houses or suitable food as an offset for unsanitary labor. A debilitated system, with such surroundings, soon leads to catarrhal conditions and dyspepsia, and eventuates in phthisis. Several persons who have been under my observation for years undoubtedly owe their existence to-day to the permanent closing of a wretchedly dirty cotton mill. Incipient phthisis had manifested itself and pulmonary hemorrhages were becoming frequent. With an enforced change of occupation came improvement in health and fewer bills for medical attendance.

With a wider application of the present excellent system of disposing of the dust, mortality tables will need considerable revising, and many so-called unhealthy occupations will be robbed of their dangers.

A most flagrant violation of all laws of ventilation was observed by me on the occasion of a visit made to one of the school-slate factories in Northampton County. We approached a low, one-story building about twenty feet square, with windows and doors all tightly closed. Before entering, I was told that I would not want to remain in there long. Upon opening the door, I could scarcely see, the air was so thick with flying particles of slate. Seated astride benches arranged around the room as closely as the expeditious handling of the material would permit, were men busily engaged with drawing-knives surfacing and edging the slates in preparation for framing. As they worked rapidly and used soft slate, free from gritty particles, the air was black with the dust which, having absolutely no means of escape, found lodgment upon rafter, ceiling, side walls and window-panes, until a dingy air pervaded the entire room. I asked one of the men if the work was not injurious? He replied: "Oh! no; not at all; but the dust from the machinery of the frame-makers is very injurious," alluding to an adjoining room, fully ventilated, in fact almost open on one side, where the frames are manufactured.

On leaving the building, my friend, an intelligent and observing clergyman, remarked that he "had noticed many cases of consumption among these slate-workers, and that very few men can work at it long without consumption showing itself."

WATER-CLOSETS.

A very few words will enable us to dispose of this subject. Proper regulations in this particular are the exception rather than the rule. In country mills the principal defects consist of wretched construction, failure to empty the vaults until they become an overflowing, offensive nuisance, too great a distance from the mill, too near the supply of drinking water, and an abominable custom of constructing them over running streams, entailing untold evils to dwellers further down the stream.

In town factories, the evils lie principally in imperfect flushing, defective trapping, uncleanliness and want of proper privacy. The importance of this matter is very great, and seems to be fully recognized by the State inspectors.

REMEDIES SUGGESTED.

Now for the conclusion of the matter. Where window ventilation is the only means obtainable, let it be the duty of some one person to preserve an equable temperature by frequent reference to reliable thermometers suitably placed about the rooms.

Let the ventilation be secured by lowering the top sash but slightly on the windward side, and further upon the sheltered side of the mill.

Have the room thoroughly aired during the dinner hour, and if possible, provide a separate room, free from dust, where dinner may be eaten by those who cannot get to their homes.

Have the windows, side walls and ceilings regularly and systematically cleaned.

Widen the application of the exhaust fans by applying them to other machinery than that in the picker-room.

The ideal mill of the future will be heated and ventilated by the forcible introduction of air, heated to the required temperature by being passed over steam coils.

Provide sanitary closets, either dry earth or flushing closets, separate and distinct from the mill buildings, and yet within a convenient distance.

And, lastly, provide suitable receptacles for sputum and saliva, which, under present arrangements, find lodgment upon the floor, and when dried, enters the air, and when tuberculous in character, endangers the health of all exposed to its influence.

The Purification of Water Supplies.*

BY C. W. CHANCELLOR, M.D.,
Secretary of the State Board of Health of Maryland.

THE subject of the purification of water, which I propose to consider in many of its details, is one of very general importance—for, next to atmospheric air, water is the first necessity of living beings.

ANCIENT AND MODERN WATER SUPPLIES.

The skill and taste of the ancients in architecture, and their knowledge of mechanics, are matters of wonder to many of the present age ; but the means which they adopted to furnish, irrespective of cost, copious supplies of wholesome water for the purpose of dietetics, health and cleanliness, excite less of surprise than it does of admiration for their wisdom and sagacity in this respect.

Pure water in abundance was regarded by them not only as one of the greatest benefits, but as indispensable to life. In the magnitude of its supply, Rome seems to have surpassed all other ancient cities. During the reign of Nerva, after the Christian era, the aggregate flow of water into the city of Rome is estimated to have been not less than three hundred and fifty millions of gallons. Estimating the city to have contained at that day one million inhabitants, the supply equalled three hundred and fifty gallons per day, per individual. The aqueducts through which the waters were conveyed from various sources, were of the most magnificent and costly construction, and such was their durability that a portion of them, spared by conquering invaders, have survived the destroying hand of time.

The Aqua Claudia, begun by Nero and finished by Claudius, conveyed to the city sixty-four millions of gallons each day. This aqueduct formed a stream of thirty miles in length, and was supported on arcades through the extent of seven miles, and such was the solidity of its construction that it continues to supply the city at this time.

The waters of the river Anio were also conducted to Rome by two different channels ; the first was carried through an extent of forty-three miles, and the latter upward of sixty-eight miles, of which six and a half miles formed a continued series of arches, many of them upward of one hundred feet in height. Compared with these, and many similar works of the ancients, the Croton, Cochituate, Fairmount, and Gunpowder Waterworks sink into insignificance. The wisdom of the ancient Romans, in the matter of a supply of pure water, is beginning to be appreciated by communities of the present day. That which but a few years since was considered to be a bountiful supply is no longer regarded as such.

In most English towns the water supply is calculated at about thirty or forty gallons for each person daily. In the United States, wherever public waterworks exist, the consumption is much greater, the average American citi-

* Read before the State Sanitary Convention at Norristown.

zen using, or wasting, more than twice as much as his London cousin. Marseilles, the only city of France with a proper water supply, will, when its projected works are completed, be able to furnish an average of 250 gallons per day, per person. Paris, with a population of 2,500,000, had, until recently, only 510,000 cubic metres of water, or about 150 gallons per day, per person, inclusive of water used for all purposes ; but works were to have been completed in 1889 which would increase the supply 140,000 cubic metres per day, giving a total supply of 650,000 cubic metres, or nearly 200 gallons per day, per person.

In New York City, with an estimated population of 1,500,000, the daily consumption of water is about 125,000,000, or an average of 83 gallons per person, per day ; Philadelphia, estimated population 1,000,000, daily consumption 88,000,000, average 88 gallons ; Boston, estimated population 400,000, daily consumption 36,000,000, average 90 gallons ; Baltimore, estimated population 500,000, daily consumption 40,000,000, average 80 gallons. The latter city has a maximum daily supply equal to about 500 gallons per person per day, which is probably the largest supply of any city in the world, except the city of Rome, which with a present population of 300,000, has a maximum water supply of 800 gallons per person, per day.

POLLUTION OF WATER COURSES.

Aggregations of population are generally found near some river, or other body of water which serves a double purpose :

1. To supply the population grouped upon it with water for domestic and public purposes.

2. To carry away the town filth, especially sewage matters.

It is with the pollution of water supplies as with diseases—" an ounce of prevention is better than a pound of cure." Many of the customs of mankind, however strongly they be recommended on the score of convenience, are open to objection with regard to their influence upon health ; and the common sense of the age has at last arrived at the conclusion that the practice of recklessly polluting water courses must be abandoned, on account of injury which may possibly ensue to the public.

Every hygienic congress that has assembled during the last decade has decided by formal resolution and solemn vote that rivers ought not to be polluted, and that all refuse likely to pollute them must be gotten rid of in some other way than by casting it into water courses ; but thus far no practical plan has been set forth by which that which is so plainly desirable can be rendered possible, unless we accept the sanitary paradox, that " all refuse likely to contaminate water courses should be passed through the soil by irrigation."*

---

* Sewage farms can only be successful when the porosity of the soil is adapted for filtration, and when the area is sufficiently large for the work it has to do ; but all sewage before being run upon the land should be treated so that secondary putrefaction cannot be set up, or the organic matter broken up into soluble and, therefore, more hurtful products. This especially is the case where the sewage is undergoing incipient putrefaction. Hence, while the effluent from an irrigation farm may be an excellent effluent, it is obviously unfit for drinking purposes, and should not be sent into a river from which the water supply of any town is drawn.

The relative wholesomeness of water is undoubtedly dependent upon the relative amount of certain kinds of organic substances which may be present, and the usual sources of depreciation may be stated as follows :

I. POLLUTION FROM MANUFACTORIES.

Many manufacturing industries yield large quantities of refuse liquid which is injurious by reason of matters either dissolved or held in suspension ; but it would plainly be impossible either to require every manufacturer to be an agriculturist, and to hold land upon which his waste liquids might be poured out, or to require every farmer to place upon his land whatever the neighboring manufacturers might choose to send him. As a matter of fact, the suspended matters of most manufacturing industries soon fall to the bottom of the stream, and the dissolved matters are soon oxidized, and, therefore, the English law, so far as manufacturing wastes are concerned, is limited to flagrant cases, or to preventing the discharge of refuse into rivers in situations where a definite mischief would be wrought before any natural process of precipitation could be completed.

No doubt the tendency of the times is to carry restrictions further than they have been carried heretofore, partly because the dwellers by the banks of rivers are becoming more and more conscious of the charms of a pure and limpid stream, partly because experience has shown that the manufacturer, when prevented from discharging his waste in the accustomed way, has more than once found means of turning it to highly profitable account, and has in the long run been the chief gainer by a prohibition which at first he regarded as a hardship.

2. POLLUTION INCIDENT TO CULTIVATION OF THE SOIL.

The influence of the cultivation of farm lands in polluting streams running through them has been the subject of some investigation, and experiments bearing on the question have been made in England, France, Germany, Belgium, Austria and other European countries. The interesting point with reference to the pollution of water courses from this source, is the small amount of rainfall which actually passes through the soil, especially during the Summer months, at which season it has been found that there is almost an entire absence of pollution from this source. If lands have been heavily manured in the Winter or Spring, and the process is followed by wet weather, the percolation and consequent escape of noxious matters into an adjoining stream would, of course, be very much greater than if the Spring season were dry. Fortunately, however, at such season there are usually freshets, which rapidly and effectually cleanse the stream and counteract ill-effects.

The depreciation of water supplies by soil pollution is generally at its minimum in the Winter, when the ground is closed by frost, so that the Winter showers and water from melting snows do not soak into the ground, but flow over the surface into the creeks and rivers.

Dr. Gilbert says : "When manurial matters have passed through a consid-erable depth of soil, there is not so much danger from ordinary agriculture as is sometimes supposed, but it should be fully understood that water largely contaminated with any kind of putrefying organic matter is always unsafe as a source of domestic supply." This view is also maintained by the Rivers Pol-lution Commission of England. They have declared that "water collected from the drains of cultivated land is invariably more or less polluted with the organic matter of manure," and that, "such polluted surface or drainage water is not of good quality for domestic purposes," but they say "it may be used with less risk to health than polluted shallow well water, if human excremen-titious matters do not form part of the manure applied to the land."

Dr. Brouardel, the distinguished Paris hygienist, in a report recently made to the Academy of Sciences of that city, has demonstrated the fact that the bacilli of typhoid fever will live during many months in the earth, and are finally carried by rains into water supplies a considerable distance from the place where they were deposited. Pasteur has shown this to be the case with the microbes of charbon and septicæmia, and his experience has lately been confirmed by Bollinger, of Germany. Dr. Charrin, the eminent French biolo-gist, has conclusively shown that the microbe of infectious pus will preserve its vitality for a long period in a cultivated soil. As we know that the fecal discharges of persons suffering from certain diseases are infected, it is easy to comprehend how the percolations of such materials into sources of drinking water may be fraught with disastrous consequences. It is indispensable to the health of communities, therefore, that the utmost care be taken to preserve the purity of their respective water supplies, and to guard them with unceasing care against every source of contamination.

3. POLLUTION FROM GRAVEYARDS.

Nitrogenous organic matter and ammonia are the dominant principles of water that has leached animal matter in a state of putrefaction, and these ele-ments, which the water sometimes takes up in large quantities, especially from human bodies that are undergoing decomposition in the ground, are not com-pletely separated by filtration through the soil. Rain water falling upon a porous soil sinks vertically, unless it comes in contact with an impervious stratum, such as clay or stratified rock, when it may flow off horizontally to a great dis-tance. If water comes in contact with vegetable matter in the soil, it will take up a certain amount of carbonaceous matter, which may not be especially inju-rious unless in large amounts ; but the case is quite different if the water should come in contact with decomposing animal matters, because the animal tissues, in undergoing putrefactive decomposition, give rise to very complex products, which are very soluble and extremely injurious to the quality of potable water. Unless the water filters through a quantity of soil, and soil of such a quality as will completely remove the products of decomposition, it is unsafe for domestic purposes, however far it may have passed under the ground before reaching the water supply.

4. POLLUTION FROM HOUSEHOLD SEWAGE.

It is obvious that infection of the soil by decaying organic matters is liable to vitiate subterranean waters and render them unsafe for drinking and culinary purposes. Depreciation of a water supply by household or domestic sewage is one of the worst forms of pollution. It not infrequently happens that waters fouled in this way contain infectious germs, and the necessity for exercising great care with reference to them is not only important but urgent. All waters, even the purest, contain some organic matter, but when it exceeds a certain limit, or has undergone putrefactive changes, the drinking of such water is attended with risk and even with danger. This is especially the case with reference to human excreta. Professor Mallet, of the University of Virginia,* has called attention to the fact that no known poison, in the diluted state, will produce the effects which have been traced to drinking water contaminated with human excreta ; in fact, there seems to be no dilution which can make such polluted waters safe. They are the culture fields for the germs of the most deadly diseases, such as cholera, typhoid fever and dysentery.

Dr. Frankland maintains that water once contaminated with excretal sewage, even if purified subsequently by filtration in the most perfect way attainable, if not positively dangerous, is still unsafe to be used. "There are," he says, "animal organisms existing in sewage matter so minute as not to be seen by the unaided eye, and we have reason to believe that they even exist outside the range of microscopic vision, and possess powers antagonistic to human life."

Dr. Macadam, of Edinburgh, who has paid great attention to the water question, says : "The line must be distinctly drawn between non-putrescent organic matter and that which is putrescent. Impregnations from household sewage form the most dreaded contamination, and yield waters which, though clear and sparkling, are yet most unwholesome and deadly."

It is true we cannot always prevent a certain quantity of household refuse from falling upon and penetrating the soil, but it is nevertheless a duty which we owe to the public health to reduce this source of pollution to a minimum. It will always be found that the increase in certain diseases is *pari passu* with the increased pollution of the water supply, no matter how abundant the flow of water may be. The annual death-rate in New Orleans from typhoid fever is only 16 in 100,000 of population. Why? Because sewage cannot pollute the water supply of the city, which is received principally from tanks or cisterns above ground filled with rain water. In Philadelphia, where the water supply is taken principally from the Schuylkill River, which drains a vast agricultural and manufacturing territory, and receives the influx of foreign matters from two large and growing cities, besides many smaller towns, and is known to be contaminated, the annual death rate from typhoid fever is said to have increased in a few years from 56 to 68, or 12.16 per cent. per 100,000 of population.

---

* Report of the National Board of Health.

It is a great error to suppose that infected matter is rendered innocuous by dilution with water. Dr. Mead Bolton, late assistant professor of bacteriology in the Johns Hopkins University, following up the experiments of Flugge, of Breslau, has shown* that the most dangerous microbes will not only live but multiply in the purest water when once introduced. The microbes of charbon, he says, will disappear in six days, but their spores, that is to say their eggs, will be preserved for twelve months. The microbes of typhoid fever have been observed to live in practically pure water for thirty days, and three months in water containing one grain of organic matter per quart of water. As to cholera bacilli, dirty water is a marvelous medium for their propagation and growth ; and even in ordinary water it has been ascertained that they will live at least seven months.

PRECAUTIONS AND REMEDIES.

The *precautions* that are best suited to preserve water supplies from contamination, and the *remedies* most appropriate to restore purity when lost, either by ordinary causes, or by those that produce epidemic diseases, may be classified as follows :

I. EXCLUSION OF ORGANIC FILTH.

Nearly all natural waters hold in solution or suspension a larger or smaller proportion of organized matter, which determines, to a certain extent, their impurity and unfitness for domestic purposes. We shall divide the organic matter present in water into the living and dead—both having their origin in the animal or vegetable kingdoms. The dead animal matter, among the natural causes of contamination, consists of the bodies of fish, insects, infusoria, etc., as also the soluble nitrogenized compounds dissolved out of these by the water. The dead vegetable substances are the remains of water plants, portions of land plants, leaves of trees, etc., which, particularly in Autumn, are found in river water in considerable quantities. As the laws of vitality have no longer any control over these substances, they become decomposed and resolved into their component elements, which combine according to the laws of chemical affinities, and yield products complex in their chemical constitution, and of a more or less dangerous or unwholesome nature.

The living organisms of animal origin found in water are fish, infusoria, insects, etc. ; of vegetable origin, water plants, and a variety of singularly organized atoms, invisible to the naked eye, known by the popular name of microbes, which are certain colorless algæ belonging to the family bacteriacæ. Insomuch as the living animal and vegetable productions are dependent upon the dead organic matter of the water for their sustenance, it follows that wherever living beings are found in water there must exist the requisite materials for their nourishment. Pure *distilled* water can neither sustain animal nor vegetable life. The existence of living organisms in water in larger nor smaller quantities, is an indication of the greater or less amount of soluble organic matter in

---

* Nouvelle Revue d'Hygiene.

the water, as also of its purity or impurity. When they exist in small quantities it follows, other things being equal, that the water must be pure. These living beings, animal and vegetable, act as depuratory, and we learn by their presence that there must exist the requisite amount and proper sort of food for their maintainance; hence their existence in water denotes a certain amount of soluble organic principles. We cannot but think, therefore, that the value of the information derived from microscopical observation of the organic impurities in water has not been heretofore sufficiently insisted on.

It is now agreed that the sewage matters of towns, including excretal and household wastes, however largely diluted, cannot with safety be allowed to flow into any source of water supply used for dietetic or culinary purposes. In order to carry off such wastes a system of closed vessels or impermeable pipes should be provided, distinct from the storm water drains, to discharge the matter at a depot or outfall independent of any river or stream, except for a practically pure effluent. The discharge, directly or indirectly, of crude sewage into any source of water supply, however remote, is a constant concomitant of epidemic diseases, while a proportionate exemption from such maladies will invariably follow the removal of the pollution. A pure and abundant supply of water is cheap at any price, and "millions" to secure it, would be better than "millions for defence." I scarcely need add that all manufactories and trades should be required to clean their own waste; not, of course, to convert it into a chemically pure water, but simply to deprive it of its power to become a nuisance to others when discharged into a public water-way.

At the International Congress of Hygiene, which assembled in Paris during the Exhibition of 1889, there was an interesting debate on the pollution of rivers. The Congress decided that the pollution of water courses or rivers by the residue of factories should, in principle, be forbidden, and that polluted water from factories should not be allowed to flow into a stream until it had been proved to be absolutely free from all injurious substances. The congress was of the opinion that the most perfect method of purification was by irrigation. This, of course, must in certain cases be preceded by such mechanical and chemical processes as would render the water fit for agricultural purposes. It was related that many manufacturers had benefited by the application of this law, as in their efforts to prevent the pollution of water courses they had made discoveries enabling them to utilize waste products. The difficulty was with the smaller manufactories—not rich enough to take the necessary measures. The congress further decided that where persistent resistance was displayed the authorities should themselves execute the work prescribed for the purification of water, and compel the persons interested to pay the cost.

2. PURIFICATION OF WATER BY ALUM.

The use of alum as a purifier of water seems to date back a long time. Particular attention was directed to its use by Jennet, in 1865, in an article published in the *Moniteur Scientifique*. He found that 2.3 grains of alum to a gallon of water rendered it drinkable, even when it was quite full of foreign matter. The time taken for this clarification was from seven to seventeen minutes. Prof. Austin, of Rutgers College, N. J., states that the amount of alum used by Jennet is unnecessarily high, and in some experiments instituted to determine what is the practical minimum limit of alum that is needed to clarify New Brunswick hydrant water, he found that 1.2 grains was about as small an amount as it seemed practical to use to get a perfect separation of the impurities. Some waters, he thinks, may require less and some may require more; but this is a matter very easily determined for any particular case which may arise. The great argument in favor of alum as a purifier of water is that it is cheap, can be obtained everywhere and is not highly poisonous.

3. FILTRATION FOR THE PURIFICATION OF WATER.

Chief among the subjects discussed at the Paris Congress, already referred to, was the purification of drinking water by artificial filtration, and some experiments were related which appear to show that noxious microbes may be removed, or at least rendered harmless, by certain methods of filtration. It was stated that guinea-pigs were inoculated with water which contained the microbe of anthrax, and that those inoculated with the water prior to filtration died with the usual symptoms of the disease, while those inoculated with the same water after filtration survived. A still more astonishing statement has been made by a London savant, viz.: That "a sufficiently careful filtration will remove most organic matters—*among others, strychnia;*" and it is said that the chemist who made this discovery was so sure of his facts that he drank, after filtration, a quantity of water in which, before it was poured into the filter, a poisonous dose of strychnia had been dissolved.

Filtration is no doubt an excellent practice, and one which, however it is accomplished, has at least the merit of rendering water more pleasing to the eye, if not to the palate; but it cannot be too widely known that some forms of filter do no more than this, and that water which is very bright and sparkling may yet contain noxious matter in solution. It would be well for the sanitarian, before extending his approval to any process of filtration, to understand explicitly the conditions which a perfect filter should be expected to fulfill, and to know that it has been subjected to adequate tests. Without this knowledge a mere belief in the efficacy of filtering may chance, in the long run, to prove a source rather of danger than of safety to the public. It is not sufficient to rely upon the sparkling limpidity or the refreshing sweetness of an effluent, because this will afford no security that the special characteristics on which the usefulness of the filter depends will be preserved in all future examples.

4. FILTRATION THROUGH CHARCOAL.

For many years charcoal held a high place as an efficient purifier of water. It has great power of absorption, but it is also capable of saturation. The experiments of Mr. Edward Byrne * deserve, in this connection, particular

---

* "Institution of Civil Engineers," May 21st, 1867.

notice. He has shown that with a filter of animal charcoal weighing 4½ pounds, through which only twelve gallons of water were passed in twenty-four hours, the purifying effect was equal to the removal of 55½ per cent. of the organic matter from the first gallon. This gradually declined until at the fourth gallon only 1.33 per cent. were removed, and already at the eighth gallon the action was reversed, organic matter being given back to the water. It has further been proved, especially by the experiments of Dr. Chaumont, that a low organic life is speedily developed in water which has filtered through charcoal, and the same effect is produced in water by long contact with this material.

The Rivers Pollution Commission of England say in their fourth report, p. 220, that "the property which animal charcoal possesses of favoring the growth of low forms of organic life is a serious drawback to its use as a filtering material for potable water." The commission found that "myriads of minute worms were developed in the charcoal and passed out with the water."

The utility of domestic filters for the purification of water intended for culinary or dietetic purposes, and the advisability or necessity of their universal adoption is strenuously insisted on by some persons and as firmly denied by others. There can be little doubt that filters are too frequently regarded as a kind of conjuring apparatus which will go on yielding to an indefinite extent pure water from dirty water, without receiving a tithe of the cleansing and attention which are bestowed on the rude sand beds of ordinary water-works. It would be well to remember that the success of any filter in the accomplishment of its legitimate work depends upon the frequency with which it is cleaned. No house filter should be used continuously for a longer period than two or three days without drawing off the contained water and allowing the air, which is much more destructive of organic matter than water, to pass freely through the filtering material for several hours. It would be well to have two filters and use them alternately every forty-eight hours. All filters in which the materials are enclosed between sides which are cemented or soldered into the case are to be avoided, as such filters are not capable of being easily cleaned.

5. FILTRATION THROUGH SAND AND GRAVEL.

From time to time considerable stir is made in scientific and popular papers and at sanitary meetings about some new device for purifying water, and consumers, terrified by the dismal pictures drawn of the condition of the town's water, frequently fall victims to sanitary "quackery," and purchase costly filters, the best of which are rarely more efficient than a common flower-pot filled with sand and gravel, while the worst are infinitely lower in the scale of utility. The simpler the construction the more effective generally will be the filter.

The artificial filtration of water on a large scale has become very general throughout Europe, where the water supply is taken from rivers, lakes or ponds. The main cause of the difficulties which have been encountered in this direction is the failure to obtain an economic system for such enormous volumes of water. This is proved by the fact that out of the numerous filtering processes, both mechanical and chemical, that have been tried not one has been generally adopted. In all mechanical filters, whether of sand or other granular beds, the impure liquid is pressed against the porous material, the surface of which should be sufficiently fine to arrest the solid impurities and allow only practically pure water to pass away. When these suspended impurities are considerable or of a slimy nature, their deposit on the filtering surface quickly becomes so impervious that the liquid is prevented from passing through the deposit to the filtering surface, even though great pressure be employed. The operation consequently comes soon to an end, and cannot be resumed until this deposit is removed. Owing to these repeated stoppages at short intervals for cleansing, such an immense amount of manual labor, and such a large number of spare machines or filter-beds are required to filter the water supply, even of a small town, as to render the cost very burdensome. It is, therefore, evident that for a system of sand filtration to be successfully employed in an economic point of view, it is necessary that these frequent stoppages be avoided. Recent experiments in this direction would seem to indicate that this can be accomplished and the filter effectually cleaned if a reverse current of water is made to pass through the filter-bed with sufficient force to agitate and separate the grains of sand to a depth of two or three inches from the top surface, thereby freeing it of the impurities which stop filtration. This process of cleaning is rendered possible by the fact that the suspended impurities are generally arrested immediately on the top surface of the sand, and never penetrate to a distance of more than two inches below the surface.

It has been stated that sand filtration is essentially mechanical, arresting only suspended matters, but experiments and observations made at the Berlin filter-beds have quite established the fact that after some hours use the beds take on a peculiar action, which modifies to a considerable extent the dissolved matters in the the water. At any rate, the filtration becomes more perfect after the bed has been in use some time. This is accounted for in two ways :

1. That certain solid matters of a chalky or mineral nature held in the water are deposited on the filter-bed and form a good filtering medium.

2. That the thin deposit which takes place on the surface of the filtering-bed is composed of minute *bacteria* which, through their depurating power, add greatly to the efficiency of the filter-bed.

No doubt these minute bodies eventually penetrate, to a greater or less extent, the entire body of the sand, and thereby improve its qualities as a filtering medium. In cleaning the filter, therefore, it is important not to disturb oftener than necessary more than a few inches of the top surface, or only so much of the surface as retains the solid matters that would stop filtration.

6. FILTRATION THROUGH SPONGY OR METALLIC IRON.

Bischoff's spongy iron has been subjected to thorough examination from several points. Besides the exertions of the inventor himself to bring the material into notice as a valuable filtering medium, it has been warmly recommended by Dr. Frankland, in the sixth report of the Rivers Pollution Commission of England. The experiments of Dr. Lewin, of Munich, however, gave results differing widely from those of Dr. Frankland. The best opportunity of witnessing the attempted application on a large scale of Prof. Bischoff's system of purifying water, which had been worked out so successfully on a small scale of domestic filters, was afforded at Antwerp, in 1883. Though correct in principle, the application of spongy iron over large areas, led after some months to the obstruction of the filter-beds, and would have compelled the abandonment of the system had it not been for the bold and radical change which it occurred to Mr. William Anderson, a civil engineer of London, to introduce. The spongy iron was removed from the filter-beds, and the reservoirs containing it were transformed into sand filter-beds, on which oxide of iron speedily forms, and plays an important part in the purification of the water passing through it.

Sir Frederick Abel appears to have suggested the application of ordinary metallic, instead of spongy iron, and Mr. Anderson seems to have worked out the idea most successfully in his application of what is known as the revolving iron purifier, which has now been in operation at Antwerp about five years. On the authority of Prof. Kemna, the distinguished Belgian chemist, it may be stated that so complete is the satisfaction given, that similar means are now in operation at Gouda, at Dordrecht, in Holland, and at the establishment Cail, quai der Grenelle, in Paris. Experiments on a large scale have also been made at Ostend, Berlin and London, and steps have been taken for its introduction into this country.

It is an interesting circumstance in connection with the purity of the water now obtained at Antwerp, and which is taken from the filthy river Nethe, that some of the steamers sailing thence to New York take in a supply of the Antwerp water for the double voyage, in preference to refilling from the Croton aqueduct for the return voyage.

A table of analysis showing the degree of purification attained is appended :

EFFECTS OF PURIFICATION BY THE ANDERSON PROCESS.

	Organic Matter.		Ammonia.			
			Albuminoid.		Free.	
	Before.	After.	Before.	After.	Before.	After.
Antwerp	77	31	0.27	0.08	0.40	. . .
Dordrecht	34	14	0.14	0.05	0.12	. . .
Gouda	151	85	0.41	0.23	0.05	0.03
Ostend (single purification)	135	76	0.58	0.22	1.30	0.12
Ostend (double purification*)	76	40	0.22	0.19	0.12	0.03
Paris	51	25	0.16	0.06	0.40	. . .

* In double purification the water is twice passed through a revolver, and twice sand-filtered.

7. THE "INTERNATIONAL PROCESS" OF FILTRATION.

This process consists in passing the water through a specially constructed filter-bed of powdered iron called "magnetic spongy carbon," or "polarite." This material is obtained from an iron ore which is found at Abercrane, in the South of Wales. It consists of carbonate and silicate of iron, together with some aluminum, calcium and magnesium. The ore is naturally very porous and absorbent. To manufacture the material (polarite) the ore is heated in closed vessels, with a limited supply of air, by which the carbonic acid and water are driven off and oxygen is taken up from the air. The resulting material is the *black oxide of iron*, which is extremely porous, quite insoluble and does not rust on exposure to air. It is to these properties that it owes its value as a good filtering material for impure water.

The material which presents the largest surface for the occlusion of oxygen in the smallest cubical space is the most powerful purifier and filtrant, provided it is composed of the proper substance. Spongy platinum fulfills these conditions best, and is consequently the most powerful purifier and filterer, and the best insoluble oxidizer known. Its enormous cost, however, shuts it altogether out from practical use, and the magnetic spongy carbon, or polarite, has been offered as a substitute. The admixture of this substance with sand forms a filtering medium which is said to purify itself by destroying organic impurities which would otherwise contaminate the beds. It is represented that the process of combustion is constantly going on in the pores of the material, and the products of that combustion are tasteless, odorless, colorless, and perfectly wholesome, creating carbonic acid, with which the water becomes charged to a limited extent, rendering it sparkling as well as palatable in the highest degree. Polluted water taken from the river Thames below London Bridge was passed through a filter composed of this material, and on being then analyzed was found to be purer than any drinking water supplied by the London water companies.

Every one of experience is aware of the disagreeable odors arising from the ordinary sand filter beds, which possess no chemical purifying action, but merely act as strainers, retaining the solid matters and filth, which corrupt and contaminate the water instead of purifying it. This, it is said, may be remedied by a layer of the "Polarite." By the use of this filtrant, properly arranged, it is not necessary to have the filtering beds half so large as is usual with the ordinary sand beds, since a bed containing a layer of polarite and sand mixed in equal proportions will do more efficient work than four times the extent of area where sand alone is used. Sir Henry Roscoe speaks very favorably of this material. He says: "The porous nature of the oxide (polarite) which is used in the filter, its complete insolubility and its freedom from rusting constitute, in my opinion, its claim to be considered a valuable filtering material."

Dr. Angell has also carefully examined the process, and reports the following experiments:

1. Ordinary domestic sewage was passed through nine inches of "polarite."

By the permanganate test it was found that 94 per cent. of the oxidizable organic matter was destroyed or rendered innocuous.

2. After passing a solution of sulphuretted hydrogen, equivalent to 4.2 grains of oxygen per gallon, it was found that not a trace of the sulphuretted hydrogen was left in the effluent.

Dr. Angell further states that "this material, though it permits the free transit of air and gases, is quite impermeable to atmospheric germs;" but the bacteria question is no doubt one which has probably still to be settled.

Taking bulk for bulk, it has been found that the following great advantages are in favor of the magnetic spongy carbon as against sand filtration :

(*a*) From an economic point of view the large filtering areas now employed would be greatly reduced.

(*b*) From a sanitary point of view the water would not be exposed in large surfaces to the unhealthy action of the atmosphere in or near large and densely populated cities.

(*c*) Lastly and chiefly, the filtration by this process has been proved to be much purer than anything obtained by the ordinary process of filtration ; in fact, we may with safety state that this material is capable of exercising a powerful effect on dissolved organic matter in water, and that it is one of the safest media in the market.

I have personally witnessed the satisfactory results of filtration through "polarite," at the sewage works of Acton, a growing suburb of London. Here the sewage of a large district is received and treated by filtration, and I found the resulting effluent to be bright, clear and free from any smell. A sample of the effluent kept nearly two months still retained its good qualities. It should be stated, however, that the crude sewage water was treated, before filtration, with a preparation of sulphate of iron known under the name of "Ferozone." *

8. PURIFICATION OF WATER BY ELECTROLYSIS.

Dr. William Webster, of England, has recently brought to the attention of the public a new process for purifying contaminated water by electrolysis, which he claims will meet all reasonable expectations as to its sanitary character. Its action, he says, if carried far enough, will absolutely eradicate all organic matters. The device, on a small scale, may be described as follows :

1. An outer vessel which may be made of iron—the sides in that case acting as negative electrodes—and an interior vessel containing a carbon electrode. By placing an oxidisable plate in the same pot as the carbon, and connecting the two to the positive pole of the current, a hyperchlorite or chloride of the metal used is produced, which further assists the resulting action. The apparatus on a large scale may be variously modified according to the strength of the solutions of chlorides acted upon, and by the use of a dynamo.

---

* For filtering potable water the company sells the magnetic spongy carbon, or "Polarite," in the form of a coarsely granular powder, and they recommend that the filtering bed should consist of a couple of inches of shingle at the bottom, then nine inches of the material, and on top of this six or eight inches of fine sand. This sand should be either partly or entirely removed at intervals and be washed and replaced.

By applying the current to a carbon filter arranged as above described, he was able to oxidise the organic matter in water. The positive pole being the porous carbon block, the nascent oxygen produced in the pores of the carbon by the electric current absolutely destroys organic matter, bacteria being killed and the filter-block itself kept clean. The action of porous carbon by itself is due to its power of absorbing noxious gases and effecting their destruction by bringing them in contact with atmospheric oxygen, but it is absolutely essential that there should be a free supply of air; how much more active the action is when nascent oxygen and even when chlorine are constantly supplied by means of the electric current can be easily imagined.

CONCLUSION.

The increasing population of large towns has made the question of water purification a very pressing one, particularly in relation to the purity of our rivers, most of which are unquestionably in a serious state of pollution. It may be that the present scientific knowledge is not sufficient to entirely and finally deal with this question; we should, however, aim at as high a standard of purification as possible; it is of no use to try half measures; but whatever the treatment may be, the nearer nature's action is approached, the nearer will we be to the solution of the difficulty. The oxidation of organic matter can only be attained by one mode—chemical action—whether it be by filtration, by the addition of chemicals, or by the force of the electric current.

Adiposity of the Breasts.

Women troubled with this accretion have usually been dosed (in Europe at least) with iodide of potassium. Kisch considers that this treatment is never efficacious except at the cost of emaciating the entire economy. He proposes the following, which he has used successfully against this condition. Cover the breasts with an ointment as follows: Deodorized iodoform, fifteen grains; vaseline, two hundred and twenty-five grains; ol. menth., one gtt. Then cover the breasts with hot cloths dipped into a solution of alum, fifteen grains; acetate of lead, seventy-five grains; aq dist., fifteen hundred grains. Impermeable paper is placed over the cloths and the dressing allowed to remain in place for eleven hours. Two dressings daily are given for several weeks. The "slack" of the skin is taken up by using frictions of aromatic alcohol. Bandages must be worn for some months after the cure is effected.

After Recovery from Measles.

Now that measles are so prevalent, it will be in order to warn parents not to permit their children to be exposed until *thoroughly* well. *Protect children getting up after measles from exposure until entirely well*, *i. e.*, until all signs of cough, and disease of the nose, throat and lungs have disappeared and the weather is such that outdoor life will be a help rather than a danger. Neglect of these precautions may make the child an invalid for life.

THE ANNALS of HYGIENE,
THE OFFICIAL ORGAN OF THE
State Board of Health of Pennsylvania.
The State Board of Health is not responsible for
anything appearing in this Journal except that
which bears the official attestation of the Board.

PUBLISHED MONTHLY. ✧ ✧

Subscription, two dollars ($2.00)
a year, in advance.

Address all communications to

The Hygienic Publishing Company,
224 SOUTH SIXTEENTH STREET,
PHILADELPHIA, PA.

EDITORIAL.

The Home of Cholera.

IN the far-eastern portions of the world cholera is always, more or less, present; as with us, typhoid fever, so with our Oriental brethren, cholera is an unwelcome resident, never entirely absent. From time to time the disease assumes unusual prevalence, and, emboldened, as it were, by the multitude of its germs (or soldiers) it sallies forth from its citadels and begins its devastating march throughout lands that are usually free from it, and, at such times, we have the startling and somewhat sensational accounts of cholera, such as we are being treated to at the present time.

Our illustration represents one of the more important of the strongholds of the disease, for, contradictory as it may seem, the traveller will find, in the centre of the holy and sacred city of Mecca, in Arabia, the eternal city of the Mohammedans, a spot that exists and is famous throughout the sanitary world as the breeding place of cholera.

Mecca is a city with a permanent, resident population of about 60,000, which is almost always doubled by the holy and dirty Mohammedan pilgrims who are continually flocking thereto from all points, the pilgrims of one season beginning to arrive before those of a previous season have all dispersed. The streets of Mecca are fairly spacious, but ill-kept and filthy, while the Mosque (depicted in our drawing), situated in the centre of the city, is much below the level of the rest of the city, the surface of which has been gradually elevated by the accumulated rubbish of centuries. In this Mosque, enclosed in one of the small buildings, in the foreground, is the famous well, "Zamzam." the "Holy Well of Mecca," from which, according to Mohammedan tradition, Hagar drew water for her son Ishmael. However sacred this water may be in the eyes of the pilgrims, it must appear evident to any reasonable, reasoning and unprejudiced mind that, receiving as it does, the drainage of the city (all of which is on a higher level and contains the accumulated refuse of centuries), it must be but little, if any, better than liquid refuse. Yet we read that this water is eagerly drank by the pilgrims, and, when poured over the body, it is held to give a miraculous refreshment after the fatigues of religious exercise. This holy water (holy and potent for good to the Mohammedan mind; most unholy, full of disease and potent for incalculable evil to the mind of the unbiased) is carried by the devout pilgrim to the most distant points, he, thereby unconsciously, but none the less surely, spreading the germs of cholera broad and far.

All about this Mosque are boarding places for the pilgrims, and the ground is as thoroughly saturated with organic refuse as it is possible for any ground to be, for we must remember that for centuries piled upon centuries, this city has been the gathering place annually for thousands upon thousands of human beings, who, remaining but a short time, have had no thought for the sanitary welfare of the locality ; while the greedy, vicious and avaricious residents of the city have had no thought beyond that of using the holy reputation of the city and its Mosque for their temporal gain.

Their greed for the money of the pilgrim has banished from their natures all the better attributes of humanity, even including the selfish one of self-preservation, for the fanaticism of the Meccan is truly an affair of the purse ; the mongrel population (for the town is by no means purely Arab) has exchanged the virtues of the Bedouin for the worst corruptions of Eastern town life, without casting off the ferocity of the desert, and it is hardly possible to find a worse certificate of character than the three parallel gashes on each cheek, called Tashrit, which are the customary mark of birth in the holy city. The unspeakable vices of Mecca are a scandal to all Islam, and a constant source of wonder to pious pilgrims.

In the centre of the Mosque we note a rude stone building, the Ka'ba, so called from its resemblance to a monstrous astragalus, or die, and in its external angle we see fixed the famous " black stone," another unconscious but terribly potent disseminator of disease. This sacred stone, kissed by all devout pilgrims, undoubtedly receives and transmits the germs of disease from one to another.

In these days of inquiry, when the penetrating mind of humanity is not satisfied with dogmatic assertions, when we want to know the "why and the wherefore," when we always endeavor to trace the relationship between cause and effect, it is but natural that we should ask from whence comes the cholera that at times ravages and devastates the civilized world.

While, of course, there are many points in the far East wherein Asiatic cholera is always present, and from where it starts on its mission of death, we imagine that there is no more prominent nor more prolific breeding place for the cholera germ than this holy and filthy well in the centre of Mecca, in far-off Arabia, receiving, as it has for centuries, the organic refuse of countless pilgrims, and being conveyed, as it is, to all parts of the Mohammedan world. Truly may it be said, that the Holy Well in the Mosque at Mecca is the home, the breeding place, the camping ground of cholera. And in these days of rapid inter-communication, when the world seems much smaller than it did to our forefathers, we must recognize that this famous well exists as a constant menace to humanity at large.

At the same time it will be well for us all to inquire (those of us who use well water) if we have not " A Holy Well of Mecca" on a small scale on our own premises. Our country is too young to have our soil so thoroughly pol-

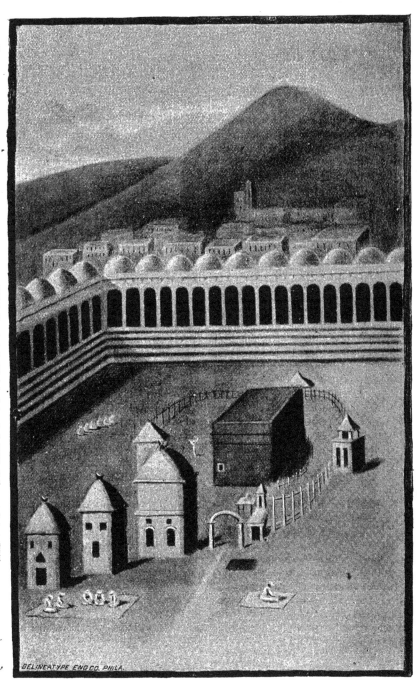

The Home of Cholera. (The "Holy Well" at Mecca.

luted with human refuse, but there are many country residents who allow entirely too much house and stable drainage to find its way into the drinking water.

Having now made some acquaintance with one of the localities from which the disease originates, it will be in order to look at the question as it to-day presents itself to us. The appearance of Asiatic cholera almost simultaneously at six different points in Spain, covering a distance of two hundred and fifty miles in a straight line, and probably four hundred by rail, indicates a very considerable survival of germs of that disease from last Summer along the shores of the Mediterranean (says Dr. Benjamin Lee in a recent report to the State Board of Health). Their wide dissemination and early maturity make a grave epidemic in that region probable, and it may be in southern Europe generally. We in this country have little to fear, however. Our quarantine stations, national, state and municipal, were never so well equipped before. That of the port of New York, which is our most vulnerable point, is fully twice as well prepared as it was when it so successfully checked the invasion of the disease at the threshold three years ago. Philadelphia, the next most likely point of attack, has a double line of intrenchments, the Lazaretto, or Municipal Quarantine Station twelve miles down the Delaware River, and the United States Quarantine Station eighty miles below, at Cape Henlopen. The latter is provided with a fumigating steamer (appropriately named the Louis Pasteur), just finished, which is capable of disinfecting the largest vessel in a few hours.

The Baltimore station is well equipped and under intelligent management. and suspected vessels for that port as well as for Norfolk, are also detained at Cape Charles by the U. S. Marine Hospital Service. The efficiency of the New Orleans quarantine has been frequently demonstrated. Its plant is the most complete and most scientifically constructed of any in the country. Should the disease pass these barriers, however, its mode of propagation is now so thoroughly understood that it will be a reproach to local health authorities if it is not at once stamped out.

It is their duty immediately to put their cities and towns into such a condition of cleanliness that the germs will find no congenial soil. The State Board of Health of Pennsylvania has in press a revised edition of its circular on this subject, which will shortly be issued.

Continuing to speak of "Hot Weather Diseases," Dr. Lee tells us that the report of yellow fever carried to Spain from New Orleans is more than doubtful. There is not more yellow fever in South America and Central America than usual at this season. Our greatest danger is from Cuba, the "ever faithful" and ever filthy isle, via Florida.

The precautions which are taken on the Plant Line of steamers and at Key West and Tampa make its introduction by that route unlikely. The fact that there were no cases of the disease in that State last Summer indicates that its germs had all perished.

Time enough has elapsed since the last epidemic to greatly improve the sanitary condition of its towns. The experience then gained will enable the authorities to meet any outbreak that may occur with entire confidence ; and the existence of a State Board of Health in that State will prevent the irregular and ill-advised action which has marked previous epidemics.

The floods in the lower Mississippi Valley have left many places along that river in a state of great destitution, and the conditions are such as will probably induce malarial fevers of such virulence that they may easily be mistaken for yellow fever. We may therefore expect false alarms. Should the disease actually appear, there will be such a concert of action between the different State Boards of Health, and between them and the United States quarantine authorities, as arranged for at their recent conference at Nashville, that it will no doubt be restrained within narrow limits without a resort to the barbarous expedient of shotgun quarantines, such as have disgraced the country in former outbreaks of this much dreaded pestilence. Thus, then, it will be seen that we are prepared to resist the invasion of epidemic disease, but, just as the most perfect army will be impotent without popular support, so will the efforts of the health authorities be robbed of much of their power if they do not have the full, free, cordial support of the people.

Atlantic City Trains. The Reading's Grand Summer Time-table.

THE new arrangement of trains on the Reading Railroad's Atlantic City line is immeasurably superior in point of number, frequency, convenience and speed to any schedule ever operated by any of the roads to the sea. Comparison will demonstrate this. On week days there are fast express trains from Chestnut Street and South Street ferries at 8.00, 9.00, 10.45 A. M. (1.30 Saturdays only), 2.00, 3.00 (3.30 Saturdays only), 4.00, "The Flyer ;" 5.00, 6.00 P. M., and accommodations at 8.00 A. M. 4.15 and 6.30 P. M. On Sundays, express trains at 4.15, 7.00, 8.00, 8.30, 9.00, 9.30 A. M. ; accommodation at 8.00 A. M. and 4.30 P. M. Up trains leave Atlantic City depot as follows : week days, express 7.00, 7.30, "The Flyer ;" 8.00, 9.00, 10.00 A. M., 4.00, 5.30, 9.45 P. M. ; accommodation 6.00, 8.10 A. M., 4.30 P. M. ; Sundays, express 4.00, 5.00, 6.00, 6.30, 7.00, 8.00, 9.45 P. M. ; accommodation 7.30 A. M., 5.05 P. M. The very finest Pullman drawing room and buffet parlor cars are run on this line.

Sanitary Legislation in Brazil.

By a decree of the Republican government which came into effect at the end of last year, medical practitioners in Brazil are compelled to notify every case of yellow fever, cholera, plague, diphtheria, smallpox, measles and scarlet fever which they may be called to attend.

NOTES AND COMMENTS.

How to Examine for Life Insurance.

Our attention has been called to a volume just issued with the above title, by P. Blakiston, Son & Co., of this city. Dr. John M. Keating, the author, is the president of the Association of Life Insurance Medical Directors, which is a sufficient guarantee, if any were needed, of his eminent fitness to issue a standard work on this subject. We have examined this book, and feel that it is just what is required by all physicians who are engaged as examiners for life insurance companies, and who are anxious to properly and conscientiously perform their duty. We congratulate Dr. Keating on the extremely satisfactory manner in which he has given to us a book for which there really was a need.

Death-Rate and Mortality of Infants in Japan.

A correspondent of the *British Medical Journal* says that the death-rate of the population of the whole Empire, as gathered from the well-edited reports of Mr. N. Sensai, the able chief of the statistical health bureau, is 19.33 per 1000, due to the low infant mortality. The Japanese have the most tender affection for their children ; and all travelers are agreed that next to the beauty of the scenery and the gentle and graceful courtesy of all classes of the population, ranks as among the most pleasurable incidents of sojourn in Japan the universal love of children and the amiable gaiety with which their pleasures are studied.

To Kill Roaches.

The following recipe from the *Druggists' Circular* is said to make a powder effective in driving away roaches. The preparation is said to be practically identical with " Peterman's Roach Food :"

	Ounce.
Borax	37
Starch	9
Cocoa	4

Early to Bed, etc.

" Early to bed and early to rise " is a motto that finds little favor with most folks nowadays, but those who have practically tested its merits stand by it and demonstrate its value by their superior mental and physical condition.

The Treatment of Corns.

Dr. C. McDermott writes to the *British Medical Journal* that a saturated solution of salicylic acid in flexible collodion is an excellent remedy for corns. The corns should be painted twice a day. It takes about twelve days for their complete removal.

Procreation of the Criminal and Degenerate Classes.

Our brethren of California are fully up to the times in matters of a social and sanitary kind. The President of the State Society, Dr. Walter Lindley, in his annual address, asks :

" Why should not every man and woman who desires a license for marriage be required, before such license is issued, to show the County Clerk a certificate from the County Physician certifying that both he and she were free from any taint of consumption, gonorrhœa, syphilis, or scrofula. I ask you, gentlemen, to give this subject, which to me seems a very important one, your serious consideration."

He further adds : " Knowing, as all surgeons do to-day, that castration and spaying are simple operations that can be performed with about as little danger as the ancient rite of circumcision, I do not hesitate to advise that the following classes be required by law to submit to this procedure : Idiots, those who commit or attempt to commit rape, wife-beaters, murderers, and some classes of the insane."

We admire the doctor's generous breadth of view in proposing to castrate the men as well as to spay the women. Fortunately, however, it is a physiological law that the degenerate classes have little procreative power and tend to die out of themselves. What society needs most, therefore, is the adoption of such ethical and social measures as will prevent the development of new vicious and criminal families.—*Medical Record.*

" Competition the Life of Business."

" Benjamin Lee M D

" Your card rec'd. There is 2 Semitary,s here (just started) & there is a fight between them to get their ground filled up and the are tearing up the old grave yards to get theirs filled up there is no other reason for it that I know of and our authoritys take no notice of it.

W. S. McD."

[The above unique communication was recently received by the Secretary of the State Board of Health.—ED.]

May a Woman with Heart Disease Marry ?

This subject being recently under discussion in a New York Medical society, the opinion was expressed by Dr. Polk that heart disease, of itself, was no bar to marriage. If the disease had progressed so far as to cause secondary disease of the liver or kidney, then the case would be different. It is not likely that a woman with heart disease would have children, hence she would not have this ordeal to pass through ; but if she should have them, it was Dr. Polk's opinion that she would be equal to the emergency.

Damages for Sickness.

We have been recently reading some portions of a lecture that was delivered quite a little while ago by Dr. C. A. Lindsley, the cultured secretary of the Connecticut State Board of Health, and we were so much impressed with the eminent wisdom of what follows that we reproduce it at length :

"The causes of, and the means of preventing infectious diseases are as well known and as readily controlled as those of railroad dangers, and yet last year in our little State of Connecticut there were permitted to occur over 2000 deaths from preventable diseases ; full 20 per cent. of the total mortality from all causes of death.

"If one-half of the care and vigilance exerted in making railroad traveling safe were also used in making communities safe from zymotic diseases, the mortality from those diseases would be reduced to less than one-quarter its present amount.

"Railroad corporations are compelled to pay damages in good money to their unfortunate passengers for injuries received on their roads ; and for loss of life, a few thousand dollars to surviving relatives. There is nothing on earth so almighty to control and direct the attention and efforts of men as the almighty dollar.

"Whenever our State legislatures get so far enlightened as to make communities responsible for the suffering of their fellow citizens by infectious diseases, and compel payment to every sufferer from the public treasury, then public hygiene will receive the attention which its importance demands. Individuals cannot alone control the spread or prevent the invasion of contagious diseases. It can only be done by the united and concerted action of communities, acting under authority. Hence communities are responsible morally for the presence and prevalence of contagious diseases, and ought to be held so pecuniarily.

"No act of the Legislature could so promptly and so surely put Connecticut in the fore front of all the States of the Union for its superior sanitary condition as the enactment of a law like the following :

"Be it enacted, etc.—

"Every legal resident, in every town in Connecticut, who shall, while residing in the town, have either of the following diseases, to wit : yellow fever, cholera, smallpox, typhus fever, scarlet fever, or typhoid fever, shall be entitled to receive from the treasury of the town $3 for each day that he is confined to his house by such sickness, or by the order of the board of health of the town, for the public safety. And in the case of the death of such person from such diseases, $25 shall be paid from the town treasury to defray the expenses of the funeral.

"And every person so afflicted shall be subject to such regulations and restrictions during his sickness as the board of health of the town shall determine to be necessary for the safety of other persons.

"There is better reason for paying such victims of disease than there is for paying damages to people who slip on icy sidewalks and hurt themselves. The town treasuries would suffer for a time. But very soon town boards of health would become an important department of town government. The members of such boards would be more considerately appointed than at present. Sanitary engineering in the way of sewers, aqueducts, drainage schemes, etc., would be going on all over the State to save the expense of paying for so much sickness, and the State of Connecticut would rival the railroad companies in the care and vigilance given to sanitary matters, and with corresponding good results.''

Disinfection of Persons, Clothing and Rooms, after Infectious Diseases.

This is a constant subject of inquiry in our correspondence, and it is worth while to keep before our readers the essential facts upon which advice is based, and the common sense of the methods advised.

The special poison of all infectious disease, is a living thing, peculiar to each disease, but all alike killed by certain agents which we use for that purpose. And this killing of the specific poison is *disinfection*. This is the strictly scientific use of the word but, in practice, we include under this process every measure which diminishes, or removes, the infection from the room, or house. Different diseases can be most successfully attacked in various ways, but there are certain rules which apply to all. These poisons agree in growing most luxuriantly in foul air, and in damp, uncleanly, ill-lighted places. *Overcrowding* helps them, not only in this way, but by aiding their direct transmission from person to person.

The first essential, then, in dealing with infectious diseases is to *forefend* them, by *cleanliness of persons' clothing, and everything in the house.* The only way to use this method is to make it a *rule of life always, before, during, after sickness.* When such diseases come and find this precaution not taken, it should not be neglected another hour, but all possible done immediately to make up for lost time. Among the means to this end, *free ventilation* is the most important. I mean "through and through" ventilation, through windows and doors. This is possible in all rooms (*including cellar*), not occupied by the patient, and should be repeated often enough to destroy the stuffy and mouldy odor peculiar to crowding. The "dusting of rooms" should be done at this time, so that the dust, the source and carrier of much foulness in the air of the house, may be taken away by the wind and oxydized and destroyed in the air of the open.

Another general fact, applicable to all eruptive diseases (*e. g.*, scarlet fever, measles, smallpox), is that "a good greasing" all over with simple ointment (one part mutton tallow to two parts lard), is always in order, almost always a benefit as a remedy, and always does more than any other measure to keep the poison, ripening in the skin, in the body clothing. The housewifely objection that it soils the clothes is true, but an advantage, as it compels more frequent change, not only of night dress but of sheets and pillow cases. *But what shall be done with them?* Put them immediately into *boiling water.* You may use a little soap if you will, but need not put in any chemical. It is the *water, hot to boiling*, which kills. Boil for ten minutes, and then treat the clothes as if they had never been infected—they are perfectly safe.

Blankets, pillows, and bed ticks may be treated in the same way, and the clothing of the nurse. *After recovery*, the warm bath, with plenty of soap, repeated as need be till the last evidence of disease has disappeared. *After death*, the body should be wrapped in a sheet saturated with a strong solution of chloride of lime and then put in a tight casket for prompt and private burial.

What is to be done with the room that was occupied by one suffering from infectious disease? Everything which can be cooked with *boiling water* is therefore safe. All else must be fumigated with *moist* sulphurous acid gas, and the room should be well steamed at the same time. This is easily done by the boiling water put in the tub, as directed, and may be helped by sprinkling the floor and walls with hot water before lighting the sulphur. After the fumigation, *thorough* "through and through" ventilation; and then hot soap-suds to the floor and to the walls if wood or painted. If papered, the paper will have suffered by the moist acid, so that it will come off all the more easily. When it is once thoroughly off, never put on any more, but paint the walls. The ceiling should not be painted, but always whitewashed with *hot* and *fresh* lime-wash.

Mind one important point, especially as respects diphtheria. After disinfecting a room, or house, see that no *moist*, damp places remain. Have *floor, walls, closets*, every bit of wood work, *thoroughly dry*, before occupation of the room again, and put off such occupation by children as long as possible.—*Public Health in Minnesota*.

Sober Railway Employees.

Considerable comment was recently created by the issuance of an order from the Reading Railroad that men who were known to be heavy drinkers, *even when off duty*, should not be continued in the employ of the company. It was felt that this was infringing upon the liberty of the individual; but to us this view is erroneous. Of course, if a man wants to drink—even to drink himself to death—he may claim the right to do so, so long as no one but himself will suffer thereby; but we hold that a railway company has no right to trust the lives of its patrons to men who, even though not habitually heavy drinkers, yet who may, if they drink at all, be sufficiently under the unnatural influence of liquor just at a critical moment as to deprive them of their *best* intelligence just at a time when it is most needed. A man who drinks at all is liable, even though he may not be drunk in the ordinary acceptation of the term, at times to have a sufficient quantity of alcohol within him to make him not the absolutely responsible individual he would be without it, and we hold that those who have charge of the lives of others have no business to consume one drop of alcohol at any time so long as they are thus employed.

Incubation of Measles.

Dr. James A. Myrtle, of Harrogate, writing to the *British Medical Journal*, February 1st, 1890, says : " In a young ladies' school with thirty-five resident scholars, a case of measles occurred ; the girl was at once removed to a cottage in the rear of the dwelling house, complete isolation secured, a nurse put in charge and all communication cut off. In twelve days the patient and nurse were sent away, and the cottage and everything in it thoroughly disinfected. Exactly fourteen days after this girl showed the disease, a second case occurred ; fourteen days after that a third, fourteen days after that a fourth, and fourteen days after that a fifth. Nos. 1, 2, 3 and 5 belonged to different classes and slept in different rooms ; Nos. 1 and 4 were sisters and slept together ; but No. 4 showed the disease eight weeks after her sister. Each case, as soon as it declared itself, was removed to the hospital. The outbreak in the first instance was supposed to have been caused by infection when away from school, but that is by no means certain, as measles was prevalent in the district. Comment on these clinical records is needless."

Hygiene and Quackery.

" . . . . It is by the judicious use of such articles of diet that a constitution may be gradually built up until strong enough to resist every tendency to disease. Hundreds of subtle maladies are floating around us ready to attack wherever there is a weak point. We may escape many a fatal shaft by keeping ourselves well fortified with pure blood and a properly nourished frame."

The above quotation is clipped from the advertisement of a proprietary article that has fabulously enriched its owners. What is here claimed for a single article is the claim made for hygiene by its advocates. This article is easy to take ; the people, therefore, buy it ; they imagine that the doctrines of hygiene are hard to take and, they, therefore, pass them by. The popularity of certain proprietary articles is due to the fact that the people are made to believe that they will prevent disease ; such, to the intelligent mind, is a delusion. No one, single article can prevent disease, but an aggregation of intelligent principles, such as constitute the science of hygiene, will and can do so.

Ice in the Sick Room.

A saucerful of shaved ice may be preserved for twenty-four hours with the thermometer in the room at 90° F., if the following precautions are observed : Put the saucer containing the ice in a soup plate and cover it with another. Place the soup plates thus arranged on a good heavy pillow, and cover it with another pillow, pressing the pillows so that the plates are completely embedded in them. An old jack-plane set deep is a most excellent thing with which to shave ice. It should be turned bottom upward, and the ice shoved backward and forward over the cutter.

Advice to Boarding Schools.

Since writing the note on "Measles and Boarding Schools," which we published in our last issue, we have learned that the disease was introduced into the school in question by a child who went home for a few days to have some clothes fitted, and in whose family the disease was prevalent. Probably 500 cases of measles can be directly laid to the criminal ignorance or careless-ness of the parents of this child in allowing her return to school. Now, the advice we would volunteer to boarding schools for their own protection is that they should positively refuse to receive any child unless accompanied by the certificate of a reputable physician that such child has not been, for at least two weeks previously, exposed to any contagious disease. This rule will, of course, apply to day as well as boarding schools. Some pupils may be lost by the enforcement of this rule, but they will be such as would have vitally dam-aged the school by the introduction of disease therein.

State Board of Health and Vital Statistics of the Commonwealth of Pennsylvania.

PRESIDENT,
GEORGE G. GROFF, M.D., of Lewisburg.

SECRETARY,
BENJAMIN LEE, M.D., of Philadelphia.

MEMBERS,
PEMBERTON DUDLEY, M.D., of Philadelphia.

J. F. EDWARDS, M.D., of Philadelphia.	GEORGE G. GROFF, M.D., of Lewisburg.
J. H. McCLELLAND, M.D., of Pittsburg.	S. T. DAVIS, M.D., of Lancaster.
HOWARD MURPHY, C. E., of Philadelphia.	BENJAMIN LEE, M.D., of Philadelphia.

PLACE OF MEETING,
Supreme Court Room, State Capitol, Harrisburg, unless otherwise ordered.

TIME OF MEETING,
Second Wednesday in May, July and November.

EXECUTIVE COMMITTEE,

PEMBERTON DUDLEY, M.D., Chairman.	JOSEPH F. EDWARDS, M.D.
HOWARD MURPHY, C. E.	BENJAMIN LEE, M.D., Secretary.

Place of Meeting (until otherwise ordered)—Executive Office, 1532 Pine Street, Phila-delphia.

Time of Meeting—Third Wednesday in January, April, July and October.

Secretary's Address—1532 Pine Street, Philadelphia.

Bureau of Registration and Vital Statistics—Department of Internal Affairs, State Capitol, Harrisburg.

State Superintendent of Registration of Vital Statistics—BENJAMIN LEE, M.D.

THE
ANNALS
OF
HYGIENE

VOLUME V.

Philadelphia, August 1, 1890

NUMBER 8.

COMMUNICATIONS

Thoughts on School Hygiene.*

BY GEORGE G. GROFF, M.D., LL.D.,

Of Lewisburg, Pa.

President of the Pennsylvania State Board of Health.

* ON the subject assigned to me papers might very properly be addressed to schoolteachers, to directors and managers of schools, and to parents. In a circular issued by our State Board of Health, I have very fully explained to teachers those matters of hygiene to which they should give constant attention, viz., to the hygienic care of the eyes, and to all that tends in school to injure these organs ; in reference to the use of drinking water ; to cleanliness in and about the school; to wet clothing; to ventilation; to proper and improper exercise; to contagious diseases; to overwork; and to the use of tobacco and narcotics. This circular may be obtained by teachers in any quantities of the Secretary of the State Board of Health in Philadelphia.

A similar circular to directors and managers of schools is contemplated, and as soon as it can be prepared, will be issued by our Board. This morning, then, only a few words to parents and friends of our common humanity in reference to hygiene as applied to school children.

After I had promised to write this paper I picked up the latest circular of our Board, " Precautions against Consumption." On the second page of the cover is a diagram of the diseases *most fatal* in a neighboring city. Out of 400 deaths in the city of Reading in 1880, 105, or more than 25 per cent., were from consumption, but examining the diagram further, it is seen that 128 of the 400 deaths, or 32 per cent., are of diseases most commonly called diseases of children, and most probably of children of school age, or below. That is, of 400 deaths in Reading in 1880, 52 per cent. are of diseases now known to be preventable, and 32 per cent. of these of children. While it is known to sanitarians that nearly every child born into the world *can* be reared to years of man-

---

* Read before the State Sanitary Convention at Norristown, Pa.

hood or womanhood, yet the fact is that in Pennsylvania, in the Nineteenth Century, from one-fourth to one-fifth of all the children born die before reaching 10 years of age. What a murder of innocents ! And in a Christian State ! !

But why this state of things ? Mainly on account of ignorance and indifference on the part of parents. These unfortunate little ones, who received the blessing of the Great Teacher, are born of parents who themselves, and their ancestors before them, have violated nearly every law which governs their physical existence. They come into homes where no welcome awaits them. They are improperly fed, improperly dressed, without proper attention as to sleep, fresh air or cleanliness. It is not alone the children of the poor and the ignorant who suffer in these respects, but in a very large degree also the children of the well-to-do, whose mothers, from improper and deficient education, as we believe, commit their helpless offspring to the tender mercies of ignorant nurses, while they, the mothers, are active in temperance, missionary, charitable, church, or society duties. Shame, shame, that this is true, and yet it is. As an illustration, I was told a few days ago of an educated woman of a neighboring town, most active and efficient in temperance work, whose own boys are growing up in the streets while she devotes her time to others.

But what has this to do with school hygiene ? This. To call the attention of teachers to the great need of educating the children, and parents, too, to the need of knowledge on these subjects. Sanitary science is a matter of first importance. It is not a branch, for while in school, "we have no time" as a principal told me a few years ago. It is imperative. We owe it to every child to teach him the plain errors of living which bring disease and death.

But people are beginning to appreciate these things. But a few days ago a matron of culture remarked in my presence : "It is no longer fashionable to have delicate children about the home." The words show that the teachings of sanitarians are beginning to bear fruit. When in home and school the known principles of sanitary science are intelligently applied, we may expect a great diminution of sickness, suffering and premature deaths, and a corresponding increase of longevity and physical happiness. Contrary to the popular opinion, studious habits, even hard study, are not injurious to the general health. Rather, in well-regulated schools, the average health of the students will be found to be above that of those of the same age out of school. This is true of both young men and women. The statement applies to private schools where the *whole time* of the pupils is controlled, rather than to public day schools.

Irregular habits (irregular eating, drinking, loss of sleep, lack of physical exercise, overwork, excitement) are the causes of failure of physical power in students as in other persons.

At present students from the farms, the shops, the mines, have, as a rule, a better physical development than the children of professional men and of the well-to-do classes, which is certainly not a favorable showing for modern culture.

In European countries school children are often seen who are underfed. The same is true in our bountiful America. Indeed, with many young girls it is just the thing to eat about half enough to supply the demands of nature, and even the tables of many well-to-do people seldom contain what growing school children need. If only a small portion of the testimony of the children of the Home for the Blind in Philadelphia was true, in reference to the dietary of that institution, there was not a child there fit to be in school and at real work. I have myself seen the school dinner of a poor boy consist of cold Indian meal mush and fried sausage ; of a child whose parents were in comfortable circumstances of bread and cold boiled potatoes, and of a rich child, bread and butter only. Children cannot grow and study on such food (unless we make an exception of the mush and sausage).

I once remarked that the young ladies in a female seminary made very little progress in their studies, when the answer quickly came, "What more could you expect, remembering what they have to eat ?" I suspect this evil is a general one in homes and schools. Bread and coffee is not enough to start the day upon if much work is to be done.

School children do not have enough sleep as a rule. For children under twelve or thirteen years, ten hours out of each twenty-four should be spent in sleep, and all other students should have at least eight hours of sound sleep each night. This is most important.

School hours are for young children entirely too long. Not over three hours for children under thirteen, and five hours for all others'.

It is generally true that the playgrounds are too small. In all small towns schools should be built in the suburbs, that large lots may be secured. If country children can safely walk two or even three miles to school through mud and snow, town children can certainly reach school having good pavements.

One of the modern innovations most to be condemned is the abolition of the recess. A prominent teacher of a neighbouring county in defending this movement remarked that "if factory children can do without a recess, certainly school children can do without it."

The eye is the organ which *first* and most generally fails in school children. This is due to overwork of the organ, to insufficient light, to poor print, to the use of the eyes when the general health is below par, as well as numerous other causes. I once visited a school room in a Pennsylvania city with windows none too large, in every window two curtains and several shelves filled with plants. I have seen school houses in which the blinds were nailed shut to save the glass from being broken. But this does not equal the cold, dark kindergarten room at the Institution for the Blind, into which sunlight is said never to enter.

Whenever the subject of school hygiene is mentioned one listens to hear something on ventilation. Bad air is bad enough, but it is given too heavy a load to carry. There are other evils much greater, viz. : The too long hours, the long terms, the lack of light, the underfed condition of pupils, overheated or under-heated condition of the room, the inaccessible and filthy privy or water closet, the system of cramming so general, the highly graded systems which bring all the children to one dead level of mediocrity in body and mind.

Our public schools furnish the means for the spread of the contagious diseases of childhood. An intelligent county superintendent of schools wrote me not long since: '' Why, I have found all sorts of contagious diseases among the pupils of our schools, and the teachers apparently never taking any notice of them. I found one child so sick with scarlet fever that she could not hold her head up ; I have heard children whooping with whooping-cough, and have seen them all spotted with measles, and right alongside of other pupils.'' This should be controlled. Directors, physicians and teachers should be able to control this matter. The principal mission of the teacher, it seems to the writer, is to instill into his pupils a reverence for their own bodies, so that a generation of strong and pure men and women may be reared for the State. The truth of sanitary science will be best instilled when the teacher himself leads a pure and healthful life. Not upon the teacher alone, but upon parents, rests the chief responsibility in reference to the physical development of school children. This responsibility the parent cannot thrust upon the teacher.

Mental Hygiene of Our Boys and Girls.*

BY ROBERT H. CHASE, A.M., M.D.,

Superintendent State Hospital for the Insane, Norristown.

It has been computed by those who have given the subject special study, that in another quarter of a century this Republic will contain a population of at least 100,000,000. The men who will then form, control and govern this mightiest of earthly powers are now being prepared in our schools and colleges for their future lives—lives which to most will prove very eventful, and to a number illustrious.

How important, then, that their future, pregnant with the greatest possibilities, should, by every means in our power, be rendered auspicious, and that when our days of usefulness are over we shall not be given to self-censure and repentance that we have not contributed, in however slight a degree, to the power and lustre of America.

This is a practical matter and not one of imagination, for every well-educated child with a healthy mind and body will add to the glory of this country, and each one who aids in its proper development will prove, though the service may be small, a true patriot.

But the systems of education as generally adopted in the United States are by no means the best for attaining the most desirable condition of mental

---

* Read before the State Sanitary Convention at Norristown, Pa.

hygiene in our boys and girls. It is a fact greatly to be deplored that mental overstrain in youth and early manhood is becoming a peril among Americans; and its disastrous results, as seen in after life, cannot be too frequently nor too emphatically proclaimed in tones of solemn admonition. This injurious influence of undue brain friction, which has its inception in our schools, will have, if allowed to continue unchecked, its termination in national deterioration and decay.

It requires but little insight of the operations of nature to discern that most of the laws of our being, as well as the blessings of Providence, are beneficial or prejudicial according to the wise or unwise use of them. The sun's rays, which are the vitalizing force of nature, may, when this principle is disregarded, produce death instead of promoting life. In like manner, education, the vitalizing force of civilization, may cause mental decay when misapplied or misdirected.

The brain, let me briefly state, is a beautiful piece of mechanism, wonderfully adapted to its purposes. It is composed of millions of "brain-cells" and "nerve-fibres," sustained in a net-work, and abundantly supplied with blood-vessels, which run everywhere through it. Its importance in the physical economy is such that it requires one-fifth of the blood of the body to maintain its vitality.

As the seemingly countless intricacies of nature's workings are reducible to the simplest forms of law, so the brain, as the mind's agent, performing such multifarious functions, follows this rule of simplicity in its construction. It depends upon the same physiological laws for its growth as other parts of the body, and, I will add, its functions are easily deranged and its powers of restoration are low. These are some of the physical properties of this heaven-endowed organ which has placed man in the scale of creation a little lower than the angels; and the proper exercise of its delicate functions in its development and training depends, in a very great measure, upon the methods of education.

Let me remind you that the natural periods of life are separate and distinct from one another, and that their duties and prerogatives should be confined each to its own term of years. Childhood, youth and manhood have well-defined limits, which precocity should not be permitted to override.

A growth which partakes of the mushroom character means early maturity, and in turn premature old age. This unyielding law is operating in all animate nature. In the vegetable kingdom, the slowly-growing forest tree is the sturdiest. It takes deepest root; it lifts its head the highest; it has the toughest fibre, and in hardihood defies the storms of centuries. So it is with the races of men and also with individual lives—deferred maturity means strength and longevity.

The brain reaches its ripeness, on an average, five years later than other portions of the human frame, and as a consequence it is more tender and susceptible in early life than generally the other organs. The chubby-faced infant in the nursery, who passes his waking hours in a ceaseless round of action, kicking, squalling and eating [blessings on him !] with all his baby force—is the picture of physical strength, but his feeble and semi-fluid brain grows slowly, as it is needed but little at this stage of automatic life. The brain gets behind in the race until the general growth of the child has advanced somewhat, and self-preservation and other necessities demand the guidance of its controlling functions.

As years creep on, waste exceeds repair ; but in youth the processes of waste and repair not only strike a balance, but there is a storing of reserve force for the purposes of growth. This surplus power, intended for brain nutrition, growth and building up, cannot be diverted from its legitimate ends without the risk of impaired vitality. The nervous, overtaxed brain, as a result of overwork, not only means ruined health in the individual, but in the succeeding generations its effects are seen in low mentality and ill-balanced minds.

That it is a defect of many of our schools of discounting the future, by forcing mental training in the young beyond healthful limits, there is little reason to doubt. Juvenile memorizing, for instance, may exhibit the handiwork of the teacher, but if carried to the extent that some zealous instructors would go, may result in mental strain, from which the victim may not recover in a life-time.

> "With curious art the brain, too finely wrought,
> Preys on herself, and is destroyed by thought !
> Constant attention wears the active mind,
> Blots out her pow'rs, and leaves a blank behind."

A well-known author says : "The endeavor to fill the minds of children with artificial information leads to one of two results. Not infrequently in the very young it gives rise to direct disease of the brain itself. In less extreme cases it causes simple weakness and exhaustion of the mental organs, with irregularity of power. The child may grow up with a memory taxed with technicalities and impressed so forcibly that it is hard to make way for other knowledge ; and, added to these mischiefs, there may be, and often is, the further evil that the brain, owing to the labor put upon it, becomes too fully and easily developed, too firm and too soon mature, so that it remains throughout manhood always a large child's brain, very wonderful in a child, and equally ridiculous in a man or woman."

The powers of growth and development are restricted in every individual, and beyond the limitations set by nature no amount of training can carry them. Mental forcing cannot go beyond the capacity of the brain, taken at its weakest point. This is especially true when hereditary tendencies are considered. There is at our disposal only a definite quantity of energy. It is transferable to some extent, and if used in one direction it is lost in another. The law applies to the whole system, and may be seen in the physical life as well as in the operations of the mind. Exhausted muscular power implies, to some degree, mental loss, and, on the contrary, violent emotion or sudden shock causes in an equal manner muscular and organic weakness. This being the case, it is plain that undue pressure in any one direction will affect the entire organism.

Do we not see in this disregard of physical laws the cause of many of the nervous complaints which now afflict the educated classes? There is reason, I fear, for humbling of national pride in the thought that there is a close connection between American nervousness, which has become proverbial, and forced education—between juvenile brain tension and adult brain debility.

Another physiological axiom that should be recognized in undertaking a course of education is that bodily and mental energies need ample time for their effective utility. Forcing always signifies great waste. To run a mile is more fatiguing than to walk five miles ; to go through in an hour what should take ten hours to complete would soon bring utter prostration ; to perform in five the work of ten years is alike disastrous to nerve tone and mental stability. Many come out apparently unscathed from such ordeals of overstrain, but, alas ! too many sink beneath the burden and become as a " bowing wall and a tottering fence." He who would bind himself to a wheel of ceaseless toil must expect Ixion's fate !

To appreciate these wide-spread dangers, let us look for a moment at the state of affairs in some of our select and public schools.

" The child," says a reliable author, " at even the tender age of five or six years, is confined in school five hours a day, on a hard seat, in a room often poorly ventilated, and irregularly heated. During the larger portion of this time he is expected to have his mind occupied with his lessons, either in actual study or recitation. A few years later, say at the age of ten or twelve years, tasks of such extent and difficulty are imposed that it becomes necessary for him to study, in addition, one or two hours in the evening."

We should ever bear in mind that the object of schooling, in a physiological sense, is to make the brain vigorous, and to strengthen its powers of endurance and stability, which can only be accomplished under the guidance of wisdom and discretion.

Various writers on mental hygiene have prescribed rules to govern the hours of study, and have set the limits to healthful brain work. One of the best authorities, in formulating a set of rules, concludes " Three hours daily of school time up to nine years of age, four hours to twelve, and not more than six hours until after the pupil is fifteen years of age."

It is essential, let me say in passing, to the school-going child that he shall have not only good, natural sleep, but that there shall be plenty of it. But, strangely enough, sleep is regarded by many as a useless waste of time, and besides an impairer of the mind, which like some honeyed temptation should be strenuously resisted and avoided. Sleep, I assert, is not a passive rest or negative state in which we lie awaiting the dawn ; but aptly may it be compared to a filter. It strains off the gross impressions which do not enrich ; or, like the farmer's fanning mill, it winnows out the superfluous materials of the day—it separates the chaff from the wheat.

If the habits of the men of letters be inquired into, it will be found that six hours a day, on an average, are quite enough for a mature mind to be engaged with advantage in study. Yet in the training of our boys and girls we find that both teachers and parents, in their blind ambition to hurry them forward, conspire in imposing tasks of such character and magnitude as to require longer hours of study than we know to be best for the adult brain.

Numerous precedents of overstudy could here be cited, and did time permit, even within my own experience, I could instance many cases of the sad effects of this abuse of education. I have heard voices that have echoed back the terrible warning in shrieks of madness, and others, again, in the low moans of a bereft mind.

" If I had written down the fierce apostrophe of a young lady of twenty on her entrance into the asylum at Morningside, at the end of a school career of unexampled success," says Dr. Clouston, "the reading of it would do more to frighten the ambitious parents of such daughters from hastening their children forward at school too fast than all the scientific protests we doctors can make. She was well aware of the cause of her illness, and with passionate eloquence enumerated the consequences of her shattered health."

Education, to answer the purposes required of it, must embrace the highest and broadest conception of the term, and be marked by a complete symmetry in all its bearings. That is, the physical, mental, and moral parts of the pupil's nature must be trained together and in harmony in accordance with the laws that govern them. His entire being must be considered as a whole ; the brain not over-stimulated at the expense of the body, nor physical training forced beyond due bounds. From this point of view, education is not mere instruction, but means the healthful development of both mind and body. A child by a hot-house system of instruction may be full of facts, and still its education but just begun.

It should be kept in view by teachers that the culture of the higher, as well as the lower, faculties is accomplished by judicious exercise and regulated activity of their functions within the bounds of health, precisely as physical training is attained by the athlete ; and, furthermore, that the same laws which control the nutrition of the body in general apply with equal force to mental food.

We are not to regard the mind as a storehouse of knowledge alone, but also as workshop, wherein, through its subtle action, ideas are elaborated and all the higher manifestations of mind are developed. Thus, by a wholesome course of education, the cultured mind is built up into a most perfect structure ; its weakest points made strong, its by-ways guarded, until it possesses all the advantages over an uncultured one which strength has over weakness, endurance over instability, and which intelligence has over ignorance, everywhere and in all the circumstances of life.

It therefore appears from the evidence adduced, that the true aspirations of parents and teachers should be to rear children with strong and healthy minds, not strained and overburdened ones. This is true, even if their ambition be of the most worldly nature; that is, to have their sons or scholars not great and good, but powerful and distinguished. For in the end, what gratification can they derive from the acquirements of a child, however precocious, who at maturity has a diseased and withered brain.

It is a fact not disputed, that scarcely one of the greatest of American generals took high rank as a student at West Point, while some of the very greatest stood low in their class. This is not said to encourage idleness, but to illustrate the point that the largest and most powerful brains require time to develop and may be blighted by too intense study during youth. The same remark applies to every one of the higher walks of intellectual life. How few of our greatest philosophers, authors, poets, statesmen, lawyers, or physicians, have been distinguished at college by close application to study. Frequently we find in reading the biographies of those whose names in our literature have become immortal, that disparaging predictions were made of their future by their preceptors because they did not overtax their minds by too arduous study.

The question of mental hygiene of our boys and girls, then, is a momentous one, both to individuals and to the nation, and upon this people, at the present time, rests the duty of solving it, as required by mercy, by justice, and by the most exalted wisdom.

Defective Vision in our Public Schools.*

BY S. D. RISLEY, M.D.,
Ophthalmic Surgeon and Chief of Ophthalmic Clinic in the Hospital of the University of Pennsylvania.

In view of the important relation which adequate vision sustains to the successful career of the pupil, there is just cause for surprise that so little attention has been given to the subject at the outset of the school life of our children. It needs no argument to show that the child who enters upon the educational process with defective vision is seriously handicapped in the struggle before him.

It is but fair to assume that the failure to inquire into the state of the vision before entering the child at school is due to ignorance of any existing necessity, rather than to the wilful neglect of a recognized obligation, since in many other directions we constantly witness the most praiseworthy attention, on the part of guardians and parents, to the welfare of the children. The very large number of children whose progress at school is impeded by congenitally defective eyes is, I am sure, not appreciated by those who have made no study of the subject. The absence of complaint is not sufficient evidence of

* Read before the State Sanitary Convention at Norristown.

good vision, for children are not prone to complain. Many a child who gets on indifferently at school, and gains a reputation for dullness or indolence, is prevented from going forward by imperfect vision—a fact of which he may himself be ignorant; for how is the child to know but that the watering eyes, the blurring page and aching head which follow any protracted use of the eyes, are not the common lot of mankind? This has always been his experience; why not that of his fellows also? So, without complaint, he struggles on, asking no relief from conditions which to him are only a part of the disagreeable duty of his school life. That these remarks are not mere idle statements finds ample demonstration in the published records of numerous observers both in this country and in Europe, who have patiently examined large numbers of eyes in the schools.

It is not in harmony with the design of this paper to give a *résumé* of this work, but a few figures are introduced which, it is hoped, will serve as a sufficient demonstration of the great need which exists for the adoption of some simple but systematic method of inquiry into the state of the vision of every pupil when entering upon the long educational process, and at every successive step in advance. For this purpose I select the statistics, collated by myself in the public schools of Philadelphia, for the reason that they are the record of conditions existing at our own door.

In 2422 eyes examined 1084 were found to have less than the normal sharpness of sight, and 1099 had more or less trouble arising from the use of the eyes at their books. While many of these were the subjects of but slight impairment of vision, and did not suffer greatly, it is nevertheless sadly true that in a large percentage of them the impairment was sufficient to unfit them for the continuation of their work without placing the integrity of the organ in peril. It is not intended by this statement to convey the impression that blindness was imminent as the penalty of continued work, but that under the imposed strain the eyes which were the subjects of these congenital anomalies became also the subjects of certain pathological conditions which not only made the performance of the school tasks painful, and thus retarded the progress of the pupil, but led up to further impairment of sight through the disturbed nutrition of the eyeball. These figures—showing, as they do, approximately 5 per cent. of eyes with less than normal vision, and, withal, troublesome from pain or other disturbance—may well cause surprise to those who have not had the opportunity to investigate the subject; but, large as are these figures, a complete expression of existing conditions compels the further statement that there still remains a large number of eyes with hypermetropic refraction, which, nevertheless, have normal acuity of vision, but perform their work at a near point, as in reading or writing, by dint of greater strain upon the muscle of accommodation than is required by the emmetropic eye, and which, sooner or later, carries them over into the group of asthenopic or painful eyes, with commencing intra-ocular disease.

In the investigation of the eyes in the schools all observers have classified the eyes into three groups, viz.: The emmetropic or model eye, the hypermetropic or shallow eye, and the myopic or near-sighted eye. The immediate object of the inquiry was to determine the relative frequency of these three kinds of eyes. It had long been known that the percentage of near-sighted eyes steadily increased with the advancement of the pupils in the educational process. To illustrate : Erisman found in the lowest classes in the schools of St. Petersburg 13.6 per cent. of myopia, which percentage steadily advanced as the higher classes were reached until 42.8 per cent. were found in the highest classes. In the schools of Philadelphia, commencing with 4.33 per cent. at 8.50 years of age, it steadily advanced to 19.33 per cent. at 17.50 years. I am anxious here to impress the fact that the myopic eye is a diseased eye, and that its increasing percentage throughout the school life is but the expression of the resulting harm from the imposed strain of the work at school, Its full significance will be comprehended when it is understood that the near-sighted eye is acquired by distention of the ball, a condition made possible only by a profound disturbance of its nutrition through diseased pathological processes. It is obvious that they must have been recruited from eyes that at the beginning of school life belonged to one of the other group of eyes, i. e., either the emmetropic or hypermetropic eyes. The investigation in the schools of Philadelphia was undertaken with a view of not only determining the percentage of the different kinds of eyes in the schools, but also for the purpose of ascertaining the relative amount of disease in all states of refraction of the eye. It was hoped by this means to discover the early stages of those forms of disease which are characteristic of the myopic eye, and thus place in our hands the facts which would reveal the cause of the myopia and the best means for its arrest. To this end a careful study of each eye was made, and all observed conditions were recorded for subsequent analysis. The condition of the general health, the hygienic surroundings of the pupils, the age, etc., were all carefully considered, as well as the state of the eyes. The result of the subsequent analysis is graphically set forth in the following percentage curves.

In Table I, the percentage curves indicate the relative frequency of the three kinds of eyes. In general terms it reveals a high percentage of hypermetropia at 8.50 years of age, which steadily diminishes as the higher classes are reached, and a low percentage of myopia which steadily increases with the advance of the classes.

Table II reveals the state of the eyes in different states of the refraction. The curve representing the percentage of disease is seen to rapidly rise as we trace it from its lowest point in emmetropia, through hypermetropia and myopia and their attending astigmatism, until the alarming point of 87 per cent. of disease is reached in myopic astigmatism. It will be observed that this disease curve starts at the already high point of 32 per cent. in emmetropia, a fact accounted for by the very unfortunate condition of a few classes of very young children, who were found at work in rooms facing the light, and in one primary class where the only light they received was reflected from the ceiling of the room, or came to them over the tops of partitions from remote windows. In this room I found it extremely difficult to read diamond type on a bright midday because of the insufficient illumination. It is almost needless to add that not a single healthy eye was found in this class. When these unfortunately placed classes are omitted, however, from the percentage curve, the starting-point for disease falls much lower, but especially was this true for emmetropia. In one class ordinarily situated in its hygienic surroundings, the percentage of diseased emmetropic eyes fell às low as 2 per cent., while in the same class the percentage of disease in myopic eyes rose to 50 per cent. I have drawn the contrast just here for the double purpose, first, of emphasizing the importance of proper attention to suitable hygienic surroundings ; and, second, because it was shown that under conditions where all suffered, the eyes having some anomaly of refraction, i. e., the defective eyes, suffered most severely.

In Table III, the steadily advancing percentage of pain is depicted in the curve marked " asthenopia," by which is meant weak, painful or troublesome eyes, headache from eye-strain, etc. The second curve displays the lowered sharpness of vision in the various states of refraction of the eye.

In Table IV, the refraction and general state of the eyes is set forth in relation to the age of the pupils. It revealed the somewhat startling truth that notwithstanding the preceding developments, the eyes grew better as the age advanced, a fact variously accounted for. In the first place many of the worst eyes had been compelled to give up the struggle. Others had been subjected to professional care, and were found wearing glasses which corrected the ocular defects, and their eyes were in a healthy condition. The most important factor, however, is the physiological one that the children were older, and their eyes better able to withstand the strain of their school work—a fact teaching, the very important lesson that the tender tissues of early childhood are relatively more liable to disease as the result of eye-strain, and that, therefore, we send our children to school at too tender an age.

I have been careful to urge the important relation which is shown by these statistics to exist between the congenital defects of the organ of vision and the harm which results during the school life, for the reason that I am convinced that any system of hygiene devised to prevent the increase of disease, which finds its expression simply in the increasing percentage of near-sight, will fail of its purpose if it does not take this primary fact into consideration. The existence of these congenital defects should emphasize the importance of attention to every detail of school hygiene, for it is even more important for weak than for strong eyes. Too much care cannot be bestowed upon it in our endeavor to secure sufficient light, appropriate seats and desks, and text books printed with clear type of suitable size, properly spaced, on good paper, etc. ; but we must understand that the utmost attention to these important details, directed by the widest experience and highest skill, will not save from injury the eye which enters upon the educational struggle hampered by an anatomical defect. We have already seen with what unerring certainty they sooner or later are forced into the category of asthenopic eyes,

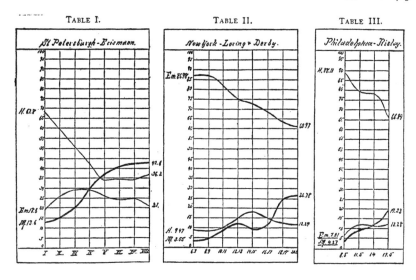

TABLE I.

TABLE II.

TABLE III.

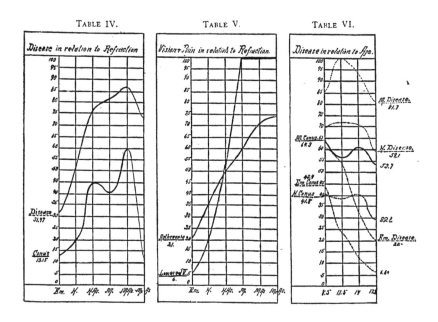

TABLE IV.

TABLE V.

TABLE VI.

In the presence of the facts revealed by these statistics, we are brought face to face with a problem of much greater complexity than we had at first anticipated. Starting, as we had supposed, to grapple with the hygiene of the schoolroom, we discover ourselves in conflict with a much broader question; one indeed involving not only a profound physiological problem, but also the problem of our readjustment to the requirements of an advancing civilization. In view of the facts which have been set forth, the conclusion is inevitable that our educational methods are not solely responsible for the resulting harm to the vision of our children. However faulty these methods may be, when viewed from the standpoint of the ophthalmic surgeon the resulting injury is primarily due to the faulty construction of the eyes of a large number of the pupils committed to the care of the schools. The task before us is, therefore, not only to devise a faultless system of instruction, under hygienic surroundings as favorable as possible, but also to provide for some simple and systematic method of examination which shall determine the visual fitness of the child to enter upon the tasks which must be imposed. I am not unmindful of the possible objections which may be urged to this suggestion, but our educators would at least have performed an obvious duty to the child with faulty vision by apprising the parents of the fact, and advising that the eyes be subjected to scientific scrutiny and professional advice. One of the first duties of science is to aid in the physical adjustment of the race to the ever-increasing complexity of our modes of life. This is particularly the function of the science of hygiene, to which this Convention is devoted. With every forward movement existing relations are disturbed and a new adjustment must be made, or the individual is ground under the wheels of the advancing car. In this country great changes in the customs and ambitions of the people have been wrought in a single century. The simplicity characterizing the mode of living which prevailed with the majority a hundred years ago, has given place to greater complexity. We look with justifiable pride upon our increase of wealth and the multiplication and expansion of our educational facilities, regarding them, quite properly, as evidence of national growth and prosperity, but we are too often unmindful of the sacrifice at which we purchase many of our best gifts. While we have in this advance secured untold luxuries, and great gratification of our ambitions, many serious difficulties have been introduced; dangers which we had not anticipated, perils unknown to our fathers. In order that we may enjoy the greatest benefit, and avoid the perils of our civilization, a wise readjustment to the new order of things is required, and in no other direction is there greater need for this, than in meeting the educational requirements of our time. The rapid increase of knowledge and its ready diffusion makes of reading the almost universal pastime. For from ten to fifteen years, many hours daily, our children are confined to their work at school, and when the school tasks are accomplished for the day, they turn to books and magazines published for their especial entertainment. Given the large percentage of congenitally defective eyes, and this almost constant demand upon the organ of vision, and we have the factors which give a sufficient answer to the inquiry which we so constantly hear ! What is wrong with our children's eyes ?   Why, we shall soon have them all in spectacles !

Briefly stated, it is but one of the numerous ways in which we are endeavoring to adjust ourselves to the new requirements.   We insist upon acquiring an education and becoming a nation of readers.   We are not models of physical perfection.   Our eyes are unfortunately equally liable with other parts of the body to anatomical distortion, and the glasses, or '' aids to read,'' are the crutches upon which we proceed.   With many individuals the existence of these visual defects makes necessary a choice between no progress, painful and injured eyes, or glasses which are designed to correct the optical defects which result from these departures from the anatomical standard of the perfect eye.

The preceding statistics have demonstrated that the normal eye bears the strain of its duties quite as well as do the other organs of the body, the increased and unnatural strain to which they are subjected ; but that when handicapped by some defect, are unable to keep abreast of more fortunate competitors, unless some artificial aid is supplied.   In a word, when the demands of life more nearly approach a state of nature, even defective eyes are sufficient for the moderate demands made upon them, but under the more severe requirements of a highly-cultivated community, the imposed strain is well borne only by the organ which approximates the ideally perfect eye.   It becomes our plain duty, therefore, as sanitarians, not only to secure the best possible conditions under which the work of the schools is to be performed, but also to stand guard over those pupils who start out, ignorantly, with eyes unfitted by nature for their important task.

The question which naturally presents itself is, how are the defective eyes to be detected?   The problem is not a difficult one, provided only that the coöperation of the proper authorities can be secured.   The necessary appliances are few, inexpensive and very simple, and can be employed by the teacher at the beginning of each term or school year.   But little skill and only a brief expenditure of time are necessary.   All the apparatus required is a table of suitably graduated test-letters, a card containing words or letters printed in clear type of a standard size, and a yard-stick or measuring tape. Instructions for their use could be printed on the back of the card of test-letters.   By these simple means the sharpness of sight for each eye could be rapidly determined for each pupil.   The facts should be carefully recorded in a properly ruled book, which, if carefully preserved, would enable the proper authorities to trace the visual history of each pupil throughout his career in the public schools, and would thus become of great scientific value.   Time does not permit me to do more than suggest the possible value of such a record in tracing the results of educational methods and various phases of school hygiene. The principle underlying the examination is very simple, and may be stated briefly as follows :   The standard eye is in a condition of health, able to distinguish objects which subtend a certain angle. Experience has shown that certain letters of the alphabet are the best test objects, but only a few of them are admissible as fulfilling the required conditions. To be distinguished, the entire letter must subtend an angle of at least five minutes, while the composing elements of the letter must subtend an angle of one minute.

Hence, in order to determine the acuity of vision it is necessary only to require the pupil to name these standard letters when placed at the proper distance from the eyes. For example : The test-letter card usually employed has upon it letters which the normal eye can see at distances varying from two or three metres to sixty metres. The large letter marked lx should be as easily distinguished at sixty metres as the line of letters marked V at five metres. The letter chart being placed in a good diffused light, the pupil should be placed six metres, approximately twenty feet, from it, and required to name the smallest letters which can be called correctly, with each eye separately. In recording the results of the examination the distance, six metres, should be used as the numerator of a fraction and the line of letters he is able to read as the denominator. Thus, number vi, is called correctly, V=6-vi. Number xxx is seen V=6-xxx. Number ix only is called correctly, V=6-ix, etc. Or it may be recorded as 1-i, 1-5 and 1-10, of the normal acuity of sight. I submit herewith a blank form as a suggestion for the ruling of the record book of such examinations. Any pupil whose acuity of vision fell much below the standard for sharpness should be admitted to the class only after the parents had been apprised of the existing defect. Vision of 6-ix, or 6-xii, is almost certain to prove a disturbing factor in the career of the pupil.

Name of School,...Section,.......................

No.............Name,..............................Age, ...Sex,................

Complexion,.............Color of Hair,....................of Eyes,...................

Condition of Health,...

Condition of Eyes,..

Vision,....................O. D.,.......................O. S.,.......................

Astigmatism,............O. D. lines at....................O. S. lines at................

Accommodation,..............p. p. O. D.,.......................O. S.,..................

Muscular Anomalies,...

Color Perception,..

Ophthalmoscopic Examination,...

One practical objection to the method suggested is the inability of the very young children seeking to enter the primary classes to call the letters, because of their ignorance of the alphabet. I am unable to suggest any other form of test object which at the same time meets the scientific requirements of a proper test. In such cases the examination could be deferred until the alphabet is learned. I had hoped that this would not prove an obstacle in the case of many children, but a brief inquiry of a few teachers in the primary schools elicited the somewhat surprising information that it was a rare exception to find a child who was familiar with the alphabet on first entering the primary department of our schools.

Arsenic in Wall Paper.*

BY F. C. ROBINSON,

Member of the State Board of Health, of Maine ; Professor of Chemistry, Bowdoin College.

It is now many years since the attention of physicians and chemists, and through them of the public generally, was called to the fact that arsenic was largely used in the manufacture of wall paper, and that numerous cases of dangerous, if not fatal, poisoning had resulted therefrom. These statements were at first denied by dealers and manufacturers of room papers. They could not deny that arsenic was present in such papers, especially in the green colored samples, but they denied most strenuously that poisoning could result therefrom unless the paper was actually taken into the mouth. Doubtless they were sincere in their denials, but it was another case of believing easily what one wants to. At this late day all doubt is removed, especially as concerning those old Paris-green papers, and they are rarely seen in the wall papers now sold. Case after case of their evil influence has been most positively identified, not only by the well-known symptoms of arsenical poisoning developed in persons occupying such papered rooms, but the arsenic has been actually obtained from their urine, and to make the chain of evidence complete both the symptoms and the arsenic have disappeared upon removing the patient or the paper from the room.

It is thus of no use for any one to contend that the use of arsenic in making wall papers is not a source of danger ; and the practical question for us here in Maine to-day is, what is our condition with reference to the matter? One thing is certain, however, and that is that even if poisonous papers are sold within our borders we have at present no redress. It is not at all against the law. We may be "ground down" by the "sumptuary law" which forbids a man from selling us rum to poison us or our children, as some think we are, but one may with impunity sell us paper loaded with Paris green, which will more surely destroy the health or lives of ourselves or children. No officer can say him nay. But are such papers being actually sold in Maine to-day, and, if so, how can we recognize and avoid them? It was to answer, and, if possible, settle this question that I began investigating the matter the present Winter, at the instance of the State Board of Health. The investigation is not yet completed to my satisfaction, and so this report is only a preliminary one. It seemed best, however, to state at this time the results already found, and the general condition of the subject, and to continue the matter in some future publication. It is hoped, too, that the spreading of the fact that such work is being done will serve to call the attention of physicians and others to the matter, and bring in cases and samples of papers which could not otherwise be obtained. And I take this opportunity to invite the co-operation of all in this most important matter to the health of the State.

* Abstracted from the Annual Report of the Maine State Board of Health.

My first work was to collect samples from different quarters of the State, and by the aid of the local health boards in Bangor, Calais, Portland and Brunswick, I soon received several hundred samples, obtained from the dealers in those cities. And I wish to say here that I found a ready wish expressed by all dealers I came in cantact with to give all aid in their power to my investigation. Of course, examination of such samples would not represent the actual condition of rooms in Maine, for they were taken from the new stock of the dealers, but by this time many of them are probably on rooms, and their examination will tend to answer one part of the question, at least, and a very important one, as to the character of the papers being now offered for sale in the State. Upwards of one hundred of these samples have now been examined for arsenic, and it is gratifying to be able to state that the vast majority of these are free from the poison or contain but the merest trace. In fact, but three only have been found which are unmistakably dangerous. But while this number is so gratifyingly small, one of them is so typical of what has been sold so largely in the past, and so dangerous in its nature, that if my investigation had succeeded only in finding it I should have regarded it as a most profitable work. It happens, too, that the paper in question was not simply obtained in sample from a dealer, but was used upon two rooms within my knowledge, and in one case caused the serious illness of children occupying the room. I am glad to say, however, that it was not a paper made in this country but imported from England ; being too poisonous for sale there it was sent like a "forced emigrant" to do its deadly work upon our shores. It was a landscape paper, made for pleasing children, representing a scene in the grape region, and the bright green grape vines and purple clusters of grapes and gay-colored clothes of the workers made truly a pleasing sight.

Temperance people will perhaps regard it as very appropriate that such scenes should be represented in poisonous pigments. The arsenic is not confined to the green parts but exists largely also in the purple, blue and drab tints. The paper contains on the average, as nearly as it can be got, 125 grains of pure arsenic, equivalent to 168 grains of arsenious acid, in every square yard. When we remember that two grains of arsenic may be regarded as a fatal dose, the astounding fact comes out that every square yard of this paper contains arsenic enough to kill seventy-five men. The bright green color is Paris-green, the blue probably London-purple, and the other shades only a little less in their amount of arsenic. But is it not harmless when securely fastened to the wall? Paint does not escape when once dried to the woodwork of a room, and how can the colors from a paper? The apparent analogy is not a real one. Paint contains oil which hardens and holds firmly any color, however poisonous. It would probably be perfectly safe to sleep in a room painted with an oil paint containing as much Paris-green as this paper. Wall paper contains no such protector. Its colors are loosely held, as every one knows. Rub your hand over most any wall paper and behold how the colors rub off ! Every disturbance or jarring of the room by walking, sweeping, or in other ways, sends into the air of it particles of these colors from the paper. From one of the rooms papered with this sample I secured a small portion of dust from under the carpet and the presence of arsenic was very manifest in it by the chemical test. It has been proved, too, that arsenic escapes from a wall paper in other ways than as dust. Some one or more of its many gaseous compounds, all very poisonous, is undoubtedly formed, especially if the room be damp so that the paste tends to mold. Now, it is well known that arsenic is not a poison which accumulates in the system as lead does. It is constantly being eliminated, especially through the kidneys. But yet if one be exposed to small doses of arsenic taken very frequently, the system becomes gradually undermined and death may result. It is well known, too, that a weakened body is more liable to contract disease than a strong one. So one weakened by arsenic may contract and die of other disease, and the agency of the arsenic never be suspected.

There is an impression among dealers and paperers that an arsenical paper can be told at a glance. While getting samples of paper for analysis, dealers informed me that they now sold no arsenical green papers, and seemed to think it strange that I should think of finding arsenic in those of any other color. But it is a well-known fact to physicians and chemists, who have had to do with such things, that the color of a paper is no guide to its character. It happened that the papers colored by Paris green were those which first caught the attention of physicians as sources of poisoning to their patients, and so the notion arose that such only were dangerous. But in every report upon the subject, in recent years at least, it has been made very clear that almost any colored paper may contain arsenic in dangerous amount. Dr. E. S. Wood, in his elaborate report on the subject, contained in the Report of the State Board of Health of Massachusetts for 1883, says : " There is absolutely nothing in the appearance of a paper by which we can form any opinion as to its arsenical or non-arsenical nature." Again, in the more recent report of D. H. Galloway to the American Pharmaceutical Association in 1889, after having examined more than 100 samples, we find the statement : " I am now convinced that it is impossible to say before examination whether a given sample contains arsenic or not." My own experience would confirm these statements in general, and yet I think I observe that the darker colored papers are the greatest sinners in this respect. It may have been simply accidental, but I found no arsenic in any of the light colored papers yet examined. One cannot help noticing, too, that the samples of arsenical paper pasted into the report of Dr. Wood, referred to above, are all dark with perhaps two exceptions. For many years past dark papers were " all the fashion," as we know, but now the light colors prevail, at least the large majority of the samples I got were light. I at first thought that my results indicated that the agitation of the matter by physicians and health boards had at last exerted that wholesome restraining action upon the manufacturers and dealers which is so desirable. I am more inclined now to think that such is not the case ; and to believe that, unless there be more positive restraint, when fashion next calls for the darker colored papers we shall see a return to the arsenical colors of preceding years.

Of course, this is not the proper place to speak minutely of the symptoms of poisoning by arsenic. Physicians will turn to their medical books and journals for detailed accounts of such. But it seems to me desirable that a few words should be said here upon the subject for the benefit of the non-professional reader especially. In the first place, it should be said that poisoning by inhaling arsenic from wall paper is rarely like, in its symptoms, that from a fatal dose taken at a given time. In this respect arsenic is like other powerful drugs ; repeated small doses of any of them differ in their effect from single large doses. We think of arsenic poisoning as accompanied by great pain and suffering ; the stomach seems burning up and nature tends to relieve herself of the destructive principle by violent vomiting and purging. Not only the physician, but everyone else knows, that something out of the ordinary course is the matter with the patient, and antidotes and the stomach-pump are at once called into service. But let the same amount of arsenic be gradually given, and no such marked and extraordinary symptoms appear. Indeed, it seems to depend upon the age and general constitution of the person as to what the symptoms will be. The difficulty in formulating any typical set of symptoms for such slow poisoning has, in the past, undoubtedly prevented its recognition even by physicians, and even to-day there seems to be no general agreement in the matter. The cases cited in Vol. CXX, Nos. 10 and 11 of the *Boston Medical and Surgical Journal* show how varied may be the symptoms in undoubted cases of slow arsenical poisoning. Some points, however, seem to be very clearly established by those and other cases, and these may well be borne in mind even by those not physicians, and the appearance of such symptoms without other apparent cause lead to a careful inspection of the wall paper in rooms inhabited by those exhibiting them. Nervous depression, with irritability and sleeplessness, derangement of the stomach, soreness of the muscles, are some of the more general symptoms observed. In addition, examination invariably shows that the kidneys are affected, albumen and even casts and blood being voided in the urine, not infrequently. In such cases, too, arsenic is always found in the urine, it being the channel by which it is most rapidly eliminated from the system.

In the case under my immediate knowledge, where the two children were affected by the landscape paper, they seemed to lose flesh, grew very pale and had occasional attacks of what seemed to be bilious sick headache They were also troubled with what they called "bad dreams," and one of them not infrequently would come into his parents' room, in the middle of the night, and say that he couldn't sleep. Their urine, unfortunately, was not examined. The children were seven and five years old. A younger child, who occasionally slept in the room, and frequently played there, grew very pale, and had a kind of "cold sore," as it was called, on his upper lip, which refused to heal for a long time, but which grew better rapidly as soon as the room was re-papered. The mother of these children, who used the room as a sewing-room at times, complained of an unaccountable feeling of depression, and was troubled consider ably by sleeplessness. There is no reasonable doubt in my mind but what one or both of these children would have been fatally poisoned if they had not been removed from that room and its objectionable paper taken off. One of the most surprising results, too, of the more recent investigations of this subject is the small amount of arsenic which seems to act deleteriously when contained in a paper. In the samples given by Dr. Wood, in 1883, all but three contained more than one grain per square yard, and those three very nearly a grain. He intimates, too, in the description of his manner of testing, that amounts much smaller than that would be too small to be considered as dangerous, but in the articles referred to in the *Boston Medical and Surgical Journal* we find a case of poisoning referred to papers containing in round numbers one-thirtieth, one-third and one-half grains per square yard respectively. And in the report of the American Pharmaceutical Society an amount equivalent to about one-seventy-fifth of a grain per square yard is thought worthy of publication as more than a trace. I must confess, too, that some of the results of such paper seem to me most surprising.

Patients exposed to it seem to be passing enough arsenic in their urine to indicate that all the arsenic contained in the paper of a whole room would be eliminated by a single person in not an excessively long time. But however apparently anomalous these results may seem, I am inclined to regard them as anomalies of analysis or figuring rather than anything else, and to believe that even small fractions of a grain of arsenic per square yard may exert a bad influence upon the health of occupants of a room, and I am perfectly convinced that the only safe way is to demand that no arsenic beyond a mere trace be allowed in the papers which are to cover our walls. Many foreign countries have laws to this effect, and it is time that the States of our Union took action in the same direction. There was no difficulty in passing a law in Maine to prevent the use of comparatively harmless glucose in our molasses, or of oleo in our butter, but the danger to our health in the use of arsenical wall paper is far greater than from either of these.

As I said at the beginning of this paper, I regard this report as only preliminary. I intend to make many more examinations in the year to come, and hope to include not only wall papers but other colored papers and articles of clothing as well, and hope for the co-operation of all interested in sending me facts and samples.

It may be of interest to state briefly my method of analysis, for although not new in principle, it is somewhat different in construction from that commonly used, and with it I am able to make more tests in a given time than in the common way, and I think with increased accuracy. I use the Marsh test, but instead of using zinc and acid, use a current of electricity from the electric light station in the town. The poles are platinum plates inserted in a U tube containing pure dilute sulphuric acid. The hydrogen is conducted through proper drying tubes and the arsenic deposited as usual. I insert the paper directly into the acid. All impurities in the zinc are thus avoided; antimony, if present, is kept back, and the gas stream is perfectly constant. The acid soon gets hot and the temperature can be kept at any desired point by surrounding the tube with water. By allowing it to be quite hot, the solution of the coloring matters is much facilitated. Of course, if the electricity had to be generated by a battery, it would be far more expensive and troublesome.

Mastication and Physical Development.

Dr. E. A. Wood, of Pittsburgh, who is an authority whose words must always command respectful consideration, thinks that we do not commence to give our children food that requires chewing early enough in life. As a result of want of use, the jaws imperfectly develop ; the arch is narrow and the teeth are crowded and irregular. Nature does not reduce the number of teeth, but she attempts to force thirty-two teeth into jaws that have only room for twenty-four, and the quality of the teeth is not up to the standard, so that they readily commence to decay. When the child has grown up it is too late to prevent the mischief. The decay of teeth is more due to insufficient nourishment than to injury or defect of the enamel.

The rational means of preventing the state of affairs just referred to is to commence early and give the child food that requires mastication. The result will be increased function of the gums, teeth and salivary glands, and of the masticatory muscles, and the full development of the lower part of the face, with a corresponding improvement in the appearance of the man. In the average family the questions of diet are relegated to the cook, whose study seems to be to provide food which is so soft as not to require to be chewed, and is accompanied by large quantities of coffee, or tea, or ice-water, which takes the place of the salivary secretions. The evil effects of this system of feeding can be seen on every hand. The remedy suggests itself.

Mastication is the most important step ; by it the food is reduced to a pulp and is thoroughly incorporated with saliva. The act of chewing also stimulates the flow of the gastric juice, and is necessary to perfect stomach digestion. General health of the body intimately depends upon digestion and assimilation of sufficient food of proper character, but no matter how a man regulates his diet he cannot overcome the evils of his early training in this direction. Just here we are confronted with a danger which strikes at the very life-blood of the nation, and is already sapping its strength.

If the proper care be observed in rearing children and giving them sound, wholesome food requiring the use of their masticatory muscles, there is no reason why a superior race of man might not be developed, just as we raise the fastest horses and the finest cattle in the world. The appeal is made to physicians especially, to see that the glorious birthright of the American citizen is not bartered away for a mess of pottage or other soft food.

By pursuing the plan adopted by the ancient Greeks, we might not only equal their achievements, but even surpass them in physical development and personal beauty.

THE ANNALS of HYGIENE, ❖ ❖

THE OFFICIAL ORGAN OF THE

State Board of Health of Pennsylvania.

The State Board of Health is not responsible for anything appearing in this Journal except that which bears the official attestation of the Board.

PUBLISHED MONTHLY.   Subscription, two dollars ($2.00) a year, in advance.

Address all communications to

The Hygienic Publishing Company,

224 SOUTH SIXTEENTH STREET,

PHILADELPHIA, PA.

EDITORIAL.

Pure Milk—Practical Sanitation.

Preaching is all very well in its way, but, if one who preaches doctrines of reform can offer to his hearers a means of putting these doctrines into practical use, a great step forward has been taken. If we can "practice what we preach," we are certainly practical reformers. We have, time and time again, impressed upon our readers the importance of pure milk. The public is now fully alive to the fact that they ought to have such milk, but they are also well aware that it is, comparatively speaking, impossible to procure it. We assume three facts :

1. The people want pure milk.
2. It is very difficult to procure such, and
3. If it could be had, the people would like to have it.

Well then, for our practical sanitation. If the people really want pure, unwatered, unsophisticated milk; if they want milk delivered to them just as it comes from good cows, properly fed and carefully tended; if they want such, they can have it. How? By asking for it. Whenever we feel that a dogma has been established in hygiene, we look about us for a practical way of utilizing such knowledge for the benefit of the people. We have been thinking a great deal about this question of a pure and wholesome milk supply, and we have solved the problem. We can give to anyone, who so desires, the facility for obtaining *truly pure milk*. But, possibly, you do not care for it. It not infrequently happens that the people raise a great outcry against an existing evil, but when a remedy is suggested they seem to care not to avail themselves of it. If such be the case with this milk question, then, of course, we have nothing further to say ; but if the people of this city (we cannot help those outside of Philadelphia, save by advice) really want pure milk, and if they want it badly enough to warrant them in dropping us a postal card asking for the information, we can tell them how they can have it delivered to their homes. We mean just what we say, staking our reputation on the purity of the article which they will receive, and we invite correspondence on the subject. Remember this applies only to those of our readers who are residents of this city.

The Hot Water Cure.

We have been asked what we think of "The Hot Water Cure." Replying, we would say, in the first place that we have no respect for any "CURE," so to speak ; that is to say, we can only condemn all particular, specific, set cures for all diseases. When the public speaks of a *cure* or a *treatment*, be it the *hot water* or the *cold water* or the *tepid water*, or the *climatic*, or any of the so-called hundreds of *cures* or treatments, we take it that they are speaking of, or have in their minds, a certain definite, particular course or routine, which is supposed to be applicable to all sexes, ages, conditions and diseases ; to be a panacea, as it were ; to be a means of relieving all the ills of humanity. With such an understanding of a *treatment* or a *cure*, we say again, we condemn them all, individually and collectively. The " Hot Water Cure" will not cure truly diseased conditions, neither will any other *treatment*. As panaceas, they are all conspicuous failures ; as adjuvants to *nature*, they are all, at the appropriate time, most glorious successes. Nature, and nature alone, can heal the disordered human frame. There are a very few diseases known to the physician in which particular drugs *seem* to have a curative effect, and these instances seem to contradict the assertion we have made, but, to one who thinks deeply, this will prove to be only a *seeming* contradiction, and our proposition that Dr. Nature is the only doctor who cures will be accepted as an axiom. Of course, nature can be assisted ; no one questions this, and all of these *cures* or *treatments* may, and oftentimes do, help greatly to aid the efforts of nature. As such, they are good ; as *cure-alls*, they are bad. A famous old atheist once said to us in conversation, " There is no such thing as evil, all things and everything is good ; some less good than others, but nothing and no one is evil." Something after this fashion might we reason about these cures ; there is some good in all of them. The drinking of hot water and eating of rare beefsteaks, while it will not cure, of itself, alone and unaided, a diseased condition of the body, is yet a harmless process, calculated to do good, unless indulged in by one whose complaint interdicts the use of large quantities of beef. So is it with all such cures. Of the " Hot Water Cure," as of all *cures* wherein drugs are not used, we can say they are harmless, as a rule, and since those who resort to them generally have great faith and confidence in their efficacy, they will, in many cases, do good, because *faith*, in the majority of cases, is, after all, the great restorer. To be more plain, the majority of those who consider themselves sick are not so ; that is to say, probably ninety out of every hundred who seek advice or treatment do not really require such. However, they think that they do. If, then, they think themselves deranged, and if, at the same time, they really think that a certain *treatment* will benefit them, it generally transpires that the expected benefit is derived therefrom. But with the remaining ten, who are truly deranged, no particular *cure* or *treatment* can be safely recommended. In these cases, those who are capable of being cured will be so only by an intelligent use and application of all the aids to nature in her work with which an intelligent, well-read and educated physician is familiar.

Delinquent Subscribers.

As a rule, our subscribers have always promptly responded to our notices of " Subscription due," and have thus materially helped to lighten our labors in building up this journal. But we have a few persons on our list who per-

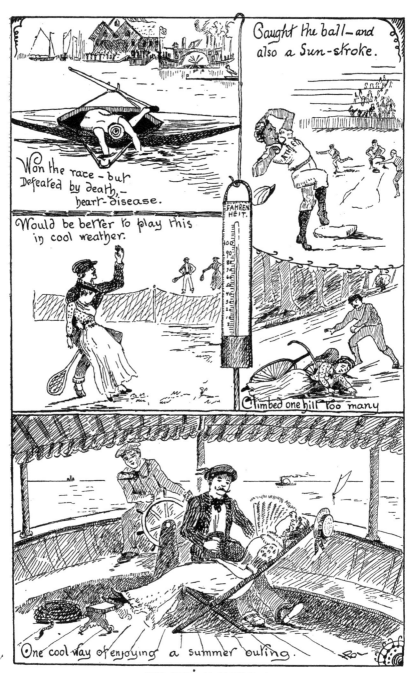

KEEP COOL IN HOT WEATHER.

sistently ignore all of our communications in reference to their indebtedness. They have received the journal, but refuse to pay for it, notwithstanding the fact that we have their written orders to send it. For the information of such we publish the following extract from a Western paper, which will enlighten them as to the law on the subject, and show them how *they* stand :

"For violating civil service law. Didn't pay for their newspapers. Cheerful news for newspaper proprietors comes from Ohio. A paper in that State recently brought suit against forty-three men who would not pay their subscription, and obtained judgment for the full amount in each case. Twenty-eight at once prevented attachment by making affidavit that they had no more than the law allowed. Under the decision of the Supreme Court they were arrested for petty larceny, and bound over in the sum of $300. Six of the defendants refused to give the necessary bonds to pay their respective arrearages, and were promptly sent to jail. This is the result of the new postal law, which declares "it to be larceny to take a paper, magazine or periodical out of the post office, and then refuse to pay for it."—*Intelligencer.*

Outdoor and Indoor Light.

The importance of light on health has never been so fully recognized as it is now. The popular conception of the degree or intensity of light is, however, very inaccurate. Most persons would say that the outside light is two or three times as strong as that within our houses. But the ratio of difference is vastly greater. Patients strolling on the seashore in sunny weather are in a light not two or three times, but 18,000 times stronger than that in the ordinary shaded and curtained rooms of a city house, and the same patients walking along the sunny side of a street are receiving more than 5,000 times as much of the health-giving influence of light as they would receive indoors in the usually heavily curtained room.

A Census of Hallucinations.

Professor William James, of Harvard University, Cambridge, Mass., requests answers from everybody to the following question : " Have you ever, when completely awake, had a vivid impression of seeing or being touched by a living being or inanimate object, or of hearing a voice ; which impression, so far as you could discover, was not due to any external physical cause?" The object of the inquiry is two-fold : 1st, to get a mass of facts about hallucinations which may serve as a basis for a scientific study of these phenomena ; and, 2d, to ascertain approximately the proportion of persons who have had such experiences. Professor James was appointed by the International Congress of Experimental Psychology, held in Paris in the Summer of 1889, to superintend this " census of hallucinations " in America, and he asks for the co-operation of all physicians who may be actively interested in the subject. It is clear that very many volunteer canvassers will be needed to secure success. Each census blank contains instructions to the collector, and places for twenty-five names, and special blanks for the " Yes " cases are furnished in addition. Professor James will supply these blanks to any one who will make application to him for them.

NOTES AND COMMENTS.

Crime vs. Hygiene.

Physicians are beginning to declare that a large amount of the crime for which punishment is inflicted is due to insanity, and that insanity is due to low physical condition, which sanitation by early physical training would remove.

The Luxury of Chamois Sheets.

Chamois sheets as soft and fine as kid are a healthy luxury indulged in by the robust as well as the invalid traveler. These are much affected by the tourists abroad, who find them a sure protection against the ills of flesh that so certainly result from sleeping in damp linen.

An Electric Flatiron.

One of the latest novelties in electricity is an electric flatiron. It consists of a hollow flatiron, in the interior of which a coil is placed, which is heated by the current passing through it. The ease and comfort derived from the use of such device, in hot weather especially, is apparent.

Earache.

Take five parts of camphorated chloral, thirty parts of glycerine and ten parts of the oil of sweet almonds. A piece of cotton is saturated and introduced well into the ear, and it is also rubbed behind the ear. The pain is relieved as if by magic, and, if there is inflammation, it often subsides quickly.

A Remedy for Tender Feet.

A remedy for tender feet is cold water—about two quarts, two tablespoonfuls of ammonia, one tablespoonful of bay rum. Sit with the feet immersed for ten minutes, gently throwing the water over the limbs upward to the knee. Then rub dry with a crash towel, and all the tired feeling is gone. This is good for a sponge bath also.

Doctored Cocoanut.

It is said there is considerable cocoanut on the market which has had more or less starch added to it. The *Grocers and Canners' Gazette* says : "Buyers will find in iodine a good detector of outside substances. Iodine will turn black any prepared cocoanut in which starch or other farinaceous substances may have been used."

A Sanitary Organization of Women.

The women of Brooklyn have united to form a Ladies' Health Protective Association, similar to the one which has for years been so useful in New York City. The lines of its work will be in the direction of such nuisances as offensive pursuits, uncared-for tenement houses, and filthy streets. The wives of physicians form a considerable proportion of the organization.

Stand Straight.

Children should be taught to stand straight, to hold up the head, with the chin down, to throw the shoulders back, and to stand on both feet; not bear all the weight of the body on one. It is excellent practice for any one to walk with a good-sized book on the head, and children are benefited by practicing it every day, gradually increasing the weight.

Cosmetics.

The president of the Chicago Board of Pharmacy asserts that the women of America spend about $62,000,000 a year for cosmetics, most of which are made of zinc oxide, calomel, water, glycerine and perfumes. This is a pretty big item for the satisfaction of artificial good looks, but it is probably small in comparison to what men spend for alcoholic poisons and tobacco smoke.

The Wise Physician.

"An Irish physician was called to see an Irish woman, and prescribed no medicine. The woman objected, and when he asked for his fee she answered, "Be jabbers, and for phwat?" His quick reply was, "Faith, and for the talk I gin ye." Were all the physicians as wise, the people would understand the doctor was worth his fee, irrespective of such medicine as he might order.

How to make a Mustard Plaster.

L. H. Cartledge (in *Medical Brief*) says: Take a thin cloth twice as long as you want your plaster. On half of it spread a thick *hot* paste made of flour. On the paste sprinkle a heaping teaspoonful of mustard to *four inches square* of the cloth. Fold the other end of the cloth over the mustard and sprinkle with warm water. Apply warm, and you have a plaster that is clean and will burn like "blue blazes."

Physicians Arrested.

Scarlet fever and diphtheria are very prevalent in the town of Highlands, near Denver, Col., and the citizens are becoming almost panic-stricken. Among other measures taken to improve the health of the community and to prevent further spread of contagion, warrants have been issued for the arrest of a number of physicians who have failed to report cases of diphtheria and scarlet fever occurring in their practice.

A Cure for Dandruff.

Dr. A. J. Harrison, Bristol, England, recommends the following :

> Caustic potash, 8 grains ;
> Phenic acid, 24 grains ;
> Lanolin ;
> Cocoanut oil, āā ℥iv. M.

This preparation should be rubbed into the scalp morning and evening. Complete cure is usually effected in one to three months.

Slept in a Coffin.

A Racine, Wis., undertaker recently made an unusual discovery when he opened his place of business. A burglar had gained entrance by breaking through a rear window. Finding nothing of value to carry away, the thief built a warm fire in the stove, moved a coffin up and then got into it and slept all night. The trimmings and sides of the interior of the coffin were smeared with blood, showing that the culprit had cut himself.

Transmission of Typhoid Fever by the Fingers.

The general public have a somewhat vague idea that typhoid fever is always caused by bad drinking water, yet we have so high an authority as Dr. Roberts Bartholow for believing that the nurse of one sick may carry the germs under the finger nail, from which they may be transmitted to the food of another, thus causing the disease, which tends to argue in favor of *disinfectant* cleanliness on the part of all those who come into contact with the sick.

Hot Water for Children.

Hot water is highly useful in the digestive disorders of children. A child will live for several days with nothing else to eat, and be in much better condition than with a demoralized digestive tract. On hot water it will live comfortably, and scarcely seem to miss the mother's milk. With a colicky baby the hot water frequently acts as an anodyne, putting it to sleep. If it seems distressed after nursing, the hot water relieves the pain, even if it be caused by an over-filled stomach.

Malaria on the Line of the Caucasian Railway in 1889.

A very grave form of malarial fever prevails along the line of the Caucasian Railway. It is often the case that every employé at the stations is attacked by it. Quinine is inefficacious. In 1888 there were 66,965 persons taken ill along the line of railway, and of these 41,069 were cases of malarial fever. In the Summer and Autumn the quotidian typhoid form and irregular intermittent fevers prevailed ; at the close of the Autumn and during the Winter, tertian and quarternian fevers.

Fruit at Meals.

As a rule, a fruit dessert in the evening and after a mixed meal ought only to be lightly indulged in, for the average stomach will but rarely tolerate a heavy influx of such cold and usually watery aliment as fruit. This is not the case if the fruit is eaten before or between the meal courses. A ripe melon eaten with salt or butter, before or immediately after the soup, can be freely indulged in. Experience teaches us that stewed or raw fruit may be largely taken between the courses. In many parts of the Continent this custom prevails ; the Germans eat stewed fruit with many meats, and in warmer climes such fruits as grapes, plums, figs, melons and sweet lemons are habitually eaten with all kinds of dishes or as palate refreshers between the courses.

The Plague in Persia.

The plague has appeared in Persia at the village of Kalé-Darapéhan, eight hours' travel from Kermanshah. A dispatch received from the Ottoman sanitary representative at Kermanshah under date of June 14th, gives the population of Kalè-Darapéhan at 280 inhabitants. Up to the date named, 42 cases of plague have been reported, Of these 26 were fatal. The symptomotolgy was as follows : Engorgement of the inguinal and axillary ganglions, temperature 40°, anthrax, and a bluish eruption on the skin.

For Tired People.

Beat two or more eggs, the whites and yolks separately, add a little sugar, and, if you wish, crumb crackers into the dish and eat it. This will often agree with the stomach when it rejects other food. It is easily assimilated, and can be taken without an appetite, without hindering the organs of digestion. Excessive mental or bodily fatigue renders the stomach incapable for the time of performing its office, and this simple dish will recuperate the strength until the person is rested enough to eat heartily.

Jack, the Ink Slinger.

A curious form of monomania has appeared in New York city recently. A quiet and apparently respectable married man developed a fondness for throwing ink on women's dresses, particularly on pretty dresses. He would follow his victim along the street, and when a favorable opportunity arrived throw the ink, which was concealed in a pipe, upon the dress. More than fifty cases of spoiled dresses were reported before the man was discovered. He was promptly condemned to six months in the penitentiary. He is a monomaniac.

The Only Rebel Hanged.

For more than a quarter of a century intelligent physicians have known that water contaminated with the stools of a typhoid fever patient would produce typhoid fever in those who drank it. A most horrible abuse of this knowledge was used to destroy the lives of Union prisoners during the war of the rebellion. Wurtz, an educated physician, arranged the prison-pen, at Andersonville, on the side of a hill ; a stream wound round the hill into the ravine below. He established the privies at the upper corner of this pen, near the river, where the soakage from these closets would run into the river, and compelled the men to get their water supply from the lower corner from this contaminated source. If any prisoner attempted to dig for fresh water, he was shot. The prison for the officers was in the ravine below, where the only water was this saturated from the privies. Wurtz's boast was that " he was killing more men at Andersonville than Lee at the front." Wurtz was the only person the Government hung after the close of the war.—*Dr. Johnson, in Brooklyn Medical Journal.*

La Grippe in India.

The *Indian Medical Gazette* says, the local names which this disease has acquired in its travels are almost as many as the countries visited. It is now prevalent in India. It first appeared in Bombay, and in Calcutta it is called the Bombay fever. Soldiers, artisans, clerks, police and prisoners have been attacked. The severe symptoms of pneumonia and capillary bronchitis which accompanied the disease in cold climates have been rare in India. Where relapses have occurred the disease has been alarming on account of the extreme debility following the attack.

Salt in Milk for Children.

Dr. A. Jacobi (*Arch. of Ped.*) says that the addition of sodium chloride prevents the solid coagulation of milk by either rennet or gastric juice. The cows' milk ought never to be given without table salt, and the latter ought to be added to a woman's milk when it behaves like cows' milk in regard to solid curdling and consequent indigestibility. Habitual constipation of children is influenced beneficially, since not only is the food made more digestible, but the alimentary secretions, both serous and glandular, are made more effective by its presence.

Juice That Won't Inebriate.

A valuable discovery, which may have an important bearing on the temperance cause, has, it is stated, been made by Dr. Jones, of Acton Hall, near Berkeley, England. It consists of a chemical process by which the juice of the apple and the juice of the grape can be manufactured into an extremely pleasant non-alcoholic beverage. Cider manufactured by this process can be kept for seven years without fermentation. But another invention of Dr. Jones' will be of more general benefit to the community. It is a method by which beef and mutton can be kept perfectly fresh for as long a period.

Max O'Rell's Coffee.

Max O'Rell, who is said to serve the best cup of coffee in London, learned how to make coffee when he was a soldier in Algeria, and this is his recipe : Take an ordinary saucepan (a small one) and pour into it as many cups of water as you require cups of coffee. Let the water boil, then put in as many table-spoonfuls of ground coffee as you have cups of water ; put in sugar to suit the taste at the same time. Wait until the coffee boils, then lift the saucepan from the fire and hold it till the bubbling subsides. Put it back on the fire until it bubbles again ; repeat this five times ; the fifth time let it remain on the fire a minute or so, when the " cream " (which seems a better word to use than froth or scum) will rise to the top ; then pour out the coffee and let it settle. Above all things, don't stir the coffee. There will be rather an unappetizing-looking sediment in the bottom of your cup when you have done with it, but if you succeed in this process as well as Max O'Rell does, you will have enjoyed a deliciously-fragrant cup of coffee before you see the sediment.

Leprosy Excluded at the Boston Quarantine.

The quarantine authorities at Boston Harbor have intercepted the importation of a case of leprosy in the person of a woman from Sweden. After the true nature of the disease had been clearly made out, the officials not only refused a permit to land, but required the Cunard Company to return the leper to her own country This was done on May 10th. It has now been learned that the diagnosis of leprosy was confirmed by the medical officials at Liverpool upon the arrival of the outcast at that port.

The Liqour Traffic and Native Races.

It is most gratifying to note that the King of the Belgians has given an audience to Dr. Hannay, of the Congregational Union, and Mr. John McKenzie, late assistant commissioner in Bechuanaland, on this subject, in which he expressed hearty sympathy with the views of those who protest against native races being demoralized and destroyed by the traffic in intoxicating drinks, and a confident hope that the conference would adopt some effective measures for the restriction of this traffic. If European nations are not strong enough to impose such restraints on their trade members in those distant regions, so much the more pity.

The Electric Railway as a Sanitary Measure.

The rapid extension of the electric street car system which has taken place (especially in this country) naturally leads to the question of the cause thereof. To have gained such pre-eminence it must be able to do not only what other systems can do, but, still more, it must be able to do it at a decreased cost. Again, removal of thousands of horses from the streets of a city, involving, as it does, the doing away with the noise and dirt, is another distinct gain to its residents. But if one goes still further, and contemplates the difference between a stable housing thousands of horses, and an electric car station of sufficient size to operate a road with the same efficiency, one is at once struck with the advantages on the side of the electric system, which, indeed, are incontrovertible. Instead of a large, ill-smelling building, whose odors are wafted for many blocks (making the tenancy of houses within half a mile almost unbearable, and involving a large depreciation of property in the neighborhood), there is a neat, substantial building, equipped with a steam plant and dynamos, and occupying hardly one-tenth the space required for an equivalent number of horses. Therefore, not only is there effected a removal of the nuisances attached to a stable, but a large saving in the cost of real estate, and the far greater amount involved in the known depreciation of the surrounding property. Besides this, the stables are of necessity required to be in close proximity to the track, whereas, the electric power station which furnishes current to the car, may be situated a mile from the track in some suitable place, as, for instance, beside a river, where, with condensing engines, power may be generated at a minimum of cost.—*Exchange.*

Cremation of Garbage.

Mr. L. T. Christian, an ardent and intelligent sanitarian of Richmond, Va., writes an earnest communication to *The Times*, of that city, urging upon the people the importance of erecting a furnace for the cremation of their garbage. We are anxious to heartily endorse Mr. Christian's efforts in this direction. In these days of sanitary enlightenment, the old, crude and dangerous methods of handling the garbage of cities must be regarded as a relic of barbarism.

American Climatological Association.

The annual meeting of the American Climatological Association will be held in Denver, September 2d to 4th, and a successful gathering is expected. The Western Passenger Traffic Association has granted a one fare for round trip rate; tickets to be bought August 31st and September 1st, and good for return till September 25th, which is open to others as well as members. One-third of the time is expected to be given exclusively to the study of Colorado subjects, and after three days' sessions the visiting physicians are to be given an opportunity personally to investigate the mountain resorts by a series of complimentary excursions.

Corrosive Sublimate Solutions.

We have occasion so frequently to recommend the use of a solution of corrosive sublimate to destroy the germs of disease, that it seems well to give some instructions for its preparation. To make a standard solution, from which the weaker solutions may be made, take four ounces of corrosive sublimate and one pound of sulphate of copper, and dissolve them in one gallon of water.

To make a solution of 1 to 500, add 8 ounces of the above to 1 gallon of water.
  " " " 1000 " 4 " " " "
  " " " 2000 " 2 " " " "

Remember that these solutions, while most effective in the destruction of disease germs, are, at the same time, highly poisonous.

Disinfection of Rooms in Boston.

The report of the Board of Health of Boston for last year, in speaking of the disinfection of rooms, says: "Our process in such cases, although not always insisted upon, is to close up the apartments to be disinfected, tightly, and to burn four pounds of sulphur to each 1000 cubic feet of space, evaporating water with the heat of the burning sulphur, and keeping the room closed for ten hours. In cases of smallpox this is all we ordinarily do; but in case of diphtheria, scarlet fever and typhoid fever, where the sputa or some other of the secretions may have become fixed and dried upon articles or surfaces in the room, and, moreover, where a stronger germicide is required for the spore-bearing germ which is likely to become so fixed, we rub the walls, floors, and other hard surfaces with a solution of bichloride of mercury—1 to 500—and boil one hour articles of clothing and bedding."

Kissing the Book.

The danger of kissing a greasy book, so often tendered in police and law courts to a witness about to be sworn, is at last appreciated by some officials and in some quarters. We see it stated that when the Duke of Fife appeared lately at Stratford in a prosecution, the Testament on which he took the oath was enveloped in some clean white paper for his use—a precaution which might with advantage be more generally adopted. Why should not the formula and method of taking the oath in English courts of justice be altered and adopted, possibly in imitation of the method adopted in Scotland, which is that of raising the hand in lieu of kissing the book?

How Diphtheria is Spread by Corpses.

In March, 1890, two corpses, woman and child of same family, dead of throat disease, certified by attending physician to be not "dangerous to the public health," were conveyed from Montmorency County to Lapeer County, Mich., where, just one week from the day the coffins were opened and the remains viewed, a person who was thus exposed came down with diphtheria. Many others would probably have been exposed except for the action of the local health officer, Dr. C. A. Wisner, who, suspecting that the cause of the deaths was diphtheria, warned the neighbors and forbade the opening of the coffins at the funeral. He promptly isolated the first case that occurred, and no epidemic resulted. This is quite different from the result of a similar occurrence at Zanesville, Ohio, last Spring, where many deaths resulted from exposure to a corpse brought from Chicago. It shows the importance of notice to the local health officer of the arrival of every corpse, so that he may take every precaution which may be necessary.

Powdered Meat.

As long ago as 1874, Dannecy, Chief Pharmacist of the hospitals of Bordeaux, prepared an excellent article of food for invalids by making a powder of meat. He took meat, chopped it very fine, and spread it upon muslin, drying it by means of a current of air. In this way he obtained a friable mass, which was easily powdered. It was administered by adding it to beef tea, or spreading it upon bread. It could also be mixed with the ingredients used for making biscuits, and this combination was found to be especially suitable for administration to children.

In the same year Yvon suggested the following method of preparing a palatable meat food : Take of raw meat (fillet of beef) 250 parts ; of charred sweet almonds, 75 parts ; of bitter almonds, 50 parts ; of white sugar, 80 parts. Rub slowly in a mortar until a homogeneous paste is obtained, adding from time to time a sufficient quantity of water to give a proper consistency for a semi-solid or a liquid mixture. In the liquid preparation the meat will settle after awhile, but may be dispersed through it by shaking. The preparation may be preserved for a long time if bottled and kept in a cool place, and its nutritious character may be enhanced by adding to it the yolks of one or more eggs.

Consumption in Cows.

The State Board of Health of Oregon has taken hold of the matter of stamping out consumption in cows. A wealthy banker of Portland, Ore., owned a herd of 158 Jerseys, which cost him $35,000, one-third of the entire sum having been paid for twenty-seven of the animals, bought in the East. A few months ago consumption was discovered in several of the cows, which led to the condemning of the animals by the State Board of Health. He was forbidden to sell either the milk or the butter made from the milk of any of the diseased animals, or others that had been in contact with them, and thirty-four of the animals were killed, others that had been exposed being placed in quarantine.

The Pollution of Streams.

There is one (among many) hygienic *dogmas* that may be asserted and should be accepted as such, namely, that the dejecta from a typhoid fever patient should never be thrown into a stream; for if a stream or river has received such discharges, it cannot be considered, at any lower point, a safe source of water supply. However pure the water may be chemically, there is no certainty that it does not contain the specific cause of this disease. The only safe thing to do with such discharges is to throttle the cause of the disease by treating the dejecta with a solution of corrosive sublimate, and then burying it, if in the country, or emptying it into the water-closet, if in the city. In this course, and in this alone, is there absolute safety.

Summer and its Dangers.

"Why is it that so many persons return to the city after a Summer's outing, and soon are taken sick with fever?" This question is often asked of physicians; and that it is so often asked implies that there is some basis for it in fact. We imagine that there are many reasons, some of which are known, and others, probably equally potent factors, which are as yet unknown.

In the first place, healthy homes are left behind for a more or less prolonged stay in malarial regions. Again, the capacity of hotels which are designed to accommodate fifty persons is stretched until more than twice that number are lodged within their walls, and the means provided for the disposition of the waste of the smaller number are so inadequate that soil-saturation and water-pollution inevitably result. Then, too, city houses are closed for months, and no provision is made for the filling of traps, the water of which gradually evaporates during the absence of its inmates, and when in the Fall the family returns, it is to a house into which, it may be, the air of a fever-infected sewer has been pouring for weeks.

Of course, the remedies at once suggest themselves to the thoughtful physician, and he should consider it his duty to advise his patients as to what they should do to avoid these dangers, not only to health, but to life as well.

Consumption of Snails.

Nearly one hundred thousand pounds of snails are sold daily in the Paris markets to be eaten by dwellers in Paris. They are carefully reared for the purpose in extensive snail gardens in the provinces and fed on aromatic herbs to make their flavor finer. One snailery in Dijon is said to bring in to its proprietor seven thousand francs a year. Many Swiss cantons also contain large snail gardens where they are grown with much pains. They are not only regarded as a great delicacy, but are reckoned as very nutritious. It is said that they contain 17 per cent. of nitrogenous matter, and they are equal to oysters in nutritive properties. Snails are also extensively used as an article of food in Austria, Spain, Italy and Egypt, and the countries on the African side of the Mediterranean. Indeed, the habit of eating snails as food has existed in various parts of Europe for many centuries.

Opium-Smoking in London.

Some startling facts are brought to light by a writer in a recent issue of the *Medical Press* concerning the increase in the habit of smoking opium in London. A gentleman who had been told that this habit was growing, determined to make some inquiries himself. After some time he learned that application for information should be made to a certain well-known medical practitioner living in the West End. The gentleman's wife wrote to this practitioner, asking information, and received in reply a copy of a pamphlet entitled "Opium-Smoking as a Therapeutic Power, according to the Latest Medical Authorities." The pamphlet describes in detail the method of preparing and smoking the opium, and recites the conditions which are said to be specially benefited by taking the drug in this form. The physician who is supposed to be the author of the pamphlet is himself a confirmed opium-smoker, and he seems to be actu-ated with a desire to drag others down to the level of his own degradation.

To Cleanse Books.

Grease spots, if old, may be removed from books by applying a solution of varying strength of caustic potash upon the back of the leaf. The printing, which looks somewhat faded after the removal of the spot, may be freshened up by the application of a mixture of one part of muriatic acid and twenty-five parts of water. In a case of fresh grease spots, carbonate of potash (one part to thirty parts of water), chloroform, ether or benzine renders good service. Wax disappears if, after saturating with benzine or turpentine, it is covered with folded blotting paper and a hot flatiron placed upon it. Paraffine is removed by boiling water or hot spirits. Ink spots or rust yield to oxalic acid in combination with hot water ; chloride of gold or silver spots to a weak solution of corrosive sublimate or cyanide of potassium. Sealing wax is dissolved by hot spirits and then rubbed off with ossia sepia (cuttle-fish bone). India ink is slightly brushed over with oil, and after twelve hours, saponified aqua ammonia, and particles of color still remaining must be removed with rubber.

Doctors and Wine.

Nothing indicates more plainly the healthful advances in regard to diet than the changes that have occurred in physicians themselves. Two hundred years ago, and even much later, doctors were notorious for their eating and tippling, and were generally very fat. Dr. Beddoes was so stout that the ladies called him their walking feather bed, and Dr. Fleming weighed 291 pounds until he reduced his weight by abstinence and eating a quarter of an ounce of Castile soap every night, and Dr. Cheyne weighed 384 pounds. It is said that it was during the seventeenth century, when doctors drank so heavily, that it became fashionable for them to write such illegible prescriptions, which were the result of their trembling hands. The man who remains abstemious where no liquor is to be had, does not deserve much credit, but the man who is temperate when the sparkling champagne stands beside his plate merits our approbation.

His Age was 7777.

An Irishman was ordered to make a coffin, which he did ; and to paint the inscription on the lid, which he did after a fashion that caused a little excitement in the churchyard. By dint of following the written copy, he managed to get as far as "Michael O'Rafferty, aged— ;" but try as he would, he could not represent the 28. At last he remembered that he could write seven, and that four sevens made 28. So he finished the inscription, which read "aged 7777." When they came to bury Michael, the coffin stood at the graveside, and the priest spoke as follows : "Ah, he was a fine lad. He's lying there so still, taken away in the very prime of life. Young as he was, too, only—" Here the priest looked down at the coffin plate to see how old Michael was, "He was only," said his reverence again, and he put his glasses on and went nearer to see how old he really was. "He was only," he continued, "seven thousand seven hundred and seventy-seven years ! "

Children's Diseases.

The impression abroad in the land to-day, that children *must* have scarlet fever, measles and the like, and that being inevitable, the sooner they have them and are done with it the better, is not only erroneous, but it is a very dangerous belief as well. In the first place there is no more necessity for a child to have scarlet fever than for an adult to have typhoid, both are equally preventable. In the second place, the longer we shield the child from these diseases, the less likely will they be to prove fatal. That is to say, with every year added to the age of the child the liability to these diseases becomes less, while, at the same time, the ability to successfully overcome them, should they occur, becomes greater. Certainly, those of us who are worthy of the name of *men* and *women* are anxious to rear our offspring, and when we tell you that the majority of those born into the world die during the first few years of diseases that we know, and you can learn, how to prevent, is this not sufficient incentive for you to familiarize yourselves with the laws of hygiene?

Finger-Nail Dirt.

The *British Medical Journal* says : The progress of bacteriology has shown that aseptic surgery means scientific cleanliness. The same lines of investigation show how very dirty people can be. Seventy-eight examinations of the impurities under finger-nails were recently made in the bacteriological laboratories of Vienna, and the cultivations thus produced showed thirty-six kinds of micrococci, eighteen bacilli, three sarcinæ and various varieties. The spores of common mould were very frequently present. The removal of all such impurities is an absolute duty in all who come near a parturient woman or a surgical wound. It is not enough to apply some antiseptic material to the surface of dirt ; the impurity must be removed first, the hand antisepticised after. It is sometimes said that the scratch of a nail is poisonous. There is no reason to suspect the nail tissue ; it is more likely the germs laid in a wound from a bacterial nest under the nail. Children are very apt to neglect to purify their nails when washing hands, and this matter is not always sufficiently attended to among surgical patients. Personal cleanliness is a part of civic duty, and, as Dr. Abbott well expressed the matter in his address to teachers, should be taught to school children and insisted on in practice.

The Hygienic Training of Women.

Mr. Frederick Treves called attention to a perfectly new branch of the work undertaken by the society with reference to physical education. Within the last few years an immense deal of attention had been directed to the matter of physical education. It had been pointed out that the education of the mind was well looked after, while the education of the body was practically allowed to look after itself. Parents did not realize that proper physical education must be conducted on as precise and as careful scientific lines as the ordinary education of the mind. Parents were quite content to send their children to gymnasiums, and when they had done this, felt that their physical education was complete. They were unaware that there was no proper control over the teachers of gymnastics and calisthenics, a large number of whom were people totally unfit for their work. The particular object of the Society had, perhaps, rather more reference to children and to women than to men and boys. As a matter of fact, the latter class was admirably looked after. No one could find much to criticize in the athletic pursuits of our public schools. When they came to the London shopboy, they found his condition had been materially changed ; he had taken to bicycling and other pursuits. When they came to schools, and especially to girls' schools, it must be confessed that the conditions were about as bad as they very well could be. They heard a good deal of the enormous advances of civilization during the last fifty or hundred years, and their marvellous improvement on the unfortunate savage, who had straight limbs, graceful carriage, and an absence of the ordinary aches and pains, and he was not disposed to be always taking tea or to be living in an atmosphere of tonics. People did not seem to be aware that by a judiciously supervised system of physical education, exercises and due attention to the development of the body it was possible to alter its proportions, to reduce redundances, and to develop deficient and feeble muscles. Motives of vanity and regard for the future physical development of their girls might so influence mothers who were indifferent to higher considerations, to see that the physical education of girls was carried out, whether in families or in schools, under persons trained, skilled, and having the requisite knowledge to make such physical training in all respects useful and in no case injurious. Neither could be said of the very limited amount of physical training now given to girls. It was pointed out that the National Health Society's diplomas would be granted to such teachers of gymnastics, calisthenics, and physical exercises as had fulfilled the necessary curriculum and passed the required examinations. The Society hoped by the institution of this diploma to encourage development of physical education in this country ; to render such training precise, effectual and scientific ; to protect the public, on the one hand, from incompetent teachers, and, on the other, to establish the position of such instructors as were fully qualified, It was intended, moreover, that the work of such teachers should be devoted and restricted to the one legitimate object set forth in the diploma, namely, physical training, and that they should not undertake the treatment of deformity or disease by "movement cures," "remedial exercises," massage and the like. The diploma would certify that the candidate had passed an examination in the art and science of physical education, had fulfilled the curriculum required by the Society, and was fully qualified to act as an instructor of gymnastics, calisthenics, and physical exercises generally.—*British Medical Journal.*

The Dangers of Dirty Streets.

In the last report of the New Jersey State Board of Health, Dr. Hunt devotes considerable space to the subject of the relation of clean streets to the health of cities. The care of the streets, he says, leads not only to the greater comfort of the citizens, but also concerns their health. He urges the necessity of good pavements and thorough drainage, and adds the following sensible advice concerning street cleaning : "Much of the surface cleansing of streets should be done at night, and even the sidewalks should not be swept in the face of those passing. Besides the discomfort, it is not appreciated what damage to health occurs from city dust. It is made up of dirty mud, of droppings of various kinds, and of various forms of decayable matter. This in a finely triturated state mingles with the air and has to go into the lungs and stomachs of the people. A very dusty city is always more unhealthy. Water sprinkling in hot days, or when there is much dust, is much the choice of two evils ; but if this has to be carried to the excess of causing undue moisture, it, too, becomes an evil. We desire to emphasize the injuriousness of city dust, and to claim its abatement as a nuisance which interferes with the health not less than the comfort of the people."

The Baths of Damascus.

An old book tells the following story of a French doctor seeking a place to begin practice, which points out a valuable hygienic lesson : "A French doctor went to Damascus to seek his fortune. When he saw the luxurious vegetation, he said : ' This is the place for me : plenty of fever.' And then, on seeing the abundance of water, he said, ' More fever, no place like Damascus !' When he entered the town, he asked the people, : What is this building ?'—' A bath !' ' And what is this building ?'—' A bath !—' And that other building ?'—' A bath !' ' Curse on so many baths ! they take the bread out of my mouth,' said the doctor ; ' I will get no practice here.' So he turned his back and went out of the gate again, and hied himself elsewhere. It would be well if every city were in respect to baths like Damascus, and all the people bathers."

A Healthy House and its Furnishings.

The *Independent* gives this picture : The healthy house will stand facing the sun, on a dry soil, in a wide, clean, amply sewered, substantially paved street, over a high, thoroughly ventilated and lighted cellar [if any]. The floor of the cellar will be cemented, the walls and ceiling plastered and thickly whitewashed with lime every year, that the house may not act as a chimney, to draw up into its chambers micro-organisms from the earth. Doors and windows, some of which extend from floor to ceiling, will be as abundant as circumstances permit, and will be adjusted to secure as much as may be through currents of air. The outside walls, if of wood or brick, will be kept thickly painted, not to shut out penetrating air, but for the sake of dryness. All inside walls will be plastered smooth, painted and, however unæsthetic, varnished. Mantels will be of marble, slate, iron, or if of wood, plain, and whether natural, painted or stained, will be varnished. Interior wood-work, including floors, will all show plain surfaces, and be likewise treated.

Movable rugs, which can be shaken daily in the open air—not at doors or out of windows, where dust is blown back into the rooms—will cover the floors. White linen shades, which will soon show the necessity of washing, will protect the windows. All furniture will be plain, with cane seats, perhaps, but without upholstery. Mattresses will be covered with oiled silk ; blankets, sheets and spreads, no comforts or quilts, will constitute the bedding.

Of plumbing there shall be as little as is necessary, and all there is shall be exposed as is the practice now. The inhabited rooms shall be heated only with open fires, the cellar and hall by radiated heat, or, better, by a hot-air furnace, which shall take its fresh air from above the top of the house, and not from the cellar itself or the surface of the earth, where micro-organisms most abound. There will be "house cleaning" twice a year.

Put into this house industrious, intelligent, and informed men and women—absolutely essential conditions—and as much will be done as at present may be done to prevent the dissemination from it of contagious disease, when an inmate brings it home from a septic house, hospital, sleeping car, school room, theatre, church, etc.

The Comparative Value of Silk and Woolen Underwear.

Dr. W. T. Stone, of St. Cloud, Minn., asks us for some information as to the comparative value of silk and woolen underwear as a preserver of health, especially in infants and children. We frankly admit our inability to *reliably* answer this question. At the last "International Congress of Hygiene," at Vienna, the great sanitarian, Pettenkoffer, made the assertion that it was, as yet, an undecided question as to whether wool or silk was the best material for underwear, from a sanitary point of view. We have no definite, accurate information on this subject, and it is, therefore, one of those questions in which each man must be guided by his own experience and observation. For ourselves, we think they are both good and doubt if there is much difference in their sanitary value.

The Secret of Health.

Don't worry. Don't hurry. "Too swift arrives as tardy as too slow." "Simplify! simplify! simplify!" Don't overeat. Don't starve. "Let your moderation be known to all men." Court the fresh air day and night. "Oh, if you knew what was in the air!" Sleep and rest abundantly. Sleep is nature's benediction. Spend less nervous energy each day than you make. Be cheerful. "A light heart lives long." Think only healthful thoughts. "As a man thinketh in his heart, so is he." "Seek peace and pursue it." Work like a man, but don't be worked to death. Avoid passion and excitement. A moment's anger may be fatal. Associate with healthy people. Health is contagious as well as disease. Don't carry the whole world on your shoulders, far less the universe. Trust the Eternal. Never despair. "Lost hope is a fatal disease." If ye know these things, happy are ye if ye do them.—*Ex.*

Encourage the Editor.

As a rule, an editor gets about one thousand kicks to one caress. Once in a while he gets a kind word and it warms and cheers his weather-beaten, storm-racked heart to the innermost core. Most people are afraid to tell an editor when he writes an article that pleases them, for fear of making him proud, we suppose, but if they find anything that does not precisely accord with their views, they will neglect their business to hunt him up, and tell him of it. Pshaw!

Dear friends, don't think you will spoil the editor by giving him an occasional word of cheer, any more than you will spoil your child by complimenting it upon a piece of patchwork it has finished. Of course you could beat the job yourself, but that doesn't deter you from heaping words of encouragement on the child. It has done its best. So you could doubtless beat the average editor at running a paper!

Of course you can. The man does not live who can't beat an editor at running a paper. The editor is willing to acknowledge that you can. He only runs it because you have not time to; but this fact need not deter you from giving him a word of encouragement occasionally.—*Danville (N. Y.) Breeze.*

Sanitation of the Campagna.

It is reported by cablegram that a syndicate of German capitalists, having $10,000,000 at command, has made overtures to the Italian government to reclaim the Campagna di Roma, on scientific sanitary principles. At present the district is a pestilential and desolate plain, a detriment to the progress of the city, and a standing menace to the health of all who are compelled to visit or reside temporarily in that region ; even the hardy peasants are not exempt from the malarial fevers that have their origin in the Pontine Marshes. This district was once well populated and cultivated, and it is thought that by the introduction of modern engineering methods of drainage and irrigation, the Campagna can again be made to blossom as the rose. If that should be done, and Rome again becomes a healthful city, it may in the end, and before many years, become a favorite health resort for winter tourists.

Bicycling for Young People.

Dr. B. W. Richardson discusses this subject in a recent issue of the *Æsclepiad*. He admits that since he first warned the public of the dangers of immoderate cycling changes have taken place in the construction both of bicycles and tricycles which materially modify the old drawbacks. He is still, however, of the opinion that cycling should never be practiced by boys and girls, since it differs from other exercises in the fact that it molds the bodily frame work, as it were, to its own mode of motion ; and riders in course of time almost invariably acquire what he calls "the cyclist's figure," which is not graceful and indicative of the possession of perfectly balanced powers. Of two things, at least, he is satisfied. They are, that the temptation of competition is to an earnest and practiced cyclist a "demon of danger," and that the systematic pursuit of cycling should never be fully commenced before the age of twenty-one.

Health Hints.

Don't contradict your wife.

Don't tell a man he is a stranger to the truth because he happens to be smaller than yourself. Errors of this kind have been known to be disastrous.

Never go to bed with cold or damp feet. Leave them beside the kitchen fire, where they will be handy to put on in the morning.

It is bad to lean your back against anything cold, particularly when it is an icy pavement upon which your vertebral arrangement has caromed with a jolt that shakes the buttons off your coat.

Always eat your breakfast before beginning a journey. If you haven't any breakfast don't journey.

After violent exercise, like putting up the stove or nailing down carpets, never ride around town in an open carriage. It is better to walk. It is also cheaper.

When hoarse, speak as little as possible. If you are not hoarse it won't do you any harm to keep your mouth shut, too.

Don't light the fire with kerosene. Let the hired girl do it. She hasn't any wife and children. You have.

Don't roam around the house in your bare feet at the dead of night trying to pick up stray tacks. Men have been known to dislocate their jaw through this bad practice.

When you see a man put the lighted end of a cigar in his mouth, don't ask him if it is hot enough. Serious injury has often resulted from this habit.— *Philadelphia Inquirer.*

The Benefit of Athletics.

" Do you believe in athletics?" was asked of a well-known business man who was found practicing with the dumb-bells at the back of the store the other day.

"Certainly I do," he promptly replied.

"Think it helps your health?"

"I know it does, and it has saved my bacon once or twice."

"Please relate."

"Well, a couple of years ago I took twenty-four lessons in boxing, and worked up a big muscle and lots of sand. I was going home one night, soon after graduating, when a man jumped out at me from the alley. In a minute he was nowhere."

"Hit him hard, eh?"

"No, I didn't hit him at all."

"Trip him up and fall on him?"

"No."

"Well, what did you do?"

"Outrun him! But for my athletic exercises I couldn't have done it."

Reforming Convicts.

The City Mission, of New York, is about to undertake a reform experiment with discharged convicts that will be looked upon with some interest. It proposes to establish trade schools in which the former prisoners are to be taught certain mechanical trades, so as to fit them to earn their living honestly. When they have learned their trades they will be expected to go to new communities where their prison record is unknown, often to earn their living by work. As prison records show that a very large porportion of convicts are without trades, and that their idle life and inability to earn a living by work is largely responsible for their downfall, there is fair ground for believing that such a school may accomplish some good in the way of reforming discharged convicts. The saving of one man a year from a career of crime would be worth the cost of a school for a hundred such— worth it not only from the standpoint of morals, but as a matter of dollars and cents. *An habitual criminal is one of the most expensive luxuries maintained by modern society.*

We are heartily in accord with this movement and thoroughly endorse the sentence which we have italicized. We would go further, however, and say that an *habitual invalid* is an even more expensive luxury than is an habitual criminal, and that if the reformation of one criminal is worth the outlay above suggested (and we believe that it is), the prevention of one invalid is worth at least equally as much. An invalid is not only an unproductive individual, but he is a burden upon the community as well.

The Secret of a Long Life.

Dr. Mark Trafton, who is a most active and vigorous man at 80 years of age, thus writes in the *American Agriculturist:* "Eternal vigilance" is not less the price of physical life than of liberty ; all organized life, whether animal or vegetable, depends for its perfection and perpetuity upon care and a strict regard for the laws of nature. "There is one Lawgiver," says high authority, and physical law is just as holy and sacred as moral law, and he who trifles with one of nature's laws is, in the sight of the Lawgiver, just as guilty as one who disregards moral law. Strange it is that one will shudder at the thought of a breach of the ten commandments and yet live in a daily disregard of the laws of physical life. It is true we must all die, but it is not true that the period of our death is fixed by divine decree. We must die under the laws of organization, like all organized beings. The fruit from bud and blossom grows, develops, ripens and decays ; so with animal organizations. Man, as other animals, develops from the embryo to the perfection of manhood, ripens and decays. There is a limit to the one as to the other, yet the startling fact stares us in the face that a large proportion of the *genus homo*, as with fruits, prematurely falls.

The law of animal organizations seems to be that all animals, of which the human is one, should live five times the period of their growth. A dog grows until two years of age ; his life period is ten to twelve years. A horse grows until five ; his period is twenty-five. An elephant grows until twenty, and his average life is one hundred years. So with man ; he grows and physically develops until twenty, and ought to live to the age of one hundred. But, alas ! a centenarian is regarded with a strange curiosity, while the death of half the human family before the age of seven excites no surprise. Should one-half of the progeny of the lower orders of animals die at or soon after birth, it would send consternation and dismay through the community ; but these young humans drop, and the mourning parents are expected to be consoled by the reflection that it is a "mysterious Providence," or that the "Giver of all Good had need of them to people heaven !" The mystery about it is that while the brutes are left to the laws of God in nature, man—this wiser animal—violates all these laws from the first moment of being.

Longevity must be rooted in infancy and early childhood. Each period of human life is probationary for that which follows, and, to a great extent, determines its character. Hence the old proverb, "The child is father to the man." I have no space to enter upon a discussion of these several points, upon each of which a book might be written, but when one sees, as often as has been seen, a mother more regardful of the laws of hygiene in the care of a favorite lapdog than in that of her infant, we can but exclaim, "O fools ! Were a moiety of the care and attention given to favorite pet animals bestowed upon infant children, there would be less mourning in households and complaint of divine dealings with men."

At the age of thirty, man has fully developed both his physical and intellectual powers, and is in full career as an active factor in life's grand enterprises. But now this is a period of especial danger to the active, ambitious person, male or female. One has a certain amount of storage power and energy upon which to draw, like so much deposit in a bank. Now the one who wishes length of days—and who does not?—must be cautious in drawing his drafts, for though indulgent nature may honor an overdrawn draft, she never fails to return them for redemption, and often they come to us to find us bankrupt. It is one's religious duty to carefully preserve physical life to its utmost possible limit, as it is to cultivate the highest spiritual life. Settle it in your heart, O man, that you can do nothing for your Creator only as you prize and honor his work. You sin against God when you sin against yourself, and you do this when you neglect or abuse your body.

In these days of rapid movement in all the affairs of life, we are constantly running into excesses which are self-destructive. We start on hearing of a suicide, but we seem to forget that there are many forms of self-murder. Not a day passes that we do not hear of some one dropping dead in the street or in his place of business. "Heart-failure," says the wise-looking doctor. Yes ; but what was the cause of this failure? If he is honest he will answer : "Some kind of excess ; his reserve power too highly taxed, and overdrawn drafts." But will business men and pleasure-seeking women heed this? I fear not ; but do not call on me to perform your funeral rites, as I shall simply say, "Died by his own hand."

Up to fifty we glide or rush along a level plateau on the summit of the hill of life, when we commence a descent into the dark valley. Our physical strength begins to weaken ; we do not take a flight of stairs with the heedless haste of former times, but find it helpful to keep one hand upon the rail. Old age is coming. Now, just here I wish to offer some practical suggestions :

First, as to clothing. Heat is life, cold is death. There is now less animal heat developed than when you were younger. Of course you must husband and save what you have. There are three points at which death directs his sharpest attacks, and which at all periods of life should be most carefully guarded—the back between the shoulders, the chest and throat, and the feet. For years past I have had my vests lined with flannel and have worn flannel undergarments and hand-knit socks. Do not sleep in cotton shirts, but woolen. Do not sleep in a cold room, but in cool weather take off the chill. Sleep all you can. Avoid all evening labor of the brain, all excitement of all kinds, and retire at an early, regular hour. Rise, not with the early bird or worm, but when you want to.

Food : For fifty years I have said, "You are killing yourselves by overeating," and have been laughed at as a fanatic ; but a recent remark of a celebrated physician in London comforts me : "More people," he says, "kill themselves by eating than by using intoxicants." And the same statement appeared in a late British magazine. I saw last Summer, when coming from the Maine woods, a Catholic priest, the picture of perfect health. Someone said to him : " I wish I could have health like yours." · "You may," replied he, " if you will live as I do. I eat but once in twenty-four hours. After my full breakfast, I eat nothing until the next morning." A lesson all persons should learn is that, when decay begins in the human system, all the organs lose vigor alike, and those organs which have been most exercised most rapidly fail. Yet people will not heed the admonitions of nature, but gormandize and cram the stomach the same as when young, and then resort to drugs, thus laying upon abused nature the double task of getting rid of 'the redundant mass of food and the poisonous drugs. Do you desire long life, a quiet, peaceful old age, with nights of soft, refreshing slumber? Cease all your excesses in eating. Remember, it is not the quantity one eats, but the amount digested and assimilated that yields strength. All beyond this is rebellion against nature.

Will you hear a bit of the experience of an octogenarian? I was a rather frail boy, flat-chested, and spent four years from. my fourteenth year bent over on a shoemaker's bench. I taught myself to perform on a clarionet, and played in a band four years, and this developed a good chest, and I have taken pains to preserve it, as above hinted. I am to-day as straight in my spinal column as a pine of my native State. At the age 'of twenty I was in the itinerant ministry of the Methodist Episcopal Church, and when I had been preaching two years a physician said to me : "You must stop preaching, or you will not live five years." He has been in his grave forty years; after this busy and exciting life of sixty years, I am here writing a word to my coevals, and "my eye is not dim, nor my natural force (much) abated." Why? Because, with the blessing of God, I have watched the operation of· nature's teaching and obeyed the teacher, and taken care of myself. For eight or nine years past I have eaten no flesh of dead animals. For many years I have eaten whole wheat, or Graham bread. My breakfast is the principal meal for the day—two soft-boiled eggs, a saucer of oatmeal mush, bread, and one cup of coffee. My dinner is bread, a slice or two, a cup of weak tea ; at night, a half-pint of milk and a slice of bread. I hardly know, from any sensation, whether I have eaten or not. I have gained in weight, and suppose, unless some accident befall me, or I slip into some indiscretion, I shall be at least a centenarian.

Sweets for Children.

Let parents try the following, and see how their children like it : Select good, sound fruit in its season—cherries, plums, peaches—just ripe and not overripe ; wash the outside and dry ; cut and remove the stones, and drain on a cheese cloth ; put into jars first two inches of very dry sugar, then a layer of fruit, followed by an inch of sugar, and then fruit ; and so on up to the top, the last being sugar, putting on a cloth and a weight for a week or so, filling with sugar as the mass settles. The sugar will absorb the moisture and keep from change.

BUREAU OF INFORMATION.

MONOCACY, PA., July 24th, 1890.

EDITOR OF ANNALS OF HYGIENE:

I am now attending five (5) children, ranging from 5 to 17 years, all in one family, besides one child who has died this A.M. They have undoubtedly typhoid fever. I am wholly unable to explain this infection, if it does not arise from the well, the water of which they have been using. This well is (they say) seventy feet deep, and within thirty feet of this well there stand the privy and pigpen. Under and around this pen is a collection of manure and filth derived from the pen. Hoping you will forward the result of your examination, I remain, Truly yours,

GEORGE HETRICH, M.D.

Examination of sample of water from Monocacy, Pa. Well seventy feet deep, within thirty feet of pigpen and manure pile. Received July 26th, 1890; examination made July 26th and August 2d, 1890, by C. M. Cresson, M.D.; reaction alkaline; condition clear. Contains:

	Grains in One U. S. Gallon.
Solid matter to dryness,	——
Lime	——
Magnesia	——
Chlorine	1.8603
Sulphuric acid	——

	Parts in 1,000,000 Parts.
Free ammonia	0.083
Albuminoid ammonia	0.083
Nitrogen as nitrites	——
" as nitrates	10.284

The microscope shows that this water contains cesspool or similar material. It carries the bacilli of typhoid fever and dysentery. It is unfit for use as a drinking water or for household use. This well should be abandoned. CHARLES M. CRESSON, M.D.

SOUTH BURGETTSTOWN,
WASHINGTON CO., PA., July 15th, 1890.

EDITOR OF ANNALS OF HYGIENE:

I send you a bottle of water taken from a well in Eldersville. Will you be kind enough to examine the water and let me know if there is anything injurious in it, or that might cause typhoid fever? A number of typhoid fever cases have recently occurred in Eldersville, and all drank water from this well. Please let me know the result of your analysis, and oblige, Respectfully,

J. C. NESBIT, M.D.

This sample was too small for proper chemical examination. This water contains a considerable amount of soluble animal matter. Microscopical examination shows that it carries great numbers of ciliata. There is no evidence of the presence of bacilli of typhoid fever or dysentery. A suspicious water. CHARLES M. CRESSON, M.D.

PUNXSUTAWNEY, PA., July 15th, 1890.

EDITOR ANNALS OF HYGIENE:

In this day's mail we have forwarded to you a specimen of our hydrant water of this town, with a view to having it analyzed, and be informed as to the result, for we are suspicious as to the fitness of it to be used for drinking purposes.

The late rains have caused this specimen to be a little worse than usual. The sending of this specimen is a private matter, and I wish to know whether or not the water is contaminated.

Please give me full particulars.

J. A. WALTER, M.D.

Examination of sample of water from Punxsutawney, Pa. For Dr. J. A. Walter, through Dr. J. F. Edwards. Received July 24th, 1890. Examination made July 24th and 31st, by C. M. Cresson, M.D ; amount of sample two quarts ; reaction alkaline ; condition opalescent. Contains :

	Grains in One U. S. Gallon.
Solid matter to dryness...................	——
Lime......................................	——
Magnesia.................................	——
Chlorine..................................	0.7442
Sulphuric acid...	——

	Parts in 1,000,000 Parts.
Free ammonia...........................	0.083
Albuminoid ammonia....................	0.274
Nitrogen as nitrites......................	——
" as nitrates.......................	Trace.

This water is badly contaminated by animal drainage, and is unfit for drinking or household purpose. As its use is condemned by the large amount of animal matter which it carries, it is not thought worth while to make a microscopical examination.

CHARLES M. CRESSON, M.D.

Care of the Teeth.

At the meeting in Berlin, last Spring, of the German Association of American Dentists, the best means of preserving the teeth were discussed, and Dr. Richter, of Breslau, said : " We know that the whole method of correctly caring for the teeth can be expressed in two words, *brush, soap*. In these two things we have all that is needful for the preservation of the teeth. All the preparations not containing soap are not to be recommended ; and if they contain soap, all other ingredients are useless except for the purpose of making their taste agreeable. Among the soaps the white castile soap of the English market is especially to be recommended. A shower of tooth preparations has been thrown on the market, but very few of which are to be recommended. Testing the composition of them, we find that about 90 per cent. are not only unsuitable for their purpose, but that the greater part are actually harmful. All the preparations containing salicylic acid are, as the investigations of Fernier have shown, destructive of the teeth. He who will unceasingly preach to his patients to brush their teeth carefully shortly before bedtime, as a cleansing material to use castile soap, as a mouth wash a solution of oil of peppermint in water, and to cleanse the spaces between the teeth by careful use of a silken thread, will help them in preserving their teeth, and win the gratitude and good words of the public."—*Boston Jour. Health.*

SPECIAL REPORT.

Minutes of the Fifteenth Regular Meeting of the State Board of Health of Pennsylvania.

The fifteenth regular meeting of the board was held at the borough hall, Norristown, May 8th, 1890, at 1.45 P.M. Present : Dr. George G. Groff, president pro tem., Drs. J. F. Edwards, J. H. McClelland, Pemberton Dudley and Benjamin Lee, secretary.

An order of business presented by the secretary was, on motion, approved as the order of the day.

The minutes of the fourteenth regular meeting, held at Harrisburg, November 13th, 1889, were read.

Dr. Groff moved that the name of Dr. J. F. Edwards be added as assisting in the inspection of the Susquehanna and Nittany Valleys, ánd that Huntingdon be substituted for Shimina in the same report.

The secretary requested to be allowed to alter the report of inspection on page 20, from Millerstown to Middletown   These suggestions were adopted and the minutes approved.

The minutes of a special meeting, held at Philadelphia, February 22d, 1890, were also read and approved.

SECRETARY'S REPORT.

The secretary then presented his report, which included the following items :

LETTER OF REGRET TO DR. DAVID ENGELMAN.

The secretary reported he had sent the letter of regret to Dr. Engelman, respecting his severance from the board, and a copy of the letter was now read, as follows :

HON. DAVID ENGELMAN, M.D. :

Sir : I am instructed by the State Board of Health and Vital Statistics of the Commonwealth of Pennsylvania, to transmit to you a copy of the enclosed resolution adopted at its fourteenth regular meeting, held at Harrisburg, November 13th, 1889.

(Signed)   GEORGE G. GROFF, M.D.,
President pro tem.,

(Signed)   BENJAMIN LEE, M.D.,
Secretary.

Resolved : That the State Board of Health of Pennsylvania desires to place on record its high appreciation of the value of the services rendered by the Honorable David Engelman, M.D., its late president, both as a member of the board and as its presiding officer for more than two years. Not only his sagacious counsel, but his urbane demeanor and agreeable companionship made his presence welcome at its deliberations. The board trusts that the severance of this official connection, which it regards with sincere regret, will not lessen the interest of their late colleague in the progress of sanitary reform in the State, or deprive the board of his valuable aid in its prosecution.

TYPHOID FEVER AT LOCK HAVEN, CLINTON COUNTY.

The secretary read a letter transmitted from His Excellency, Governor Beaver, reporting an epidemic of typhoid fever at Lock Haven. The secretary had communicated with Dr. Groff, who visited and inspected the district. He reported much sickness, as many as from 300 to 400 cases of fever having been reported to him. He had conferred with the physicians there, many of whom thought the worst of the sickness was over, had inspected the reservoir, a sample of water from which he had submitted to the secretary for analysis. He found the June flood had partially filled the water pipes with mud, and that they had only very recently been flushed. In accordance with the suggestions contained in Dr.

Groff's report, the secretary had addressed a communication to His Honor, Mayor Mason, strongly urging that all water for domestic purposes be bottled before use, that pipes leading from the reservoir be opened and flushed, and that the flushing be repeated as often as necessary to keep them clean.

The report was accepted and referred for publication.

DIPHTHERIA AT WEATHERLY, CARBON COUNTY.

The secretary's attention was recently called to a serious outbreak of diphtheria at Weatherly, Carbon County, by the Rev. A. M. Masonheiser. Dr. Charles McIntire was instructed to make an inspection. He reported the population to be about 3500. The authorities had been fighting against the disease for several years. He considered the chief cause of the epidemic to be the carelessness of the people. A statistical report of the causes of deaths for three years showed the disease to have been exceptionally prevalent and fatal, causing nearly one-half the entire mortality. Founded upon this report, the secretary had addressed a letter, which he read, containing suggestions with regard to the proper measures to be taken to check the spread of 'the contagion, to the *Weatherly Herald* for publication. This had produced favorable results, as the epidemic had rapidly diminished.

The report was accepted and action approved.

TYPHOID FEVER AT JOHNSTOWN.

The secretary presented a report from Dr. George W. Wagoner, Assistant Deputy Medical Inspector at Johnstown, demonstrating that the epidemic of typhoid fever in that city was not a result of the flood of June last. The disease was imported into the town by a milkman, the first cases having occurred at the suburb of Moxham, which was entirely out of reach of the waters. The sanitary condition of the town was in no way responsible for the disease, which had soon diminished, never having been very serious.

The report was accepted and referred for publication.

DEFECTIVE DRAINAGE AT NATRONA, ALLEGHENY COUNTY.

The secretary had received a complaint that the drainage of Natrona was defective, and that sickness had resulted therefrom. Dr. J. R. Thompson, of Pittsburgh, was requested to make an investigation. He reported the complaint to have arisen from a stream in a foul condition, running through the heart of the town. It was putrid with human excreta and filth and the offal of a slaughter house. He suggested that the only plan to effectually abate this nuisance was for the railroad company to divert this run or stream into another channel. The secretary had addressed a communication to the secretary of the railroad, suggesting a new culvert, but the reply of the company was to the effect that to do so would be antagonistic to their charter, and on these grounds they declined to accede to this request. The secretary had further instructed the slaughter house proprietors to deposit no more refuse in this stream.

The report was accepted and further action upon it deferred.

PREVENTION OF THE SPREAD OF LEPROSY.

The secretary reported that at the last meeting of the American Public Health Association, he had submitted a resolution relative to the prevention of the spread of leprosy in the United States. It was adopted by the Association, and copies distributed throughout the country. As a result of this action, the Supervising Surgeon-General of the U. S. Marine Hospital Service had issued a regulation, which makes it incumbent upon the medical officers at the U. S. quarantine stations to examine emigrants for evidences of this disease, and if any are discovered to be suffering from it, to return them at once to the port from which they came.

The report was accepted and approved, and the regulation ordered to be printed in the annual report of the board, as also the resolutions of the California State Board of Health upon the same subject.

DEFECTIVE DRAINAGE AT MANSFIELD, TIOGA COUNTY.

Acting on a complaint of defective drainage at Mansfield, the secretary had ordered an inspection by Dr. E. D. Payne, who reported that the matter was not of such a nature as necessitated the board's interference. The secretary had reported this to the borough authorities. The report was accepted.

TYPHUS FEVER AT NEW YORK ON STEAMSHIP WESTERNLAND.

The secretary reported that the Secretary of the New York State Board of Health had recently communicated with him, stating that six cases of typhus fever had been discovered among the steerage passengers of the steamship Westernland, from Antwerp. He furnished a list of the steerage passengers for information. The Secretary had had copies of this list prepared and distributed among the boards of health in Pennsylvania. No further outbreak had been reported. The communication and report were accepted.

DEFECTIVE DRAINAGE AT DEVON INN.

The secretary had in hand correspondence between Mr. Howard Murphy, C. E., and Mr. Russell Thayer, C. E., relative to a proposed plan for abating the nuisance arising from the drainage of the Devon Inn. Mr. Murphy had approved the scheme proposed, subject to certain conditions, and suggested that further action be suspended until the scheme could be tried, which suggestion had been adopted. Report and action of secretary approved.

TEST FOR DIAGNOSIS OF TYPHOID FEVER.

The secretary submitted a test for diagnosis of typhoid fever, which had been brought to his notice by Dr. Thomas F. Wood, Secretary to the North Carolina State Board of Health. Resolved, that the communication of Dr. Wood be received with thanks, and referred for publication in the annual report.

INSPECTION OF WATER SUPPLY AT BERWICK, COLUMBIA COUNTY.

In response to a request from the Jackson Manufacturing Company, at Berwick, Columbia County, the secretary had instructed Dr. William Leiser, Jr., to examine the proposed new source of water supply for that village. Dr. Leiser's report, which was now read, was to the effect that the source was not entirely free from risk of pollution, but that certain precautions being taken, it would not be seriously objectionable. A copy of this report had been sent by the secretary to the company. The report was accepted and referred for publication.

DIPHTHERIA AT LEHMAN, LUZERNE COUNTY.

The secretary reported a recent epidemic of diphtheria at Lehman, Luzerne County. The physicians in the district were communicated with by Medical Inspector L. H. Taylor, who reported about thirty-five cases and ten deaths. Circulars had been freely distributed and the epidemic had abated. The report was accepted.

DIPHTHERIA AT EAST STROUDSBURG.

In consequence of a rumor that diphtheria was epidemic at East Stroudsburg, the secretary had directed Dr. Charles McIntire, medical inspector, to investigate. He had placed himself in communication with the resident physicians, who reported that the epidemic had nearly spent itself. He had also visited the district, and had suggested the foundation of a local board of health.

The secretary had addressed a communication to the chief burgess on the importance of these matters, which he read. The report was accepted.

The secretary read a report of Dr. L. H. Taylor, medical inspector, on an alleged epidemic of diphtheria at Pittston, Luzerne County. The report was accepted and ordered to be filed.

The secretary had received a complaint from the school board of Stowe Township, McKee's Rocks, that certain persons dumped manure and refuse near the public school, which created a serious nuisance. Dr. J. R. Thompson, medical inspector, had been ordered to investigate, and he had declared this condition a nuisance.

The secretary had sent orders to each person making such deposit of manure to cease and abate the nuisance forthwith. The report was accepted and ordered to be filed, and action approved.

ALLEGED CASE OF YELLOW FEVER AT WOMELSDORF, BERKS COUNTY.

A somewhat alarming report appeared in the *Press* of March 25th, that a case of yellow fever had terminated fatally at Womelsdorf. The secretary had instructed Dr. Murray Weidman, medical inspector, to make full inquiries, and to interview Dr. F. Sallada, who had had the case in charge. On receiving the inspector's report he had detailed the symptoms in a communication to a yellow fever expert in Florida, who denied the accuracy of the diagnosis, considering it rather a case of pernicious malarial fever. The report was accepted, and ordered to be filed.

CASE OF LEPROSY IN PHILADELPHIA.

The secretary reported the discovery of a recent case of leprosy in the person of a Chinaman in a Philadelphia hospital. He has addressed communications to secretaries of all local boards in Pennsylvania. and to secretaries of all State boards, reporting the case, his object being to arouse the profession to a sense of the importance of being on the lookout for that disease. The report was accepted, and action of secretary approved.

INSPECTION OF NEW QUARANTINE STEAMER FOR STATION AT MOUTH OF DELAWARE BAY.

The secretary submitted a report of an inspection of the fumigating steamer Louis Pasteur, together with cuts showing the special designs and engines and apparatus for disinfecting vessels and cargoes on a large scale. The report was accepted, and the matter of publishing the cuts in the annual report was left to the discretion of the secretary.

TRI-STATE SANITARY CONVENTION AT WHEELING, WEST VIRGINIA.

The secretary reported that he had attended the Tri-State Sanitary Convention at Wheeling, West Virginia, on February 27th and 28th last, held for the purpose of considering the problems which confront the sanitarian as a result of great floods, the States interested being Pennsylvania, Ohio, and West Virginia. Many valuable papers were presented which have already appeared in the ANNALS OF HYGIENE. The proceedings and papers were largely reported in the daily press, and much good would no doubt result. The report was accepted, and papers ordered to be published.

DIPHTHERIA AT OXFORD AND LINCOLN INSTITUTE, CHESTER COUNTY.

The secretary read communications from Dr. S. W. Morrison, Health Officer of Oxford on "Diphtheria at Oxford, and Lincoln Institute." Dr. W. B. Atkinson, medical inspector, had been directed to investigate. He reported that careful precautions were now being taken, and apprehended no further spread of the disease. The report was accepted.

INSPECTION AT GREENSBURG, WESTMORELAND COUNTY.

The secretary reported that at the urgent request of the borough authorities of Greensburg, he had directed Dr. W. E. Matthews, medical inspector, to visit and make an inspection of that borough. Dr. Matthews reported that the most serious obstacle in the way of sanitary improvement of the borough, which was greatly needed, was the lack of the necessary grant of power in its charter of incorporation. The report was accepted, and action deferred for further consideration under the head of new business.

DISINTERMENT AND TRANSPORTATION PERMITS.

The secretary reported that authority had been given to disinter and transport the bodies of the following, due notice having been given to, and permission having been obtained from, authorities interested : George L. Bowen, buried two years, from North East, Erie County, Penna., to Savanna, Illinois; cause of death, diphtheria. Dr. H.

Schell, from California to Pennsylvania; cause of death, phthisis. Twenty-nine bodies of persons identified, and a general permit for the unidentified, from or about the district of Johnstown, Pennsylvania; cause of death, drowning. The report was accepted, and the action of the secretary approved.

INSANITARY CONDITION OF HAZLETON, LUZERNE COUNTY, AND TARENTUM, ALLEGHENY COUNTY.

The secretary reported that private complaints had been received of the insanitary con dition of Hazleton and Tarentum, Pennsylvania. The usual printed letter requiring ten persons to unite in the complaint, had been sent, and nothing further had been heard. The report was accepted.

PROPOSED BOARD OF HEALTH AT MIDDLETOWN, DAUPHIN COUNTY..

The secretary reported that he had been in communication with the Burgess of Middletown with regard to a board of health being established there. The report of Dr. Hartman at the last meeting of this board showed that it was greatly needed, but the people evidently preferred to get the State Board of Health to do the work for them. Report accepted, and referred to new business.

COMPLAINT OF TYPHOID FEVER AT ROCKWOOD, SOMERSET COUNTY.

The secretary reported that he had recently received a complaint from one of the resident physicians at Rockwood, that typhoid fever prevailed there. He had instructed Dr. C. L. Gummert, medical inspector, to make an inspection. His report led the secretary to conclude that the complaint was founded upon jealousy between the local physicians, and no further action had been taken. The report was accepted.

WATER SUPPLY OF MUNCY, LYCOMING COUNTY.

The secretary reported that with regard to proposed source of water supply for Muncy, he had written to the authorities as directed. A copy of the letter was read, warning the council to be cautious in accepting a water supply of doubtful purity.

REQUEST FOR REPORTS OF MORTALITY IN THE STATE HOSPITAL FOR THE INSANE, NORRISTOWN, PA.

The secretary reported that at the request of the Norristown Local Board of Health, he had addressed a communication to the Board of Trustees, State Hospital for the Insane, Norristown, requesting them to furnish copies of the monthly reports of that institution to said local board. The request was complied with. The action of secretary was approved.

A copy of the letter to his Excellency, Governor Beaver, declaring the nuisances in the Valleys of the Juniata and the West Branch of the Susquehanna abated was now read. The action was approved.

In response to a request from the Pennsylvania Forestry Association, the secretary reported that he had addressed communications to the chairman and members of the committee appointed by Congress, on Forestry, to aid in obtaining an Act of Congress for the better protection of forests. One reply had been received, which was read. The report was accepted.

ANNUAL REPORTS OF BOARDS OF HEALTH.

The secretary placed before the board the annual reports of the boards of health of Altoona, Oil City and Reading, Pa. Ordered that the reports be read by title, and abstracts from same be printed and published in the annual report.

POWERS OF BOARDS OF HEALTH IN BOROUGHS.

The secretary had been in correspondence with the Attorney-General relative to the powers of boards of health in boroughs. The opinion of the Attorney-General was now read by the secretary. The secretary further reported an interview with Dr. H. H. Whitcomb, secretary of the Norristown Board of Health on this subject. The board was of the opinion that in case a local board was inoperative, through lack of power, the State Board could aid by ordering an abatement of any nuisance.

The report of the secretary was accepted and action deferred.

APPOINTMENT OF SPECIAL MEDICAL INSPECTOR FOR THE PENNSYLVANIA RAILROAD CO.

The secretary reported the appointment of Dr. E. C. Town as special medical inspector for and at the request of the Pennsylvania Railroad Company, with power to act with regard to sanitation of Broad Street and other stations in and near Philadelphia.

The action of the secretary was approved and the appointment confirmed.

STATISTICS ON PAN-DEMIC OF INFLUENZA AND RESULTS OF TOBACCO SMOKING.

The secretary reported the results of answers to circulars sent out to the physicians in Pennsylvania on the subjects, to date as follows :

Number of physicians reporting	265
Number of cases	37,275
Adults	26,302
Children	10,973
Number of cases nervous	6,913
" " " catarrhal	16,434
" " " inflammatory	5,829
Number of deaths directly caused	56
" " " indirectly caused	205
Immediate cause of death, bronchitis	8
" " " " pneumonia	117
" " " " phthisis	42
" " " " nervous	21
Number of circulars sent to date	4,500

The report was accepted.

TRANSPORTATION OF DEAD BODIES.

Revised regulations on the disinterment and transportation of dead bodies.

PRECAUTIONS AGAINST CONSUMPTION.

Circular No. 28, on Precautions against Consumption. The secretary presented copies of these circulars, and reported that they had been distributed throughout Pennsylvania to physicians, boards of health, borough councils, newspapers, medical journals and undertakers. The report was accepted.

FINANCIAL REPORT.

The secretary reported that as treasurer his disbursements, since last meeting, amounted to $1435.92. The report was accepted.

The secretary reported that the number of written communications received since last meeting were 978 ; number sent, 1037; cyclostyle letters sent on influenza, 4500, and on the inveterate smokers of tobacco, as regards tuberculosis, 4500; books added to library, 11 ; pamphlets added, 70. The report was accepted. Reports of committees being next in order.

EXECUTIVE COMMITTEE'S REPORT.

The executive committee reported that it had held three meetings since the last meeting of the board, at which accounts represented by vouchers Nos. 305 to 359 had been audited and approved, the amount expended having been $1435.92. The report was accepted and approved.

REPORT OF COMMITTEE ON VITAL STATISTICS.

Dr. Lee, chairman of committee on vital statistics, reported that the register of the physicians of Pennsylvania was now going through the press, and would be ready for the board's next annual report. The committee also desired to present for consideration of the board a system nomenclature to be followed by physicians and registers in making returns of diseases and deaths, a copy of which would be sent to each member for his individual criticism and suggestions. The report was accepted.

PROPOSED FORM OF BLANKS.

Dr. J. H. McClelland moved, and it was

Resolved: That this board recommends all boards of health and health officers to adopt a uniform blank for reporting " Causes of Death," and would recommend the use of the following form in describing the " Causes of Death," viz.: Predisposing or Complicating, Immediate or Determining.

REPORT OF COMMITTEE ON TRAVEL AND TRAFFIC.

Dr. J. F. Edwards, chairman, reported that he had had prepared special resolutions of thanks to Dr. Benjamin Lee, secretary, and George G. Groff, President pro tem., for their arduous services in connection with the flood of May 31st, 1889. The resolutions were read and accepted.

REPORT OF COMMITTEE ON ADULTERATIONS, POISONS, ETC.

Dr. Pemberton Dudley, chairman, reported that Professor Henry Leffmann had proposed to make certain analyses and examinations without cost to the board. The report was accepted.

REPORT OF SANITARY CONVENTION COMMITTEE.

Dr. J. F. Edwards, chairman, reported that the arrangements were now completed, and presented the preliminary announcement and programme. Several conferences had been held with the committee of the Norristown Board of Health, and invitations had been extensively circulated among physicians, borough authorities, boards of health and school teachers. The report was accepted and the committee discharged.

The board now adjourned to meet at 7.30 P.M., at the Montgomery House.

The board reconvened at the Montgomery House at 7.30 P.M.

NEW BUSINESS.

New business being in order, the subject of the nuisance from open drain at Natrona was called up.

Dr J. H. McClelland was appointed a committee to lay the matter personally before the receiver of the Allegheny Valley Railroad, and to urge an abatement of the nuisance, and the secretary was instructed to address an official communication to the railroad authorities on the subject.

SANITARY CONDITION OF GREENSBURG, PA.

In reference to the request of the authorities of Greensburg, Pa., the secretary was authorized to offer and extend to the authorities of Greensburg all assistance to the extent of the board's legal powers in improving the sanitary condition of the town.

NUISANCE AT MIDDLETOWN.

The secretary asked for instructions as to the course to be pursued in regard to the nuisances reported by Dr. Hartman, as existing at Middletown, Dauphin County.

This matter was referred back to the secretary, with power to act according to his judgment and discretion.

ADJOURNMENT TO SANITARY CONVENTION.

The board then adjourned to meet at 8 P. M., Friday, May 9th, to listen to the annual address before the board, to be delivered by Prof. A. Arnold Clark, of Lansing, Michigan.

The board reconvened at 8 P. M., Friday, May 9th, according to adjournment, to hear the annual address, which formed a portion of the proceedings of the State Sanitary Convention. The subject of the address was :

ANNUAL ADDRESS AT SANITARY CONVENTION.

It was a masterly exposition of the subject, and riveted the attention of the large and intelligent audience. Excellent music was furnished for the occasion by the orchestra of the State Hospital for the Insane of the South-Eastern District.

At 2 P. M. the day following, Saturday, May 10th, the board accepted the kind invita. tion of the trustees of the above-mentioned hospital, to visit their institution and inspect its drainage system. At the conclusion of the inspection, the Hon. S. T. Davis, M.D., offered a resolution thanking the trustees, resident physicians and steward for their courtesy, and expressing the gratification of the board at the care bestowed upon the sanitary arrange. ments of the Hospital.

The board then adjourned *sine die.*

(Signed)　　　　BENJAMIN LEE, M.D., *Secretary.*

State Board of Health and Vital Statistics of the Commonwealth of Pennsylvania.

PRESIDENT,
GEORGE G. GROFF, M.D., of Lewisburg.

SECRETARY,
BENJAMIN LEE, M.D., of Philadelphia.

PEMBERTON DUDLEY, M.D., of Philadelphia.

J. F. EDWARDS, M.D., of Philadelphia.	GEORGE G. GROFF, M.D., of Lewisburg.
J. H. McCLELLAND, M.D., of Pittsburg.	S. T. DAVIS, M.D., of Lancaster.
HOWARD MURPHY, C. E., of Philadelphia.	BENJAMIN LEE, M.D., of Philadelphia.

PLACE OF MEETING,
Supreme Court Room, State Capitol, Harrisburg, unless otherwise ordered.

TIME OF MEETING,
Second Thursday in May, July and November.

C. R. WOODIN, President.　　　　　　　WM. F. LOWRY, Treasurer.
C. H. ZEHNDER, Vice-Pres't and Gen. Manager.　　　FREDERICK H. EATON, Secretary.
H. F. GLENN, General Superintendent.

THE JACKSON & WOODIN MAN'F'G CO.

BERWICK, COLUMBIA CO., PA.

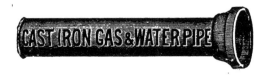

FREIGHT CARS, CAR WHEELS, BAR IRON,

SPECIAL CASTINGS.

THE
ANNALS
OF
HYGIENE

VOLUME V.

Philadelphia, September 1, 18ço

NUMBER 9.

COMMUNICATIONS

The Restriction and Prevention of Dangerous Diseases.*

BY HENRY B. BAKER, M.D.,

Secretary of the State Board of Health of Michigan.

MR. PRESIDENT, LADIES AND GENTLEMEN :—One of the first questions suggested by the subject assigned to me is : What diseases can be restricted or prevented ? So far as relates to the class of diseases the answer is easy. The diseases which can be restricted are those which are *communicable.* The " communicable" diseases include those which are contagious, those which are infectious, those which are in any way communicated or spread from one person to another—such diseases as smallpox, scarlet fever, diphtheria, measles and whooping-cough.

Then an important question is, whether any of the most dangerous diseases which have not heretofore been considered communicable do really belong to that class, and can therefore be restricted or prevented. To this question we can now answer "yes." At least one of the most dangerous of all diseases, namely, consumption, has in recent years been found to be a communicable disease and a preventable disease. There is considerable evidence now tending to prove that pneumonia is a communicable disease, and that probably many deaths from that disease could be prevented by the general adoption of measures which recent investigations have revealed.

THE IMPORTANCE OF THIS SUBJECT.

The importance of the subject of the restriction of the dangerous diseases cannot easily be estimated. Let us see what aid the vital statistics can give us. The statistics of deaths in Michigan are not perfect, but the relative importance of the several diseases is probably shown with approximate accuracy. The diagram which I exhibit, and copies of which are distributed in

---

*An address before the Sanitary Convention, Charlevoix, Michigan, August 15th, 1890.

this audience, is accurately drawn to scale, and correctly represents the deaths reported to the Secretary of the State. The diagram shows the relative importance of the several dangerous communicable diseases. It shows that in Michigan every one of the diseases named in the diagram is much more important than smallpox as a cause of death, and that when compared with diphtheria, and especially when compared with consumption, smallpox is insignificant, or at least that it was so during the twelve years 1876–87. If the diagram included pneumonia it would appear between " diphtheria" and "typhoid fever," and then the five diseases which cause most deaths in Michigan would be shown in the diagram. The five diseases which cause most deaths in Michigan, named in the order of their importance, are : Consumption, diphtheria, typhoid fever and scarlet fever.

We thus gain some idea of the vast importance of this subject—the restriction and prevention of the dangerous communicable diseases which include all the most important causes of deaths in Michigan. Especially do we appreciate the importance of this subject when we consider that we absolutely know that a large proportion of the cases and deaths from the most of these disease are *preventable*, and we believe that this is true of all of these diseases.

CO-OPERATION NECESSARY FOR THE RESTRICTION OF DISEASE.

For their prevention, however, it is necessary that all the people shall co-operate. No one can fully protect himself so long as others do not understand the subject and act accordingly. Therefore, the only way these most important causes of deaths can be most completely avoided by any of us, is by increasing the proportion of the people who know how to restrict and prevent them. If we except smallpox, which may, by vaccination, be avoided by each person for himself, this statement is true relative to each of the dangerous communicable diseases. For the restriction of each there is required general diffusion of knowledge, and general co-operation of all classes of people. That is a good reason why " the restriction and prevention of the dangerous diseases" is given so prominent a place on the programme of every Sanitary Convention.

HOW THESE DISEASES ARE SPREAD.

But these diseases are not all spread in the same way ; and it is necessary that the people generally shall know how each one is spread in order to know how to restrict each disease. In each disease something goes from a sick person which is capable of causing the disease. It goes from that part of the body in which the disease is located, and generally it thrives best when it reaches that same part of the body to which it goes. In consumption that part is generally the lungs ; and the specific cause of consumption goes out with the sputa and is scattered about not only wherever the moist sputa goes, but also wherever the dust from the dried sputa goes. And as the dust of the air is breathed in with the air inhaled, there is opportunity for the specific cause of consumption to go at once to the part of the body in which it is usually found.

This indicates what is the most important measure for the restriction of consumption, namely, the *destruction or disinfection of all sputa from every consumptive person.*

But this subject will be sufficiently dealt with by the speakers who are to follow me.

TYPHOID FEVER.

Typhoid fever causes about ten times as many deaths in Michigan as small-pox does—probably about one thousand deaths per year—and most of these deaths should be prevented. The greatest number of deaths from typhoid fever is of persons in the prime of life, and this should prompt to greater efforts for the prevention of this disease.

The most common modes of spread of typhoid fever are not the same as of smallpox and consumption, consequently the measures for its restriction and prevention are not the same. The pamphlets on this subject issued by the State Board of Health, and freely distributed here, contain plain directions how to prevent typhoid fever, and how to restrict its spread. It is now believed that typhoid fever is most frequently spread by means of the drinking water, that the microscopic cause of the disease is probably reproduced in the bodies of persons who have the disease, and that this specific cause gains access to the drinking water by filtering through the soil, and sometimes by being washed into wells or streams from which the drinking water is drawn. The noted instance at Lausanne, Switzerland, where the discharges from typhoid fever patients were thrown into a small stream, which disappeared by sinking into the earth and gravel, and reappeared about a half mile distant as a mountain spring, the clear water of which caused typhoid fever in 144 persons, is instructive, and is useful for us to hold in mind as illustrative of how the disease may be spread. The most usual mode of spread is probably by way of the privy vault and the neighboring well. The facts concerning the outbreak at Lausanne prove (and the same has been indicated in other instances) that the cause of typhoid fever sometimes passes great distances by way of the underground water flowing through strata of gravel.

We must not forget, however, that typhoid fever may be spread through the air, that the supposed "germ" of the disease is not destroyed by simply freezing, and is not yet known to be destroyed by ordinary drying. We know that the microscopic "germ" of consumption is most dangerous when dried and floating in the air we breathe. It may be that the specific cause of typhoid fever is dangerous in the same way.

The prevention and restriction of typhoid fever requires the disinfection of all bowel discharges from those sick with such disease, and constant watchfulness of the sources of supply of water for drinking and culinary purposes. All water from a suspected source should be boiled before its use. Numerous instances are reported where typhoid fever has been spread by the rinsing of milk cans with water apparently pure, but really infected with the germs of typhoid fever, capable of infecting the milk. This teaches us the importance of having water free from typhoid infection for all household purposes.

Typhoid fever is a disease which, in my opinion, it is important that citizens of every village should understand, because of the nature of the soil and earth underlying villages and the surrounding country from which the milk supply comes. Sooner or later there will come a time when no ordinary well in such a place can be safely relied upon to supply water free from the specific cause of typhoid fever.

But the general water supply of cities and villages is a matter of the greatest concern, and it should be procured from places where there can be no probability of immediate or remote contamination. The well-known outbreak of typhoid fever at Plymouth, Pa., where over a thousand cases and 114 deaths occurred, is apparently an illustration of how great a calamity may follow the fouling of a *general* water supply by the specific cause of typhoid fever.

There is not time at my disposal to give all the evidence proving the enormous saving of human life from the ravages of typhoid fever which in recent years has been accomplished because of such knowledge as this to which I have just alluded, but I wish briefly to refer to some of this evidence. In a pamphlet published by the Michigan State Board of Health, and entitled, "The Influence of Sewerage and Water Supply on the Death Rate in Cities," Mr. Erwin F. Smith shows conclusively very great reductions in the mortality from typhoid fever in many of the great cities in this country and in foreign countries, the reductions in the typhoid mortality following the introduction of systems of sewerage and general water supplies. For instance, in the city of Munich the death rate from typhoid fever in the period from 1854 to 1859 was 24.2 per ten thousand inhabitants, while in 1884 it had declined to 1.4 per ten thousand inhabitants; that is, before the city was sewered, and while it was supplied with water from wells, the mortality from typhoid fever was about seventeen times as great as it was after the city was well sewered and had a good general water supply.

To give you a mental image of this important subject, I have had copies made of two diagrams prepared by Mr. Erwin F. Smith to illustrate his paper, and they are here for distribution to such of you as will study them.

If there should be in Michigan such a reduction of the mortality from typhoid fever as was secured in Munich through better sewerage and water supply, there would be a saving of over 900 lives per year and over 9,000 cases of sickness per year. To point out how such favorable conditions for healthful existence may be secured, is one of the objects of such sanitary conventions as this.

Let us pass now to the consideration of diseases which are fatal chiefly to children.

DIPHTHERIA.

About 85 per cent. of all the deaths from diphtheria are of children under 10 years of age. Grown people have diphtheria, but it is usually considered only as an ordinary sore throat, and proper precautions to prevent the spread

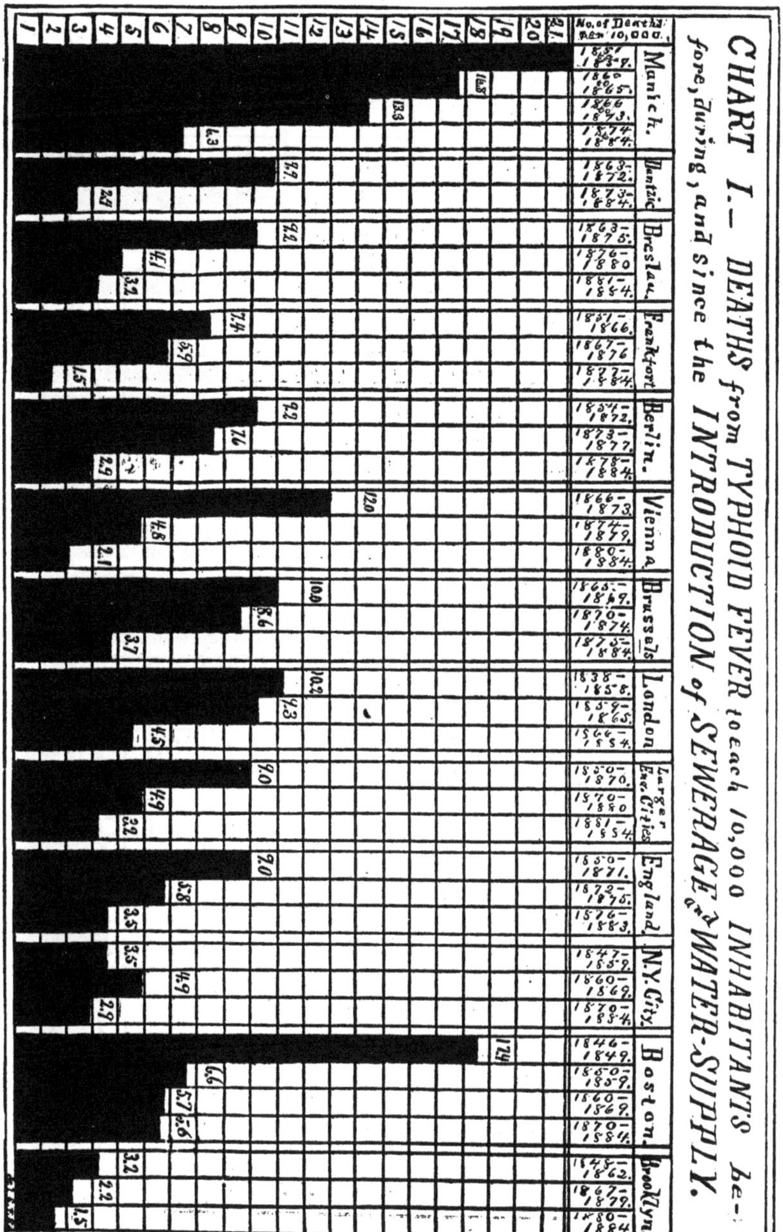

CHART I.— DEATHS from TYPHOID FEVER to each 10,000 INHABITANTS before, during, and since the INTRODUCTION of SEWERAGE and WATER-SUPPLY.

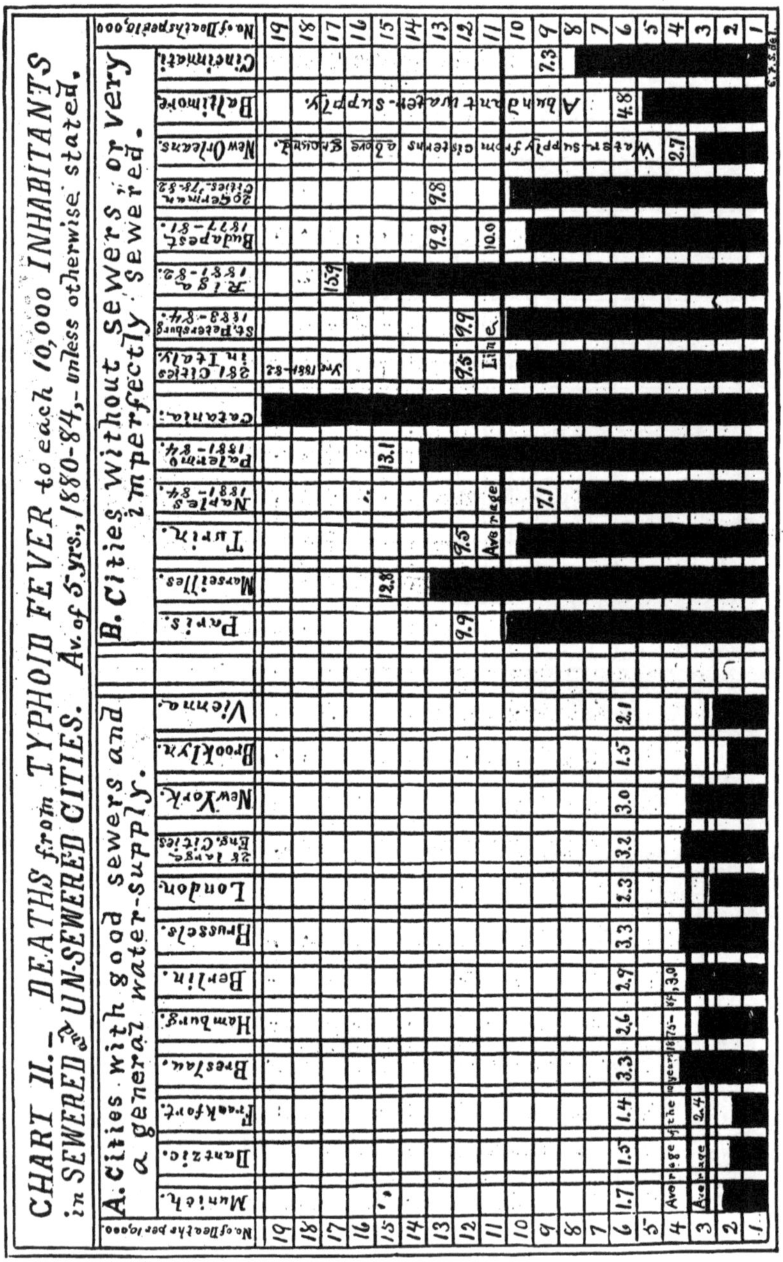

CHART II.— DEATHS from TYPHOID FEVER to each 10,000 INHABITANTS
in SEWERED and UN-SEWERED CITIES. Av. of 5 yrs., 1880-84,- unless otherwise stated.
A. Cities with good sewers and a general water-supply.
B. Cities without sewers; or very imperfectly sewered.
No. of Deaths per 10,000.
Munich.
Dantzic.
Frankfort.
Breslau.
Hamburg.
Berlin.
Brussels.
London.
25 large Eng. Cities.
New York.
Brooklyn.
Vienna.
Paris.
Marseilles.
Turin.
Naples 1881-84.
Palermo 1881-84.
Catania.
281 Cities in Italy.
St. Petersburg 1883-84.
Riga 1881-82.
Budapest 1877-81.
20 German Cities, '78-82.
New Orleans.
Baltimore.
Cincinnati.
Average of the 10 years 1875-84, 3.0
Average
Average Line
Water-supply from cisterns above ground.
Abundant water-supply.
1.7
1.5
1.4
3.3
2.6
2.9
3.3
2.3
3.2
3.0
1.5
2.1
2.4
9.9
12.8
9.5
7.1
13.1
9.5
9.9
15.9
10.0
9.2
9.8
2.7
4.8
7.3

of the disease are not taken. This ought to be generally known, and many more lives can be saved when all our people come to understand the facts.

In Michigan diphtheria causes about seventeen times as many deaths as smallpox does. I think that it is probably more contagious than smallpox, because the spread of diphtheria is not so easy to trace, and yet we know that diphtheria is contagious, because it is sometimes very easy to prove this, and to trace its mode of spread. Diphtheria seems to be more frequently spread by indirect means than smallpox is ; because if it were not, we ought to be able to trace the spread of diphtheria as easily as we do the spread of smallpox. But whether diphtheria is more or less contagious than smallpox, one important reason why we suffer so very much more mortality from diphtheria than from smallpox is the fact that for diphtheria we have no such preventive measure as vaccination.

Diphtheria is prevented by keeping away from where the disease is, and from everybody and everything that has been near the disease ; keeping away until everything has been disinfected. In order that this shall be possible, it is essential that every place where diphtheria is shall be promptly reported and plainly placarded. The law requires the local board of health to " give public notice of infected places," and to " use all possible care to prevent the spreading of the infection." Another law requires the health officer to " give public notice of infected places by placard on the premises, and otherwise if necessary." Common humanity requires of every person that he do his utmost to fulfill the letter and spirit of all such laws for the public safety against such a terrible disease as diphtheria.

The law was amended at the last session of the legislature, and its provisions should be generally known. Every householder, hotelkeeper, keeper of a boarding-house, or tenant is required to report to the local health authorities, diphtheria and any other disease dangerous to the public health, and whoever fails to do this is liable to a fine, and to imprisonment if the fine is not paid. Physicians are required to report, and if the physician reports the householder is excused from that duty. Health officers, unless otherwise ordered by the local board of health, must take prompt, thorough and efficient measures to stamp out the disease ; and if they neglect their specified duties they are liable to a fine, and to imprisonment if the fine is not paid.

But however good the laws may be, their execution depends upon the enlightened public sentiment of the locality, upon the people themselves, from whom the prompt notice should go to the local health officer, upon intelligent and faithful local officers who should perform duties which are of the highest importance to the people.

SCARLET FEVER.

Scarlet fever is a disease to be dreaded on account of the mortality which it causes, and also on account of the permanent injuries which result from it. Thus, as an instance, of 263 pupils in the Michigan School for the Deaf, at

Flint, during the years 1887–88, who became deaf since their birth, the loss of hearing of 16 per cent. is attributed to scarlet fever.* Of the 114 pupils in the Michigan State School for the Blind, at Lansing, during the two years 1887–88, who became blind since birth, 6.1 per cent. lost their sight from the effects of scarlet fever.†

In Michigan, scarlet fever causes about nine times as many deaths as smallpox does. The only *preventive* is to keep away from the disease, and to allow no person or article infected with the scarlet fever contagion to come near a person susceptible to that disease.

For its restriction, except that there is no vaccination, all the measures proper in the case of smallpox are proper in scarlet fever.

Inasmuch as scarlet fever causes nine times as many deaths as smallpox does, the importance of prompt notice to the health officer is at least nine times as great as it is in smallpox.

All the other measures should be promptly and thoroughly executed. I will not stop to give you details. They are published in our pamphlets here for distribution.

PRACTICAL RESULTS IN RESTRICTING SCARLET FEVER.

At the close of the year 1887, the statistics published by the State Department showed that the mortality from scarlet fever in Michigan had been reduced in the years when the measures recommended by the State board of health had been, to some extent, fulfilled, so that over 5,600 persons had lived who, under the old mortality rate, before the board began its work, would have prematurely died. This is an average saving of 400 lives per year—rather more than a life every day for fourteen years—saved from that dread disease, scarlet fever.

But we have other evidence than the mortality statistics showing the great saving of life which it is possible to have in Michigan through such measures for the restriction of scarlet fever as I have briefly outlined. The experience of the local health officers in restricting scarlet fever in this State is reported each year to the State Board of Health; and a compilation of these reports shows that in those outbreaks in which isolation and disinfection were neglected there were about five times as many cases and about five times as many deaths as in those outbreaks in which they were enforced.‡

This is about equivalent to saying that four-fifths of the cases and deaths from scarlet fever are known to be preventable through measures which we can describe in three words—*isolation and disinfection.*

PRACTICAL RESULTS IN RESTRICTING DIPHTHERIA.

While on the subject of the saving of life in Michigan, I may mention that the experience of the health officers in restricting diphtheria in this State is also reported each year to the State Board of Health, and the compilation of

---

* Eighteenth Biennial Report of the Board of Trustees of the Michigan School for the Deaf.
† Report of the Superintendent of Public Instruction, Michigan, 1888, pages 78–80.
‡ The evidence for one year, 1888, is shown in the diagram, page 455 of this journal.

Scarlet Fever in Michigan in 1888:-Exhibiting the average
numbers of cases and deaths per outbreaks- in those
outbreaks in which Isolation and Disinfection were
both Neglected; and in those outbreaks in which both
were Enforced. (Compiled in the office of the Secretary of the
State Board of Health, from reports made by local health officers.)

Scale for cases and deaths.	Isolation and Disinfection neglected. Average.			Isolation and Disinfection enforced. Average.	
	Cases.	Deaths.		Cases.	Deaths.
11	11.87				
10					
9					
8					
7					
6					
5					
4					
3					
2				2.22	
1					
0		.54			.08

these reports shows that 833 lives were saved and 4374 cases of sickness prevented from diphtheria in Michigan during the year 1886, and that in the year 1887 518 lives were saved and 2371 cases of sickness prevented ; during 1888 416 lives were saved and 3292 cases prevented.

Thus, during the three years 1886–1888 over ten thousand (10,037) cases were prevented and more than seventeen hundred (1767) lives were saved from diphtheria in Michigan. Or another way of stating this is to say that during the last three years the *known* saving of life in Michigan from diphtheria has averaged one and a half persons per day.

You may be interested to know the method of estimating the number of cases prevented and lives saved by means of isolation and disinfection. It is as follows : "Multiply the *whole number* of outbreaks by the average number of cases and deaths in the *neglected* outbreaks, and the product is the probable number of cases or deaths which would have occurred if *all* outbreaks had been neglected. Deduct from this number of cases the deaths which actually occurred, and the remainder is the indicated number of cases of sickness prevented or lives saved by the efforts made to restrict the disease.

As the local health officers report to the State Board of Health the number of cases and deaths in outbreaks of diphtheria, and also report just what was done (in each outbreak) to restrict the disease, we are thus supplied with the data necessary to learn the success which attends any line of action which is taken.*

PRACTICAL RESULTS IN RESTRICTING SMALLPOX.

The statistics collected and published by the Secretary of State of Michigan—taken in connection with the facts on record in the office of the State Board of Health—prove that in Michigan, through such measures as I have outlined, the mortality from smallpox has been reduced, and that if it had continued at the same rate as before the State Board of Health was established, more than one thousand five hundred persons in Michigan *would* have died from smallpox that have *not* died of that disease. This was true at the end of the year 1887, and since that time the mortality from smallpox in Michigan has not increased. The statistics now cover so many years that we think there can be no doubt of the reliability of their evidence.

The success which has already been achieved in dealing with scarlet fever, diphtheria and smallpox should encourage all to more thoroughly co-operate for the restriction of those diseases, and also to enter vigorously upon the work of restricting typhoid fever and consumption. The relative importance of these diseases can be seen by the diagram which is exhibited here.† I believe that one hundred lives per year have been saved from death from smallpox. The diagram is accurately drawn to scale, and correctly represents the relative mortality in Michigan from these important diseases which, we believe, are largely

---

* The diagram on page 457 of this journal exhibits graphically the experience in restricting diphtheria in Michigan in 1888.

† Printed on page 459 of this journal.

ISOLATION AND DISINFECTION RESTRICT DIPHTHERIA.

Diphtheria in Michigan in 1888:- Exhibiting the average numbers of cases and deaths per outbreak:- in those outbreaks in which Isolation and Disinfection were both Neglected; and in those outbreaks in which both were Enforced. (Compiled in the office of the Secretary of the State Board of Health, from reports made by local health officers.)

Scale for cases and Deaths.	Isolation and Disinfection neglected. Average.			Isolation and Disinfection enforced. Average.	
	Cases.	Deaths.		Cases.	Deaths.
15	15.50				
14					
13					
12					
11					
10					
9					
8					
7					
6					
5					
4					
3		2.38			
2				1.74	
1					.53
0					

preventable. You can see for yourselves the tremendous opportunity which there is for life-saving work for the restriction and prevention of the dangerous communicable diseases in Michigan. I do not see how one can have a better field or a nobler work, and I trust we shall all do what we can in this direction to forward the work. There is certainly room for all classes of workers, because

THIS SUBJECT INCLUDES ABOUT ALL THERE IS OF GREATEST IMPORTANCE IN SANITARY SCIENCE.

Let us glance at a few of the many ways in which progress can be made in this work :

1. Is it not true that the subject of "water supply" is of importance chiefly with reference to one or more of these five most dangerous diseases?

We may grant, if you please, that some deaths and sickness other than from these five diseases may result from impure drinking water, or if not actual deaths, uncomfortable sickness may result ; but we must all admit, with Prof. Clark, that "The most uncomfortable thing which can happen to a man is to die," and so the most important reason why we should labor for pure drinking water is to prevent death from that disease (due to impure water) which causes the most deaths. Briefly, we need a pure water supply chiefly to prevent deaths from typhoid fever, one of the five diseases which cause the most deaths in Michigan.

2. Is it not true that the subject of "ventilation" is of importance chiefly with reference to these five most dangerous diseases? We may admit that headache and many other discomforts may result from the breathing of bad air ; but that "most uncomfortable thing" death, which comes through lack of ventilation or bad ventilation, is, I believe, most frequently due to one of those same five diseases which cause most deaths in Michigan. Excepting typhoid fever, which itself has sometimes been caused by bad ventilation, or rather might have been prevented by good ventilation, all the other four diseases are most prevalent during or following the cold weather, that is, the season of the year when ventilation is the poorest. Every one of these diseases is believed to be caused by a specific particle, usually called a "germ." These particles, given off from the sick person, are now known to be liable to cause disease to be contracted somewhat in proportion to the number of them which gain entrance into the bodies of susceptible persons. Most of these germs get into our bodies by the way of the air passages. They go in with the air we breathe. The better the ventilation the less the danger of contracting each of these diseases to all persons who come into a room in which there is one of these diseases. Proper methods of ventilation are especially important for the restriction of consumption. This disease being most frequently spread by the dried germs which have been coughed up, spit upon the floor or handkerchief, become a part of the dust of the room, and, as such, breathed in and lodged in their favorite location, if all such dust can be prevented from rising into the nostrils or mouths of

DEATHS IN MICHIGAN, 1876-'87.

- CONSUMPTION.
- DIPHTHERIA.
- TYPHOID FEVER.
- SCARLET FEVER.
- WHOOPING-COUGH.
- MEASLES.
- SMALL-POX.

occupants of the room, much will be done to restrict consumption. It is, therefore, of extremely great consequence that all opera houses, school-houses, and other public assembly rooms shall have such a good system of ventilation that the current of all air in the room and the dust which it contains shall be downward and out at the floor level, and not upward from the floor into the nostrils of persons in the room.

Ventilation is of much importance with reference to this one greatest cause of deaths, that "great white plague" which is the cause of about one-eighth of all the deaths in Michigan. Ventilation is chiefly of importance with reference to those diseases which cause most deaths—the most dangerous communicable diseases.

3. Is it not true that "the hygiene of schools" should be chiefly concerned with those diseases which cause most deaths? The diseases which have been most considered as spread in schools in recent years at least, are: scarlet fever, diphtheria, measles, whooping-cough, etc. To these we should now add consumption, and probably pneumonia, and, by reason of the drinking water and perhaps by reason of the disposal of excreta in or near school houses, we may also add typhoid fever. This completes the list of the most dangerous communicable diseases.

4. Is it not true that "the disposal of excreta and waste" is of most importance with reference to those diseases which cause most deaths? Here, however, we come to a subject which is most closely related to that disease which has been partially excepted from relation to some of the other subjects; I refer to typhoid fever, that disease which annually causes in Michigan a thousand deaths and ten thousand cases of sickness, most of which we believe are preventable, chiefly through proper disposal of excreta and the obtaining of unpolluted water supplies.

5. Should not the "duties and compensation of the local health officer" relate chiefly to these dangerous communicable diseases? The State law says "yes;" and you may be surprised to know that the law does not directly confer upon the health officer power to abate any nuisance, but it contemplates vigorous action for the restriction of "diseases dangerous to the public health." But as that subject is to follow this immediately, I will not elaborate this thought.

6. Should not the "ideal summer resort" be most secure from those most dangerous communicable diseases?

7. I believe I have mentioned every theme upon the programme of this convention, except the opening addresses, the prayer and the music, and I maintain that all these were good; but I am going to claim, or at least to ask you to admit that, as far as relates to this world, their utility relates chiefly to the extent to which they tended to aid progress in restricting and preventing the dangerous communicable diseases, those diseases which cause most deaths in Michigan, and which, named in the order of their importance, are: consumption, diphtheria, pneumonia, typhoid fever, and scarlet fever.

The Relation of the Church to Sanitation.*

BY REV. THOMAS R. BEEBER,

Pastor First Presbyterian Church, Norristown, Pa.

The wise man says :

"A prudent man foreseeth the evil and hideth himself; But the simple pass on and are punished."—Prov. xxii, 3.

The church is an assembly of Christians. The relation of the church to sanitation is therefore the relation of Christians.

A Christian is a man who accepts the principles of the Bible as the law of his life. A sanitarian is a man who aims to keep the body in health by perfecting its physical conditions.

Our question therefore comes to this : What is the relation between the Christian and the sanitarian ?

In the light of Egyptian history, it is too much to say that Moses was the first sanitary legislator.

In the light of Greek and Roman history, of the writings of Hippocratés, and the work of the civil engineers of the Eternal City, it is also too much to say that Moses was the inspiring leader of all sanitarians since his time.

But I think this can be demonstrated : That a Christian ought to be a sanitarian. He ought to be at least where an obedient Jew was 1500 years before Christ.

The principles of the Word of God will make the Christian a sanitarian. Take the reverence for the body that the Bible emphasizes.

The emphasis on this truth by the Old Testament is seen in its ceremonial code for the cleansing of eleven kinds of impurity, in its things allowed and forbidden in men's diet, and in the remarkable fact that so long as the people obeyed they were the longest-lived nation of the past.

The New Testament inherits the same emphasis.

The martyr father of Origin used to kiss the breast of his sleeping child, saying with the profoundest reverence, "It is the temple of the Holy Ghost." The heart of Christianity was in the act, for the sacredness of the body is one of its leading teachings.

While one school of contemporary philosophy was teaching that the body had no value, was to be pinched by voluntary fastings, bruised by whips and macerated by self-inflicted penances, and that the best men treated these things with indifference ; and while another held that the body was to be put in the first place, and its needs to be met at all hazards, and its motto, "Let us eat, drink and be merry, for to-morrow we die," Christianity was teaching that the body was to be held in honor and reverence, that men were to provide things needful for the body, not neglecting it with the Colossians, nor dishonoring it with the Romans ; that the body was for the Lord, and the Lord for the

---

*Read before the State Sanitary Convention at Norristown.

body; that the body was the temple of the Holy Ghost; that men were to glorify God in their bodies, were to present them a living sacrifice; that the body of man was a holy and a sacred thing, and made forever hallowed by this: That God Himself condescended to take upon Him the form of a servant and to be made in the likeness of men.

This is the principle. Now for its application.

If the bodies are so sacredly to be used, to be held in such reverence, the inference is clear and direct that every Christian man will utilize every well-approved means to keep these bodies clean, pure and strong, and at their highest range of physical life. No means are better adapted to this end than pure air and in great abundance, pure water applied externally and internally, and digestible food well cooked.

These are the well-recognized sanitary forces to-day. And since sanitation means the setting in motion of all these forces, the enlightened Christian will certainly be a sanitarian. His full reception of the principle of the sacredness of the human body will make him such. It must. There is no other issue.

A second principle that makes the Christian a sanitarian. It is this: The following of the example of his Lord.

Let the Christian think of his Lord's acts of healing. See how He here touched the leper, and there the blind man; here saying to the palsied man, "Arise and walk," and there to the devils possessing men and tearing children, "Come forth;" and how, wherever he went, he healed all that were sick of whatsoever disease they had.

And what will follow? This that has followed. The medical missionary will walk among the diseased and suffering heathen, and put upon them the touch of healing. And the Christian at home will have the same spirit. He will yield to the inspiration of his Lord's example, and will take his stand for all things that heal the sick and cure the diseased. And this principle will carry him on from the effort to heal to the effort to prevent sickness. And hence, once show to the Christian that such and such conditions of life forestall disease, and he stands for those conditions; that is, he becomes a sanitarian. He must. Again, the principle that makes him a healer makes him a preventer of disease.

Another principle makes the Christian a sanitarian. It is this: The value of human life that the word emphasizes. In all clearness the Bible teaches that life is a sacred thing; that no man has a right to kill his brother or himself. "The Eternal has fixed His canon against self-slaughter." It condemns murder of all kinds and by all methods, whether by the poison of arsenic or the poison of the death-dealing germs that abound in the foul air, foul water and unwholesome food.

Saul, Ahitophel and Judas committed suicide by the sword and the rope. But not a whit more are they suicides than the man who knowingly puts himself in contact with the life-destroying conditions of pestilential swamps, of imperfect sewage, or of the fetid and deadly stench of· filthy alleys, rotting garbage and the offal of slaughter houses.

Hence, show the Christian such facts as these : That in Europe, in four years of the Fourteenth Century, the black death, springing from the filthy conditions of life, destroyed 40,000,000 people, and that now, by sanitary laws, this appalling plague has been banished from the continent ; that in 1852, in Munich, the death rate from typhoid fever was 24 for every 10,000, and that since the establishment of the hygienic laboratory there, and the sanitary legislation resulting, the death rate from this cause has steadily decreased until, in 1884, it was only a little over 1 for every 10,000 ; that in England 120,000 deaths occur annually that might have been prevented, and 1,200,000 cases of preventable sicknesses occur ; that the death rate in the Peabody buildings of London is 16 per 1000, and in the immediate vicinity it is over 30 per 1000 ; that in Michigan it is estimated that one-half of the persons who sicken and die annually might have been kept in health by proper sanitary precautions ; that in New York city the mortality is 55 per 1000, when, if fitting sanitary conditions were created, it would be but 15 out of 1000, and that half the sicknesses annually come from filth ; and that sanitary laws, strictly enforced, would practically add one-third to the population of any place by lengthening out the years one-third. Show these and similar educating facts to the Christian, and he will first be astounded and horrified, and then he will set himself to establish the forces that prevent this awful and wicked degradation and waste of human life. He becomes a sanitarian. He is driven to this position by Christianity's teaching of the sacredness and worth of human life.

Another principle of the word makes a Christian a sanitarian. He is under the most sacred obligation to consider the well-being of his fellow man, physical as well as spiritual. He is his brother's keeper. Strong, he ought to bear the infirmities of the weak. "Noblesse oblige" is his law. He is to love his neighbor as himself. He is under the Golden Rule.

The Christian in the first centuries felt this responsibility and acted upon it.

St. Basil builds a hospital at Caesarea in the Fourth Century.

St. Cyprian, at Carthage, when in the midst of the plague the heathen were casting out their dead to rot in the streets, is organizing what is practically a sanitary commission.

The Christian of to-day feels the same pressure in other than sanitary directions. He is building hospitals and establishing eleemosynary institutions of all kinds. And the same principle will carry him on to the standpoint of a sanitarian. Once show to him that the poison of unsanitary conditions is affecting the health and destroying the life of his brother, and this principle of responsibility for his fellow-man's best interests will make him a sanitarian. The moment he sees that disease and death lurk in the drain or cesspool or garbage barrel he will strive to abolish these things. And as he does it for himself the Golden Rule will make him do it for others. The man's activity will be exactly proportioned to his knowledge.

Further, the peculiar aim of the Christian will make him a sanitarian.

The aim is to found and build up the Christian life in the soul. There is the most intimate and interdependent relation between the body and the soul. And one of the greatest hindrances to effective Christian work among the tenement population of our large cities is the filthy and disease-breeding conditions of their lives.

An earnest student of this problem of carrying the Gospel to the masses, Prof. Blackie, of Edinburgh, tells us that "heathenism is caused and aggravated by crowded dwellings, want of ventilation and the means of cleanliness, by want of training in domestic economy, and generally by habits of thriftlessness and untidiness. And those who are concerned for the regeneration of these lapsed classes cannot but seek to assail these social evils, or to have them lessened by means of weapons which the civil authorities are able to wield against them."

And every Christian who seeks to evangelize the people surrounded by these unsanitary conditions must stand with Prof. Blackie, and see that they are in the way of the efficient action of the moral and spiritual forces he is trying to bring to bear, and must also see the necessity of removing them if his aim is to be reached, and a symmetrical Christian life to be built up.

In one word, the well-informed and wisely-working Christian will recognize the interdependence of soul and body, and feel that he influences the most the first when he surrounds the second with the best possible conditions of life. He will say with Bishop Stevens, of the Episcopal Church : "Public morals are so interlaced with the general principles of sanitation, are so akin to purity of life, that whatever enlightens and instructs the people on the matter of public health will indirectly advance the cause of pure and undefiled religion before God, and in the light of men." He will say with Bishop Mallalieu, of the Methodist Episcopal Church : "One of the most important functions of Christianity in the immediate future will be to prevent disease."

And he will catch the meaning of this experience of a sanitarian minister : "Twice of late have I been called to spiritually medicate poor souls who fancied that they had committed the sin against the Holy Ghost, but whom two weeks of careful diet, rest and good medical care released from the horror of that unpardonable sin."

The precedents of Christianity in these days make a Christian logically a sanitarian.

The Christian is necessarily a philanthropist. Prof. Ely, of Johns Hopkins University, says : "A man who claims to be a Christian and is not at the same time a philanthropist is a hypocrite and a liar."

Now, Christian philanthropy may be remedial or it may be preventive in its action. Preventive philanthropy is gaining great prominence. It is establishing reform schools whose methods and influence are directed to prevent incorrigible children from becoming criminals. It is legislating against drunkenness by preventing the sale of liquors to minors. It is establishing school laws to prevent the children from growing up in ignorance ; factory laws to prevent children from being dwarfed and diseased as they grow up from long hours and unsuitable labors. And other laws to compel manufacturers to fence in dangerous machinery, and railroad companies to use every means to prevent the loss of life.

I need not stop to specify other preventive measures of Christian philanthropy. The point is this. The principle that originates these will originate all others that are needed. The past development of the principle commits the Christian to stand for the same preventive measures in the matter of sanitation. Once convince a Christian of the damage done by unsanitary conditions, and every precedent will make him a sanitarian.

The word of "Ecce Homo" will stand: "No man who loves his kind can in these days rest content with waiting as a servant upon human misery, when it is in so many cases possible to anticipate and avert it. Prevention is better than cure, and it is now clear to all that a large part of human suffering is preventable by improved social arrangements. Charity will now fix upon this enterprise as greater, more widely and permanently beneficial, and therefore more Christian than the other. When the sick man has been visited, modern charity will go on to consider the causes of his malady. What noxious influences besetting his life, what contempt of the laws of health in his diet and habits may have caused it, and then to inquire whether others incur the same dangers and may be warned in time." Ecce Homo, 211, 212.

And now lastly. The Christian's leading examples to-day make him a sanitarian.

The leaders of Christian progress are chosen of the Lord to a certain work. They stand alone in advance of their generation.

But the next generation comes up to where they stood.

The leaders of Christian philanthropy are calling the Christian to-day to sanitary effort.

John Howard, the founder of modern philanthropy, calls. His sanitary work at Cardington changes it from the abode of disease and death from its sourroundings, to one of the healthiest villages in England.

William Wilberforce calls. Nearly a hundred years ago he founded a "society for bettering the conditions of the poor," whose ruling aims were the prevention of sickness, poverty and suffering of all kinds.

Sydney Smith repeats the call.

Charles Kingsley also. A very prince in his advocacy of sanitary reform, and a brave battler with the diphtheritic scourge that smote his little village of Eversley, both curing the disease and removing the causes.

These are the men who, with their compeers, Arnold, of Rugby, Robertson, of Brighton, and Augustus Hare and Sir John Chadwick, and a host of others, found England a country where 30,000 or 40,000 people died annually from causes that might have been removed. And who, by introducing the forces, moral, legislative and personal, that removed the dead from the dwellings of the living, drained the cities, supplied pure water in copious abundance, tore down the old tenements and built new ones, lessened epidemics, increased the duration of human life, and made their native land, after Sweden and Denmark, the healthiest spot in Europe.

George Peabody calls. Giver of a million for the Peabody tenements in London. Florence Nightingale from Constantinople, and Agnes Jones from Liverpool.

And the calls of all these Christian philanthropists are the calls of the leaders. They are the planting of the colors on the line where, sooner or later, all Christians will take their stand. Their inspiring examples make the Christian a sanitarian. They emphasize the word of Loring Brace in his " Gesta Christi :" . " Reduced mortality from pestilence is due to pure religion begetting sanitary progress."

I conclude. The Christian is under obligation to be a sanitarian, from the principles of Christianity, from its aims, from its history and from its inspiring leaders in preventive philanthropy. There is but one thing he needs—education.

By educating the Christian conscience, you have in the past made him an enemy of the lottery, of slavery, polygamy, of gambling and liquor selling.

Educate the conscience of the Christian to-day, and you will have an enemy of foul air and foul water, and a supporter of all sanitary forces and laws.

Educate the Christian and you will find him saying, with one of our profoundest students of social science, and in the deepest reverence : " It is as holy a work to lead a crusade against filth, vice and disease in the slums, and to seek the abolition of disgraceful tenement houses in American cities, as it is to send missionaries to the heathen."

Ocular Hygiene in Myopia or Nearsightedness.

BY J. WALTER PARK, M.D.,

Of Harrisburg, Pa.,

Late Clinical Assi·tant Royal London Ophthalmic Hospital, London, Eng.

As this article is not intended for the specialist in ophthalmology, but for the general practitioner in medicine and for the public in general, I will confine myself to as few professional technicalities as possible, in order that all who may read it will readily understand. It is a visible fact that myopia, or nearsightedness, is daily increasing to such an alarming extent that it is an urgent necessity to inaugurate certain measures for its prevention. This subject is now attracting the attention of the public in general throughout America and Europe, and its prevalence in the two great continents is such as to demand compulsory laws as regards the construction and illumination, regulation of studies, hours of work, etc., in the various schools, colleges and manufacturing establishments, with a view of decreasing the percentage of myopic people.

A definition of the term myopia may be of aid to a great many readers who may not understand its meaning, and will further aid them to fully comprehend what is meant when I speak upon its causes and preventive treatment.

Myopia is that state of refraction of the eye where the retina is situated behind its principal focus. Its optical axis is elongated, due to a lengthening of the antero-posterior diameter of the eyeball. Very frequently this elongation of the optical axis is accompanied by a backward protrusion of the coats of the eye, in the region of the optic nerve entrance, and a high degree of myopia must follow. These results frequently follow where the eyes have been put upon a long and continuous strain at near work.

Hyperopic, or farsighted people often become myopic, following a long and continuous strain upon their eyes at near work. A few statistics upon this subject seem to confirm what I have just stated. According to Erisman,

Scholars who study 2 hours per day, 17 per cent. are myopic.
      "   "   " 4   "   " 29   "   "   "
      "   "   " 6   "   " 40   "   "   "

Tschering finds that in comparing professional men with merchants, mechanics, day laborers, etc., the highest percentage (32.38), exists among the former. Burschuck finds that children who go to school and work in knitting mills at the same time, that 5.4 per cent. more of them are myopic than an equal number who go to school, but do not work in the mills. It is also an established fact that convergence of the visual angle causes a great pressure upon the eyeball through the external and internal recti and inferior oblique muscles, thereby lengthening the antero-posterior diameter of the eyeball, and myopia is the result. The question is frequently asked, Why is it that so few watchmakers are myopic, whilst it exists to about 45 per cent. in lithographers? This query is readily answered. Watchmakers fix upon their work with one eye mostly, and then generally through a magnifying lens, whilst lithographers fix with both eyes, and thereby require constant and continuous convergence ; this combined with a stooping forward position of the head and body causes an active and passive congestion of the eyes, and nearsightedness necessarily must follow.

M. Motais, in making his report to the Academy of Medicine of Paris, in November, 1889, says that the numerous researches made in the schools of Germany and Switzerland have demonstrated the dangerous influence of excessive study upon vision to an alarming extent, and to be sure upon the subject, he made an examination of 5000 scholars in the French colleges and lyceums, and came to the following conclusions : In rhetoric and philosophy classes of the ordinary colleges and lyceums he found 46 per cent. of the pupils myopic. In Germany there were 57 per cent., and in Switzerland 50 per cent. in similar classes. In the lowest grade classes he found no myopia ; in third grade classes 17 per cent., and in the same grade of philosophy classes 35 per cent.

Three-fourths of the myopes examined showed serious complications. Myopia is a serious question throughout France, on account of its army rules and regulations, which forbids any of its officers or privates wearing eyeglasses or spectacles. Ocular hygiene is there becoming compulsory.

Preventive Treatment.—It is to close eyework, small size of objects, type and insufficient illumination that I attach the most importance in the preventive treatment of myopia. The infant departments of all schools should be supplied with books having large, coarse letters printed upon yellowish-tinted paper. Their blackboard exercises should all be in large letters. They should be compelled to write a large hand and use heavy strokes in forming their letters. Drawing, fine sewing, crochetting, knitting work, etc., should not be taught until after the years of childhood have elapsed. They should be compelled to sit in an erect position. School desks should be so constructed as to fit the back of the child, and not the child's back the desk. The object looked at, or work to be done, should be directly in front of the eyes and at an angle of about forty-five degrees ; hence the importance of not sitting too low in comparison to the object looked at. All work requiring close observation, such as reading fine print, all kinds of fine fancy work, worked by hand or machine, etc., should not be continued for a longer period than a few hours at a time before changing it to some other playful or light employment. Students working hard all day trying to master some difficult problem which requires a constant concentration of their eyes upon the work engaged in should not then take up some novel as a recreation, but should adopt some exercise which will give rest and relief to their eyes. When reading, myopic people should invariably cast their eyes from their book or paper to some other object at least every twenty or thirty minutes, thereby relieving the convergence, intense strain and temporary congestion of the eyes, and thus lessening the tendency of stretching the several coats of the eyes, which is otherwise sure to follow if excessively indulged in. They should always be advised by their family physicians not to select occupations or professions which have a tendency to increase their myopia. Illumination is another great factor to be considered in the prevention of near-sightedness. Of all the various methods there are none that equal the light of the sun, and all the work of myopes should be done by daylight as much as possible. All flickering lights should be avoided to read or do work by. The steady light of an Argand gas burner is preferable to most others. According to ''Landolt,'' the non-flickering electric light is nearer like the rays of the sun in brightness than any others. The intensity of illumination should also be regulated so as to exclude all excessive rays of bright light by different colored glass suitable for different-colored lights ; as, for example, daylight being a bright light, smoked or colored glass lessens its intensity. Blue glass absorbs all red, yellow and orange rays. All objects should be well defined on suitable backgrounds. There would be fewer dressmakers complain of their eyes if they were allowed to use white thread on black goods, and *vice versa*. All typographical matter should be of such a size as not to be fatiguing to the eyes. All near-sighted people should never do straining work in a stooped position, or any physical exercise which has a tendency to produce a strain upon the eyes. Myopia should be corrected as soon as detected, by properly-adjusted glasses. Too great stress cannot be laid upon their proper adjustment, and should only be entrusted to those skilled in their profession. Glasses properly fitted generally prevent any further progress of myopia, but when improperly fitted they generally produce more myopia, and very often progressive malignant myopia is the result. The last-named form of near-sightedness requires very strict hygienic treatment, and should only be entrusted to the care of skilled oculists. They should be regularly, carefully and frequently examined, and should be advised as to what and what not to do in the use of their eyes in their daily work; for preventive measures in such a serious disease are of the utmost importance. This subject is of such vast importance that laws should be enacted requiring compulsory examination and treatment of all pupils in schools, and the working class of people employed in the various manufacturing establishments requiring fine work done, such as silk mills, knitting factories, etc. By the observance of at least a few of my remarks, a great amount of good will result upon one of the most important and alarming ocular subjects of the day, and I hope the time is not far distant when someone will present to our legislatures such preventive measures for them to consider which, when passed and carried into effect, will at least lessen this constantly-increasing near-sightedness among the American people.

700 N. Third Street.

The Harmonious Development of the Physical with the Mental Powers.*

BY C. E. EHINGER, M.D.,

Of Norristown, Pa.

THE moral and intellectual nature of man has, from the earliest civilization been considered the chief object of training and development; and while we may seriously question the methods sometimes employed and results obtained, it is impossible to gainsay the interest and thought bestowed upon the problems involved in the attainment of intellectual vigor and moral rectitude.

In the days of simpler living, the question of the harmonious development of mind and body did not, from the condition of things, present itself, or at least with the same urgency, as it does to-day. The occupations, habits and environments of our forefathers were such as to make the question one of minor importance. But the ushering in of this new era of telegraph and rail-

---

* Read before the State Sanitary Convention at Norristown.

way, the increase of urban inhabitants, more intense competition, the eager scramble after wealth and position, with the high brain tension and general nervous strain accompanying, has wrought a wondrous change, and developed in America a nervous type of people presenting peculiarities quite unique in history.

Within the last decade so much has been said upon these phases of American character that it seems quite unnecessary to dwell upon them at length. Suffice it to say that among the competent observers it seems to be almost universally conceded that the present high-pressure mode of life, in connection with the improper or over-education of our youth, is largely responsible for this unfortunate state of affairs.

I am aware that it seems to be rather the fashion of the day to decry our educational methods, and that it is equally the fashion in certain quarters to hold up the typical American as a lamentable wreck and fearful example of what misguided energy and mistaken ideas of success mean. I confess that an extended and exclusive study of the evils of our educational methods and the darker side of our social and commercial life presents a most startling picture, and one calculated at first sight to give anything but an encouraging view of our future. I do not wish, however, to array myself with that already too numerous class of criticizing malcontents and evil prophets who so delight in dwelling upon the weaker spots in our social fabric, and must at the outset disclaim all desire to be sensational in my remarks.

Sir William Grove justly remarks, "that civilization begins by supplying wants and ends in creating them, and each new supply for the newly-created want begets other wants, and so on."

We congratulate ourselves upon the prodigious strides which we have made during the present century, and point with pardonable pride to the almost miraculous achievements wrought by means of the successful utilization of steam and electricity ; but we seem to forget that these changed conditions, this supplying of wants, has induced others which we have not as yet sufficiently regarded.

With the higher cerebral development, more finely organized nervous systems, there necessarily follows greater danger of disturbance of the delicately adjusted organism, and as a result a whole list of new maladies confront us that demand relief. Without asserting that the intellectual and moral sides of us have been given all the attention they should, it is, at least, not saying too much to declare that the third principle in this great triune which constitutes the human being has received proportionately less attention, and is at present the weak member.

To what extent these evils are to be accounted for by climatic influences I am not prepared to state. Nor do I believe it possible for anyone to answer with certainty, though there seem to be numerous and excellent reasons for supposing this to be a potent factor in the case. S. Wier Mitchell, in his admirable little treatise, "Wear and Tear," was, I believe, one of the first to call attention to these points. In the first edition of his work, published in 1871, he dwelt at some length upon this matter of our climatic peculiarities, and insisted that it accounted for much of the so-called "American nervousness." In the fifth edition, published fifteen years later, he found no reason to change these views, but on the contrary had seen much to strengthen his belief. While more extended observation is necessary to give full credence to this theory, we find even now much to confirm it, and believe it is by no means one of the least factors in the problem, though it is, perhaps, the only one which is entirely beyond our control. Still, a general recognition of this fact might do much to alter our methods of living, and so induce in the best manner to adjust ourselves to the existing conditions.

A fitting prelude to what is to follow may be the quotation of a paragraph from Dr. Mitchell's little treatise explanatory of his title : "Wear," he says, "is a natural and legitimate result of lawful use, and is what we all have to put up with as the result of years of activity of brain and body. Tear is another matter : it comes of hard or evil use of body or engine, of putting things to wrong purposes, using a chisel for a screwdriver, a penknife for a gimlet. Long strain or a sudden demand of strength from weakness causes tear; wear comes of use ; tear of abuse."

It is just this "putting things to wrong purposes" which has wrought such havoc with the mental and physical well-being of our American people. The boundless opportunities, the unfettered customs and climatic stimulus have made America and Americans the wonder of the world ; but this rapid and resistless march has only been made at great sacrifice, and the time has arrived when it behooves us to slacken our pace and count well the cost of such advance in the future.

The apparently disproportionate increase of nervous affections among Americans makes the subject of the "harmonious development of the physical with the mental powers" one of peculiar interest and paramount importance. To say that nervous diseases are on the increase is but equivalent to saying that we are degenerating physically ; and that one side of us is being overused, exhausted and perverted to such a degree that Dame Nature sounds a warning note with no uncertain voice.

Nervous exhaustion, hysteria, insanity, chorea, epilepsy, heart failure and kindred affections tell the story only too plainly. But where shall we begin to correct the evils, and what is the remedy ? The question is one of such vital moment that to attempt to answer without the most searching inquiry and profound thought seems but a presumption. Broadly speaking, the answer lies in the one word "education." Such generalisation however, signifies but little, therefore to be a trifle more specific, there seems reason to believe that the prefixing to this great term of the adjectives "judicious physical" would be contributing a suggestion worthy of trial. Since the physical is prior in order of development, reason would seem to demand that we grant it the foremost place in education.

A suggestive writer has said : "The first requisite to success in life is to be a good animal," and Herbert Spencer pithily adds, "and to be a nation of good animals is the first condition of national prosperity." How to become "a good animal" is clearly a question which greatly concerns the American of the future. If we are to remedy the evils noticed, arrest the tendency to physical deterioration, we must look to this "first condition of national prosperity." In the words of Dr. Nathan Allen, this will be : "When our educators become thoroughly convinced that physical development as a part of education is an absolute necessity—that a strict observance of the laws of physiology and hygiene is indispensable to the highest mental culture—then we shall have vital and radical changes in our educational system. The brain will not be cultivated so much at the expense of the body, neither will the nervous temperament be so unduly developed in proportion to other parts of the system, often bringing on a train of neuralgic diseases and exposing the individual to the most intense suffering which all the advantages of mental culture fail not infrequently to compensate. . . . . . The whole system of education, especially in early life, must be based more and more upon the systematic training and development of the body. . . . . . Then, in all matters pertaining to mental improvement, to the progress of society, to every phase in civilization and the various developments of Christianity; the sanitation of the body and of the mind must be paramount to every thing else."

The powers of the human system must find expression through two great channels, the muscles and the nerves ; and in proportion as these mediums are perfectly developed and harmoniously related is our power enhanced or retarded. Perfect adjustment, the even balance of the co-ordinate functions of nervous and muscular systems is what we term health ; any deviation from this balance we characterize as disease. The interference with or preponderance of either nervous or muscular power results in abnormal sensations in disease. The demands of modern life place undue stress upon the nervous energies, and we habitually disregard that proper adjustment so essential to growth and perfect nutrition. The interdependence of mind and body seems not to be recognized, or if recognized almost wholly disregarded. It is strange, notwithstanding what has been said and written on the harmonious development of mind and body, from the time of Pluto to the present day, that even now in practice and the course of ordinary thought, we persist in considering mind and body as independent principles, not answerable to the same laws, and in a measure antagonistic in their nature and development. Our literature is overflowing with maxims concerning the maintenance of health, such as the often quoted one : "A sound mind in a sound body." The final injunction of departing friends to "Take good care of yourself," is but a popular attestation of at least a superficial knowledge of the importance of a healthy mind and body. But our disregard of these maxims is as total as maxims are numerous. The preservation of health, hygiene, we have known but as a name. Listen to what that eminent authority, Dr. Parkes, has to say of it : "Taking the word hygiene in the largest sense, it signifies rules for perfect culture of mind and body. It is impossible to dissociate the two. The body is affected by every mental or moral action ; the mind is profoundly influenced by bodily conditions. For a perfect system of hygiene we must train the body, the intellect, and the moral faculties in a perfect and balanced order." On the fatal tendency of this prevailing evil of looking upon man as a two-fold nature, the components of which are in constant antagonism, let me quote the pregnant words of that greatest of physical educators, Archibald Maclaren : " For there is no error more profound or productive of more evil than that which views the bodily and the mental powers as antithetical and opposed, and which imagines that the culture of the one must be made at the expense of the other. The truth is precisely the reverse. . . . . . Mind and body should be viewed as the two fitting halves of a perfect whole, designed in true accord mutually to sustain and support each other, and each worthy of our unwearied care and unstinted attention, to be given with a fuller faith and more reverent trust than they have who would argue that He who united us in our two-fold nature made them incompatible, inharmonious, opposed. No, no ! even blind and blundering man does not yoke two oxen together to pull against each other. Mind and body can pull well together in the same team if the burden be fairly adjusted. . . . . They seek to sever what were bound together in the very planning, if one may so speak on such a subject of a living man ; they disunite them and complain that the dissevered halves are of unequal value ; they take the one and cultivate it exclusively, and neglect the other exclusively, and then make comparisons between them ; forgetting that their fitness, each for the other, lay in the fair nurture of both, and in their mutual cultivation."

The opinion of competent authorities on the value and need of physical training is well summed up by Dr. Hartwell, of Johns Hopkins University, in the following words : " It seems to me evident that muscular exercise deserves more attention than educators in this country have ever been willing to give it, and that when properly chosen, regulated and guided, it makes a boy into a better man, in many respects, than his father was, and enables him to transmit to his progeny a veritable aptitude for better thoughts and actions. Herein lies the power of the race for self-improvement, and the evolution of a higher type of man upon the earth."

Physical educators, specialists in various branches, and intelligent people generally, who have taken the time, and had even moderate advantages for experiment and investigation, are fully awake to the necessity of introducing some rational system of physical culture into our schools. But school authorities seem slow to appreciate its importance, and where the subject is given any consideration it is usually dismissed on the score of cost. The most progressive and intelligent of our educators show a disposition to accept the verdict of sanitarians that the lighting, ventilation and drainage of school buildings *must be the best regardless of cost*, and that in the end the expense is insignificant as compared with the incalculable saving in sickness and loss of life. Now let them devote a little attention to this other phase of sanitation, and in a few generations we will cease to deserve the oft-repeated saying that we are a nation of dyspeptics and neurasthenics.

The really strange thing about this matter of physical culture is that it should require any argument to demonstrate its need and immense value when properly employed, and the wonder is still greater that it should need any defence among intelligent people. Yet its introduction is most frequently opposed with a bitterness quite surpassing comprehension. The consensus of opinion of those who have seen it fairly tested, and among the abler members of the medical profession, is so overwhelmingly in its favor as to make its tardy introduction seem well-nigh incredible. The abuse of gymnastics and athletics is too frequently brought forward as an argument against physical culture, but this is on a par with the railings of some misguided persons against the church because it is sometimes used for worldly or unworthy ends.

I do not believe there is to-day in America a single prominent teacher of physical education who is not combating with all his power the abuses which have crept into gymnastics and athletics, and discouraging the tendency to specialism and professionalism. Let any one read the papers annually presented before the American Association for the Advancement of Physical Education, or those presented at the recent Physical Training Conference, at Boston, and then judge. Nothing will give a better idea of the character of the men and women who are devoting their life's work to this "New Profession," and of the work they are endeavoring to do, than a careful perusal of the many scholarly and practical papers presented at these meetings.

But there is another side to the subject which is well worthy of serious attention, and which has not received a tithe of the consideration it deserves. The educational value of physical culture—aside from mere muscular development—has not been appreciated. To set the point clearly before you, let me quote a little from an address delivered at Berlin, in 1881, by the eminent physiologist, Dubois Raymond. He says: "By exercise we usually understand the frequent repetition, seconded by the aid of the mind, of some more or less complex action of the body, for the purpose of attaining perfection in that exercise, or, it may be, the exercise of the mind alone. In physiological text-books we generally seek in vain for information upon exercise, and if any is vouchsafed at all, it is with regard to bodily exercises, and these are considered solely as exercises of the muscular system. Now, it is of course true that for such exercises as gymnastics, fencing, swimming, riding, dancing, skating, etc., a certain degree of muscular force is requisite, but we may very well imagine an individual with muscles like the Farnese Hercules, and yet unable to either stand or walk. This we see when we deprive him of the power of regulating and co-ordinating his movements, by giving him chloroform or making him drunk. It is plain, therefore, that every motion of the body depends, not so much upon the force of the contractions of the muscles, as upon the harmony of their action. . . . Since the nerves are merely organs for the conduction of impulses originating in the motor cells, it follows that the actual mechanism of every complex motion must have its seat in the central nervous system. . , . All species of bodily exercises, therefore, are not simply muscular gymnastics, but nerve gymnastics, too.''

To again quote Dr. Hartwell: ''The functional improvement of the nervous mechanism which represents any movement, whether it be simple or complicated, reflex, automatic or voluntary, is the most important effect of muscular exercises; or, in other words, muscular training which fails to develop brain power falls short of its aim.''

We seem to forget that the mind acts through a material organ; that all mental processes depend upon the harmonious development and perfect integrity of the brain. We recognize in a loose way that the exercise of the brain involved in education results in strengthening and amplifying the mental powers; in short, in growth of the brain. Every well-informed person has learned that the brain in civilized races is larger and more perfectly developed than in savage races. It is less obvious, however, or at least more generally overlooked, that the brain is not the exclusive seat of intellection, or perhaps better, that it is not occupied solely or mainly with thought, volition and the emotions. It is in reality as indispensable an organ for the performance of voluntary movements as for the more purely intellectual processes. Every movement—not reflex—brings it into action.

The influence of sensory and muscular impressions upon the brain is so great that it demands some special attention. Different sensations are received, interpreted and recorded in different portions of the brain. This greatest of the nerve centres may be likened to a collection of organs rather than a single one. Every portion, or each subordinate organ, must receive its proper development, or failing to, affects the general symmetry. Not only does it influence the portion neglected, but indirectly the whole brain by reacting injuriously upon the other portions.

Every exercise of a muscle reacts upon the nerves and nerve centres with which it is in connection, producing a change in the cells and fibres. Each repetition of such a movement increases the facility for originating and transmitting stimuli. While such changes are not visible to the eye, as in the case of the muscle, it is highly probable—yes, almost certain—that the changes which take place in the grey matter of the brain, for the purpose of inducing muscular action, influence the nutrition of the portion of the brain involved quite as markedly as contraction of the muscle influences its growth.

Luys and other observers have recorded observations which seem clearly to substantiate the foregoing conclusions. It has been found that the amputation of a limb causes certain parts of the grey matter of the brain to gradually undergo atrophy, and that the cessation or diminution of certain movements also cause the same result in those centres which control the movements. It seems, therefore, naturally to follow that portions of the brain which control voluntary movements are developed just as certainly by muscular action as other portions of the brain which preside over the intellectual operations are by mental exercise.

We may sum up those conclusions in the physiological law that "function makes structure," and the corollary added by a recent writer, "the cessation of function leads to the disappearance of the structure."

There is a striking analogy between the muscular and mental work ; the same physiological laws govern nutrition and activity of both muscular and nervous tissue. Every voluntary bodily exercise involves a two-fold expenditure of force ; that of the muscle in contracting, and that of the brain in animating the contraction, thus warranting the saying that "the brain works when the body acts."

Who can fail to see the important bearing which the application of the advanced but generally recognized principles of physiology may have on our educational methods. The appreciation of these truths, perhaps empirically at first, accounts for the increased popularity of object teaching, the kindergarten and manual training systems. It is the application of the same principles in slightly different fields which is creating so much interest and producing results surpassing the most sanguine expectations in the training of our defective classes. Feeble or deranged minds, stunted and perverted moral natures, find their most ready expression, if not their sole cause, in abnormal bodies and undeveloped or irregularly developed cerebral structures.

The result of experiments undertaken in the State Reformatory at Elmira, N. Y., to determine the effect of systematic physical culture upon the criminal dullard furnishes eloquent pleas for the more general adoption of this humane, rational and eminently successful method. Mere restraint and appeal to the emotions of the criminal can do but little to abolish crime. Valuable as physical culture is in this sphere it is not, however, so much in the light of a corrective measure as it is prophylactic, that it should be regarded and here it goes hand in hand with sanitation of which it is, indeed, a branch.

I touch upon these phases of the subject because they are comparatively new and somewhat different from the generally implied results of muscular training, though they are in perfect accord with what has been accomplished in the department of education to which physical culture has heretofore been assigned. The direct effects of exercise upon the muscular system are so obvious that it seems hardly worth the while to enumerate them to an assembly of this character.

I can hardly do better in closing my remarks than to quote the testimony of Amherst College, since it was the pioneer in physical education. The following is from a collection of Dr. Nathan Allen's essays on Physical Development. Dr. Allen, himself a graduate of Amherst, took a leading part in the introduction of physical education in that institution, and has been styled the god-father of this department. He was a trustee, and for over twenty years served on the gymnasium committee. The doctor's life-long study of physical culture and degeneracy, hygiene, heredity and kindred topics, eminently qualifies him to speak with authority on the subject under consideration. I refer mainly to that portion of his remarks bearing upon increased health of the students. He says : " It can, we believe, be safely stated that no large literary institution in this country or Europe, has for a quarter of a century conducted physical education so successfully and so thoroughly as this college. One of the secrets of this success has been that the department, at its very start, was placed upon high ground ; was treated with an importance and character equal to the classics, or mathematics ; and like these, its exercises were made obligatory, and its results, like these also, entered into the merit roll of every student. But a stronger argument still, was that the students themselves became from year to year so convinced of the great advantages of their physical exercises in improving their health and perfecting their scholarship, that they would not give up on any account. . . . A careful account has been kept every year of the sickness or loss of time from every kind of complaint of the students, and it has been found to be steadily diminishing ; but what is more striking, less and less in each class. The freshman class have the most, the sophomore not so much, the junior still less, and the senior the least of all. Thus year by year each class steadily improves in health, showing the immediate benefits of such exercises. This is the reverse of what occurred thirty forty, and fifty years ago."

This is strong evidence, and the schools and colleges throughout our country can make no mistake in following the example of Amherst.

When our educators come to realize the importance of physical education in its larger sense ; when they look carefully to the proper lighting, heating, ventilation and drainage of the school building ; when they minimize the worry and strain incident to examinations, limit the hours of admission, hours of study and number of branches pursued ; exercise a general care over the pupils' health by appointing medical inspectors ; in short, when they watch over and educate the *whole child*, we shall have made a long stride toward the harmonious development of the physical with the mental powers.

On the Necessity for the Early Diagnosis of Communicable Diseases and their Immediate Report to the Health Authorities.*

BY PEMBERTON DUDLEY, M.D.,
Member of the State Board of Health of Pennsylvania.

HISTORICAL references to communicable diseases in their various forms run parallel with the history of the race and almost coextensively with it. Marked, as these diseases were, in times past with a malignancy unknown in our day—sweeping the fair earth as with consuming flames, and carrying black death and frightful disaster to families and cities and nations—it is little wonder

---

* Read before the State Sanitary Convention at Norristown.

that men turn away in horror from the perusal of their history, and shudder at the thought of what our modern world has escaped, and escaped so narrowly.

Yet the history of the world's epidemics, rightly read, is both interesting and instructive. Interesting, in that it shows from what a depth of darkness the knowledge of pathology and sanitary science has lifted us ; instructive, as exhibiting the fact that men, always and everywhere, have acted, in reference to these diseases, in a manner consistent with their own conceptions regarding their nature and causes, and which we, with all our present enlightenment, must respect as rational, however misjudged and misdirected we now know it to have been. If the ancient methods of dealing with a plague were absurd, it was because the cause and quality of the malady were either wholly misunderstood, or, if understood, were found to be beyond the control of the scourged inhabitants. If fathers and mothers fled in affright from their infected children, if unguided or misguided children walked into scenes of peril, if men and women stood still and waited in listless apathy for the coming of inevitable death, it was because that death was hurled upon them by the gods whose wrath they could not conciliate and whose power they could not oppose—a comet or a planet whose course they had no means to control, or a demon whose malignant purpose they could not thwart. In the light of their knowledge, or utter lack of it, we may say that their methods and measures were futile, but we dare not call them irrational.

And what of ourselves? Knowing, as we do, or as we might, all about the communicability of scarlet fever, we take our children by the hand and deliberately lead them into the presence of pestilential death, to bend above the peril-environed form, perhaps to kiss the death-laden lips, and, when they, too, are laid low, to seek comfort in the almost blasphemous thought that we suffer under the will of Providence, and go out to invite our neighbors' children to the funeral. When we—and there are a hundred thousand of us in this enlightened Commonwealth to-day—when we, either through ignorance or perversity, are capable of thus wantonly sacrificing our own and our neighbors' children, is it not high time that some authority shall step between us and our purpose, and, with the strong hand of law, prevent its consummation?

To modify the old proverb a little : "Familiarity breeds contentment." Even in our enlightenment we tolerate numerous evils that, but for our daily familiarity with their presence, would be mercilessly suppressed, and communicable disease, at least in some of its forms, is one of them. It is inconceivable that a thoughtful people could otherwise meet, face to face, upon their streets and in their public conveyances, a foe that daily and hourly threatens their dearest interests and their own lives, and not make most determined efforts to vanquish it.

But, really, can these communicable diseases be thus contended with and conquered? As regards at least some of them the question is easily answered. During the sessions of this convention there have been assembled here many of the most distinguished sanitarians in the United States, any one of whom will tell us that even with our present knowledge an epidemic of Asiatic cholera or of yellow fever, of typhoid fever, of scarlet fever, of diphtheria or of small-pox need not be. They can be prevented or else arrested in their course always. In certain countries of Europe to-day smallpox is practically unknown. Why? Simply because the governments of those countries have determined not to tolerate it. During the year ending November 1st, 1889, the State Board of Health of Pennsylvania was called upon to combat more than a quarter of a hundred epidemics of various forms. With the counsel and aid of distin-guished sanitary experts, located here and there throughout the Commonwealth, the Board, in the brief time required to obtain control of the circumstances, defeated and stamped out these epidemics in every instance. Other boards of health, State and local, are meeting with like uniform success. If an epidemic can be arrested at ,its one-hundredth case, why not, and much more easily, at its first case?

But the prevention or suppression of epidemics cannot be accomplished by preaching or by teaching, or by the administration of medicine (though all these may be effective auxiliaries), but by legal authority, and by legal authority backed and supported by a hearty co-operative public sentiment. Here we may be wise to remember that public sentiment is composed of a large number of private sentiments. If what we have said respecting the suppressibility of epidemics is true, then, while an invasion of disease may be a misfortune, an epidemic is a crime. And what more appropriate than that a crime should be dealt with by legal authority?

There are probably few occasions arising in connection with the adminis-tration of government, when there is greater necessity for the exercise of large powers and for prompt and vigorous action than in the presence of an outbreak of a serious and virulent epidemic. In the face of so grave a public danger, no temporizing and no half-way or half-hearted measures can be considered. Ineffective sanitation is no sanitation. The gate half closed might as well be wide open. Doubtless it is this view that has prompted our legislature to vest such broad powers in the hands of our health authorities, knowing that with-out it their efforts for the public defense must fail of success.

But if the action of the health authorities must be prompt in order to be effective, it follows that those whose duty and interest it is to secure this action must be equally prompt. Just here it is that health officers, left without public co-operation, find themselves almost powerless. Here it is that they are com-pelled to rely upon the wisdom and fidelity of the physician, in order to obtain prompt and accurate information upon which to base their action.

The importance of an early diagnosis, with a view to an early official report, of a case of grave communicable disease, can hardly be overstated. And this we say, notwithstanding the involved liability to make even serious mistakes in diagnosis. I am not unaware of the fact that physicians are fre-quently subjected to vexatious and expensive lawsuits, and sometimes mulcted in heavy damages, because of a false diagnosis leading to the isolation of a patient in a smallpox hospital for what has afterward proved to be a case of measles. And I also know that the fear of such a sequence has induced many a physician to withhold a final and formal diagnosis a whole day, or even longer, to the increased jeopardy of the community. But it is quite likely that as the necessity for prompt action on the physician's part becomes more generally recognized, law will provide more ample means for his protection in the exercise of this high public duty, while at the same time the safety of the unfortunate subject of his possible mistake will be absolutely guaranteed.

It may, perhaps, be asked, Wherein consists the necessity for reporting a case of infectious disease to the health authorities at all, except in cases intended for removal to a hospital? Well, there are several reasons why such reports should be made. First, because the case is a public menace, and the authorities ought to be informed of the exact location of every such danger point even though it may not be necessary to take any action thereon. Secondly, because the physician may need the moral support of a law officer to enable him to secure compliance with his sanitary orders. Patients and their friends are sometimes not only ignorant, but likewise perverse. Thirdly, because in every densely populated community there are those who are unable to apply, or even to obtain, the means necessary for the proper sanitation of the premises. Fourthly, because it frequently happens that not only the premises occupied by the patient, but those also of his neighbors, together with the surrounding streets, lanes, etc., need the attention of the sanitary officers. Fifthly, because upon the subsidence of the disease, the proper disinfection of the house and its contents may require the direct supervision of a sanitary expert.

Such are some of the reasons, and others of scarcely less importance might be added, why all cases of grave communicable disease should be reported to the health officers as soon as possible after their nature is ascertained. It is a first and absolutely necessary step toward the prevention or suppression of an epidemic of communicable disease.

Advice to Suckling Women.

In the *Petit Journal de la Santé*, Dr. Sully gives the following advice to suckling women: Abundance of substantial food, which should be easily digested. This food should contain a considerable quantity of albumen, also of salts of lime, of soda, and of potash. On this account, lentils deserve the preference. After having tried alcohol in all its forms, the author concluded that every variety of alcoholic drink is injurious as much to the mother as to the child. It is true that the absorption of a glass of beer or porter increases the afflux of milk to the breasts, but this milk is watery, poor in nutritive principles, and not at all comparable to that which is produced by the digestion of substantial nourishment.

ᴛʜᴇ ᴀɴɴᴀʟs of ʜʏɢɪᴇɴᴇ,

THE OFFICIAL ORGAN OF THE
State Board of Health of Pennsylvania.

The State Board of Health is not responsible for anything appearing in this Journal except that which bears the official attestation of the Board.

PUBLISHED MONTHLY.

Subscription, two dollars ($2.00) a year, in advance.

Address all communications to

The Hygienic Publishing Company,
224 SOUTH SIXTEENTH STREET,
PHILADELPHIA, PA.

EDITORIAL.

Walking, Riding, Driving and Running.

Now are we fast approaching the season of the year when out-door life assumes its greatest charm. The sun, so warm in Summer, now just tempers the coming frost so as to give us what is really the most pleasant quarter of the year. During the coming three months, nature, by the combined magnetism of a delicious atmosphere and a lovely and changing foliage, invites us to an out-door life, so conducive to health. Let us not be slow to accept the invitation, but let us do so with prudence and judgment. Let us remember that running as an exercise is not only not beneficial, but absolutely injurious. We care not what may be said in favor of running by college boys and ardent athletes ; it is a form of violent motion well calculated to injure the heart, and has nothing special to commend it. Riding is, unquestionably, a good form of exercise, as is also driving, but they are both indulgences that entail expense. Good, plain, old-fashioned walking is a form of exercise than which none is better, and that is within the reach of all. The thought has recently entered our mind that it is really a man's business to preserve his health ; that it is and should be considered just as much his business to preserve his health as to pursue his daily business avocations. If this thought be correct, then we hold that a man should make it his business to devote a certain portion of every day to healthy exercise. There is not a man living who could not find one hour out of the twenty-four to devote to his health, and as one could walk from three to four miles in this hour, we know of no more valuable piece of advice to offer our readers this month than that they should resolve (and keep the resolution), that hereafter one hour's walking will constitute a part of the routine of each day's life. Do not, however, tramp through the monotonous streets of a city. Those of you who live in the country have the proper walking track at your door ; those of you who live in the city can for a few pennies be transported three, four or more miles into the country, where, alighting, you can walk back. Take our word for it, if you will faithfully walk the distance suggested in the country every day during the coming three months, you will be ready to cheerfully say that this little piece of advice alone has been worth to you more than you will pay for this journal during the rest of your life. The experiment we suggest will cost nothing, is equally applicable to men, women and children, and is well worthy of a trial.

January, 1890, Issue.

If any of our subscribers do not intend to preserve their volumes, we would thank them if they will kindly mail to us the issue for January, 1890, for which we will pay twenty cents.

Second-Hand Street Car Tickets.

The good people of Washington, D. C., are, at the present time, justly exercised over what may be righteously termed a . disgusting and dangerous practice of the street car companies. It seems that fare tickets are sold in packages. When one is received from a passenger, the conductor punches a slip which he carries, while the tickets pass into his pocket and are subsequently turned into the office, to be again sold, thus becoming, in time, not only *second*, but *tenth*, *twentieth*, and even *fiftieth* hand. The dirt and probable disease with which these tickets become, in time, encrusted is marvellous to behold. Certainly, the saving to the companies must be very slight and not at all a justification of a practice which we must conscientiously say is not only opposed to the teachings of hygiene, but is antagonistic to the very dictates of decency itself.

Dyspepsia—The Diet and the Humors.

The answer of the wife of the good-natured husband to that of the ill-natured one, was, if coarse and blunt, also philosophical. When asked how she managed to keep him so good-natured, she answered, "I feed the brute." Lauder Brunton in his Lettsomiam Lectures, quoting Sidney Smith, said: "Happiness is not impossible without health, but it is very difficult of attainment. I do not mean by health merely an absence of dangerous complaints, but that the body should be in perfect tune, full of vigor. and alacrity. The longer I live the more I am convinced that the apothecary is of more importance than Seneca ; and that half the unhappiness in the world proceeds from little stoppages, from a duct choked up, from food pressing in the wrong place, from a vexed duodenum or an agitated pylorus. The deception as practiced upon human creatures is curious and entertaining. My friend sups late ; he eats some strong soup, then a lobster, then some tart, then he dilutes these esculent varieties with wine. The next day I call upon him. He is going to sell his home in London and retire to the country. He is alarmed for his eldest daughter's health. His expenses are hourly increasing, and nothing but a timely retreat can save him from ruin. All this is the lobster ; and when over-excited nature has time to manage this testaceous incumbrance, the daughter's health recovers, the finances are in good order, and every rural idea effectually excluded from his mind. In the same manner old friendships are destroyed by toasted cheese, and hard salted meat has led to suicide. Unpleasant feelings of the body produce corresponding sensations in the mind, and a great sense of wickedness is sketched out by a morsel of indigestible and misguided food. Of such infinite consequence to happiness is it to study the body."

NOTES AND COMMENTS.

Salt for Headaches.

An English doctor reports over thirty cases of headache and facial neu-·ralgia cured by snuffing powdered salt up the nose.

Boston Cars and Boston Sewers.

W. R. Nichols, of Boston, found more than twice as much deadly carbonic acid gas in the air of passenger cars than in the Berkeley Street sewer.

Removal of Ashes and Garbage.

There is no earthly reason why the scavenging of our cities should not be done at night. The dripping swill cart and the wind-scattered ashes would be less of a nuisance at this time than when the streets are full of people.

A Substitute for Handcuffs.

A French policeman arrested three prisoners, and not having the handcuffs to secure them, he just cut off their suspender buttons. Their hands were thus occupied, and they couldn't run away, so they were marched safely to prison.

A Dangerous Hugger.

There is said to be a girl in Genesee County, New York, whose strength is so great that when she hugs a man she always breaks one or more of his ribs. When she drives with a young man she is always asked to take the lines.

Prescription for Tramps.

R.   Bark of dog, ...   ℥ij.
    Commercial lead, ...   ʒvij.
Sig.   In pills.   One every minute till disappearance.
                                    —*Druggists' Bulletin.*

Essay on Man.

At ten, a child ; at twenty, wild ;
At thirty, tame, if ever ;
At forty, wise ; at fifty, rich ;
At sixty, good, or never !

An Ideally Healthy Locality.

The conversation had turned on the healthfulness of two localities.

" In our village," said one, " we don't average over a death a year."

" Why, that's a terrible mortality," replied the other ; "in our town we only had one death in five years, and that was the doctor."

" Couldn't he cure himself ?"

" No, poor man ; he died of starvation."

The Cost of "La Grippe" in England.

The cost to England of the influenza epidemic is estimated at $10,000,000, about one-half of this amount having been paid by insurance companies and friendly societies, and the remainder representing loss of wages and disorganization of business.

Wholesome Food for Russian Soldiers.

The medical department of the Russian Ministry of War has decided to establish movable laboratories of toxicological chemistry and bacteriology attached to each army corps. In these laboratories all food supplied to the troops will be analyzed.

Tonsorial Disinfection.

The authorities at Nordhausen, in Saxony, at the suggestion of the district medical officer, have issued an order to barbers to disinfect their brushes and other implements immediately after use and before they are applied to the hair or beard of another customer.

He Retired from Business.

A strong man, under forty, was accustomed during the four months of Winter to leave home at 6 A. M., and return from business at 11 P. M. "In about three years his body grew so tired that it retired from business to a quiet place under the sod, where it is now taking a long rest."

Sweating of the Hands.

A lotion composed of four ounces of cologne water and half an ounce of tincture of belladonna, is highly recommended as a cure for the disagreeable sweating of the hands and feet, from which many persons suffer. The affected extremities should be rubbed two or three times a day with the lotion.

Malignant Scarlet Fever.

Recent observations seem to show that inflammation of the ear and other grave complications which often arise in scarlet fever, are due to secondary infection, that is, self-infection by the patient. This fact emphasizes the importance of thorough cleanliness, ventilation and disinfection in this disease.

Influence of Pure Air.

A dairy at Frankfort-on-the-Main made the following valuable observations. They kept in a standard stable eighty Swiss cows, extraordinarily well fed and treated. In the years 1878 to 1879, prior to the introduction of a ventilation system, the same yielded on an average per cow, 3,700 liters in 1877, same amount in 1878, and 3,716 liters in 1879. Subsequent to the introduced ventilation the amount of milk yielded, the food being the same, was as follows: In 1880, 4,050 liters milk per head; in 1881, 4,152; in 1882, 4,354 liters.

Contagion by Kissing a Corpse.

The following simple, yet wonderfully eloquent paragraph needs no comment; it carries its lesson so plainly that he who runs may read:

"A woman in Ohio recently lost her child by diphtheria, and forced her other children to kiss the dead body. The latter also sickened and died."

Diet in Diseases of the Kidney.

According to Dujardin-Beaumetz, the nourishment should consist chiefly of hard-boiled eggs and such vegetables as beans, peas, lentils and potatoes, which may be made into a thick soup. Green vegetables may be used and also mush made from corn, barley, or oats. Fruit may be eaten freely. The drink should consist of milk.

Spurious Cloves.

Spurious cloves are reported from Germany. They consist of a paste of wheat flour and ground oak bark, with a small proportion of genuine clove, pressed into metal moulds and roasted. In general external appearance they approximate closely the genuine. In the mouth they soften to a gritty paste, color the saliva brown, and have a remarkable bark flavor.

To Clean Lamp Burners.

To clean lamp burners, take a piece of sal soda the size of a walnut, put into a quart of soft water, put your lamp burner in it (an old tomato can is good enough), set it on the stove; after boiling for five minutes remove the burner, and when put back on the lamp will be as good as new. All the carbon on the old burners should be removed once every month.

Comparative Value of Cows and Steers.

Three and a half pounds of milk are said to be equal to one pound of meat; and if we estimate a cow to give but 4000 pounds of milk in a year, her product would be equal in food value to 1000 pounds of meat, which would require a steer, under ordinary feeding, four years to produce; so that the cow produces as much return for her food in one year as a steer does in four.

Perpetual Paste.

A correspondent of the *Br. and Col. Dr.*, gives directions for making a paste which will keep twelve months. Dissolve a teaspoonful of alum in a quart of warm water, cool, stir in flour to give it the consistence of a thick cream, carefully breaking up all lumps; then stir in as much powdered resin as will lie on a sixpence, and half a dozen cloves to give it a flavor. Have on a fire a sauce-pan with a teacupful of boiling water. Pour the flour mixture into it and stir well all the time. In a few minutes it will be of the consistence of porridge; then pour it into a jar, let it cool, cover it and keep it in a cool place. When any is needed, take out a small portion and soften it with warm water.

Rest.

Rest, as well as exercise, is indispensable to health and life. *Good health,* says a retired manufacturer, watching the strife from which he has withdrawn, tells of five business men under forty-four, in the circle of his personal acquaintance, who within one year died of brain or kidney disease, or went to the madhouse, all from overwork.

Laws of Health.

TRAMP—"Thankee kindly, mum ; I'd no hope of gettin' sich a fine supper to-day, mum. May heaven bless ye !'' HOUSEKEEPER—"As you've had a good supper, I think you might chop some wood." "Yes, mum ; but you know the old adage, 'After a dinner rest a while ; after supper walk a mile.' I'll walk the mile first, mum."

Elastic Mucilage.

Dissolve 1 part of salicylic acid in 20 parts of alcohol, add 3 parts of soft soap and 3 parts of glycerine. Shake thoroughly and add the mixture to a mucilage prepared from 93 parts of gum arabic and the requisite amount of water (about 180 parts). This mucilage keeps well, and when it dries remains elastic without tendency to cracking.

Perfumery as a Detective.

The well-known detection of a crime in Diplomacy, through the perfume of a woman's glove, was reproduced by a recent occurrence in Paris. A man who found his room robbed of all his jewelry perceived a peculiar perfume, and a few days later noticed it again when passing two well-dressed women in the street. They were arrested and found to be the thieves.

Removing Indelible Ink.

Physicians are often asked how to remove indelible ink, and they sometimes cannot quite remember, so the *Medical and Surgical Reporter* mentions the following method : First moisten the stain with tincture of iodine, and, after a few minutes, remove the iodine stain with a solution of hyposulphite of soda. Finally wash in clean water. Repeat if necessary.

The Influence of Diet on Character.

The *Dietetic Gazette* says : " By searching we might find that the egotism, conservatism, and tenaciousness of the Englishman are as much the results of his beef and ale as is his gout ; that the sparkling *bonhomie* of the Frenchman comes from his *cuisine* and bubbling champagne, as do also his mercurial disposition and his passionate life ; that the maccaroni and fortified wines bestow song and art on the Italian, as do beer and *sauerkraut* stamp solidity and patriotism on the German. America, ever able to give the world a lesson, contributes rush and dyspepsia as the production of hog and whisky.

What can a Vegetarian Eat?

In a letter to the *Medical Press* the secretary of the Vegetarian Society says that there is more or less confusion in the minds of many people as to what constitutes the dietary of a vegetarian. It does not consist in an exclusively vegetable diet, for the vegetarian may eat, at his option, all animal products that have-not possessed animal life, *e. g.*, milk, butter, cheese, eggs, honey and the like.

Free Love and Cesspools.

Free love, as between you and your neighbor's wife, may be very agreeable to you ; but, as between your neighbor and your wife, is sure to be disagreeable to you. So, a cesspool on the back end of your lot, under your neighbor's dining-room window may be convenient for you, but a cesspool on your neighbor's lot, under your dining-room window, is not entirely satisfactory to you.
— *Wight.*

The Influence of Light on Development.

An English scientist has been making experiments to determine the important part which light plays in the development of animal life. A dozen tadpoles were confined in a box, from which every ray of light was excluded. The result was that only two of them developed into frogs, and those were short lived. The others increased considerably in size, but never left the tadpole form.

Scarlet Fever.

A bright little girl four years old died of scarlet fever recently in Maine, and the secretary of the local board of health writes that the infection was taken in playing with old clothes or a doll where they had been in a chamber since the same disease was in the same house more than a year ago. It is dangerous to let a single infected article escape a thorough disinfection during and after the prevalence of this disease.

Drugging Crying Children.

A young mother remarked to us recently that her babe had been quite restless at first, but now she always gave it "drops," and this made it rest. This mother, with thousands of others, is making the sad mistake of putting her child to rest by drugging it. The "drops" of which she speaks, contain opium, in one or the other of its various shapes, and thus a stupor is induced in the child which may dull its natural brightness for life, possibly making it a half idiot. Little children seldom cry unless they have pain. They get pain by being fed to excess. The normal, common sense method of relieving the pain and stopping the crying, is not by drugging the child, and dulling or destroying its sensibility, but by feeding it less at a time and more frequently.
—*National Educator.*

Hygienic Breakfast Cakes.

One pint of fresh oatmeal, one quart of water ; let it stand over night. In the morning add one teaspoonful of fine salt, one tablespoonful of sugar and the same of baking powder, and one pint of Graham flour. If above proportions make a batter too stiff for griddle cakes, add more water. If gems are preferred instead of cakes, the addition of a little more flour is all that is required to produce an extra article.

The Latest Banquet Feature.

At Paris dinner-tables the latest feature for dessert is the practice of putting on the table small receptacles called marmites, or " pots," in which are inclosed nuts, bonbons, and any other trifle that the hostess pleases. Each guest takes a pot, and before opening it trades it for that of some one else. The fun comes in when the results of the trades are known, and some are found to have swapped a pot filled with candy for one containing something of value.

Meteorology and Disease.

There would seem to be good reason for believing that there are certain definite relations between certain meteorological conditions and the prevalence of particular diseases. What these relations are we, as yet, know very little about. But it would seem as though this was a promising field for research. If we can definitely ascertain what atmospheric conditions favor the production of a certain disease, we are in a fair way to learn how to antagonize the onslaught of such a malady.

Buttering Bread by Machinery.

The latest and most unique electrical invention is a machine for buttering bread. It is used in connection with a patent bread cutter, and is intended for use in prisons and reformatory institutions. There is a cylindrical-shaped brush, which is fed with butter, and lays a thin layer on the bread as it comes from the cutter. The machine has a capacity of cutting and buttering 750 loaves of bread an hour. The saving of butter and of bread, and the decrease in the quantity of crumbs is said to be very large.

Hurried Dinners.

When a crude mass of inadequately crushed muscular fibre, or undivided solid material of any description, is thrown into the stomach, it acts as a mechanical irritant and sets up a condition in the mucous membrane lining that organ which greatly impedes, if it does not altogether prevent, the process of digestion. When the practice of eating quickly and filling the stomach with unprepared food is habitual, the digestive organ is rendered incapable of performing its proper functions. Either a much larger quantity of food than would be necessary under natural conditions is required, or the system suffers from lack of nourisment.

Chocolate and Cocoa.

Chocolate and cocoa, according to Dr. A. N. Bell, are much less potent as disturbers of the nervous system, and are proportionally more wholesome as a beverage than tea or coffee, besides possessing specially nutritive qualities, which render them much more sustaining; and there can be little question but that a general substitution for tea, especially of that cheap, oversteeped, second-edition kind, which is the too common beverage of overworked women in various avocations of life, would be promotive of health.

A Warning to Chloroform Inhalers.

A man in New York recently met with death because he did not understand the simple principle of capillary attraction. He had been in the habit of taking chloroform to quiet his nerves. One night he dipped a towel in the anæsthetic and placed it over his face when he went to sleep. But one end of the towel reached to the end of the bowl containing the chloroform, and gradually absorbed the liquid and carried it up to the sleeper's face. In the morning the bowl was empty and the man was dead.

Brandy Drops.

The artificial lives led by so many of our city girls of this day and generation prove such a tax upon their vitality that some artificial stimulant seems to them a necessity. Hence have the confectioners come to manufacture a chocolate drop, containing each a small quantity of brandy. If we spur a jaded horse, he will be stimulated into action, and if a jaded girl refresh herself with brandy, she, also, will be freshened into artificial life, but, in both instances, the ultimate result will be premature and irremediable physical prostration.

The Vaccination Controversy in a Nut-Shell.

An infant was once brought to a hospital with eyes irrevocably put out and dark for life. The great surgeon to whom it was brought was helpless. All he could do was to find out how such a tragedy had happened. Some such dialogue as the following transpired :

Surgeon : How came the child to lose its eyes?

Mother : It had smallpox, Sir.

Surgeon : How came it to get the smallpox? Was it vaccinated?

Mother : No, Sir ; it was not vaccinated.

Surgeon : Why was it not vaccinated?

Mother : The child before this had very sore arms and I determined I would have no more children vaccinated.

This is the vaccination controversy in a nut-shell : Sore arms against boils, carbuncles, ulcers, impaired health, blindness, hideous disfigurement—the frequent sequelæ of smallpox—and enormous loss of life ; an utter loss of the sense of proportion, and a perverse preference for the greater of two evils.

Test for Cotton-Seed Oil.

There is no reason why we should not use cotton-seed oil in lieu of olive oil, so far as health is concerned. However, if you wish to know whether that which you are using as olive oil contains any cotton-seed oil, the following process will settle the question : Mix 1 part of pure nitric acid with 2½ parts of the oil to be tested. Place a clean copper wire in the mixture, and stir thoroughly with a glass rod. The oil, if it contains cotton-seed oil, will turn red in the course of half an hour.

Valuable Liquid Glue.

Liquid glue possessing great resisting power, and particularly recommended for wood and. iron, is prepared, according to Hesz, as follows : Clear gelatine, 100 parts ; cabinet-makers' glue, 100 parts ; alcohol, 25 parts ; alum, 2 parts ; the whole mixed with 200 parts of 20 per cent. acetic acid and heated on a water bath for six hours. An ordinary liquid glue, also well adapted for wood and iron, is made by boiling together for several hours 100 parts glue, 260 parts water and 16 parts nitric acid.

Good Health and Good Citizenship.

Good health not only conduces to longer life and public wealth and happiness, but to good citizenship, says the *Iowa Monthly Bulletin*. It is not a great boon nor benefit to anyone, nor to the public, for a person simply to *live ;* but to live and to be in good health makes the fortunate possessor a benediction to all, since every one, however humble, in no insignificant sense touches every other person within the State. Hence, whoever contributes anything to the promotion and maintenance of good health is a public benefactor ; and whatever of law or deed lessens the danger from preventible diseases and accident is a public benefaction.

Amniol for Disinfecting Sewage.

Mr. Woolheim, a Londoner, is said to have discovered a disinfectant which far surpasses anything now applied for that purpose. This is "amniol," a gas which, when introduced into a sewer, rapidly destroys the microbes of putrefaction and of disease. The odor in the sewer pipe is almost instantly displaced by that of the gas introduced, and in less than an hour the sewage thus treated is deodorized and sterilized.

Dr. Klein has in part confirmed the claims of the discoverer, in so far that one sample of sewage examined by him was found to be absolutely sterile after having been treated by the amniol method.

It is to be hoped that further experiments will soon be made with this agent, which will enlighten us as to how long the putrefactive processes can be delayed by it, and the character of microbes it is capable of destroying. If all that is claimed for "amniol" be true, then we will have a new boom in sanitation.—*New Orleans M. and S. Journal.*

An Easy Way to Raise a Reputation.

A South Carolina physician, asked why he located at Monclova, said : " It is a first-rate place for a doctor. If a man is sick all you have to do is to tell his friends (no matter whether the affair is serious or not) to go to a priest and have him confessed and prepared for death. If he dies they will say : ' What a good doctor he is, he knew he must die, and so had his spiritual interests attended to.' If he recovers they will say : ' What a capable physician he must be. The man was in the last extremity and prepared for death, and he cured him.' So in either event it is a first-rate place in which to achieve a medical reputation."

Rights and Lefts.

Dr. Louis Jobert has published a work on the cause and frequency of left-handedness. No purely left-handed race has ever been discovered, although there seems to be a difference in different tribes. Seventy per cent. of the inhabitants of the Pendjab use the left hand by preference, and the greater number of the Hottentots and Bushmen of South A'frica use the left hand in preference to the right. Dr. Marro, as a result of his study of criminals, has found that from 14 to 22 per cent. of those who have been convicted of crime were left-handed, the highest ratio among people of all classes being only nine in the hundred.

How to be Miserable.

An excellent recipe for being completely miserable is to think only of yourself, how much you have lost, how much you have not made, and the poor prospect for the future. A brave man with a soul in him gets out of such pitiful ruts and laughs at discouragement, rolls up his sleeves, sings and whistles and makes the best of life. This earth never was intended for paradise, and the man who rises above his discouragement and keeps his manhood will only be stronger and better for his adversities. Many a noble ship has been saved by throwing overboard the valuable cargo, and many a man is better and more humane after he has lost his gold.

Transmission of Consumption in Married Life.

M. Leudet has occupied himself with collecting some statistics on the question of whether a wife can give consumption to her husband, or a husband to his wife. He has taken 111 widows or widowers, whose husbands or wives, respectively, have died in undoubted consumption. Out of these 7 were consumptive ; but several of them had facts in their previous history, before marriage, showing a consumptive tendency. His inference was, therefore, that the transmission of consumption in married life must be very rare ; even more rare in the upper classes than in the middle and lower. In 80 out of these 112 cases there was a family history which he could follow ; and 27 of these showed some members who were consumptive.— *The Practitioner*.

Falsification of Wine in Brazil.

It appears, from a small pamphlet referred to in the *Lancet* by Dr. Campos da Paz, of Rio de Janeiro, that the manufacture of the imitations of wines and liquors flourishes unchecked in Rio, and forms a more or less important industry. The replies, based on analyses, which were returned by the local official chemists to inquiries submitted by Dr. Campos da Paz and Dr. Freire, show that extensive and systematic falsification of a kind likely to be seriously injurious to public health is practiced. Indigo-carmine, dinitro-cresylate of potassium, aloes, chloroform and the compound ethers of valeric, butyric and caproic acid, oxalic acid and amyl alcohol are among the ingredients used in this branch of misapplied chemistry.

The Advantages of a Sea Voyage.

The benefit to health following upon a sea voyage is, according to Dr. Burney Yeo, due to the following causes : 1. Perfect rest and quiet, a thorough change of scene, and perfect and enforced rest from both mental and physical labor. 2. The life in the open air, and the great amount of sunshine enjoyed, it being quite possible to spend fifteen hours every day in the open air. 5. The purity of the sea air, no organic dust or impurities—the air of the open sea being the purest found anywhere. 4. The great humidity of the atmosphere and the high barometric pressure, which are considered to exercise a useful sedative influence on certain constitutions. 5. The exhilarating and tonic effects of rapid motion through the air—the sea-breezes are constantly blowing over the ship. These breezes increase evaporation from the skin, and impart tone to the superficial bloodvessels.—*The Nineteenth Century*.

Diphtheria Conveyed by Cats.

A physician of Kansas writes that last Winter he was called to attend a little 3-year old girl suffering with diphtheria. Upon careful inquiry it was found that she had not been exposed to the disease, although there were some cases within a mile of her father's house. He incidentally learned that there was a sick cat in the house, which had been fondled by the little girl some days before. The cat died shortly after its playmate became sick, and a second cat also became sick and was killed. Suspicions were aroused that the disease was conveyed by the cat, and inquiry revealed the fact that one farmer had lost seventeen cats, and another fifteen, with some throat trouble. One of the farmers stated that he had examined the throats of some of the cats, and found them covered with a white membrane. The little girl died and her little brother a few days later had a severe attack of the same disease. Cats are disposed to run from house to house at night, and one diseased cat may be the means of carrying diphtheria to half the cats in the neighborhood, they in turn carrying it to the children whom the parents are taking every means to protect from danger. It is well to keep an eye on the cats in times of diphtheria.

Constituents of Food.

The amount of solid matter in the different kinds of food used should be kept in mind as completely as possible. The following table exhibits the proportion of solid matter and water in 100 parts each of the following articles of diet :

ARTICLES.	Solid Matter.	Water.	ARTICLES.	Solid Matter.	Water.
Wheat	87	13	Pork	24	76
Peas	87	13	Codfish	21	79
Rice	86	14	Blood	20	80
Beans	86	14	Trout	19	81
Rye	86	14	Apples	18	82
Corn	86	14	Pears	16	84
Oatmeal	74	26	Carrots	13	87
Wheat Bread	51	49	Beets	13	87
Mutton	29	71	Milk	13	87
Chicken	27	73	Oysters	13	87
Lean Beef	26	74	Cabbage	8	92
Eggs	26	74	Turnips	7	93
Veal	25	75	Watermelon	5	95
Potatoes	25	75	Cucumber	3	97

The Gospel of Soap.

One of the most gifted and practical of sanitarians was the late Sir Edwin Chadwick, of London, who recently died at the age of 90. What faith is to the Christian religion, soap and water are to the Gospel of Health. He believes that the immunity that nurses and internes of hospitals have from infectious diseases comes largely from their daily baths. He said lately ; "I cannot tell you how strongly I believe in soap and water as a preventive of epidemics. If an epidemic were to occur I would proclaim and enforce the active application of soap and water as a preventive."

Dr. Chadwick states that by this simple means he has been able to greatly reduce the mortality of the Indian army, and that the death rate has been reduced from sixty-seven to twenty per thousand.

He has rather a novel theory in regard to air purification, which is highly endorsed by M. Eiffel, which consists in the erection of lofty towers in the cities by means of which the life and health-giving ozone of the upper regions may be pumped down so as to exert its beneficial influence upon the inhabited strata of air.

It is said that while there is plenty of ozone at the summit of St. Paul's cathedral there is none at the base. He thinks that hygiene so taught in the schools as to *impress* upon the children and the coming generations the advantages of soap and water as applied regularly and frequently to the body, would be vastly more important to the world than time spent in acquiring a knowledge of the dead languages.

We heartily concur in this opinion, and reiterate the declaration so often made, that the greatest, and almost the only essentials to good health, are pure air, pure water, pure soil and clean bodies.

Filling for Old Nail Holes.

The following method of filling up old nail holes in wood is not only simple, but is said to be effectual. Take fine sawdust and mix into a thick paste with glue, pound it into the hole, and when dry it will make the wood as good as new. One correspondent says he has followed this for 30 years with unvarying success in repairing bellows, which is the most severe test known. Often by frequent attachment of new leather to old bellows frames the wood becomes so perforated that there is no space to drive the nails, and even if there was the remaining holes would allow the air to escape. A treatment with glue and sawdust paste invariably does the work, while lead, putty and other remedies always fail.

Gingerette.

A popular cold weather beverage abroad is prepared as follows :

Simple syrup,	½ gal.
Acid solution,	2½ fl. ozs.
Soluble essence of ginger,	1½ fl. ozs.
Soluble essence of lemon,	2 fl. drs.
Essence of vanilla,	3 fl. drs.
Essence of capsicum,	20 drops.
Caramel, or coloring,	1 fl. oz.

To one quart of syrup add the acid solution and all the essences and coloring; well mix by agitation. Add remaining quart of syrup, and shake well together, and, if necessary, pass through flannel bag, when it is ready for bottling. Color, deep sherry.

Drugs versus Hygiene.

That delightfully concise and expressive paragraphist, Oliver Wendell Holmes, is credited with having said, "Give me opium, wine and milk, and I will cure all diseases to which flesh is heir," from which wise remark we might infer, did we not already know that Dr. Holmes is not an ardent advocate of drug-dosing. No more is any intelligent, thoughtful physician. There are certain drugs, with a specific action, each peculiar to itself, which at times are absolutely essential, but it would be better for humanity were most of the drugs that are described in our bulky books devoted to this subject left to the obscurity from which commercial enterprise has dragged them. We must clearly understand that drugs cannot cure ; they possess a potency, and since they do not cure, this potency must in very many cases do harm. Nature alone can cure, and the remedies which nature uses are the remedies suggested by the sanitarian ; *they are not drugs.* As it is at present, the public demand drugs and the physician must, therefore, order them or be set down as an ignoramus and lose his patients. Just as soon as the people are willing to be treated by natural remedies and to stop *drug-dosing*, just so soon will the physicians conform to their wishes. It is a gratifying sign of increasing intelligence among the people that this happy period is fast approaching.

Food for Children.

In those cases where we have an irritation of the stomach and bowels, evidenced by a looseness of the bowels, perhaps some vomiting, unhealthy-looking passages, and, it may be, want of appetite, the following diet will prove very useful :

Wheat, ... 1 tablespoonful.
Oatmeal, ... ½ "
Barley, ... ½ "
Water, ... 1 quart.

This is to be concentrated by boiling to one pint, strained and sweetened. The result is a mucilage readily taken by children. The patient should be given small quantities of this mucilage at frequent intervals, and no other food administered until the passages assume their normal color.

Be More Careful.

There is too much carelessness in letting children visit other children who are sick before it is definitely known whether they have an infectious disease or not. Even when it is announced of the sick child that "it is nothing but a slight sore throat," the prudent mother should hesitate before sending her child to the sick chamber and into a possible danger lying in ambush. Scarlet fever and diphtheria sometimes put off their characteristic appearance and masquerade in the form of a "slight sore throat," retaining, however, their capability of communicating infection which may reproduce the diseases in their more usual and more frightful forms. The truth of this is emphasized every year in the histories of outbreaks in our own State. A word to the wise is sufficient, it is said, but we find that the word needs frequent repetition—*Sanitary Era*.

The National Museum of Hygiene.

Under the auspices of the Medical Department of the United States Navy, there is located in Washington a "Museum of Hygiene," regarding which Medical Inspector Wells says that the experience of the past year has demonstrated more fully than ever the necessity and value of a museum of this character. The health reports of States and cities received at this office indicate the widespread interest taken in sanitary science. The increase of visitors and applicants for special hygiene reports, the addition of sanitary appliances by inventors, the visits of students from the colleges and universities for study and observation, the contribution of books and pamphlets, are all evidences of the growing influence of the museum. During the year a circular letter was sent to every large hospital and asylum in the country, calling attention to the collection being made of waste-pipes long in use, and this has brought some very interesting specimens, particularly from insane asylums. Such a museum constitutes a most valuable "object lesson" in hygiene, and we have always felt that every large city should harbor a similar institution.

Statistics of Leprosy in the United States.

In view of the general impression that leprosy is spreading in this country, it is desirable, in the interest of public health, to obtain accurate information on this point. The undersigned is engaged in collecting statistics of all cases of leprosy in the United States, and he would ask members of the profession to aid in this work by sending a report of any case or cases under their observation or coming within their knowledge. Please give location, age, sex and nationality of the patient, and the form of the disease—tubercular or anæsthetic, also any facts bearing upon the question of contagion and heredity. Address   Dr. Prince A. Morrow,

66 West 40th Street, New York.

Relative Mortality in Certain Cities as Influenced by Influenza.

A study of the table of total number of deaths in Berlin, Vienna, Amsterdam and Paris, in December, 1889, and January, 1890, admits of important conclusions as to the proportion of the influenza epidemic in the four cities, the increase of mortality having been conditioned upon the complications and consecutive diseases of influenza. It is shown that the disease was mildest in Berlin, stronger in Vienna, very violent in Amsterdam, and most intense in Paris.

The following table exhibits the number of deaths in each thousand of the inhabitants of the four cities during the months of December, 1889, and January, 1890:

	Berlin.	Vienna.	Amsterdam.	Paris.
December 1–7, 1889	19.9	23.5	18.97	25.09
December 8–14, 1889	26.2	26.3	21.16	28.32
December 15–21, 1889	31.6	29.5	25.94	31.19
December 22–28, 1889	36.5	45.6	24.52	54.60
December 29, 1889, to January 4, 1890	31.2	42.6	26.97	62.47
December 5–11, 1889, to January 4, 1890	26.1	34.6	46.71	47.79
December 13–18, 1889, to January 4, 1890	22.8	26.3	61.54	34.34
December 19–25, 1889, to January 4, 1890	22.9	27.6	38.97	26.38
January 26 to February 1, 1890			30.45	24.06
February 2–8, 1890			22.84	24.54

Causal Theories Concerning Choleraic Outbreaks.

The French Society of Hygiene has received from Dr. Tholozan, honorary member of the society, some precise information with regard to the outbreak of cholera in Mesopotamia. He asserts that cholera lingered in this region during the Winter in a light, sporadic form, to break out with violence with the first heat of Summer, and that, in view of this fact, "the theory that choleraic epidemics can be controlled and subdued by restrictive measures must be abandoned."

The unexpected appearance of cholera in certain small localities in the province of Valencia, Spain, is also fatal to the "tradition which makes all cholera epidemics originate on the banks of the Ganges." The partisans of a theory which reigned supreme from 1867 to 1887, and which was affirmed by every international congress of hygiene and by the academies of sciences and of medicine, will find it difficult to deny that the cholera which appeared in the village of Puebla de Rugat was an epidemic of local origin—a revival of the great choleraic epidemic which in 1884 and 1885 prevailed in Spain, and especially.in the province of Valencia.

In 1875 Dr. Tholozan showed, by authentic reports, "that many epidemics of cholera and plague originate on the spot from germs previously deposited in the soil."

At the conference of Rome, and at the Congress of Hygiene of Vienna, the French delegates urged the establishment between the several states of the two hemispheres of an international treaty directed against pestilential diseases (cholera, yellow fever and plague). Among the fundamental terms of this treaty an "international sanitary inspection of vessels entering the Suez Canal" was proposed.

In his last study of cholera Pettenkofer demonstrates, from the history of choleraic epidemics, that general prophylactic measures, based on the theory of contagion, measures costly and impossible of application have proved their complete inutility in the past, and that they will be equally inefficacious in the future.

On the other hand, Dr. Mahé, sanitary physician of France at Constantinople, in a paper on "The Progress of Asiatic Cholera from the East Indies Westward During the Past Decade," asserts "That all choleraic epidemics which have descended upon Europe have come, some by direct irradiation of the epidemic from Hindoostan, some by importation into the Hedjaz and Egypt."

Sir Joseph Fayre, in an article presented to the Medical Society of London, entitled "Natural and Epidemiological History of Cholera," arrives at the following conclusions :

"The theories of contagion and propagation by human means do not explain the spread of choleraic epidemics, since their frequency and direction, and the rapidity of their propagation, bear no relation to the development of the means of communication.

"Epidemics, although a constant condition of the life of man, are not unavoidable and are subject to common sense and the laws of hygiene."

Dr. Kelsch, of the *Val du Grace*, in his remarkable work, "Considerations on the Etiology of Cholera," after an impartial review of the rival theories which have disputed the ground during the past half-century—the theory of importation, supported by Fauvel, Rochard and Proust, and the theory of evolution, supported by Jules Guérin, Tholozan and Didiot—sums up the discussion with this practical conclusion :

"The prophylaxis of cholera belongs primarily to local and individual hygiene."

In 1884 Dr. Jules Rochard, in a report on cholera in Toulon, read before the Academy of Medicine, asserted that "cholera can reach us only by way of the Red Sea. The Suez Canal is the only dyke which protects Europe against this scourge. Whenever it shall be broken a destructive flood will sweep over Europe."—*Abstract of Sanitary Reports.*

Common-Sense Breakfast Menus.

Oranges.

| Moulded Farina. | Sugar and Cream. | | Smothered Beef. |
| Stewed Potatoes. | Pulled Bread. | Cocoa. |

Shaddocks.

| Oat-meal. | Sugar and Cream. | Broiled Tomatoes. | Cream Sauce. |
| Gluten Gems. | Coffee. |

| Boiled Rice. | Sugar and Cream. | Broiled Steak. | Water Toast. |
| Baked Apples. | Wafers. | Coffee. |

| Gluten Mush. | Sugar. | Broiled Fish. | Baked Potatoes. |
| Stewed Prunes. | Zwieback. | Coffee. |

MRS. S. T. RORER.

Curious Food.

The lion is eaten by some African races, but its flesh is held in small esteem. The Zulus find carrion so much to their liking that, according to the late Bishop Colenso, they apply to food peopled by large colonies of larvæ the expressive word "uborni," signifying in their uncouth jargon "great happiness." David Livingstone, that keen and accurate observer, reminds us that the aboriginal Australians and Hottentots prefer the intestines of animals. "It is curious," he says, "that this is the part which animals always begin with, and it is the first choice of our men." On this point I may remind the civilized reader that the woodcock and the red mullet or sea woodcock are both eaten and relished without undergoing all the cleansing processes which most animals used for food among us generally experience to fit them for the table, so that our aversion to the entrails of animals is not absolute, but only one of degree. The hippopotamus is a favorite dish with some Africans when they can get this unwieldy and formidable river monster, and when young its flesh is good and palatable, but with advancing years it becomes coarse and unpleasant. The Abyssinians, the amiable people to whom, according to the Italian Prime Minister, his countrymen proposed to teach wisdom and humanity, find the rhinoceros to their taste ; so they do the elephant, which is also eaten in Sumatra. Dr. Livingstone describes the elephant's foot as delicious, and his praises will be echoed by many travelers in lands where that sagacious monster still lingers in rapidly decreasing numbers. "We had the foot," wrote the doctor, "cooked for breakfast next morning and found it delicious. It is a whitish mass, slightly gelatinous, and sweet like marrow. A long march to prevent biliousness is a wise precaution after a meal of elephant's foot. Elephant's tongue and trunk are also good, and after long simmering much resemble the hump of a buffalo and the tongue of an ox, but all the other meat is tough, and from its peculiar flavor only to be eaten by a hungry man."

The Influence of Ventilation on the Micro-Organisms Floating in the Air.

According to Dr. Stern, it is *à priori* to be expected that the influence will depend very much on the character of the ventilation. His opinion, being founded on direct experiments, will bear a value proportionate to the known reliability of the experimenter. He found that when the air was still the germ-bearing dust rapidly fell to the ground, so that in the course of an hour and a half the air was practically free from germs. Lighter material—wool, the spores of fungus, etc—required a longer time to settle down. The most powerful ventilation in ordinary use—that in which the air of a room is renewed three times in the hour—did not make the air more rapidly free from germs than simple settling. One more powerful is scarcely possible without creating a draught, but it becomes gradually more effective in proportion to its strength. Its action in removing germs rapidly becomes effectual when a rapidity of six or seven renewals of the air of the room per hour is reached. It was not observed that the rapid entrance of fresh air removed, to any extent, the germs from the floor, carpets, furniture or clothes. Steam was not successful in producing a rapid deposit of the suspended germs—at least not to any great extent. *Zeitschrift für Hygiene.*

What Water Costs.

From a profusely illustrated article on "The New Croton Aqueduct," by Charles Barnard, in the *Century*, we quote the following: "It is a curious commentary on the demands of modern civilization to observe the effect of building this dam. The million people in the city need a reserve of drinking water, and twenty-one families must move out of their quiet rural homes and see their hearths sink deep under water. The entire area to be taken for the reservoir is 1471 acres. Twenty-one dwellings, three saw and grist mills, a sash and blind factory and a carriage factory must be torn down and removed. A mile and a quarter of railroad track must be relaid and six miles of country roads must be abandoned. A road twenty-three miles long will extend around the two lakes, and a border or 'safety margin' 300 feet wide will be cleared all around the edge to prevent any contamination of the water. This safety border will include a carriage road, and all the rest will be laid down to grass. As the dam rises the water will spread wider and wider over fields, farms and roads. Every tree will be cut down and carried away. Every building will be carted off, and the cellars burned out and filled with clean soil to prevent any possibility of injury to the water. Fortunately there is no cemetery within the limits of the land taken for the reservoir. Had there been one it would have been completely removed before the water should cover the ground. Fifty-eight persons and corporations, holding 111 parcels of land, will be dispossessed in order to clear the land for the two lakes and the dams, roads and safety borders.'"

The Regulation of Sleep.

Insomnia is rightly regarded as one of the marks of an overwrought or worried nervous system, and conversely we may take it that sound sleep lasting for a reasonable period, say from six to nine hours in the case of adults, is a fair test of nervous competence. Various accidental causes may temporarily interfere with sleep in the healthy ; but still the rule holds good, and a normal brain reveals its condition by obedience to this daily rhythmic variation. Custom can do much to contract one's natural term of sleep, a fact of which we are constantly reminded in these days of high pressure ; but the process is too artificial to be freely employed. Laborious days with scanty intervals of rest go far to secure all the needful conditions of insomnia. In allotting hours of sleep it is impossible to adopt any maxim of uniform custom. The due allowance varies with the individual. Age, constitution, sex, fatigue, exercise, each has its share of influence. Young persons and hard workers naturally need and should have more sleep than those who neither grow nor labor. Women have by common consent been assigned a longer period of rest than men, and this arrangement, in the event of their doing hard work, is in strict' accord with their generally lighter physical construction and recurrent infirmities. Absolute rule there is none, and it is of little moment to fix an exact average allowance provided the recurrence of sleep be regular and its amount sufficient for the needs of a given person, so that fatigue does not result in such nerve prostration and irritability as render healthy rest impossible.—*The London Lancet.*

Physical Troubles of the Great Folks.

"Uneasy lies the head that wears a crown" appears in these days to be true not only from the cares of royalty, but also from their inherited or acquired bodily ailments. The Czar of Russia is said to be hypochondriacal and terribly shaky in the nerves. The Czarina is even worse, and is subject to attacks of intense nervous prostration. The Emperor of Austria is physically healthy enough, but in consequence of the suicide and the sad circumstances attending the death of his son is a melancholy, heart-broken man, while his wife is said to be a martyr to sciatica, rheumatic fever and melancholia. She belongs to the same family which numbers among its members the crazy kings of Bavaria. The North Germans declare that the King of Wurtemberg is more than half demented. King Milan of Servia is haunted by a dread of assassination, and the Sultan of Turkey is in constant fear of the fate of his predecessor. The physical defects of William II. of Germany give him almost constant pain, and are well known. The King of Holland is paying the penalty of a dissipated life. The King of Italy suffers from chronic gastric derangement, said to be the result of excessive smoking of green cigars. The infant King of Spain inherits from his father weaknesses which will probably make his life miserable. The King of Belgium is lame. The Queen of Roumania is troubled by hallucinations. Queen Victoria may be physically well enough, but she is an irascible old lady, and notoriously difficult to manage. The list might be continued still further.—*Medical Record.*

London Past and Present.

Sanitarians have watched with considerable interest the coming of each annual mortality report of London, for we have the instructive example of the largest of the cities of the world showing a death-rate lower than that of almost any other city of considerable size, and a mortality rate which is constantly coming down. .

And yet we are told by Dr. G. V. Poor, in a lecture before the Sanitary Institute last January, that "there can be no doubt that down to the commencement of the present century London was a veritable fever bed, the cause of death being largely malarial fever, spotted or typhus fever, plague, smallpox, measles, scarlet fever and whooping-cough, the two latter being comparatively recent introductions."

"The difficulty of rearing children is referred to as evidence of the unsanitary state of old London." Of the children of James I., three out of five died under 3 ; of the children of Charles I., the ages of death were 29, 26, 20, 15, 4, 1 ; of eleven children of James II., by two wives, one (the old Pretender) attained the age of 78, and of another the age is doubtful, but eight died under 4, and two others died at 11 and 15 ; of the six children of Anne, one reached the age of 11, and the remaining five died under one year.

The Transmission of Typhoid Fever by the Air.

It has come to be generally admitted that the transmission of typhoid fever takes place principally, if not exclusively, through the water supply. Experience, indeed, has proved this to be the case, but it must not be overlooked that other ways may exist, notably by the breathing of air contaminated with the spores of the typhoid bacillus. Some observations by Dr. Chour, of an epidemic of typhoid fever among soldiers, commented upon in the *Revue Scientifique*, serve to show the importance of not concentrating one's attention too exclusively upon any one vehicle in the endeavor to prevent the spread of the disease. Two regiments stationed at Jitomir, and supplied with drinking water from the same source, suffered in a very different degree from the disease. The soldiers belonging to the regiment which suffered most severely were quartered in various barracks, and it was remarked that at one particular locality the men were attacked in far larger proportion than their fellows who were located elsewhere. In December, 1886, the buildings were evacuated and thoroughly cleansed and disinfected, whereupon the mortality fell to 1.7 per 1000 in 1887, and *nil* in 1888. In the other barracks, which had not been thus dealt with, the mortality rose to 22 per 1000 in 1887, and 33 per 1000 in 1888. It occurred to Dr. Chour to institute an examination of the dust from the infected barracks, and he found therein an average of 14,000,000 microbes per gramme, among which the typhoid bacillus was easily detected. The evacuation of the rooms and their thorough disinfection promptly put an end to the epidemic.—*Medical Press.*

The Science of Prevention Applied Only to Epidemics.

There seems to be an almost universal coincidence of opinion, not only among lay, but professional persons as well, says Dr. Mann, of Alleghany, Pa., that so long as any one disease does not assume a distinctly and overwhelming epidemic form, there is no reasonable excuse for attempting in any way to limit the spread of preventable diseases. Or, in other words, the function of preventive medicine is to stand idly by, with folded hands, waiting listlessly until some terrible scourge fastens itself upon the community, before attempting even the simplest hygienic measures. Perhaps this opinion is not openly expressed in words, but general apathetic inaction speaks louder than any set phrase, and the responsible parties must either acknowledge this sentiment, or plead guilty to the equally bad alternative of having been negligent in the case of the lives entrusted to them.

_____

Sanitary Regeneration.

It would be well if all of our cities would, as speedily as possible, follow the wise example that has been set before them by the city of Nashville, Tenn. Roused from its insanitary lethargy by the ravages of the cholera in 1873, a sanitary survey of the city was made to learn wherein deficiencies existed. Based on this survey, a sanitary regeneration was begun, the result of which may be thus stated : In 1877, Nashville occupied an area of scant three miles, with a population of 27,000, and a death rate of 34.55 per 1000 yearly. Now it has an area of 4021 acres, or six and one-third square miles, with a population of 68,531, and a death rate of 15.31. Certainly these facts plainly prove that sanitation _does pay_. There are but few, if any, cities in our land that are in a proper sanitary condition. The appointment of a competent commission to inquire into the sanitary needs of a locality and the fulfilment of their recommendations, would, in every instance, produce the same gratifying results that have followed similar wisdom in Nashville.

_____

State Board of Health and Vital Statistics of the Commonwealth of Pennsylvania.

_____

PRESIDENT,
GEORGE G. GROFF, M.D., of Lewisburg.

SECRETARY,
BENJAMIN LEE, M.D., of Philadelphia.

PEMBERTON DUDLEY, M.D., of Philadelphia.

J. F. EDWARDS, M.D., of Philadelphia.	GEORGE G. GROFF, M.D., of Lewisburg.
J. H. MCCLELLAND, M.D., of Pittsburg.	S. T. DAVIS, M.D., of Lancaster.
HOWARD MURPHY, C. E., of Philadelphia.	BENJAMIN LEE, M.D., of Philadelphia.

PLACE OF MEETING,
Supreme Court Room, State Capitol, Harrisburg, unless otherwise ordered.

TIME OF MEETING,
Second Thursday in May, July and November.

THE
ANNALS
OF
HYGIENE

VOLUME V.

Philadelphia, October 10, 1890

NUMBER 10.

COMMUNICATIONS

The Climate of our Homes, Public Buildings and Railroad Coaches, a Leading Factor in the Production of the Annual Crop of Pulmonary Diseases.*

BY R. HARVEY REED, M.D.,

Mansfield, Ohio.

Health Officer, Member American Public Health Association, American Climatological Association, American Medical Association, British Medical Association, National Association of Railway Surgeons, Ohio State Medical Society, Honorary Member D. Hayes Agnew Surgical Society, Philadelphia, Texas State Sanitary and Medical Associations, Surgeon Baltimore and Ohio Railroad, etc., etc.

WHILST the word climate in the broad sense of the term is usually applied to the peculiarities of the seasons of a given latitude as regards the temperature, moisture, prevailing winds and sunshine, as well as the local influences affected by the cultivation and consequent changes in the soil and its products, yet, in a more circumscribed sense, it is also just as applicable to the variations in temperature and qualities of the air in our homes, public buildings and railroad coaches, as it is to the more extended area of a country or any particular region of the same.

The climate of a country is the legitimate result of certain natural causes, producing consequent effects, which may be modified in a degree by artificial conditions.

The climate of our homes, public buildings and railroad coaches is largely the direct result of artificial causes followed by their corresponding effects.

When this association was organized in Washington, in 1884, it adopted for its object "the study of climatology and hydrology, and diseases of the respiratory and circulatory organs," and a great deal has been said in its transac-

---

*A paper read before the Seventh Annual Meeting of the American Climatological Association, held at Denver, Colorado, September 2d, 3d, and 4th, 1890.

tions of the various climates of this and other countries regarding their good or bad effects on certain diseases.

A great variety of opinions have been expressed as to which locality and what particular conditions of climate are most congenial to the restoration of lost health in the greatest number of cases of a given disease. As a rule a change of climate is seldom sought for the prevention of disease, but more generally for its supposed curative effects after certain diseases have been contracted.

That the purity of the air, the regularity of the temperature and the hydromatic conditions of the atmosphere play an important part in the production of a healthful climate and the prevention of certain diseases, stands without a question. That it is better to prevent disease than to cure it is a self-evident fact.

In order to prevent disease, it becomes a necessity that we know at least the chief causes that lead to its production. For brevity and convenience we will divide all pulmonary diseases into two general classes; 1st, those of tubercular origin; 2d, those of non-tubercular origin.

Each of these have their predisposing and exciting causes. I believe it is pretty generally conceded now that the bacilli of tuberculosis exist in a latent form in the physical organism of every person, but only become developed under favorable circumstances; and that anything that tends to reduce or devitalize the general economy leads to the development of these latent tubercles into active ones.

From this we arrive at the legitimate conclusion that among the predisposing causes of pulmonary tuberculosis is congenital predisposition or the so-called tubercular diathesis; the reduction of the vitality by syphilitic poison, which may often be as remote as the third and fourth generations; illy ventilated rooms, poor or insufficient nourishment or prolonged mental depression; all of which lead directly to a general reduction of the vital forces, which soon creates a fertile field and puts it in a high state of cultivation for the development of a productive crop of active tubercles.

Among the exciting causes of pulmonary tuberculosis is the introduction into the system of active bacilli from persons suffering from the advanced stages of phthisis; the incomplete oxidation of the blood by the constant inhalation of impure air; extreme and sudden changes of temperature; exposure to drafts of air and great variations in the moisture of the atmosphere.

In the non-contagious pulmonary affections, the leading predisposing causes are constitutional weakness, chronic alcoholism, the continual inhalation of air laden with fine dust or obnoxious gases. Age is another cause; the very young and the advanced in years are more apt to contract non-tuberculous pulmonary affections than those in the prime of life.

The chief exciting causes of non-tuberculous pulmonary diseases are sudden and extreme changes of the temperature, the exposure of one part of the body to a very warm and the other to a much cooler temperature, sudden changes from a moist to a very dry atmosphere, or the opposite ; exposure to drafts of cold air, and the inhalation of impure air.

With these few preliminary remarks we will first proceed to investigate the climate of our homes, public buildings and railway coaches, and try to ascertain in what respect they become leading factors in the production of the annual crop of pulmonary diseases ; and second, how said causes which lead to the production of said pulmonary affections can be so modified, and their climates so improved as to avert to a great extent these disastrous results.

"Our homes" cover a great variety of architecture, all possible shades of comfort, every imaginable method of heating, from the open fire-place to the most improved air warmers of the age, and form no provision whatever for changes of air to complete scientific ventilation.

From personal investigations continued for years in quite a number of our northern states, I find that but few homes are blessed with perfect methods of heating combined with complete scientific ventilation. The homes that suffer the most for the want of pure air and proper heating are the tenement houses and "flats" of our cities ; farmhouses and ordinary city residences rank next, and lastly the palatial residences of our capitalists.

Time and space will not permit our going into the details, and consequently we will confine ourselves to a discussion of the conditions of heating and ventilation found in the average houses of our average citizens, which constitute by far the great majority of "our homes," and therefore cover the "rank and file," so to speak, of our population.

Among the farmers of our country and laborers of our cities, the average living room is the kitchen, which seldom exceeds 14 by 10 feet with an 8 foot ceiling, giving a total of 1792 cubic feet of air, or scarcely enough of air to supply one adult for two hours. This room usually has from two to three windows and one or two outside and inside doors, and as a rule is located at the rear of the main building, and is generally the poorest finished room in the entire structure. It is usually heated with a common cook stove, and is used for a cooking department and a dining and sitting room combined. In short, the entire family live in this room when in the house, except during the sleeping hours.

There is no provision for ventilation outside of the doors and windows, which are usually very loosely fitted and furnish numerous drafts of cold air from nearly all sides of the room, which is usually the only source of fresh air supply, while the cook stove furnishes the main exit for the foul air, or rather the chief source for any circulation of air whatever.

Allowing five members as the average number of an ordinary family and 1000 cubic feet of air for each person per hour the average amount of fresh air which should be supplied, and they will require 5000 cubic feet of air an hour, and consequently would breathe all the air in the room in less than twenty minutes. A room under these conditions, after making a most liberal allowance, would not receive to exceed 500 cubic feet of fresh air an hour from the cracks in the windows and doors, or but one-tenth of the actual amount necessary, unless a door is opened or a window raised or lowered, which is seldom the case, especially when the temperature is low, and when done is a very objectionable method of ventilating at best, particularly in cold weather.

The temperature in a room heated and ventilated like this will vary from 20° to 40° F. between the floor and the ceiling and the more remote parts of the room. I have seen water freeze in one part of a room like this with a red-hot stove in the other, and the thermometer registering 75° F. on the wall at the level of the head. Again, I have seen as high as 35° difference in such rooms between the head and feet while sitting on an ordinary chair, and yet people wonder how they "catch cold" and contract pneumonia, pleurisy and acute bronchitis, or suffer from nasal catarrh and frequent attacks of quinsy.

Nor is this all. Go with me to the sleeping rooms of these same people and here you will generally find an 8 by 10 or 10 by 12 room with an 8 foot ceiling, or not to exceed 960 cubic feet of air—a scanty supply for one person for a single hour—but those rooms usually contain two inmates and not infrequently three or four. In the former there would be just pure air enough to supply the two persons half an hour. These rooms are seldom heated, and less seldom the windows are either raised or lowered to admit fresh air, which must find its way in around the crevices of one or two windows and a single door. We will make a liberal estimate and allow 100 cubic feet per hour for each window and door when closed, which in the case of two windows would amount to 300 cubic feet per hour—less than one-third the requisite amount for one person, and less than one-sixth the amount for two, or an average of 150 cubic feet of fresh air per hour to each person, with no provision whatever for the escape of foul air except by the same channels—the doors and windows. Is it any wonder they get up in the morning with headache and have frequent attacks of throat and lung diseases? The wonder is there is not more.

Let us leave "our homes" for the present; go with me to our public buildings, of which the schoolhouse is the most important. It has been my privilege to make personal inspections of hundreds of schoolhouses and scores of churches, courthouses, hospitals, almshouses, jails, several State and provincial capitals, a few penitentiaries and asylums, and one National capital, which combined form the basis of my personal information on this part of the subject before us; and with few exceptions, when weighed in the balance with approximately perfect heating and ventilation, they were found wanting.

In the large majority of our public buildings there is a variation of temperature existing in the same room in ordinary cold weather of from 15° to 35° F. between the floor and the ceiling and those parts of the room most remote from the heating apparatus; whilst the fresh air supply is either inadequate or absent altogether. Generally there is no provision made for the escape of foul air whatever; occasionally there is an open grate or stove with open doors which allow a portion of the foul air to escape, but usually in these cases there is no provision outside of the windows and doors for the supply of fresh air.

By the usual methods of steam and hot-water heating, there is neither provision for the introduction of fresh air or the escape of foul air. I have seen scores of schoolrooms with from forty to sixty scholars in them and no provision for heating except a stove, and no provision for fresh air outside of an open door, window or transom, in which case some scholars must sit in a draft of cold air, others in a part of the room which is too hot, and the rest in a part that is just as much too cold. I have seen scores of schoolrooms heated by furnaces which only supplied from two to six thousand cubic feet of "red-hot" air per hour for forty-five scholars, or not to exceed 150 cubic feet of air an hour for each scholar (instead of at least one thousand or fifteen hundred cubic feet of warm air for each child for the same length of time) without any provision, except the doors, windows or transoms, for the escape of foul air.

Just imagine from six to ten scholars being restricted to the use of only air enough for one scholar, and while they are being starved for pure air they are being tortured by extremes of temperature, whilst their brains are being taxed with long lessons and burdensome tests. Is it any wonder that after twelve or fifteen years of this kind of torture they finally succumb to pulmonary tuberculosis and fill a premature grave?

Next to the homes and public schools there are, perhaps, more people living in passenger coaches than in any other class of structures, take it the year round. Let us see what kind of a climate they furnish the great army of the traveling public. After a series of systematic inspections on four of our trunk line railroads, and the inspection of some thirty passenger coaches of all classes, from the smoking car to the palace Pullman coach, I have found a variation of temperature between the floor and the level of the head while sitting in an ordinary seat, in each car examined, which ranged from 12° to 30° F., in first-class coaches.

The coach referred to in the first instance was a ladies' coach heated with hot air, whilst the temperature outside the car was only 15° above zero : and in the latter case the car was a Pullman sleeper heated with hot water, with a coil of pipe under each seat and extending around the sides of the car, with the outside temperature 12° above zero. In the coaches heated with common stoves, hot water or steam, there are no provisions whatever, except the windows, doors and transoms, for the admission of fresh air or the exit of foul air (except when stoves are used a little foul air escapes through the stove), and these sources are not only exceedingly unsatisfactory and incompetent, but positively dangerous to the health and lives of the passengers. In the coaches heated by hot air, the supply of fresh air used is not only irregular but insufficient, and varies with the direction of the wind and the velocity with which the train is running ; none of these coaches are supplied with foul air exhausts outside of the draft in the stoves, the doors, windows and transoms.

The average number of passengers found in the thirty coaches inspected was thirty to a coach, varying from seven to fifty-seven people in each car ; this would require on the average of at least 20,000 cubic feet of warmed air to the car every hour, and the proportionate exhaustion of foul air to keep the atmosphere of the car in a practically pure condition. We also found from 4.41 parts of CO^2 in 10,000 parts of air in the summer time, with the doors and windows open and only eleven passengers in the car, to as high as 18.33 parts CO^2 in the winter season, with fifty-seven passengers in the coach.

By these series of researches we have found that from the cradle in our homes to the public schools, from the schools to the churches and public buildings, and from the quiet cottage or busy counting room of everyday life to the whirling palace car, we are bathed in one continuous impure atmosphere.

From the moment they are born until they draw the shroud around them for their last sleep, the great army of people who live indoors are breathing impure air. They send their children to school where they breathe and rebreathe the air over and over again ; nay more, the putrid breath of the syphilitic and tuberculous child is inhaled by the child with rosy cheeks and a sound constitution from the beginning to the end of the school year. You would scorn the idea of having but one handkerchief, tooth brush or tooth pick for each school room and having your children all compelled to use them daily in common with the rest of the scholars, but you sit with folded hands and peaceful conscience while your children violate sanitary laws a thousand times worse by the inhalation of millions of cubic feet of foul and even putrid air from their diseased classmates or daily associates each school year.

Again, the fond mother sits her helpless child on the floor and tries to have it amuse itself with toys, while the whole body is bathed in an atmosphere of from 15° to 25° colder than the body of the mother, and then wonders why it cries and is discontented and fretful, and is in a perfect quandary as to how it ever contracted pneumonia.

If it survives this, it is sent to school, and not only bathed in a poisonous atmosphere but subjected to drafts of cold air from windows and transoms in one part of the room, or overheated in another, while as a rule its feet are bathed in a stratum of cold air from morning until night.

How many of us, who in our younger days played the rôle of a school teacher, cannot recall the frequent and familiar plea of "please, may I go up to the stove and warm my feet?" and recall the sickening cough, cough, cough of the child with "only a cold," or picture the flannel-bound necks of the children with sore throats, and point in our mind's eye to the flushed cheeks and watery eyes of the child with the "splitting headache" vainly striving to get out a lesson for the coming recitation ; and yet, with all these melancholy facts staring us in the face, like ghosts from the graves of the martyrs, from bad heating and ventilation, we have gone on and on for years with little or no improvement for the relief of these conditions which cause the death and daily suffering of countless thousands of our rising generation.

Is it any wonder their constitutions are undermined and their health broken down at the age of 20, and before 25 a large percentage of them fill the consumptive's grave? Is it any wonder that countless thousands of children die of acute lung trouble before they reach the age of 5 years, when we rehearse the facts we have tried to set before you regarding the heating and ventilation of our homes? Is it any surprise that pneumonia so frequently claims the business man as he turns the age of 40, and hustles him off to meet his God with scarcely a moment's warning?

Oh, no! my fellow practitioners, these are only the legitimate results of physical causes and the direct violation of sanitary laws; and just so long as we continue to heat and ventilate our homes, our public buildings and railway coaches as we do at the present time, just so long may we expect to find the annual crop of pulmonary diseases to stand at the head of the mortality list in all our annual health reports. Just so long as cause is followed by effect, and just so long as the great masses of our people are exposed to one continued bath of impure air, complicated with great extremes of temperature in our homes, public buildings and railroad coaches, just so long may we expect consumption to stand at the head of the annual mortality list, and the remainder of our pulmonary diseases generally to hold their present rank in mortuary statistics. Iron, cod liver oil and foreign climates must yield to common sense and sanitary reforms in our homes, our public buildings and railway coaches first, before we can hope or legitimately expect to see any reform in the mortuary statistics of pulmonary diseases.

We have tried in vain for centuries to "cure" consumption. People by the thousands and hundreds of thousands have flocked from one health resort to another vainly seeking to free themselves from the lion grip of pulmonary consumption; they have, figuratively speaking, soaked themselves in cod liver oil and clad themselves inside and out with iron; they have loaded their poor stomachs with the hypophosphites and been pumped with the pneumatic cabinet and injected with carbonic acid gas; but the end was all the same; it was only a question of time until the funeral knell sounded the requiem of their departed spirits.

These are undeniable facts, and as such should claim not only our attention as physicians and surgeons, but our united efforts in search of relief. The law compels our railroads to guard its city crossings, and in many States to stop all trains at the junctions, besides a dozen and one other things for the physical protection of their passengers. School boards quarrel over the kind of text-books, the style of seat, or particular form of architecture they shall adopt; while our fellow-countrymen waste their physical and mental energy to have a pretty home painted and papered in the latest style. But scarcely one of them spends a moment of time or a dollar of money to secure perfect heating and ventilation, which are a thousand times as important to their physical prosperity and length of days as the guarding of a street crossing, the selection of a text-book, or the architectural beauty of a home.

The question naturally arises, How shall we heat and ventilate our homes, public buildings and railroad coaches with practical perfection? In answer to this question, I will say there are three prime factors that must be carefully considered. They are : 1st. A practically uniform temperature should be obtained through each room or car ; 2d. From 1000 to 1500 cubic feet of pure air warmed to about 70° or 75° F. should be supplied each person hourly who is occupying a given room or car ; 3d. The prompt removal of all foul air from each room or car as fast as it is produced.

While securing these prime factors it is also necessary to observe four other important features in the selection of the apparatus and system for heating and ventilation. They are : 1st. Safety ; 2d. Economy ; 3d. Durability ; 4th. Simplicity. To accomplish the required results in compliance with the above requisitions, an air warmer should be used with sufficient radiating surface to simply warm the required amount of air to the requisite temperature without the air having to pass at any time over a red-hot surface of iron, or be heated so hot as to materially deprive it of its natural amount of moisture. This may be done by three principal methods : 1st. By passing it over pipes heated with steam ; 2d. By passing it over pipes warmed by hot water ; 3d. By passing it over the heated plates or through the air flues of a furnace or stove.

The first and second methods are what is known as indirect heating and ventilation, and when properly constructed and in good order give fairly satisfactory results. The objections to this method of heating are : 1st. It is much more costly to secure the necessary plant, and from a fourth to a third more expensive to run than the direct system of heating ; 2d. In climates where the temperature falls under 12° or 15° below zero, the indirect system is a practical failure, as the condensation in the steam pipes is greater than the expansion, while the water pipes cannot be kept sufficiently warm ; 3d. The danger of explosions, even with low pressure, and in the hot water system makes these methods more or less objectionable ; 4th. The expense of repairs and the replumbing of a part or the whole of the heating apparatus every few years makes another objectionable feature to these methods of heating and ventilation.

The third method is what is known as the warm air or direct method of heating and ventilating, and is not only the least expensive to commence with, and by far the most desirable, but decidedly the safest and most efficient method of heating and ventilating yet discovered.

A furnace should be so constructed as to have a large heating surface without escape of dust or gas from the fire, and at the same time economize the fuel by utilizing all the heat possible by transmitting it directly to the air to be warmed.

In no instance should the air pass over red-hot iron, or only a portion of the air be heated very hot and allowed to cool off by mingling with the cold air of a room ; but the entire quantity of air required for a building, or any part of it, should be heated only sufficient to maintain a temperature of about 70° or 75° F., when it is distributed through a room, and, at the same time, retain its natural moisture. Whenever a furnace or stove requires an evaporating pan to keep the air moist, it is high time such a stove or furnace should be removed and a modern furnace or stove become its successor.

After the air has been properly warmed, the next important question is, where shall the fresh warm air enter the room, and where shall the foul air be allowed to escape ? Time and space will not permit me to enter into the details of this part of the subject and give you all the reasons for the faith within me. Suffice it to say that the method which gives the best results, everything considered, is the one which brings the warm air in at the floor, at the side of the room least exposed to the external elements, and exhausts the foul air at or near the windows, or, in other words, at the side of the room most exposed to the weather, and afterward returning it in tight conduits under the floor, delivers it to the ventilating shaft.

By this method the cold foul air is immediately exhausted through the ventilating shaft, which keeps the air in the rooms pure and of an even temperature. I have repeatedly examined rooms heated and ventilated by this method, and have failed to find more than from $3°$ to $5°$ F. between the floor and the ceiling, or the warmest and coolest parts of the room. My own house is heated and ventilated after this method, and is open for inspection by any person who is interested enough to do so in proof of the assertions I have just made.

The old method of putting a register at the top of the room for the escape of the foul air is neither economical nor scientific, and it wastes your heat, cools off your room and leaves the cold foul air as its legacy. It may be said, for people in moderate circumstances, that this is too expensive. In that case, I would recommend them to get improved heating stoves made to carry out this general plan, and which are provided with an air chamber that is supplied with fresh air from the outside of the room or building, which in turn is warmed and delivered to the room to be heated and ventilated ; while the foul cold air can easily be exhausted through a double chimney, with an opening at the floor on the one side for its escape, all of which can be done for less than would pay the doctor's bill for one case of pneumonia.

It has cost thousands and tens of thousands of dollars to practically demonstrate the few condensed facts I have just given you in this paper, besides years of experimenting and repeated investigations to detect and eliminate the defects, and develop and establish the correct principles of heating and ventilation and put them on a practical basis ; and to that ingenious, persevering, energetic and progressive sanitary engineer, Mr. Isaac D. Smead, of Toledo, Ohio, this country and the world at large owes more than to any other living man for the practical development of the most economical and scientific method of heating and ventilating our homes and public buildings which has yet been developed.

But you very properly ask me, How are you going to improve the heating and ventilation of our railway coaches, which may be called portable houses, and must be supplied with portable heating apparatus, and be duly provided against currents and counter-currents of air produced by the running of the trains ? I will answer you that the same general principles of introducing the warm air at the floor and exhausting the foul air at the same level, will hold good in the railroad coaches just the same as in a private room or a public building.

In order to accomplish this, the windows and transoms must be kept closed and the fresh air of each car supplied by an air pump from the engine, which air supply, when necessary, should be warmed by being passed over the radiating surface of steam or hot water pipes, or some form of safe, portable furnace before entering the car. By this method a regular supply of fresh warm air could be supplied to each car regardless of the outside zephyrs or the direction or speed the car was running, whilst the same gentle but regular air pressure would constantly facilitate the escape of the cold foul air and keep the floor of the car comfortably warm and the air of the coach practically pure day and night. .

That these methods of heating and ventilating our homes, public buildings and railroad coaches are a practical success, especially in the first two instances, is now beyond a peradventure, and that they will remove the foul air from a room has been proven by repeated chemical analyses ; while the hydrometer has shown that the natural moisture of the air is practically retained and the thermometer has determined the regularity of the temperature thus obtained, which shows but a trifling variation in any part of a room.

Who can deny that an abundance of pure air of a regular temperature and moisture, is not a preventive to pulmonary disease ? That is just what we seek to find in our health resorts for the relief of pulmonary affections—a regular climate, which is neither dry nor too moist and never too cold nor too hot, and which is supplied with oceans of pure air the year round.

Are not these the conditions of climate we have just shown you can be produced in every home, public building and railroad coach throughout our land, if properly heated and ventilated ? Then can an Italy, a Florida, a California or even a Colorado boast of more ? But even granting they can furnish the invalid all of these conditions of climate in their perfection, only a limited few of the surging masses of humanity can afford these natural blessings, while the preventives I have just prescribed are within the reach of all, whether rich or poor, high or low, from their childhood to matured old age.

We dare not deny that the production of a regular climate of pure air in our homes, public buildings and railroad coaches such as we have suggested, although the production of art, will aid materially in reducing the annual crop of pulmonary affections ; neither can we deny that the opposite conditions which we have shown you now exist in by far the large majority of homes, public buildings and railway coaches, have and do aid very materially in increasing the annual crop of pulmonary diseases throughout our land.

Our laws throw their protecting arms around the swine in our pig-pens and the cattle upon a thousand hills, and say to the contagious diseases that affect them, thus far shalt thou go and here shalt thy destroying arm be stayed. Are not the health and lives of our fellow-citizens, nay, I will put it, your daughter or my son, worth [even as much as those of the dumb brutes in the field ? And yet the laws of our land are practically as silent as the statue of Liberty in New York Bay on the question of a bountiful supply of God's pure air in our homes, public buildings or railroad coaches.

Our prohibition friends have organized and maintain a third political party, and spend millions of dollars annually to prevent the suffering and premature death of the inebriate, which only constitutes a fraction of the premature deaths produced by the ravages of pulmonary affections throughout the length and breadth of our land each year. I doubt if they have ever turned a hand or spent a dollar to secure a reform in the heating and ventilation of our homes, public buildings or railway coaches, and thereby aided in preventing a far worse and much more fatal affection of the human family than even chronic alcoholism, and at the same time, one, that to a large extent, can be prevented by compelling and maintaining, if need be by law, a genuine supply of God's pure air, properly warmed in the cold season, to every home, public building, factory, workshop, store, office and railroad coach throughout our land.

Then, and not till then, can we ever expect to see the dawn of a sanitary millennium in the reduction of the mortality statistics of pulmonary affections to a common level with other ordinary diseases.

Mansfield, Ohio.

The Ventilation of Cities, or the Sanitary Value of Interior Open Spaces.*

BY J. M. ANDERS, M.D.,
Of Philadelphia.

LARGE cities cannot afford to be systematically neglectful in regard to sanitary matters. Human life and public health are too valuable to be estimated in dollars and cents. Wherever human beings congregate, a plentiful supply of fresh pure air in constant movement is necessary to the preservation of sound health. A stagnant air is slowly but surely mortal. Among the sanitary needs of a city, good ventilation ranks second to none. In this connection, the question of open spaces in cities is far-reaching in its relation to the cause of many of the more commonly prevailing as well as most fatal diseases ; and it also involves a consideration of the ill effects of overcrowding, which is caused largely by the tenement system of building houses, by high buildings, narrow streets, and by small counting-rooms.

It is to be noted that the rate of increase in population of cities, and their growth in area are not, as a rule, in equal ratio. As pointed out by Professor E. R. L. Gould, "they grow rapidly in height, but not so fast in length or breadth." The comparative growth of urban and non-urban populations

---

*From the *Medical and Surgical Reporter*.

during thirty years is also mentioned by Gould, who writes : " In the United States, in 1850, the inhabitants of cities amounted to 12.5 in each 100 of the total population ; in 1880 the number had advanced to 22.5, an increase of 80 per cent."

For the last quarter of a century there has been observed an increasing popular sentiment in favor of small parks. This favorable change of public opinion is due largely to the fact that, wherever open spaces have been created in populous centres, they have proved of incalculable benefit in a great variety of ways.

No member of the medical profession, knowing the importance to sound health of pure fresh air and sunlight, can reflect upon the unfortunate state of society as met with in some of the worst quarters of large cities, where persons are often packed together without the slightest regard to the proper cubic air-space per head, and escape the conviction that something ought to be done speedily to bring relief to all who are exposed to these pernicious influences. That the powers of the human system are intolerant of the baneful effects of overcrowding is no new fact in medical science. Massing a population unduly lowers the general vitality and favors the development of such diseases as rickets, anæmia, phthisis, and others. There is also a group of infectious and contagious diseases—more especially measles, scarlatina, diphtheria and typhoid fever—for whose propagation densely populated districts, where natural ventilation is defective, furnish a good breeding-ground.

All sanitary authorities agree that the cubic air-space per head should not be less than one thousand cubic feet, and that the air of this space should be thrice renewed every hour, if we would prevent undue accumulation of noxious organic substances which are given off in respiration and by the skin. Perhaps all except our best homes fall short of this hygienic requirement ; and certain it is that in the homes of the poor the average cubic space per head is reduced to less than one-third of that mentioned as necessary.

Wilson,* speaking with special reference to society as found in European cities, states that among the poorer classes the cubic space for each person, instead of approaching to one thousand feet, in number of cases does not amount to two hundred feet. In the tenement houses of New York City and Brooklyn we have the most impressive example of the evil consequences of the massing of a population to be found in the United States. One of the wards in New York City has over 290,000 persons to the square mile, and several have a population of 200,000 to the same area. One-half of the whole population, indeed, live in these houses, while more than 75 per cent. of all deaths occur here. In view of the hygienic truth that the mortality rate increases with the density of the population, the fact that not many years since the death rate in New York City was 28 in 1000 per annum will excite no surprise. And we need not wonder at the declaration of an eminent authority

*Text-Book of Hygiene, p. 252.

when he states that there is no third generation in many New York tenement houses.

Time was when the chances of life were twice as good in the rural districts of England as in Liverpool and Manchester,* and less than half a century ago the mortality rate of nearly all great cities bore to sparsely populated rural districts about the same ratio.

Within the last twenty-five years, however, all this has been greatly changed ; the annual average death rate in many of the older cities has already been reduced by nearly one-half. To some extent this has been occasioned by the enforcement of better sanitary rules and regulations, more especially such as pertain to the drainage, on the part of local and state boards of health, and also by a better knowledge of hygienic principles and the spreading of that knowledge among the people. But it has been clearly observed that, in consequence of having created new interior open spaces and public parks and having widened their thoroughfares, thereby securing a better system of outdoor ventilation for the people, many of the older European cities have greatly assisted in lowering their mortality rate.

The sanitary importance of ventilating the home is universally acknowledged. But a perfect system of ventilation implies that the air admitted to our dwellings shall be pure. Now this cannot be the case in districts where the buildings are high, the streets narrow and tortuous, often near alleys and occupied by a dense population, and with light and fresh air practically excluded. Surely under these conditions foul air is abundantly generated and filth especially accumulates. In cities, an efficient system of indoor ventilation must go hand in hand with an efficient system of outdoor ventilation, the one always implying the other. In order to secure a proper air movement and a plentiful supply of fresh air, the streets should be wide, and frequently-recurring small breathing spaces should be introduced, especially in overcrowded parts ; thus to some extent scattering the population, on the one hand, and admitting sunlight and fresh air on the other.

Open spaces act as powerful ventilators of large cities, not only by diluting any impurities that may be present, but also by their favorable influence in promoting mild wind-currents. This is especially true where public squares communicate with wide avenues or streets open at each end. With a view of showing the great importance of interior open spaces to the best interests of the inhabitants of large cities, we have the testimony of Dr. T. Newell.† This author, speaking with reference to London, a city liberally provided with park areas, says : "Reckoning the population of London at 4,100,000, the reduction in the death rate during the last two hundred years shows a saving of 91,020 lives for the year 1886, more than two-thirds of the population of Providence, R. I. The extravagant employment of 'fresh air' and 'elbow room' has doubtless been the most important factor in bringing about this desirable change."

---

*Twenty-fifth Report of the Registrar General.
†Interior Open Spaces in Cities, 1889.

As showing the favorable influence of wide streets over the prevalence of consumption, we also have the results of the very interesting observations of Dr. Arthur Ransome upon the cause of this disease, in Manchester, England. He writes : " The longest and widest streets in the district were Jersey Street, with ten deaths, and George Street, with eight deaths ; but the number in these streets is approached by the mortality of eight deaths in Hood Street, which is only half its length, but which is a mere lane, blocked at each end, so as to obstruct free ventilation. Again, Henry Street, which is a long thoroughfare, has only four such deaths, while Boord Street, a narrow *cul-de-sac* only a quarter its length, has seven." Dr. Ransome's investigations furnish fresh evidence of the fact that some of the most fatal as well as most prevalent diseases are to a great extent within human control, and that these would lose much of their terror if more decided measures were adopted to prevent them.

So much for the sanitary effects of city air-holes as mere open spaces ; much might be said concerning their hygienic value when treated of as spaces filled with growing vegetation. The salutary influence of living plants upon the air, however, having received a good deal of attention during the last decade, will here be dismissed with the mere enumeration of a few well-established facts. The effect of a space filled with growing trees and shrubbery is to increase slightly the local degree of saturation and to maintain its equability ; to increase the ozonizing power of the atmosphere, thus rendering it safer and purer ; to furnish grateful shade, which also has a cooling effect upon the air in Summer, and to exercise a well-known moral of æsthetic influence.

This question also has its humanitarian aspects. Every large city has its toiling multitude, which cannot get a change of air during the heated term—cannot even, for want of means and time, reach the larger parks and pleasure grounds, which may be but a few miles distant from the scenes of their daily labor. For this large class, as well as the sick children of the workingmen, numerous open spaces, at short distances from each other, though they are small, would, as before stated, be of incalculable benefit as places in which to spend a brief period for refreshing and healthful recreation.

The members of this Society may be interested in knowing what provision has been made by certain leading foreign and American cities in the direction of public parks for the people. The subjoined tables show the park acreage as well as the proportionate population per acre.*

From a glance at the following tables it will be seen that there is great diversity in the extent of the park area in proportion to the population. Among the cities having the smallest park surface are Providence, Brooklyn, Cincinnati, Savannah, and Pittsburgh, the last named having only one and one-third acres, and, although it may appear strange, this small open space is said to be difficult to locate. I may be excused for stating that it is a disgrace to Pittsburgh that it cannot afford more play-grounds for the children and breathing spaces for

---

*Dr. T. Newell, Interior Open Spaces.

their parents. The inhabitants of this enterprising city should remember that to continue to disbelieve in fresh air will inevitably lead to physical degeneration.

PARK ACREAGE OF CITIES IN THE UNITED STATES.

	Population.	Park Acreage.	Population per Acre.
Providence	123,000	123	1,000
Boston	400,000	0,200	200
New York	1,839,000	4,902	375
Philadelphia	971,363	3,000	323
Brooklyn	665,600	940	639
Chicago	704,000	3,000	234
St. Louis	400,000	2,232	179
Washington	205,000	1,000	205
Baltimore	355,000	832	439
Cincinnati	325,000	539	603
San Francisco	270,000	1,181	211
Buffalo	202,000	620	326
Detroit	175,000	740	204
Minneapolis	129,200	808	159
Savannah	33,000	60	550
New Haven	80,000	384	208
Bridgeport	40,000	240	170
Worcester	68,000	280	243
Pittsburgh	156,389	1.25	120,299

FOREIGN CITIES.

	Population.	Park Acreage.	Population per Acre.
London	3,832,000	22,000	174
Paris	2,270,000	58,000	37
Berlin	1,122,000	5,000	229
Vienna	1,103,000	8,000	138
Brussels	380,000	1,000	380
Amsterdam	350,000	800	437
Dublin	250,000	1,900	131
Montreal	120,000	550	218

Dr. Gould,* in a recent article, has formulated a table giving a classification of open spaces as to size, together with the largest open space in acres for certain American cities. What will strike the reader of this table most is the tendency in cities to large parks and the absence of a liberal number of small open spaces in the squalid portions in which the population is densely herded together, and where light and air are most needed.

In conclusion, it should be pointed out that some of our leading American cities are making provision for new open spaces. Indeed, there is scarcely a representative city—excepting Pittsburgh, of course—in the Union which is not to-day bestowing some attention upon the subject of its interior adornment by means of parks and other open spaces, as well as wide and long park-ways ; and this is not a question demanding the attention merely of physicians and leaders in social reform, but of all citizens also.

Washington can boast of an ideal park system, with which that of no

---

*Park Areas and Open Spaces in America and European Cities. Reprint from publications of the American Statistical Association.

other city can be compared. In 1866 Chicago began to take decided steps toward creating public parks, and it now ranks next to Washington in point of desirable features in the arrangement of its interior open spaces. In Boston the subject has been before the people for many years, and the excellent results accomplished there are well known to students of municipal history ; and the same thing is true of St. Paul, Minneapolis, and of Providence. In New York the movement began in 1881, and already much has been done in the direction of opening up new pleasure grounds. As late as May, 1888, Philadelphia was awakened to the necessity of creating additional park areas through the influence of a few public-spirited men and women, who about the same time formed the "City Park Association." This is an active organization which has already achieved excellent results and has been the means of giving Philadelphia five new and valuable public parks.

The Conveyance of Disease by Corpses.*

BY B. FRANK KIRK,
Of Germantown, Pa.

ANY of us may inhale the germ, but if the conditions of our body are not predisposed, it does no harm. Doctors do not yet agree just in what the predisposition consists. It is not a pleasant piece of news to be told how the germ gets into the air. This is the formulas. The masses of tissue loosened and expectorated by consumptives become dried, ground up in many ways, and rise into the air by every disturbance, and they can be caught upon the clothing and carried with us to be spread by the winds. Handkerchiefs used by the sick become dry. The patient may carry his money in the same pocket with his handkerchief. He pays his butcher with a note ; the jolly butcher claps the note between his lips while he makes the change. He pays his grocer, who in turn gives his wife the boodle to buy headgear. She instinctively places the money in her bosom as the safest place and nearest to her heart, and her infant child sucks its nutriment and bacilli at one and the same time. We can conjecture a hundred ways more in which the poison can be handed around. Bank notes certainly are a ready vehicle in transmitting disease. They are most fitly titled as filthy lucre. It occurs at this moment to present a case not unusual in our experience. A young gentleman in business at Panama returned home and died of yellow fever. In preparing the body for burial we found a belt, inside of which was a large sum of money. The sufferer in his agony had perspired so freely that the notes had absorbed the moisture from his body to the extent of almost reducing the notes to a pulp. We spread them to dry while we finished our duties, and then gave them to the young

* Abstract of an address delivered before the Funeral Directors' Association of Pennsylvania at Erie.

man's father. Every piece of clothing, all the bedding and the curtains around the chamber were carried out and burned, but the precious all potential and welcome boodle, to the amount of over a thousand dollars, was most dexterously and unceremoniously dropped in the capacious side pocket of the now half-consoled father. We received our pay out of this money, and how many others got a share the Lord only knows. Had the conditions and surroundings been such at that time as to have been susceptible of receiving the poisonous germs, we might have cultivated a little crop of yellow fever. We have received money from smallpox patients in the same pleasant manner. The fact that germs of disease can readily be distributed and carried about is absolutely proven, and cannot be ignored. It certainly becomes a duty, a very peremptory duty, to intelligently study how to avoid planting the more malignant epidemics that appear at intervals and run their course. But by the superior knowledge of the physicians of to-day, and the co-operation of intelligent undertakers, with sensible and effective sanitary rules, these outbreaks can be confined to a small territory. Undertakers have not failed to notice the sinful carelessness of persons in letting loose the demon of disease and death. A few circumstances might be mentioned, which in themselves are only too common to us, but seldom thought of by the people.

But see, for instance, milk is declared by competent authority to be the best absorbent known of the bacilli of typhoid and scarlet fevers and other diseases, and it has been established to a certainty that scarlet fever and diphtheria have been thus transmitted. Some time ago we had charge of a typhoid case just outside the city limits. We found the corpse resting upon a long table in a large room. In that room, upon a series of shelves, there stood at least twenty shallow tin basins containing milk, all open to the contaminating atmosphere of the room, so placed that the cream might rise to the surface to be distributed in the early morning to their city customers. At one end of the room lay the soiled clothing just removed from the corpse, as well as a portion of the foul bedding. We at once called the family's attention to the danger of such an exposure of the dead body and soiled clothing in proximity to the milk, but were most decidedly assured that the matter gave them no uneasiness at all, as they intended to send it all to the city for sale the next morning and not use it themselves. And so they did, and then placed the next day's supply in the same place. And this was a family by no means ignorant, but simply indifferent. At another place, a person also died of typhoid fever, we found in the rear of the house a large filthy cow stable. Ten yards off a water-closet of the worst character, and in the line between them a shallow well, but we were kindly cautioned against drinking the water, as it was only used to supply the cows with drink and to wash milk pans. To our certain knowledge typhoid fever did prevail in two families where these people served milk, and we suppose you think we co-operated in sharing the benefit of this crime, as we had two profitable funerals. We had a dear friend, a pious old lady, who, moved by the best of motives, but ignorant of the nature of infection or contagion, used to visit poor families where sickness prevailed and loan picture-books and magazines to the afflicted, no matter what the disease. The more terrible the nature of the ailment the more daring she would be, knowing full well, just as we know, that combined poverty and loathsome disease are not interviewed by gilt-edged charity. She considered it her sphere of duty to thus let in one ray of beautiful sunlight by pious attention upon the noisome hovels easily found, but not sought for. She carried a lot of these books from a house where two children had died of diphtheria to a home a few blocks away, where some light sickness had attracted her notice. We asked her if she did not think it a dangerous proceeding to thus carry her books around and spread disease. She answered, "The Lord directed every good work." As she seemed to think she had the co-operation of the Lord, we simply waited until our services were needed at some of her new calling places. A wealthy lady, whose little boy we carried to the tomb, after it had died of scarlet fever, requested us to carry in our wagon a large bundle of its clothing to a poor family not far away. When we meekly suggested that the articles had better be disinfected first, she seemed hurt, and with a look of ineffable scorn repelled the imputation that any disease lurked in the habiliments of her precious babe. But we must do the lady the justice due her big kind heart, and testify to the fact that she contributed quite largely to the expenses attending the burying of two children of the poor woman whose little ones soon wilted and perished of scarlet fever after receiving the package of fine clothing. Almost on top of this instance we placed a victim of smallpox in his coffin, and a person who was very officious and aided us with a will to do the work, went straight to a social gathering without changing his clothes or washing his hands, but it was all right, nevertheless, for the body was placed in the coffin in strict conformity with sanitary rules, while the clothes and bedding were heaved out upon the shed roof for the benefit of an appreciative and curious neighborhood.

Is Life Worth Living?*

BY D. H. BECKWITH, M.D.,
Of Cleveland, Ohio.
President of the Ohio State Board of Health.

Is life worth living?

If life is not worth living, we need not concern ourselves about prolonging it. Under that condition, we might better seek after "the art of shortening life."

Well, suppose we decide that life is worth living. We know the inexorable law of nature : that life must end in death. We know, also, that a wise man said : "Our years are threescore years and ten," expressing thereby the physiological limit set to the life of man.

* Abstract of an address delivered before the Ohio State Board of Health.

Do you know that this estimate, made many thousands of years ago, shows a wonderful knowledge on the part of its author? Since his day science has taken hold of the question, and the result of the most elaborate and careful observations has been to place the physiological limit of human life just where this wise Jew placed it—threescore years and ten.

The death of man comes, with the death of all living things, as a law of nature. He is worn out, and ceases therefore to continue.

The nature and causes of the death of the body are questions that lie within the province of natural science. Now what does science say? It says: "Every form of life has its special type of existence," from the tiny object that sports a short hour in the sunbeam, and then dies, to the ponderous elephant, whose life covers more than a century. We have, I say, between these a myriad of beings, each class of which follows its own type, has its definite limit of existence, and, like man, "dies when its time comes."

Gentlemen, this is the source of the unity and harmony of nature.

Only in this way can nature maintain an equilibrium of existence among the innumerable creatures that swarm the surface of the earth.

I believe that the love of life is instinctive in every human being. Only by some dreadful catastrophe, whether it be like the explosion of the dynamite or like the insidious and fatal work of dry rot, only until calamity or decay has done its worst, does the largest or the most insignificant soul lose its love of life.

> "When all the blandishments of life are gone
> The coward sneaks to death."

But one more nobly sings:

> "Tell me not, in mournful numbers,
> Life is but an empty dream."

Loving it, what more natural than its continuance should be, if possible, preserved? Ah! gentlemen, this was the wild dream centuries ago; when Ponce de Leon crossed unknown seas in search of the fountain that would give eternal youth, he was driven by the breath of many ages, whose sighs for immortality have been flowing across centuries. De Leon has many successors, who, not daunted by his failures, still pursue the ever-eluding "ignis fatuus."

The old alchemist who, in the privacy of his cell, sought for that touchstone that could turn all baser metals to gold, kept his eye always on the possibility of finding that wonderful something which would forever cheat old age and death. The most modern exemplification of this hope, which has never quite died out of the human breast, was the almost universal craze in the use of Dr. Brown-Sequard's Elixir of Life. Scarcely had he whispered it in the air before the swift telegraph carried it to the bounds of civilization, and, not waiting to learn the exact conditions of his methods, thousands of physicians—educated and experienced men, whom we might suppose knew something of the laws of pathology and physiology—seized upon the idea with the zeal of men living in the dark ages, and vainly attempted to defeat the laws of nature by giving to hopelessly diseased and wornout bodies a new and indefinite lease of life.

But while we find with great frequency persons of 75 or 80 years, we never fail to note that they are always "in the sere and yellow leaf."

In years gone by they bravely mounted the rising hill of life, youth and ambition giving wings to their feet, until, like the sun, which rose in grandeur and swept upward from horizon to zenith, they stand at the summit of life— the highest type of all that is glorious on earth.

• We all find much in the world to admire, but we seldom find a man who in his heart, at times, does not think that if he had his hand on the throttle of the engine of the universe, he could run things after an improved plan.

In quite another sense this question of living has an important practical bearing. Let us for a moment address ourselves to it. The American nation is based upon this grand principle : "Life, liberty and the pursuit of happiness are the inalienable rights of man." The right to live belongs to every child, born or unborn. He is entitled to live until he dies of old age. But what do our statistics show in Cleveland ?

That in the past year, in that city alone, over 1600 children died under the age of 1 year, over 2300 children died under the age of 5 years, and over 2500 between the ages of 5 and 10 years. This death rate, that is so fearful all over our beautiful State, could be lessened at least one-half if sanitary laws were better understood by those who have the care of children.

What is human life worth? Ask the god Mars when he leads his battalions to war ; ask the pestilence when it sweeps over the land ; ask the cyclone ; ask the mad conflagration. They will tell you life is cheap. But, gentlemen, with advancing civilization the value of human life is steadily appreciating.

We have awakened to a realizing sense of our duties in saving life. Sanitary science is born—the noblest daughter of the Nineteenth Century—and she is now nobly laboring to save the human race from premature death. Already she has done a great work, and yet she is but just begun.

Would you prolong life ? Give sanitary science your ardent support. She builds a great wall of safety around your happy homes, and she hovers like a protecting angel over the cradle of your children.

There was a time when doctors alone were expected to know anything about sanitation. Against their own interest, in the matter of dollars and cents, they have worked hard to develop and spread abroad the knowledge of the laws of health and the prevention of disease. All this knowledge is now given to the world. Books, pamphlets and addresses have been printed and freely given without money and without price.

If men who spend years in making money would only spend a few hours in studying hygiene, they might perhaps live to enjoy what they have made. If books on sanitary laws, on rearing children, caring for the home, food, ventilation, dress, exercise and other sanitary topics were in all libraries and on centre tables, what boundless profit it would be to mankind. Ten, twenty and a thousand-fold it would return to you.

But now, in conclusion, gentlemen, "that life is long which answers life's great end."

> "We live in deeds, not years; in thoughts, not breaths;
> In feelings, not in figures on a dial.
> We should count time by heart-throbs. He most lives
> Who thinks most, feels the noblest, acts the best."

Feet.*

> "A plump little foot, as white as the snow,
> Belonging to rollicking, frolicsome Joe,
> In a little red sock, with a hole in the toe
>   And a hole in the heel as well.

> "A trim little foot, in a trim little shoe,
> Belonging to sixteen-year-old Miss Sue,
> And looking as if it knew just what to do,
>   And do it in a way that would tell.

> "A very large foot in homely array,
> Belonging to Peter, who follows the dray,
> So big that it sometimes is in its own way,
>   And moves with the speed of a snail.

> "Ah! a very big thing is the human foot,
> In dainty-made shoe, or in clumsy boot;
> So 'tis well there are various tastes to suit,
>   And that fashion can't always prevail.

> "The plump little foot, a beautiful sight,
> And the trim little foot, so taper and slight,
> And the very large foot, though much of a fright,
>   Are travelling all the same road.

> "And it matters but little how small, or how great,
> So they never grow weary of paths that are straight,
> And at last walk in at the golden gate
>   Of the city whose Builder is God."

But when encased in shoe-leather, whether it be thick or thin, tight or loose, good or bad fitting, the foot must receive considerable attention, else it will become "weary of paths that are straight" as well as of those that are crooked. The fact that nearly everyone confesses to the torture of corns is direct evidence that this attention is not forthcoming, for with proper care the feet may be kept in as presentable and healthful a condition as the hands. Corns are the direct result of long-continued friction, uncleanliness and neglect —a broad statement, but nevertheless true. The shoe prevents the free circu-

* From the *Sanitary Volunteer*.

lation of air and the evaporation of the natural moisture of the foot, and the high heel and pointed toe cause a constant friction of the toes against the leather and against each other.

Corns are of three varieties : (1) Laminated corns, in which the hardened cuticle is arranged in layers; (2) fibrous corns, having an imbedded peg of hardened cuticle, and (3) the soft corn, which occurs between the toes, most commonly caused by the pressure of the joint of the little toe against the adjacent fleshy part, which has been allowed to remain bathed in perspiration (for the hard, dry foot is seldom thus afflicted) and the part scalded, and although the cuticle thickens, it does not become hard.

If the corn has already formed and become inflamed and tender, the first point is to reduce the inflammation. Thoroughly cleanse the foot by allowing it to soak in quite warm water, made soft with ammonia or Castile soap ; then apply any good stick salve on a piece of linen, and remove all pressure, if possible. Allow the plaster to remain a day or two, and again soak the foot well. The plaster may now be removed, and the cuticle will be found to be soft and white. Now with a pin (the point of a needle might break) gently raise a layer of the skin, beginning at the outside edge of the corn, and thus remove layer after layer until no hardened cuticle remains. If the corn is still tender, it may not be possible to "cure" it at once, and it should not be made to bleed. After it has once been reduced so that the cuticle over the part is of no greater consistency than on other parts of the foot, keep it so. After every bath look to the place, and if the cuticle is found to be thickening, remove a layer, and do not neglect it until forced to cry out with pain. A saturated solution of salicylic acid in flexible collodion is recommended to reduce inflammation, painting the corn twice a day, after which the cuticle may be peeled off; but it will stay *cured* only with regular and frequent attention, so long as the cause remains. Soft corns will yield to the same treatment.

Cutting the corn with any sharp instrument is a pernicious practice, and should never be indulged in, for while it may give temporary relief, it perpetuates the evil. This treatment would appear to be quite common, from the fact that the itinerant scissors-grinder, when asked to put a fresh edge upon a pocket-knife, inquired, in a very matter-of-fact way, "How will you have it sharpened, mum, for parin' corns, or rippin'? "

Longevity in Single and Married Life.

BY ISAAC FARRAR, M.D.,
Of Boston, Mass.

IT has been the opinion of those who have paid attention to the subject, that marriage, in both sexes, is conducive to long life, if happily married. A European philosopher has recently made observations which renders the fact indubitable. His researches, together with what was previously known, give the following remarkable results : Among unmarried men between the ages of 29 and 46 years, the average number of deaths per annum is twenty-eight in a hundred ; but of married men, at the same period of life, the deaths are only eighteen. While forty-one bachelors attain the age of 40, there are seventy-eight married men living. As age advances, the difference becomes more striking. At 61 there are only twenty-three unmarried men alive, for ninety-eight who have enjoyed the benefits of matrimony. At 70 the proportion between the bachelors and married men is eleven of the former for twenty-seven of the latter, and at 80 there are nine married men for three single ones. The same rule holds good in nearly the same proportions with regard to the other sex.

Married women at the age of 31 may expect to live thirty-seven years longer, while for the unmarried the expectation of life is only thirty years and six months. Of those who attain the age of 45, there are seventy-three married women for fifty-three spinsters. These estimates, it must be understood, are based on *actual facts*, by observing the difference of longevity between equal numbers of individuals in single and in married life.

We believe marriage is conducive to longevity more through *mental* and *moral* than the physical system. To the man, the quietude of domestic life (when properly united), its peaceful cares, and the calm sense of virtuous affections, would be likely to prevent the soul from wearing out the frame too soon. The course of a married man's life is (or should be) regular. His wife's influence tempers his masculine character and makes him often forget care, and he is less adventurous. He feels that he is not exclusively his own property, and therefore is not as careless in regard to his health. Surrounded with a family, he is in better spirits, and does not hurry himself into vicissitudes, whether of good or evil fortune. If he is an *honest* man, and desires to live a *proper* life, he has bidden adieu to all feverish passions. His health is exposed to far less peril than before, and in sickness or accident he has the tenderest of nursing. Yes, he totters a long way down into the vale of years, becomes supported by a careful arm (so *careful* that it more than makes up for the *strength* of man), when he otherwise might sink. Let us compare such a life with the ill-regulated and reckless course of too many unconjugated men, and here is at least *one* cause for the briefer span of the latter class. This reasoning is, to a *certain extent*, applicable to the unmarried women, who are subject to the same laws as men.

Tin Canned Foods.

BY BENJAMIN LEE, A.M., M.D,
Secretary of the State Board of Health of Pennsylvania.

ONE of your subscribers makes an inquiry as to the healthfulnesss of "tin-canned goods." He also adds the statement that articles have appeared in print asserting "that the solder in its chemical action was particularly injurious to the kidneys."

Premising that preserved articles of food, meats, vegetables or fruit, can never afford quite the wholesome nourishment that the fresh articles supply, and that, therefore, they should only be used as a substitute for the latter, when they cannot be obtained, and not as a mere matter of economy (and this is especially true as regards fish and meats), I would say, in reply,

First. That, cases of poisoning by food preserved by hermetically sealing in tin cans are usually acute, taking the form of severe indigestion and cholera morbus. My attention has never been called to chronic poisoning arising from this cause, and I doubt whether it has been observed.

Second. The danger from the solder would be from the lead which it contains. This could not be injurious to the system unless it were dissolved by an acid. No food which did not naturally contain an acid or had not undergone acid fermentation, therefore, could be contaminated by it.

Third With the improved method of manufacturing tin cans at the present day, there is very rarely any opportunity for the food to come in contact with the solder, and it probably rarely does so.

Fourth. While it is true that in chronic lead poisoning, albumen is found in the urine, thus indicating that the kidneys are affected, there are other symptoms which would be present, prominent among which is "wrist-drop," or paralysis of the muscles which support the hand when the arm is stretched out.

Fifth. Physicians are rather inclined to attribute the occasional cases of poisoning which fall under their notice as the result of eating articles thus preserved, to the fact that decomposition had begun before the articles were sealed up. The decomposition of meats, cheese and fish results in the development of powerful poisons known as "ptomaïnes," which produce the same train of symptoms as those usually met with in these cases.

Sixth. If such decomposition has taken place in any given case, or if the sealing has not been perfect, leading to putrefactive changes, there will usually be a development of gas in the can. The result of this will be that the top of the can, instead of being concave (slightly depressed), will be convex (slightly bulged out or rounded). The can should, therefore, always be examined in this respect, and if the top bulges, it should not be used.

Seventh. Any article which has been cooked in a copper vessel may contain a poisonous salt of copper. This is true, of course, of old-fashioned preserves and pickles as well as of canned goods.

Eighth. Canned goods certainly deteriorate by age, losing their nutrient properties, if not becoming actually deleterious or poisonous. It is important, therefore, to obtain them from reliable dealers and as fresh as possible.

Ninth. Every State should pass a law requiring the date of the sealing of the cans in which such food is preserved. Indeed, it is a question whether, inasmuch as these goods are shipped all over the United States, Congress would not have a right to legislate upon the subject, as a matter affecting interstate commerce.

Tenth. In conclusion. The preservation of food by hermetically sealing is a most important means of varying the dietary and of providing for cases of emergency, such as long voyages, etc.

Such food, if not kept an inordinate length of time, is palatable and nutritious. Cases of poisoning from its use are very rare in comparison with the immense quantities consumed. Such poisoning is usually acute, not chronic, and there is no reason to suppose that the kidneys are especially affected by it. A can with a bulged end should always be promptly rejected.

Night Terrors in Children.*

BY G. L. ULLMAN, M.D.,
Of Albany, N. Y.

The condition of an attack of night terror is an agonizing idea which transiently occupies the mind of the sufferer. To illustrate, I will rehearse two typical cases.

A little boy about 8 years of age exhibited a true case of this terrifying distress. A few hours after falling asleep he awakened suddenly, started up crying out loud, screaming, struggling and exhibiting all signs of violent terror. During this condition he failed to be soothed with kind words, by stroking the forehead with cold water or by the inhalation of bay rum, but continued to arouse the household with his loud cries and expressions of evidence that a man with a large head, preposterous in size, was there in his room ready to bite him. He continued these lamentations again and again, with the terrible thought that an attack was surely and immediately imminent from this object of vast size and growing larger and larger with an expansion of colossal greatness, there, ready to swallow him or take him away, which was the cause of his struggling alarm and great terrifying persistence in begging aid to have it taken away. He convulsively clung to his mother's arm and gown, which he clutched with great tenacity. It became, for the time, utterly impossible to convince him that the object in question was nothing real, but imaginary. He quivered all over in a state of nervous exhaustion, with a staring and anxious expression of countenance, panting and covered with cold sweat. Several minutes elapsed while in this condition of screaming and receding from the great object that was about to seize him. His manner of violent fright was pitiful, and his freak of disturbed fancy curious. The attack was of short duration, for it was only a few minutes more when the little fellow had recovered composure, brushed away his tears, had taken a drink of water, turned around and kindly walked to his bed, and after covering himself up was soon asleep and sighing.

It was only a few nights ago that I was called about 10 o'clock by a hasty

* From the Albany *Med. Annals.*

summons to see a little girl 4 years of age, it being thought a convulsion would result during one of these nocturnal paroxysms. She was trembling with great fright and crying continuously. Her imagination was that a side-bracket globe was a hideous object—an animal—and continued to develop to an amazingly large size. Her fears were overcome after about fifteen minutes of exhausting terror, and she sobbed herself to sleep. I was informed by her parents that this was her third night successively, each attack lasting longer and being more severe, and her exclamations each night of a different nature and exhibiting alarm.

In neither case was the health of the patient apparently impaired ; both seemed to enjoy good health, and on my visiting them the next morning, their recollections of the unpleasant event of the previous night was a real blank to them. Such has been my observation in other cases.

In all probability the attack was the result of a vivid impression made in the daytime, and reproduced in distorted nocturnal horror.

The victim of night terrors, or *pavor nocturnus*, experiences an awful, unpleasant, terror-stricken disturbance of the mind, and it takes considerable soothing before tranquillity is restored. The annoyed condition of the little sufferer in his terrific expressions of alarm before awaking fully to the realization of where he is and how well all is, requires a good temper and the exercise of patience in those who are with the child, particularly when the paroxysm is of frequent, yet irregular occurrence, as it usually is.

I knew a person whose boy had at irregular intervals attacks of night terrors, who went through the corporal punishment act as regularly as the paroxysms appeared, but little satisfaction was derived, and the irate father afterward regretted his violent feeling at the time, which was caused mainly from being aroused from his own slumbers by the boy's wild expressions in these attacks, which he inappropriately termed " crazy spells." The lad has grown up and has acquired genteel night demeanor, and knows nothing of his past behavior.

The great exhaustion of the wild and frightened unfortunate is distressing. The nervous system of a child so affected is morbidly susceptible to various exciting causes, such as violent exercise and mental excitement, which have a tendency to bring on indigestion or even constipation ; also the presence of worms, causing intestinal irritation, may excite an attack ; eating a full evening meal, a distention of the bladder, dentition, or ghost stories may be named as causes.

Dr. Pepper says : " In children it evidently needs but a vivid impression upon the mind in the waking state to produce in the course of the following night, and sometimes for many nights afterward, the dream which is to cause all the phenomena of the severest night terror. The child may be in perfect health, and yet the mind shall in sleep so act as to reproduce in full or exaggerated force the terrors which have been first felt in the waking state, and perhaps whilst the child was in full, happy play. Children predisposed to this condition by some unusual activity of the brain, have the attacks whenever their health is deranged in any way, as by indigestion or by febrile disturbances from any cause."

Search for the cause, which may come from a variety of circumstances ; and treat each as the case indicates. My inability to detect any cause other than the result of an active mind and high-strung nervous system leads me to instruct the mother to use suitable discretion in giving a light supper to the little one ; to have it void its urine on retiring ; if it is restless and talks during its sleep, to change the position ; then I always endeavor to impress upon the parents the idea that much good can be done with kindness and soft words ; reasoning with the patient is of but little benefit ; he begs pity, and should not be harshly spoken to. Harshness and violence are harmful means, and aggravate and prolong the distress. Offer kind words of cheer, soothe and encourage. Though some effort will be required to pacify the unfortunate terror-stricken little one, relieve the frightened child by caresses rather than treat with a douche of cold water or by placing him out in the cold hall to shiver in fear with more fright, and begging for help. This kind of treatment is not advisable. The charming advice of good nature, coupled with time, always meets my expectations admirably.

Hunting for Money.

A burglar who had entered a house at midnight was disturbed by the awakening of the occupant of the room he was in. Drawing his knife, he said, "If you stir, you're a dead man. I'm hunting for money." "Let me get up and strike a light," said the other, "and I'll hunt along with you."

Open-Air Medical Consultation.

We know that we usually consider medical men asses, yet we are all too willing to consult them on the least indisposition. One of my friends, who resides in a city in the interior of France, is often annoyed by persons stopping him on the street and asking for advice, for which they never expect to pay. He lately devised an original scheme to rid himself of open-air consultants. When one meets him on the street and complains of some obscure malady, he cries out : "The devil you say ! Show me your tongue." After glancing up and down the street the consultant timidly extends a small portion of his lingual organ. "I tell you to put out your tongue !" exclaims the doctor, angrily ; "I can only see the end of it. Stick it out, I say. How can I make a diagnosis without seeing the tongue? Stick it out farther. Ah ! there. Now close your eyes—that's right." The patient submits with closely shut eyes and his tongue hanging out several inches. This is the occasion the doctor desires, and he disappears with lightning-like rapidity around some corner. The open-air patient always attracts a crowd.—*St. Joseph Med. Herald.*

** THE ANNALS of HYGIENE,** ✣ ✣

THE OFFICIAL ORGAN OF THE

State Board of Health of Pennsylvania.

The State Board of Health is not responsible for anything appearing in this Journal except that which bears the official attestation of the Board.

PUBLISHED MONTHLY.

Subscription, two dollars ($2.00 a year, in advance.

Address all communications to

The Hygienic Publishing Company,
224 SOUTH SIXTEENTH STREET,
PHILADELPHIA, PA.

EDITORIAL.

Why we Should All be Familiar with Hygiene.

WE trust that we will not be prejudged as giving utterance to the vaporings of a "*crank*" when we assert that every human being should be familiar with the teachings of hygiene, *because such knowledge is the only knowledge that is, in reality and reflectively, worth having.* We crave a suspension of sentence on our assertion until we have brought forth the evidence upon which it has been based. In the first place, we hold a much broader view of the meaning of the word hygiene than is usually accorded to it. We are not willing to have it defined simply as "the prevention of disease," broad, glorious, beneficent and divine as even such a definition really is. We do not understand that hygiene is merely synonymous of pure air, pure water and pure food, as so many now suppose. We go much further, and maintain that hygiene should be defined as that knowledge which gives health, contentment and happiness to all who follow its teachings.

Now, let us ask, in these days of materialism, for what purpose the material man exists ? To answer our question, we must recognize that there are several types of man. We have the selfish man, whose whole thought seems centered upon self ; we have the unselfish man, whose whole life is passed in the service of others ; we have the single man, passing through life, uncaring and uncared for, dependent upon no one and none depending upon him ; we have the family man, *ideally*, he who is naturally the head of a family, and we have the family man, *artificially*, who, in name only, is the father of the household. Thus, then, we find many types, but, in all, we venture the assertion that the main thought in life, from a materialistic point of view, is the securing of as much happiness as is possible during the brief period of life vouchsafed to each individual.

Some of those in whose minds religion is the guiding star will take issue with this assertion, because they will claim that the dominant motive in this life should be the securing of happiness in the next, but by the very fact that doing here that which they believe will secure for them happiness hereafter, they are doing according to conscience, does not this very fact bring them happiness here ? The man who believes that death means annihilation will secure for himself, while alive, the greatest measure possible of happiness here ; the man who believes that death means but a translation to a higher sphere, will, by the very acts which will make this translation a possibility be securing for himself happiness and contentment on this earth. So that, whether we view the question from a purely religious or from a purely materialistic standpoint we are forced to the conclusion that the chief aim of humanity is the acquisition of happiness. Will the study of law, of medicine, of theology, of astronomy, of mathematics, of philology, of zoology, will an intimate knowledge of chemistry, of anatomy, of Latin, Greek, Arabic, Hebrew or German, bring happiness to the individual who, because of an ignorance of hygiene, is a confirmed invalid? Did any of our readers ever see a *thoroughly healthy man* who was an unhappy man, even though his ignorance of artificially acquired knowledge might be as dense as that of the inhabitants of the jungles of India? Health and unhappiness have not even a "nodding acquaintance;" they will not mix any more than will oil and water. It may be accepted as an axiom that it is absolutely impossible for a thoroughly healthy man to be for a moment unhappy. Our non-professional readers may not be prepared to wholly accept this statement, but, take our word for it, it is dogmatic truth; our professional friends will bear us out in our doctrine that since happiness is a mental production, and since all mental productions are the results of physical actions, the happiness will be partial or complete just in proportion to the integrity or deficiency of the physical acts which have given rise to the mental production. An unhealthy body cannot make complete happiness for its possessor any more than you can develop the greatest measure of steam in an old and worn-out boiler.

But, you may say that the thoroughly healthy man, made so by nature, has no need for hygiene; and I will ask you in reply, whether the well-made locomotive engine has no need of care? As the perfect machine will become imperfect by neglect, so also will the perfect body become deteriorated for want of care.

We may accept it as an incontrovertible truth that just so far as an individual cares for himself, just so far will he enjoy health, and that just so far as he is healthy, just so far will he be happy.

If, then, health means happiness, and if happiness is the chief aim of life, can it be questioned that the knowledge which vouchsafes health is the only knowledge worthy of acquisition? The study of theology by the *ardent* theologian is, in reality, a pursuit of hygiene, because the very pleasure which any particular study will give to one who is fond of it, this very pleasure will be a promotor of health. So is it with all lines of study and work. The pursuit of that *which is congenial* is conducive to health. If our idea be grasped, it will be seen that hygiene is the broadest of all sciences. It includes all other sciences and arts; it covers every walk in life; it is the friend of judgment and the enemy only of impulse. Humanity is endowed with reason, and it is the design of nature that we should be guided by reason, and he who once properly understands this fact will become thoroughly obedient to the science of hygiene. It is the man who allows impulse to control reason, who violates the teachings of hygiene or of nature, and it is the impulsive man who is the frequently unhappy man. If we will but cultivate reason and "weed out" impulse, we will become better, healthier and happier individuals ; we will soon come to learn the all-pervading application and beneficence of hygiene, and we will be cheerfully ready to admit and enthusiastically to proclaim that the only really, practically valuable knowledge in this world is a knowledge of hygiene.

Pure Air was Needed.

It not infrequently happens that physicians base their advice to patients, at least in part, upon the latter's financial condition. A case in point : A friend tells me that his daughter consulted a physician, and the latter, having satisfied himself as to the trouble, suggested a trip to the Yosemite. "But my father cannot afford that," said the young lady. "In that case," the doctor replied, "ask him to buy you a pony and a village cart, and take a long drive every day." "I am afraid," said his patient, "that papa could not afford that, either." The doctor was equal to the occasion. "Then take a good, long ride in an open horse-car every day," he said ; "it will do you just as much good." My friend's daughter is now engaged in exploring the suburbs by open street cars, and is improving rapidly under this "treatment," which costs just ten cents daily.

The United States and its Doctors.

There is certainly no more curious social phenomenon than that of the extraordinary popularity of the medical calling in this country as a means of securing a livelihood.

The subject is one that is often dwelt upon, but we doubt if many even yet realize the grotesque misproportion which medicine in the United States holds to other bread-winning occupations. Here are some of the naked facts in the matter :

France has 38,000,000 of population, 11,995 doctors, while it graduates 624 medical students in one year.

Germany has 45,000,000 of population, about 30,000 doctors, and graduates 935 students in one year.

The United States has about 60,000,000 of population, nearly 100,000 doctors, 13,091 medical students, and graduates 3,740 students in one year.

Germany, which has relatively less than half as many doctors as America, is already groaning over its surplus. When one compares France with this country, the excess of medical men here seems most astonishing. A comparison of the United States with European countries, in whatever way it is made, leads one to think that there is something almost morbid in our medical fecundity.

NOTES AND COMMENTS.

Removal of Freckles.

Freckles are said to be easily removed by a lotion of equal parts of lactic acid and glycerine.

A Curious Delusion.

A Birmingham man, while under the influence of drink, knocked off his great toe with a hammer, imagining that he was cutting his throat with a carving-knife.

The Hygiene of Infancy.

The Paris Academy of Medicine has voted to offer a prize of 1000 francs for the best essay on the hygiene of infancy. It is open to all comers, and will be awarded in March, 1891.

Don't Kiss the Baby.

It would not be amiss if every mother would attach to her baby a placard with the above words in bold relief. The skin and mucous membranes of infants are exceedingly delicate and susceptible to poisons and diseases which make little or no impression upon adults.

For Chapped Hands.

The following preparation is said to be excellent for chapped hands, lips, etc. : Dissolve one part of boric acid in twenty-four parts of glycerin ; add to this solution five parts of lanolin, free from water, and seventy parts of vaseline. The preparation may be colored and perfumed.

Earache.

Take five parts of camphorated chloral, thirty parts of glycerine and ten of sweet almonds. A piece of cotton is saturated and introduced well into the ear, and it is also rubbed behind the ear. The pain is relieved as if by magic, and if there is inflammation, it often subsides quickly.

Baldness and Dandruff.

A solution of chloral hydrate, five grains to the ounce of water, will clear the hair of dandruff and prevent its falling out from that cause. In many instances where the patient is nearly bald, the application of the above-mentioned solution will restore the hair.

Arnica oil is also an admirable remedy to promote the growth of hair. A small quantity well rubbed into the scalp three or four times a week can be tried with expectations of benefit.

An Unprofitable Field for the Patent Medicine Manufacturer,

There is a law in Bulgaria to the effect that if a patent medicine, which is advertised to cure a certain malady, fails to do so, the vendor of the remedy is liable for damages, and may also be sent to prison for a limited period of time as a punishment for publishing an untruth to the injury of the public.

Cooking Eggs.

How many women know how to prepare a perfectly fresh egg so that an afflicted stomach can eat it ? Pour boiling water over the egg (in its shell), let it stand on the tank in the water for five minutes. The egg will be nearly as smooth as custard, and is almost as easily digested as a raw one, while its flavor is something delicious.

The Wisdom of Nature.

It may be received as a rule, that the habits and customs of a country are those which are best suited to it. Dr. Seymour has concluded that the houses of the Japanese, built of wood, are better suited to their country than the brick and stone structures erected there by Europeans. The wooden houses dry quickly. Infant mortality is very small among the Japanese.

She Took no Stock in it.

Omaha Pater-familias—" It is remarkable what a large number of doctors claim that diseases are transferred by kissing, and——"

Miss Ethel—" What kind of doctors, pa ? "

O. P.—" Why, the allopathic doctors."

M. E.—" But, pa, you know we're homœopaths."—*Omaha World.*

Street Conveniences.

The French show their good sense in providing ample conveniences for individuals in their cities. The Department of Public Comfort is equipped in a way that might be well imitated here. The establishment of urinals along our streets would not only conduce to the sanitary improvement of the city, but would be as potent a temperance promoter as the high license law.

Religious Dogs.

The famous St. Bernard dogs are very carefully trained. A traveler, who visited some of the monasteries of the monks of St. Bernard a few years ago, found the monks teaching their dogs from the earliest stages of puppyhood. Not only is physical and mental training included in the teaching, but spiritual culture is by no means neglected. At meal-time the dogs sit in a row, each with a tin dish before him containing his repast. Grace is said by one of the monks ; the dogs sit motionless with bowed head. Not one stirs until the "Amen" is spoken. If a frisky puppy partakes of his meal before grace is over, an older dog growls and tugs his ear.

To Get Rid of Flies.

People in the country who are annoyed by flies should remember that clusters of the fragrant clover which grows abundantly by nearly every roadside, if hung in the room and left to dry and shed its faint fragrant perfume through the air, will drive away more flies than sticky saucers of molasses and other fly traps and fly-papers can ever collect.—*New York Tribune.*

Hygiene in Germany.

During the past few years the subject of hygiene has received marked attention from the German government. In nearly all the leading universities there are now hygienic institutes, thoroughly equipped in every way. Recently the new Hygienic Institute in the University of Halle was opened. The institute has a lecture-room and also special chemical, physical and bacteriological laboratories.

Practical Teaching of Hygiene.

Hygiene is taught in Paris by Professor Proust, and the manner in which he conducts his courses is certainly commendable. Besides his didactic teachings and practical demonstrations, he invites the students to Saturday afternoon excursions to visit some caserne, factory or similar establishment, and there commends the good points or calls attention to the defects of the building and its hygienic management.

The Plumber and His Patrons.

It is all well enough to talk of educating the plumber, but an equally important matter is the educating of the public up to a proper understanding and appreciation of good plumbing. The great majority of our plumbers—all real, genuine plumbers are educated, but the ignorant public keep on employing men who know nothing about plumbing to save a few dollars at the expense of health.—*Sanitary News.*

A Peculiarity of the Figure 9.

Did you ever notice the peculiarity of the figure 9? When an error has arisen from any transposition of figures the difference between such transposed numbers is universally a multiple of the numeral 9. For an instance: Suppose an error occurs in bringing out a trial balance or cash settlement, or that the sum short can be divided by 9 without any remainder. If it has occurred in this way there is a strong probability that the mistake has been made by transposing figures; at any rate, if such mistake takes place by reason of transposition, the sum in question will always divide by 9 without remainder. To illustrate this: If 97 has been put down as 79 the error will be 18, or twice 9, exactly. If 322 be set down as 223 the error will be 99, or 11 multiplied by 9, and so on between any transposed numbers. Try it and prove it. —*St. Louis Republic.*

Scented Cake Suspicious.

A practical baker says : If a cake is scented with something pleasing to the smell, you can make up your mind that the cake was thus scented to kill the odor of bad materials. I have seen as many as six bad eggs put into a large cake. The scent used killed the smell. Tainted meat is also used by some conscienceless bakers in mince pies, where the high spicing and liquoring disguises the putridity.

Lung Expansion.

We have seen men and women increase their lung power by five minutes' exercise morning and night. Stand up straight on the balls of the feet, head thrown back, and inhale deeply, first inflating the lower part of the lungs, and then the upper. Then expire slowly, letting the chest sink first and then the lungs. Do this fifteen times, morning and evening, and our word for it, you'll spend less money on colds and catarrh.

Chicken Lunch.

Dark meat of cold roast chicken is the coolest lunch on a hot day, says a New York epicure, and gravely adds a word of commendation for the drum-sticks, in order to quote the comment of an irate restaurant cook who had just received an order for three chicken legs : "I can't help that," snapped the cook, "I can't cut more than two legs off one chicken. Ask them do they want the earth? Do they think fowls are centipedes?"

Look to Details.

Health, like success in life, is to be gained by paying attention to details. It is better to try to keep from catching cold than to be always trying to avoid infection. More can be done to check cholera by keeping houses clean than by using tons of disinfectants. Nature gives health. It is a man's perversity in departing from nature's teaching that leads to disease. Nature intended all to have fresh air, sufficient plain food, uncontaminated water and exercise. Let us accept nature's bequest, if we prefer health to disease.

Perspiring Feet.

A "Surgeon" who had used alum, belladonna, bismuth and boracic acid for the above, with little good result, wrote to the *British Medical Journal*, and received the following replies: 1. Wear low shoes, wool socks, and dust the feet over twice a day with iodol ; they will soon be as hard, sweet and comfortable as one could wish. 2. Wash the feet at night with very hot water, put on white cotton socks, and immerse the feet, thus covered, in methylated spirit poured into a basin. Wear the socks all night ; they will soon dry in bed. During the evening wear cotton socks and common felt slippers, and keep the socks constantly saturated with spirit. In a week the cure will be complete.

Palpitation of the Heart.

Dr. Nabo says (in *Journal de la Santé*) that an excessive palpitation of the heart can always be arrested by bending double, with the head down and the arms pendant, so as to produce a temporary congestion of the upper part of the body. In almost all cases of nervous palpitation, the heart immediately resumes its natural functions. If the respiratory movements be suspended during this action, the effect will be only the more rapid.

Apes as Cashiers.

The ape is in great request among Siamese merchants as a cashier in their counting houses. Vast quantities of base coin obtain circulation in Siam and the faculty of discrimination between good money and bad would appear to be possessed by these gifted monkeys in such an extraordinary degree of development, that no human being, however carefully trained, can compete with them. They put the coin in their mouth, immediately spitting it out if bad.

Mad Dogs.

In case of bites from dogs suspected of being mad, it is of importance to determine as soon as possible whether the dog is really rabid or not, says the *Sanitary Inspector*. If he is not, the proof of the fact is worth much to the person bitten ; if he is, the early proof of this fact is of vast importance with reference to treatment. A dog biting as the result of rabies is doomed to death within a few days as the natural termination of his disease ; therefore, to determine whether he is mad it is only necessary to confine him securely for a few days.

Kidney Disease and Garden Rhubarb.

A correspondent of *The Lancet* writes concerning a little "local epidemic" of kidney complaints. The majority of the patients had frequent urination, several of them had bloody urine, and all of them complained more or less of pain in the loins and of general indisposition. After some consideration it was found that they were eating delicious rhubarb tarts ; indeed, several of the patients were indulging in them morning, noon and night, and, in addition, they were drinking hard water rather copiously, as the weather was very hot. With these facts before him, the production of the epidemic was quite easy of explanation. The rhubarb supplied plenty of oxalic acid, and the hard water an abundance of lime ; so countless minute calculi of oxalate of lime, easily seen in the urine with a magnifying glass, were manufactured in the system, and caused the symptoms complained of. From that day to this he has been on the lookout for kidney complaints in the spring and summer, and he frequently finds them and the cause of them. Gooseberries when eaten freely often produce symptoms similar to rhubarb, and so do acid unripe apples. In the production of these kidney affections lime seems to be an almost necessary ingredient.

In Time of Sickness.

The following will be found to be a cheap and pleasant fumigator for sick rooms, and diffusing a healthful, agreeable and highly penetrating disinfectant odor in close apartments or wherever the air is deteriorated. Pour common vinegar on powdered chalk until effervescence ceases, leave the whole to settle, and pour off the liquid. Dry the sediment and place it in a shallow earthen or glass dish, and pour into it sulphuric acid until white fumes commence arising. This vapor quickly spreads, is very agreeably pungent, and acts as a powerful purifier of vitiated air.

Prejudices about Foods.

In his address before the Chemical Society of Washington last January, Mr. Edgar Richards called attention to the objections some people have to food liked by others.

A large proportion of the articles suitable for food and produced in all countries, he said, is wasted annually because of people's prejudice against them. The old saws, "What is one man's meat is another man's poison," and "There is no accounting for taste," are trite, but warranted by the facts. We do not object to eating a live oyster, but prefer all our other meats dead, and undergoing putrefaction to a slight extent, in order to get rid of the "toughness," as it is generally called, produced by the *rigor mortis*. Some people like to let the putrefaction proceed further until the meat is "gamey." The Texan cowboy eats goat's meat in preference to that of the cattle and sheep he is herding. Young puppies, rats and birds' nests are considered delicacies by the Chinese. Frog's legs and snails are among the highest priced dishes served at Delmonico's. Except the bones and hide, every part of an animal slaughtered for food is eaten by most civilized nations—the brain, tongue, blood in the shape of black pudding and sausages, the liver, heart, lungs, stomach as tripe, the pancreas, thyroid and sublingual glands, which are called sweetbreads, and considered a great delicacy; the feet in the way of jellies, and pickled; the intestines as sausage covering, etc. In the markets of Paris there is a steady demand for horse-flesh as food. The Arabs and other nomadic tribes prefer mare's or camel's to cow's milk. Many people would as soon eat a snake as an eel, yet the latter commands a higher price than most fish in many parts of the world. Lobsters, which are the scavengers of the sea, are eaten by people who would not touch pork. The Eskimo, who eats blubber and other solid fats, and the native of the tropics, who "butters" his bread with a liquid vegetable oil, have the same object in view, viz., to supply a concentrated form of fuel. The squirrel is considered a great delicacy in many parts of this country, but is not eaten in England. The vain efforts of Professor Riley some years ago to induce the starving people of Kansas to eat the food they had at their doors—grasshoppers, sorghum, and millet seeds, and squirrels—himself setting them the example, will be recalled by many present.
—*Science*, 1890.

The Japanese Stoop.

In *The Medical Record*, February 8th, there occurs an item relative to Dr. Kidera Yasuatsu's conclusion of an inquiry into the cause of the habitual body-stoop of the Japanese, which attributes it "to their excessive politeness, the bent posture being considered one of deference." Dr. A. S. Ashmead, late Foreign Medical Director Tokio-fu Hospital, Tokio, Japan, writes to the same journal, stating that he thinks this is an error, It is due rather to their habitual use, from infancy, of the elevated wooden sandal, whose stilt-like effect on the body's equilibrium makes it difficult to maintain a perfect perpendicular, and to their habit, when walking, of keeping the arms folded, with hands pocketed in opposite sleeves.

Heart Failure.

This is the fashionable and delusive, and hence dangerous, term used in many cases of death from diphtheria. As an illustration of the danger arising from such a misleading term, we notice the following from a communication from the Secretary of the State Board of Health of Ohio :

A child 13 years of age died from diphtheria at Ravenswood, Ill., on December 6th, 1889. On the 8th, the corpse was taken to Zanesville, Ohio, accompanied by the parents and their four children. The coffin was opened and viewed by the family of the dead child on December 8th. On the 13th these four children and their mother were stricken with the disease, and four days later three of the children of the family in which they visited, and one other child contracted the disease. Nine cases from one centre of infection—four of them resulting fatally. The cause of death of the child brought from Chicago is said to have been given as heart-failure and blood poisoning, and the casket was marked for transportation "non-contagious."

Dr. J. H. Rauch, the eminent secretary of the Illinois State Board of Health, to whom the above communication was sent, in his report to the board at its last session says :

The history of this case is another illustration of the contagiousness of the disease of diphtheria, the necessity for strictly private funerals and the danger of transporting the bodies to distant places for interment of those who die from contagious and infectious diseases. In this connection I would suggest to the board that instructions be issued to local health authorities not to accept certificates where the cause of death is said to be "heart failure." This term has recently become fashionable, but for sanitary purposes amounts to nothing, as nearly all die from that cause.

We heartily second the suggestion of Dr. Rauch. As a sequel to the above and as illustrating more fully the dangers to the public from those dead of contagious diseases, we furnish the following from a late issue of the Chicago *Herald* relating to the same body. Here we find nearly thirty *fatal* cases of diphtheria, all traceable to the shipment of a corpse from Chicago. The testimony in the case shows that the attending physician first reported the case as dying from "heart failure" resulting from diphtheria. Finding there would be difficulty in obtaining transportation for the corpse the doctor, anxious to accommodate the friends, suppressed the fact of its relation to diphtheria, and reported it simply as "heart failure." —*Monthly Bulletin.*

Horses in Dark Stables.

The pupil of a horse's eye is enlarged by being kept in a dark stable ; he has a harness put on him and is suddenly brought out into glaring sunlight, which contracts the pupil so suddenly as to cause extreme pain. By persevering in this very foolish and injudicious, as well as cruel practice, the nerve of the eye becomes impaired, and if continued long enough loss of sight will ensue. To see how painful it is to face a bright light after having been in the dark, take a walk some dark night for a short time till the eyes become used to the darkness, then drop suddenly into some well-lighted room, and you will scarcely be able to see for a few moments in the sudden light. You know how painful it is to yourself, then why have your horses to repeatedly bear such unnecessary pain ? asks *Field and Farm.*

Stammering and Deafness.

Stammering has hitherto been supposed to be purely a nervous defect. Some experiences recently acquired by the surgeons connected with the Ear Hospital, Soho Square, tend to call this view more or less in question. In carrying out certain operations to cure children of deafness, it was found that in several successful cases the operators had also simultaneously cured the patients of stammering. This fact attracted special attention and study, and the outcome has been the firm conviction that stammering, in the majority of cases, does not proceed from a nervous malady, but from some obstruction or defect connected with the organs of hearing. In a number of cases selected purposely from the public schools this fact has, it is said, been abundantly demonstrated.—*St. James' Gazette.*

Effect of Exercise.

Dr. Thomas M. Bull, in the *New York Medical Journal,* says : The high grade of general health which a proper amount of exercise tends to develop is the best possible safeguard against the encroachments of morbific germs. This is shown well in the case of ordinary colds. I have repeatedly seen people who, before taking exercise regularly, were afflicted with colds nearly all the time, but afterwards had a great many fewer or none at all. And right here I should like to mention a little plan to avoid taking cold when exposed to a draught. Many of us are frequently exposed to draughts when we are in company and cannot avoid them. If a person in this position would rapidly and strongly contract the large body muscles, or opposite plates of those attached to the limbs, by means of which a great deal of force may be exerted and but little motion caused, he will have no fear of draught producing a chill. By contracting in this way the muscles which cause adduction of the arms while the arms are at the side, I can in a short time produce a very comfortable state of perspiration, and certainly ward off any bad effects of a draught.

Where Travelling is not Altogether Pleasant.

Travellers on the Eastern Bengal Railway have placed before their eyes on entering the stations of the road a placard containing the following cheerful information : " Passengers are hereby cautioned against taking anything to eat or drink from unknown persons, as there are many who live by poisoning travellers. They first of all court acquaintance with passengers in a *sarai* or some other place, and then gain their confidence on the plea of being fellow-travellers going to the same place. When they reach a place convenient for the purpose, they poison the water or food of the passengers, who become insensible, and then they decamp with all their property. They also at times poison the passengers' water when being drawn out of wells, or sweetmeats brought from the bazar, or food when being cooked."

The Doctor's Harvest.

The man who first made use of the proverb, " It's an ill wind that blows nobody good," knew what he was talking about. Yesterday afternoon I called on a young doctor on Lexington Avenue. One of the principles of this young doctor is that he never buys anything until he is ready to pay cash. Since last winter he has bought and presented his wife with a pretty and cozy dwelling, and yesterday when I called I heard the notes of a sweet-toned piano. "You are succeeding admirably." I said to the doctor. " I congratulate you."

" Do you know to what we owe all this ?" asked his wife, as she turned around from the piano.

" What ?"

" La grippe," she answered.—*New York Star.*

Prevention of all Infectious Diseases.

The science and practice of medicine and surgery are undergoing a revolution of such magnitude and importance that its limits can hardly be conceived. Looking into the future, in the light of recent discoveries, it does not seem impossible that a time may come when the cause of every infectious disease will be known ; when all such diseases will be preventable or easily curable ; when protection can be afforded against all diseases, such as scarlet fever, measles, yellow fever, whooping cough, etc., in which one attack secures immunity from subsequent contagion ; when, in short, no constitutional disease will be incurable, and such scourges as epidemics will be unknown. These, indeed, may be but a part of what will follow discoveries in bacteriology. The higher the plane of actual knowledge, the more extended is the horizon. What has been acknowledged within the past ten years, as regards knowledge of the causes, prevention, and treatment of disease, far transcends what would have been regarded, a quarter of a century ago, as the wildest and most impossible speculation.

Poison Ivy and Poison Sumach.

Four things need to be committed to memory to insure safety against our poison-sumachs :

First.—The three-leaved ivy is dangerous.

Second.—The five-leaved is harmless.

Third.—The poison-sumachs have white berries.

Fourth.—No red-berried sumach is poisonous.

Both the poison-ivy and the poison-sumach, though unlike in appearance of foliage, have similar white berries growing in small slender clusters from the axils of the leaves. In all other sumachs the berries are red and in close bunches at the ends of the branches, and, far from being dangerous, yield a frosty-looking acid which is most agreeable to the taste, and wholesome withal. With these simple precepts fixed in the mind, no one need fear the dangers of the thickets.

What Constitutes a Nuisance.

The Board or its members are oftentimes asked what constitutes a nuisance, and therefore it may not be amiss to define the term. This would hardly be necessary were it not for the fact that many people seem to regard it as one of their inherent rights to do as they please, so long as they do not trespass upon the domain of others. Very often such people seem to forget that there is any difference between the sanitary condition of the town and the city. It does not occur to them that there must be vast differences in the social compact between the farm-house with its wide-spread acres, and the house-lot in the city that is measured in square feet, and that conditions that might constitute a nuisance in the one place might be of importance as a necessary adjunct to the other.

Strictly speaking, any use of property annoying to another's rights is a nuisance. Still, two things are necessary—a right and an injury. To illustrate : No matter how much your refined taste may be violated by the architectural structure of your neighbor's house, it is not a nuisance because no right is violated. So one may not like the looks of his neighbor's pig-pen, still one can look the other way; but so soon as that pig-pen gives off offensive odors, as it will in hot weather, it is a nuisance, because every person has a right to pure air.

The nuisance need not be injurious to health ; it is enough that it is annoying and offensive to the senses.

Most nuisances may be classified as violations of our right to pure air and pure water, the practical inferences being that in the management of our own affairs we should not be unmindful of the rights of our neighbors ; and we would add that in no place can the golden rule be better applied than in matters relating to the sanitary conditions of local districts in a small city.-
Report Board of Health, Concord, N. H.

Mortality Among Artificially Fed Infants.

Dr. Bertillon recently, on the basis of statistics prepared by Dr. Richard Boëckle, made a report on this subject to the Société de Médecine Publique (*Revue d' Hygiène Thérap ; Med. Age*, March 10th). He demonstrated that the mortality of infants fed on artificial food or reared upon the bottle, all things being equal, is six to seven times as great as among infants nourished at the breast. The statistics also prove that neither the age of the babies, their legitimacy or illegitimacy, nor the social condition of their parents, is able to explain or modify this discrepancy. The very considerable difference in the mortality found between the two categories of infants (forty-five to seven per thousand living in each category) is wholly due to the difference in alimentation. Although the mortality among illegitimate infants in Berlin is generally double that of the legitimate, yet this is quite consistent, as the former are far more often nourished by the bottle than the latter.

Cats, Chickens, and Diphtheria.

I would like to narrate three cases of diphtheria that occurred in one family in my practice about three years ago (says Dr. J. E. Sayre in the *Med. Record*). On May 6th, 1887, I was called to see a little girl two years of age who was taken with malignant diphtheria. She lived five days and died a horrible death. Isolation, disinfectants, and all other precautions were used to prevent the remaining three children from taking the dreaded disease, but notwithstanding all this, only a few days elapsed before it had marked a boy of 8 years for its victim, and in five days he died. Not long after this the third child, 4 years of age, was taken with the same disease, and he lived two weeks and died with paralysis. Different physicians were called in consultation in these cases, but all our efforts would not check the onward march of the disease. As it manifested itself in such a malignant form, the father and myself thought we would search the cellar and yards for the cause. Nothing was found that aroused our suspicions excepting some damp and decayed boards in the cellar and a dead cat under the piazza.

A few days after this the father read and showed me an article in the *New York Times*, in reference to the fatality of diphtheria when contracted from the lower animals. He then related to me the following story ;

"Previous to my children's sickness they had a pet cat of which they were very fond. It was taken sick very much as my children were with swollen throat and running at the nose, and as it wandered away we saw it no more. Thinking it was dead I immediately got another cat for the children, and that was taken with the same symptoms and soon died. Also some chickens in the back yard were found dead."

After hearing this story I was not long in deciding the origination of the disease as far as the children were concerned, as the first child was taken only a few days after the death of the cats and chickens.

The New Surgeon-General of the Army.

Surgeon-General Jedidiah H. Baxter, United States Army, recently so appointed to succeed Surgeon-General John Moore, retired, is and has been for upward of twenty-five years, so favorably known to all who have taken interest in the medical corps of the Army, as to give no occasion for comment save to express the general satisfaction with which his appointment is received.

While it is true, as alleged by some of the contestants for the position, that Dr. Baxter has not had as much active frontier service as some who would urge that as a qualification, it is difficult to see the force of it, as compared with such familiarity with the duties of the office as Dr. Baxter's long service as Chief Medical Purveyor, with headquarters at Washington, has afforded him. But, besides this, the faithful and meritorious services of Dr. Baxter, both during and since the war, add to the justness of his preferment.—*The Sanitarian.*

Water for Babies.

The following, which is a fact, illustrates a common occurrence : A physician being called upon to visit a sick child, found the babe in apparently good health, but crying and struggling continually as though suffering extreme pain and anguish. The mother stated that the child was desirous of nursing continually, and in order to quiet it she had been obliged to let it nurse as often as the crying paroxysms came on. When that failed to quiet it, paregoric or soothing syrup had been administered. "When did you give the babe a drink of water last?" inquired the physician. "I don't remember," replied the mother. "I seldom let him drink any water. Does he need it?" "Need it!" exclaimed the doctor. "Why should he not need it as much as you? The child is suffering from thirst—nothing more." He called for cold water, gave the infant a few tablespoonfuls, and it immediately ceased crying and fretting, and soon went peacefully to sleep, enjoying a long refreshing slumber, the first for many hours.

Why Thunder Storms Affect Milk.

During electrical disturbances it seems that cream and milk are put into a condition to sour easily. The probable cause of this, the editor of the *Cultivator* (Albany) explains as follows : The effect of an electrical discharge is to decompose a portion of the atmosphere, by which ozone is produced. This substance has peculiar properties from its intense activity as an oxide of oxygen, and its action is often believed to be the cause of the souring of milk, beer and fresh wine during what are known as thunder storms. The ozone is diffused through the air, and is believed to be the cause of the strong acid odor which prevails after the storm is passed. No doubt if the milk is submerged in water, and access of air is prevented, no result of the kind need be apprehended ; and as the more milk is exposed to the air the more it will be affected by the ozone, the milk in open pans will be acidified more readily than that in deep pails, although these may be open. In our long experience, however, the writer adds, we have never had any milk affected in this way, either in shallow pans or deep pails, and we are of the opinion that heat of the air preceding thunder storms is more directly the agent in the souring of the milk than the ozone that may exist in the air after the storm is passed. Carefulness to maintain a proper temperature, by closing dairy houses and cellars against the outer atmosphere, will be a means of safety.

The Hygienic Aspect of Marriage.

There can be little doubt that marriage, which is the natural, physiological condition of man- and woman-kind is the state most conducive to health, happiness and longevity. But by marriage we mean all that the word, rightly understood, implies ; we mean the normal union of two congenial persons, not the linking together of two names or two fortunes solely for material or worldly reasons. Therefore do we favor and recommend the marriage of our young men and women. Celibacy, while it may be well in certain cases, yet as a rule, is not the natural condition of humanity, hence is not to be encouraged. Marriage can be supported by countless arguments ; celibacy by very few ; that is to say, when we speak of these states as a rule. That wise and illustrious man, Dr. Benjamin Rush, writing on this subject towards the close of his long life, very aptly said : "Celibacy is a pleasant breakfast, a tolerable dinner, but a very bad supper. The supper is not only of a bad quality but, eaten alone, no wonder it sometimes becomes a predisposing cause of madness."

Consumption Among Firemen.

As the result of a statistical investigation, Dr. Thomas J. Mays, of Philadelphia, tells us, in an article published in the *Medical and Surgical Reporter*, that consumption is, as one might suppose, very prevalent among firemen. Liable to be called out at any time, their life is in great part one of perpetual excitement. The sudden transition from a warm room to active duty on a cold winter's night—sometimes the urgency being so great that they are compelled to finish their toilet *en route* to the fire ; the daring, the excessive and almost superhuman exertion demanded in battling with the flames ; the extreme oscillations of temperature to which their bodies are subjected—bathed in perspiration one moment and drenched and chilled by an icy stream of water the next ; the necessity during emergencies of wearing and even sleeping in wet clothing from one fire to another, are burdens which no human constitution can long successfully withstand, and are unquestionably some of the most prominent causes which undermine the health of these self-sacrificing men, and make them so vulnerable to the disease under consideration.

The Streets of Berlin

Thsse streets compare very favorably, in the matter of cleanliness, with those in most American cities. This is in large measure to be attributed to the fact that many of them are paved with asphalt, and can thus be easily swept by the gangs of street-cleaners. These latter are armed with rubber scrapers and follow the watering carts, gathering all the mud and manure into little heaps along the curb, which are then carted away before they have had time to dry and be spread again over the street.

English Death Rates.

Dr. D. R. Drysdale says that at present the average age at death among the nobility, gentry and professional classes in England and Wales is 50 years; but among the artizan classes of Lambeth it only amounts to 29; and while the infantile death-rate among well-to-do classes is such that only eight children died in the first year of life out of 100 born, as many as 30 per cent. succumbed at that age among the children of the poor in some districts of our large cities. The only cause of this enormous difference in the position of the rich and poor with respect to their chances of existence, lies in the fact that at the bottom of society wages are so low that food and other requisites of health are obtained with too great difficulty.

Bogus Coffee-Beans and Spices.

The *Pacific Record of Medicine and Surgery* appears to be responsible for the following :

"That is not coffee," said the reporter.

"Who said it was?" replied the jolly, rosy-cheeked grocer. "Are there any marks on to indicate that it is coffee?"

"No, not particularly ; but it certainly looks like coffee, and tastes entirely different."

"Ah, you have hit the nail on the head," continued the grocer, with a smile. "It would not do to let everyone know it, as it might shake people's confidence in their grocey store. That bag, a few beans from which you have just tasted, contains an imitation of coffee. It is nothing more than flour, and poor flour at that, which has been shaped like a coffee bean, and baked down. If you will take a genuine coffee bean in your hand and put it alongside the imitation, you can see that there is a difference in the color. The shape is also different, but this is nothing, as the various kinds of coffee vary in shape and size. The flavor, of course, is not there, but the way the imitation is sold does not require its presence. The grocer is not a foolish man. He does not sell these flour beans for cofiee. This would give the business away. But when trade is dull, and the grocer must have something to occupy his mind, it is a pleasant recreation for him to mix a quantity of the flour beans with the genuine coffee. Then it cannot be easily detected. Only just enough of the flavorless bean is used to make a little profit. This is not quite one-half. When the honest housewife who buys the whole coffee so as to get it pure grinds up this mixture, and the odor steals out from the mill, her eyes snap, and she laughs at the people who are foolish enough to buy the coffee which is ground at the store, and can be easily adulterated. The taste of this compound is not unpleasant, and it will not injure anyone. Even the babe can take it with impunity. If the coffee were drunk plain its weakness would be noticeable, but being usually taken with milk and sugar, the fraud is not detected. Years ago all the coffee was ground in the grocery, but adulteration was carried on so extensively that the practice was established of buying the whole bean. This led some inventive Yankee humanitarian, who believed that too much coffee is bad for the nerves, to bring out the flour bean.

" Here is something else interesting. See these beautiful samples of cloves and peppers? Imported? Well, no, not exactly. They are home-made to suit the trade. They look good, but there is little flavor to them. Someone thought it was a shame to waste the beautiful and nourishing cocoanut shell, and conceived the idea of heating it, and then grinding it to a fine powder. This, when artistically mixed with various kinds of oils, makes a good spice for pies and other good things. It is a growing industry, and well patronized. Some of this powdered shell, after being flavored and made into a stiff paste, is pressed through moulds into the shape of peppers and cloves. These, when mixed with a quantity of the genuine article, give about all the flavor that it is safe for a person to take, and the grocer does not lose anything, but goes on paying his pew rent and building rows of houses, the same as if there were a little sugar in the glucose, a small quantity of cream in the cheese, and a taint of butter in the oleomargarine."

Rules for Bathers.

Avoid bathing within two hours after a meal. Avoid bathing when exhausted by fatigue or from any other cause. Avoid bathing when the body is cooling after perspiration. Avoid bathing altogether in the open air, if, after having been a short time in the water, it causes a sense of chilliness and numbness in the hands and feet. Bathe when the body is warm, provided no time is lost in getting into the water. Avoid chilling the body by sitting or standing undressed on the banks or in boats after having been in the water. Avoid remaining too long in the water ; leave the water immediately if there is the slightest feeling of chilliness. The vigorous and strong may bathe early in the morning on an empty stomach. The young, and those who are weak, had better bathe two or three hours after a meal—the best time for such is from two to three hours after breakfast. Those who are subject to attacks of giddiness or faintness, and those who suffer from palpitation and other sense of discomfort at the heart, should not bathe without first consulting their medical adviser.

BUREAU OF INFORMATION.

WELLS AND TYPHOID.

SALEM, OHIO, Sept. 22d, 1890.

JOSEPH F. EDWARDS, M.D.:

By express to-day I send you two samples of well water for analysis. I have a case of remittent fever at one place, and at the other have a convalescent from typhoid, with one other member of the family sick with the trouble, and possibly a third will be. Both wells are shallow affairs, with the slope of the ground from the privies toward the wells.

Please send me the result of the analysis, and greatly oblige, yours fraternally.

T. T. CHURCH, M. D.

Examination of sample of water from shallow well. Slope from cesspool toward well. Marked "No. 1." From Dr. T. T. Church, Salem, Ohio. Sent by Dr. J. F. Edwards. Received September 24th, 1890. Examination made September 24th–26th, 1890, by C. M. Cresson, M.D. Reaction alkaline. Contains:

	Parts in 1,000,000 Parts.
Solid matter to dryness	——
" " to redness	——
Lime	——
Magnesia	——
Chlorine	36.036
Sulphuric acid	——
Free ammonia	0.055
Albuminoid ammonia	0.220
Nitrogen as nitrites	——
" as nitrates	10.254

This water is unfit for drinking purposes. It carries cesspool drainage, and probably household drainage also. The microscope shows the presence of ciliata and epithelial scales and great numbers of micrococci. No bacteria indicating disease were found.

CHARLES M. CRESSON, M.D.

Examination of sample of water from shallow well. From Dr. T. T. Church, Salem, Ohio. Sent by Dr. J. F. Edwards. Marked "No. 2." Received September 24th, 1890. Examination made September 24th–26th, 1890, by C. M. Cresson, M.D. Contains:

	Parts in 1,000,000 Parts.
Solid matter to dryness	——
" " to redness	——
Lime	——
Magnesia	——
Chlorine	70.856
Sulphuric acid	——
Free ammonia	0.137
Albuminoid ammonia	0.274
Nitrogen as nitrites	——
" as nitrates	2.056

This water is badly polluted, probably with cesspool drainage, as well as that from kitchen wash. It is unfit for drinking purposes. The microscope shows the presence of ciliata and micrococci in great numbers, and of that character which indicates pollution by animal matter. The bacilli indicating disease were not found.

CHARLES M. CRESSON, M.D.

SUSPECTED WATER.

Examination of sample of water from A. P. Hull, M.D., Montgomery Station, Pa. Sent by Dr. Edwards. Received October 11th, 1890. Examination made October 11th-15th, 1890. Contains:

	Parts in 1,000,000 Parts.
Solid matters to dryness	——
" " to redness...................	——
Lime..	——
Magnesia...... :.............................	——
Chlorine.................................	3.543
Sulphuric acid	——
Free ammonia	0.081
Albuminoid ammonia	0.135
Nitrogen as nitrites......................	——
" as nitrates......................	3.359

This water contains a few large ciliata, but there are no evidences of the presence of bacilli which indicate the carriage of typhoid fever. Except that this water contains nearly the allowable maximum of soluble organic matter, it would be classed as a fair water for household use. Many waters which contain similar amounts of organic matter are in constant daily use.   CHARLES M. CRESSON, M.D.

The Faith and the Mind.

Charles Dudley Warner says the difference between the "faith cure" and the "mind cure" is that "the mind cure" doesn't require any faith and the faith cure doesn't require any mind.

How the Vanderbilt Children are Trained, Dressed, Fed and Educated.

It is one of the rules in all the houses of the Vanderbilts that the children shall go to bed early and rise early. The little boys and girls are up before 7 o'clock in the morning. Their nurses immediately take charge of them, see that they are properly bathed and dressed, and then they go down to breakfast, which is served at 7.30 o'clock. It is an unpretentious meal, with plenty of fresh milk, eggs, oatmeal, and a bit of steak or a chop that will add strength to their physique and color to their cheeks.

After breakfast there is an hour of study. There is something for these little ones to do at all times during the day. They go through their studies systematically, and then about 9.30 are taken out for a walk. They are allowed to romp in the streets and in the parks to their hearts' content. At 11 o'clock they are brought home, and a light luncheon of milk and bread is served, after which there are more studies—either French, German or drawing—then another breathing spell—it may be horseback riding, or a drive through the park and along the country roads. Back they all come about 4 o'clock, and there is another hour of study, and then they are through for the day. They are allowed to do just as they please until tea time, when, after their meal, they spend a pleasant hour or so with their fathers and mothers. Promptly at 8 o'clock they are all in bed to sleep soundly.—*Ladies' Home Journal.*

SPECIAL REPORT.

Special Meeting of the State Board of Health of Pennsylvania.

SPECIAL MEETING AUGUST 30TH, 1890.

A special meeting of the Board was held at the Executive office, August 30th, 1890, for the purpose of auditing accounts for general routine business. Present: Dr. Geo. G. Groff, president, in the chair; Dr. Pem. Dudley, Dr. J. F. Edwards, and Dr. Benjamin Lee, secretary.

Mr. Howard Murphy arrived just after adjournment, having been detained by the failure of his train to make the usual connection.

The Secretary stated that Dr. S. T. Davis had written expressing his regret at being unable to be present.

AUDIT AND APPROVAL OF VOUCHERS.

The Secretary presented bills amounting to $189.92, and covering vouchers Nos. 387 to 391, which had been audited and found correct by the Executive Committee. They were approved.

PROPOSED SCHEME OF NOMENCLATURE, AS A GUIDE FOR BOARDS OF HEALTH.

The Secretary presented on behalf of the Committee on Vital Statistics printed copies of the scheme of nomenclature of diseases, intended as a guide for all boards of health in the State in making returns, referred to at the last meeting. He begged that the members would give it careful consideration, and send him as soon as possible any suggestions or criticisms that might occur to them.

CIRCULAR TO CLERGYMEN. PUBLIC FUNERALS IN CONTAGIOUS DISEASES.

The Secretary laid before the Board copies of the new Circular No. 29, addressed to clergymen, on the "Dangers of Public Funerals in Infectious Diseases," and announced that copies were being distributed as ordered at the last meeting.

REVISED EDITION OF CIRCULAR NO. 27.

A revised edition of Circular No. 57, " Precautions against Cholera, Cholera Morbus, Cholera Infantum, Summer Diarrhœa and Dysentery," which had also been partially distributed.

The circulars and the action of the Secretary were approved.

CIRCULAR TO TRUSTEES OF PUBLIC INSTITUTIONS.

The Secretary presented and read a copy of the proposed circular letter to the Trustees of Public Institutions, on "the Disposal of the Sewage of Public Institutions," which the Board had instructed him to prepare at the last regular meeting.

It was approved.

INSPECTION OF STATE LUNATIC ASYLUM AT HARRISBURG.

The Secretary reported that at the request of the Trustees of the State Lunatic Asylum at Harrisburg, he had visited that institution in order to examine its drainage system.

The authorities of the Asylum were anxious to be advised, and were willing to adopt any reasonable plan recommended by the Board. In the absence of the chairman of the Committee on Drainage the matter was referred for subsequent consideration.

POLLUTION OF WATER AT HORATIO AND PUNXSUTAWNEY.

The Secretary read two letters describing the pollution of the water supply at Horatio, Jefferson county (from Dr. Charles G. Emst, of Punxsutawney), and asking for an official investigation by the Board.

On motion the Board directed that Dr. Emst be requested to forward the usual formal complaint with affidavits, and that on receipt thereof an inspection be ordered.

ALLEGED POLLUTION OF BEAVER RIVER BY SALT AND OIL RESIDUUM.

The Secretary presented a complaint from citizens of Beaver Falls with regard to the pollution of Beaver River by salt and oil from oil wells.

The Secretary was directed to instruct Dr. J. R. Thompson to make an inspection of the polluted stream, and to obtain, if possible, the assistance of Dr. J. H. McClelland in prosecuting the investigation.

NUISANCE FROM A CHEESE FACTORY AT BUTLER.

A complaint has been received of a nuisance from a cheese factory at Butler, Alleghany County. Dr. J. R. Thompson had inspected the factory. He reported a nuisance from decomposing whey and a filthy hogpen. The proprietor had promised that no swine should be kept on the premises after the coming Fall.

The Board directed that notice be served on the proprietor to keep the pens and premises in proper condition.

ALLEGED POLLUTION OF THE LOYALHANNA RIVER AT SALTSBURG.

A complaint of contamination of waters of the Loyalhanna River at Saltsburg was on investigation by Dr. J. R. Thompson found to be correct. The polluted water had killed many fish. The pollution was supposed to be caused by a chemical (perhaps sulphite of soda) from the paper manufactory establishment of James Peters & Company. It did not appear, however, that the poisonous material affected the water supplies of Pittsburgh and Allegheny as had been charged. The complaint was dismissed.

ALLEGED POLLUTION OF STREAM AT POTTSTOWN.

The Secretary reported the receipt of a similar complaint from a fish warden of Montgomery County, stating that large numbers of fish had been killed either by poison or dynamite in a mill race near Pottstown. The Board was of the opinion that the powers of the fish warden were sufficient in the premises.

COMPLAINT OF POLLUTION OF STREAM AT ALTOONA.

The Secretary presented a complaint from Dr. S. C. Baker, alleging that a stream which passed through his property was being seriously contaminated by the sewage of Altoona. A letter on this subject from the School Board of Altoona was also read, stating that Dr. Baker had refused to pay the assessment necessary for constructing a sewer. An investigation was ordered.

REPORTS OF INSPECTIONS AT EDGE HILL AND SHARON HILL.

Dr. W. B. Atkinson's reports of inspections at Edge Hill, Montgomery County, and Sharon Hill, Delaware County, were also read. In each case the nuisance had been abated after receipt of order from the Secretary.

The action of Secretary was approved.

On motion the meeting then adjourned.

Minutes of the Sixteenth Regular Meeting of the State Board of Health of Pennsylvania.

THE sixteenth regular meeting of the Board was held at the Supreme Court Room, Harrisburg, July 10th, 1890, at 4 P. M. Present : Dr. George G. Groff, Dr. P. Dudley, Dr. Samuel T. Davis, Dr. J. H. McClelland, Howard Murphy, C. E., and Dr. Benjamin Lee, *Secretary.*

ORDER OF BUSINESS.

An order of business presented by the Secretary was adopted as the order of the day.

The Secretary announced that Dr. J. F. Edwards had expressed to him his regret at being unable to be present, owing to sickness in his family.

CONFIRMATION OF MINUTES OF FIFTEENTH REGULAR MEETING AND OF SPECIAL MEETING.

The minutes of the fifteenth regular meeting, held at Norristown, May 8th, 1890, were read and approved. The minutes of a special meeting, held at the executive office, May 28th, 1890, were also read and approved.

SECRETARY'S REPORT.

The Secretary then presented his report, which included the following items:

PERMIT FOR DISINTERMENT AND REMOVAL OF DEAD BODY.

In response to a request, by telegraph, for permission to disinter and remove the body of Theresa E. Maratta from Rochester, Beaver County, to Minneapolis, Minn., the Secretary had replied that the permission of the health officer of Minneapolis must first be obtained. This was done, and the Secretary then directed the authorities at Rochester, after assuring themselves that all the requirements of the Board have been complied with, to issue the necessary permit.

The action of the Secretary was approved.

RESOLUTION OF THANKS TO HOSPITAL TRUSTEES AND OTHERS.

The Secretary reported he had sent a special resolution of thanks to the following persons at Norristown, for their courtesy to the board at the late sanitary convention: Dr. Robert H. Chase, Superintendent, Male Department, State Hospital for the Insane; Dr. Alice Bennett, Superintendent, Female Department, State Hospital for the Insane; President and Trustees of the same institution; the leader of the orchestra of the insane asylum band; County Commissioners of Montgomery County; the Board of Health of Norristown, and the Borough Council.

REPORT AS DELEGATE TO NATIONAL CONFERENCE OF STATE BOARDS.

The Secretary reported that he had attended, as delegate, the National Conference of State Boards of Health, held at Nashville, Tenn., May 19th and 20th last, and presented a detailed statement of their proceedings. As chairman of a committee on the subject of the contagiousness and spread of leprosy as affecting the United States, he had read a report and presented resolutions calling for a stringent enforcement of the quarantine against that disease.

The report was accepted with thanks.

INTER-STATE QUARANTINE ACT.

A copy of the Inter-State Quarantine Act passed at Washington during the present Congress was presented, and ordered to be included in the annual report.

PUBLIC FUNERAL IN CASE OF DEATH FROM SCARLET FEVER.

A communication had been received from Dr. H. A. Arnold, Ardmore, former President of the Montgomery County Medical Society, stating that a public funeral had been held at Catasauqua in the case of a death from scarlet fever, and that he had been called to see a child who had contracted the disease on that occasion. The Secretary had at once addressed the authorities of Catasauqua on the great danger of public funerals in contagious diseases, and had sent circulars on scarlet fever to the minister who conducted the service and other persons implicated.

The action of the Secretary was approved.

INSPECTION OF A DRAIN AT UNIONTOWN.

Dr. C. Gummert, Medical Inspector of the Southern Tier District, had recently inspected a mill race or drain at Uniontown, which he found to constitute a nuisance. The citizens had requested him to superintend the abatement of the nuisance. The Secretary had replied, declining to allow Dr. Gummert to superintend the abatement in his official capacity as medical inspector, and warning him against making himself or the board liable for any expense. He had also sent notices declaring the drain a nuisance, and ordering an abatement. The general opinion of the board was condemnatory of medical inspectors accepting compensation for superintending the abatement of a nuisance, so declared by the State Board.

The action of the Secretary was approved.

CIRCULAR TO CLERGYMEN ON PUBLIC FUNERALS.

Mr. Howard Murphy suggested that a circular be printed and sent to all the clergymen in this State, asking their aid and co-operation in the prevention of public funerals where the death was from a contagion of epidemic disease.

After some discussion the matter was referred to New Business.

CORRESPONDENCE WITH STATE ANATOMICAL BOARD.

The Secretary had received a communication from Dr. William H. Parish, Secretary of the State Anatomical Board, stating that it had been reported to him that the State Board made a charge of fifty cents for each body delivered to the Anatomical Board from a State hospital. The Secretary replied denying this, and pointed out that a local board had the right to make a reasonable charge for a transportation permit for each body so delivered, and that this charge had probably been so made. This Dr. Parish afterward found to be the case.

The report was accepted.

MILK INSPECTION AND DUTIES OF A HEALTH OFFICER.

The Secretary had received a request from the health officer of Scranton (Dr. W. E. Allen), to explain to him the course generally adopted in regard to milk inspection and the powers of a local board to assign new duties to a health officer. He had replied, stating that the laws of Pennsylvania made the specific gravity test legal and the basis for prosecution, and naming the most modern instrument for milk inspection (Fogliabue's lactometer). He also stated that the chief milk inspector of Philadelphia would gladly explain his system to any officer.

The report was accepted.

SMALLPOX IN PITTSBURGH.

A notification of the occurrence of a case of smallpox in Pittsburgh had recently been received. The Secretary had notified all the State Boards of this, and also the health boards in Pennsylvania.

The report was accepted.

APPOINTMENT OF DELEGATE TO STATE SANITARY CONVENTION.

The Secretary reported the receipt of a communication from the State Board of Health of Delaware to the effect that a delegate from that Board would in future attend the meetings of the Pennsylvania State Sanitary Convention. He had replied acknowledging the courtesy and promising to give the board due notice of the next convention.

PROPOSED ORDINANCE FOR THE PROTECTION OF MILK IN PHILADELPHIA.

The Secretary laid before the Board a copy of the proposed ordinance for the protection of the milk supply of Philadelphia. He suggested that such ordinance be inserted in the next report of the State Board, together with the explanatory pamphlet of Dr. Ford, president of the Philadelphia Board.

The suggestion was adopted.

INSPECTION AT DEVON INN, AND STATE NORMAL SCHOOL, MILLERSVILLE.

The Secretary reported that together with the members of the Board he had inspected the sewage purification system at the Devon Inn, Berwyn, on the 27th of June, ult. Also the drainage of the State Normal School at Millersville, Lancaster County, on June 28th, the day following. A report on these inspections would be received from the Committee on Water Supply, Drainage, Topography and Mines, which made it unnecessary for him to go into detail.

MORTALITY RETURNS OF WILLIAMSPORT.

The Secretary presented the mortality returns for the year 1889 of the city of Williamsport, and suggested that they be inserted in next annual report.

The suggestion was adopted.

NUISANCE FROM STAGNANT PONDS AT BRIDGEPORT.

A communication had been received from Mr. Howard Murphy, stating that a nuisance existed at Bridgeport, Montgomery County, from stagnant ponds. He had addressed a communication to Mr. Young and to Mr. J. Andrews ordering an abatement of the same, and to Mr. Coates, the complainant, informing him that this action had been taken.

COMPLAINTS OF MINOR NUISANCES.

The Secretary reported the receipt of complaints of minor nuisances from Apollo, Armstrong County; Blairsville, Indiana County; Springdale, Alleghany County; McKees Roads, Allegheny County; Valley View, Easton, Northampton County; Swedeland, Montgomery County; McKeesport, Allegheny County; Burgettsown, Allegheny County; Bridgeport, Montgomery County; Mont Clair, Montgomery County. In all of which the complainants had failed to respond to the circular letter which had been sent in each instance, requiring the affidavits of ten householders before any action can be taken.

The report was accepted and action approved.

EPIDEMIC SORE THROAT AT STATE COLLEGE.

The Secretary reported the receipt of a complaint from State College, Centre County, that much sickness prevailed in that institution, and asking for an investigation. Dr. Groff, at the Secretary's request, stated he had visited the institution in answer to a telegram from the President. He recommended that the cases of acute sore throat which he found be isolated and treated as epidemic; that the building be thoroughly disinfected, and confirmed the request for an inspection.

The Secretary read the report of D. C. B. Dudley, who had been instructed to inspect the college, which stated that he had made inquiries by telegraph, and learning that the epidemic of sickness had abated, had not visited the college in person. The Secretary stated that further instruction would be sent to Dr. Dudley.

SECRETARY'S REPORT ADOPTED.

On motion the Secretary's report be adopted in full as the Report of the Board, the recommendations contained in the same approved, and the report ordered for publication in the annual report.

REPORT OF COMMITTEE ON VITAL STATISTICS.

Dr. Lee, Chairman of the Committee on Vital Statistics, reported that in connection with the recent census, he found that some doubt had arisen among physicians with regard to the propriety of giving information as to physically or mentally defective classes. He had communicated with Hon. Robert P. Porter, Superintendent of Census, on this subject, and Dr. John S Billings, of Washington, D. C., in charge of special statistics, both of whom assured him that all such communications would be treated confidentially and at once destroyed after being used to correct the returns of enumerators. He had conveyed the correspondence through the press to all physicians in Pennsylvania.

The report was accepted and approved.

REPORT OF COMMITTEE ON DRAINAGE, WATER SUPPLY, MINES, ETC.

Mr. Howard Murphy, C. E., reported that the Committee on Drainage, etc., had recently inspected the drainage purification system of the Devon Inn, Berwyn, and the drainage of the State Normal School, Millersville, Lancaster County. With regard to the former, as the system had evidently not had time to become perfect, the committee recommended that after reasonable time had elapsed a complete set of analyses be made to obtain the exact results of the process, after which a further report will be submitted by the committee.

As regards the drainage of the State Normal School at Millersville, the committe regards it as almost superfluous to enlarge upon the conditions which prevail, as it was about the filthiest stream the committee ever saw, and they recommend that proper action be taken in this case at the present meeting.

The report was accepted.

REPORT OF COMMITTEE ON SANITARY LEGISLATION.

Dr. Samuel T. Davis reported that the next legislature would soon meet, and it would be for the Board to decide what matters would require to be introduced in the coming session.

The report was accepted.

NOMINATION OF A PRESIDENT.

Nomination of a President being next in order, Dr. J. H. McClelland nominated Dr. George G. Groff, president for the ensuing year. The Secretary was directed to cast a single ballot, and to act as teller. The Secretary reported that five ballots had been cast, unanimously in favor of Dr. Groff, who was now declared duly elected president.

NEW BUSINESS.

New business being next in order, the following points which had been discussed during the reading of the Secretary's report were called up for action. It was moved by Mr. Howard Murphy

CIRCULAR TO CLERGYMEN.

That a circular be addressed to all clergymen in Pennsylvania, asking for their influence and co-operation with the Board in preventing public funerals of those who die from contagious and infectious diseases. The Secretary requested to be allowed to introduce in such contemplated circular the paper on this subject read at the recent Sanitary Convention by the Rev. S. Bridenburgh, of Norristown. This was complied with, and the preparation of the circular referred to the Committee on Sanitary Legislation, Rules and Regulations.

NUISANCE AT SUNBURY.

The disposal of the complaint of a nuisance from a drain at Sunbury was left in the hands of the Secretary.

NUISANCE FROM DRAINAGE AT STATE NORMAL SCHOOL TO BE ABATED.

The Secretary was authorized to declare the drainage of the State Normal School at Millersville, Lancaster County, a nuisance, and to recommend to the trustees of the institution, in the most urgent manner, that it be promptly abated.

The meeting then, on motion, adjourned.

The French Society of Hygiene

Will award in 1891 a gold medal of 200 francs, also a silver medal, and two bronze medals, to the authors of the best essays on the following subject : '' What is to be done, before the arrival of the doctor, in case of a street accident, or accident in a factory.'' Further information, 30 Rue du Dragon, Paris.

Adulterations in New Jersey.

The report of the State Dairy Commissioner shows 2507 analyses of foods, of which more than 45 per cent. were found adulterated. Of 1072 drugs analyzed, about 65 per cent. were found adulterated or below standard of these various articles. Of those which gave the highest percentage of adulteration, or not standard, the percentages of each were as follows :

Oleomargarine .... 57 per cent.
Imported canned goods 88   "
Ground coffee................................. 80
Spices 45   "
Extracted honey ..,........................... 74
Maple syrup................................... 50
Vinegar 64
Pickles....................................... 73
Baking powder................................. 81
Sausage......................................100   "
Dried apples..................................100
Jellies and jams 76

Copper was found as chief adulterant, used for giving a green color to vegetables. The report is interesting, and contains valuable results for the chemist.

State Board of Health and Vital Statistics of the Commonwealth of Pennsylvania.

PRESIDENT,
GEORGE G. GROFF, M.D., of Lewisburg.

SECRETARY,
BENJAMIN LEE, M.D., of Philadelphia.

PEMBERTON DUDLEY, M.D., of Philadelphia.

J. F. EDWARDS, M.D., of Philadelphia.   GEORGE G. GROFF, M.D., of Lewisburg.
J. H. McCLALLAND, M.D., of Pittsburg.   S. T. DAVIS, M.D,, of Lancaster.
HOWARD MURPHY, C.E., of Philadelphia.   BENJAMIN LEE, M.D., of Philadelphia.

PLACE OF MEETING,
Supreme Court Room, State Capitol, Harrisburg, unless otherwise ordered.

TIME OF MEETING,
Second Thursday in May, July and November.

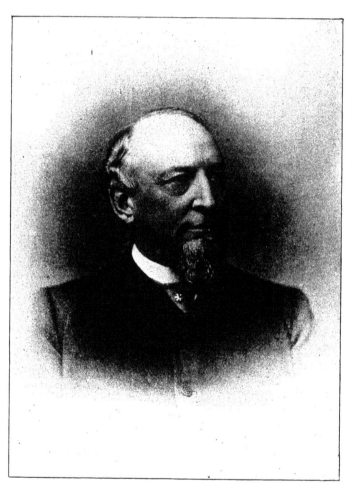

HONORABLE EDWIN H. FITLER
MAYOR OF PHILADELPHIA

THE
ANNALS
OF
HYGIENE

VOLUME V.

Philadelphia, November 1, 1890

NUMBER 11.

COMMUNICATIONS

The Lesson of Mayor Fitler's Life.

AMONG the varied arguments that are oftentimes adduced against the value of hygiene, we are not infrequently confronted with the statement that "hygiene" is all right for the rich, but that the poor man cannot avail himself of its teachings. Such an idea, of course, is never advanced by one who has given thought to the subject, for he really knows that the laws of hygiene are but the laws of nature, and that it is just as easy for the man with only a dollar a day to obey the laws of nature as it is for the man with many millions to do so.

But a very general impression prevails that, as we have said, only the rich can care for their health, and that the poor man must take his chances.

To correct this erroneous impression, better than mere argument could do it, let us lay side by side the life of a rich man, with all the possibilities of health that his wealth can vouchsafe to him, and that of the day laborer, and learn how much alike, so far as the preservation of health is concerned, these two lives can be made.

Desiring to point this tale with a name so well known that a record of his life would prove interesting reading, we have selected the Hon. Edwin H. Fitler, Mayor of Philadelphia, because, since he is interested in the subject of hygiene, his inclinations would lead him towards an observance of her laws, while his great wealth places within his grasp all the possibilities of the science.

First, we all know that change, variety, is a sauce that gives piquancy to life and promotes good health.

Three times in the course of every year does this wise Mayor of ours change his residence. During the days of Winter, when he knows that it is conducive to his health to mingle in society, to meet and to be met by his fellow men, then is he to be found located in the handsomest house, in the most centrally located and fashionable portion of our city. Here he gathers about him the most prominent and intelligent of our people, and the Winter months are passed in the most delightful of social intercourse.

But, all this time, Mr. Fitler's servants are tending to his magnificent farm at Torresdale, a few miles from the city, and daily does he receive at his city home the·pure and choice and nutritious farm products. After a while the sprouting trees on the street warn our Mayor that the days of Spring are at hand. Then comes the carpenter, and boarding up the windows and doors of his city mansion, Mr. Fitler and his family, *hurry* (no, we will not say *hurry*, for Mr. Fitler is too wise ever to hurry ; he knows that nothing is ever gained by hurry, and that health is often lost thereby) they leisurely move to his magnificent country home, already referred to.

This farm is so located that Mr. Fitler can use either the steam-cars or the steamboat (on the Delaware) in his daily trips to and from the city.

But, let us stop for a moment and answer the question that we hear being asked : "How can the clerk or the laborer have such places as you have described as belonging to your Mayor." He cannot ; neither does he require them, nor are they essential to his health. Contentment with one's lot in the world is the first prime requisite of health ; a *discontented man cannot be a healthy man*. Having established this proposition, we would ask whether it is necessary for every man to have Mr. Fitler's wealth and his elegant homes in order that he may be contented ; far from it ; contentment must come from within, and it cannot be produced by extraneous surroundings. All the wealth of the world and all the palaces thereof, cannot, of themselves alone, produce contentment. A philosophic reasoning with oneself, a cultivation and exercise of one's will power alone can bring contentment ; a realization that *discontent can do no good* will bring about that contentment so essential to health.

Look for a moment upon the portrait of Mayor Fitler, which we publish ; did you ever see a more contented, satisfied expression upon any face ; yes ; you may say, that is true, but then he has everything to make him so ; but, I tell you in reply, that he did not always have such gorgeous surroundings ; yet he was always a contented man ; for the lines of discontent that imprint themselves on the face of a discontented man are ineffaceable. Throughout his life Mr. Fitler has had the wisdom to be contented ; always ambitious, always active, always anxious to rise until he has reached his present exalted position, yet each day found him not discontented with his position of that day.

Having then demonstrated the importance of contentment, and that it is as possible to the pauper as to the millionaire, let us see how the man who is earning $10 per week can enjoy the same advantages to health that are vouchsafed to Mr. Fitler.

If he be a clerk or a book-keeper, or a day laborer, he does not require a city residence. The duties devolving upon the Mayor of a great city require him to reside at the seat of government at least a portion of the year ; not so with the ordinary individual. Let him go out into the country (to Torresdale if you please) and rent or buy a little house and an acre of ground. He can have the same air and the same water that the Mayor enjoys ; a strip of ground, worked in the evenings, will give him the same pure vegetables, while a cow

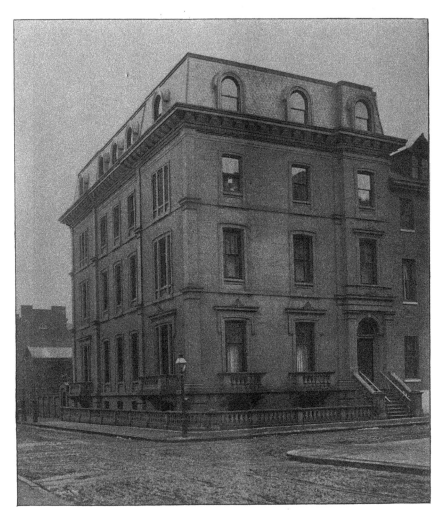

PHILADELPHIA RESIDENCE OF MAYOR FITLER
16th and Walnut Streets

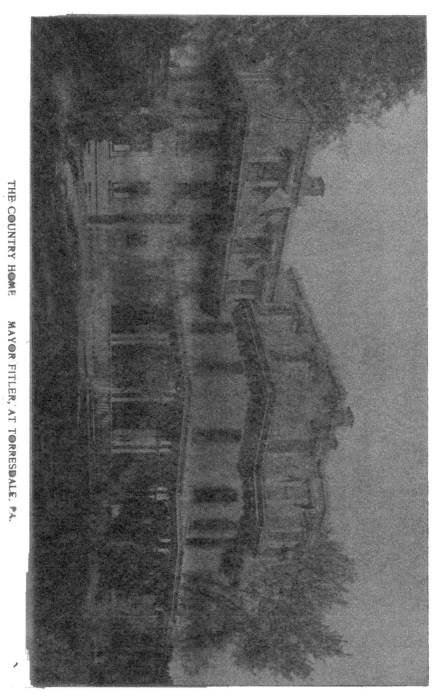

THE COUNTRY HOME   MAYOR FITLER, AT TORRESDALE, PA.

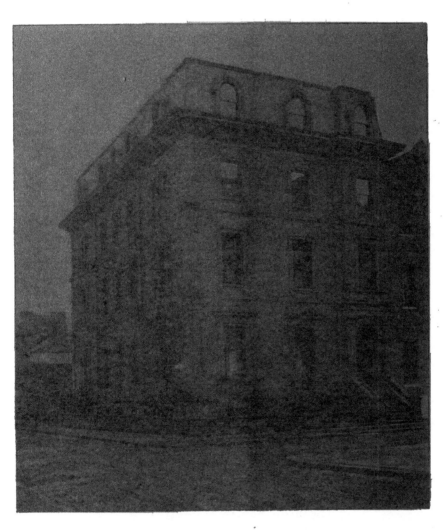

PHILADELPHIA RESIDENCE OF MAYOR FITLER
16th and Walnut Streets

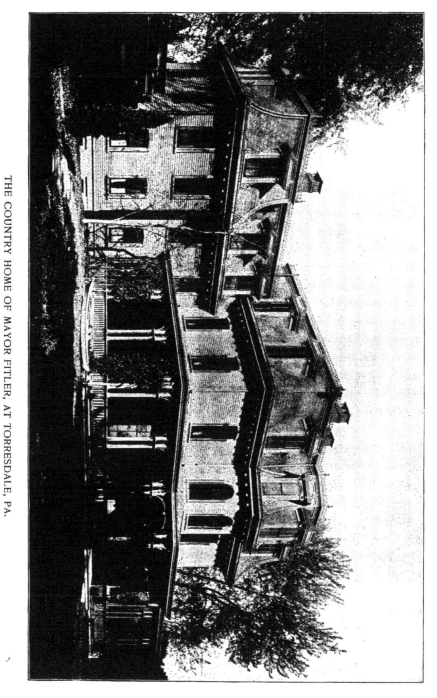

THE COUNTRY HOME OF MAYOR FITLER, AT TORRESDALE, PA.

and a few chickens will give him milk and eggs just as good and pure as Mr. Fitler, with his millions, can procure.

The various companies that have been organized for the purpose make it within the reach of any one to own such a home, while the frequent train service and cheap fares make it perfectly feasible for one laboring in the city to reside in the suburbs. We have advanced thus far, where we can say that "Contentment," "Pure Air," Pure Water" and "Pure Food" are essentials to healthy life, and have we not made it clear that these four factors are as accessible to the clerk as to the millionaire.

It is not the mere possession of so much wealth and that which it renders possible that makes Mr. Fitler such a healthy, happy-looking man, but it is his *contentment* that vouchsafes to him the health and happiness that he enjoys.

To go back from our digression. After a while the hot days of Summer are upon us, and then we find our Mayor located in his palatial residence on the edge of the sea at Long Branch; a house so magnificently beautiful that it is a pleasure to gaze thereon.

Can the $10.00 a week clerk go to Long Branch ; yes ; if he so wishes. Excursion rates are now so cheap and our seaside resorts are so full of boarding houses at reasonable prices that almost any one can enjoy the health-giving atmosphere of the seashore for a time.

It is true that he cannot surround himself with the luxuries enjoyed by Mayor Fitler, but then it must be remembered that while such surroundings are all very well for one who has the wealth to possess them, yet they are not at all necessary to health.

Mayor Fitler is a great friend of the working-man, and in conversation he heartily coincided with our idea, that while it would, of course, be entirely out of the question for any ordinary individual to possess that which belongs to him, yet there was and is no earthly reason why the poorest laborer should not enjoy the same hygienic advantages that are accessible even to the Mayor of this great city. Mayor Fitler thoroughly believes in hygiene, and in this fact we recognize that he is abundantly endowed with that rarest of all senses, "Common Sense," for we have always maintained that there is pre-eminently the savor of common sense attached to all the teachings of hygiene.

There is one point in connection with hygiene that we have always had a desire to see demonstrated, namely, the possibility of plumbing, when an intelligent plumber was given "carte blanche" by a man with whom expense was no consideration. This problem has been demonstrated to us by Mayor Fitler's experience with his three homes. When he first purchased these truly palatial mansions, it was not uncommon for both His Honor and Mrs. Fitler to suffer more or less with ill-health. Believing thoroughly, as we have already stated, in the efficacy of hygiene, and recognizing that good plumbing is one of the foundation stones of our science, Mayor Fitler called into requisition the services of an intelligent plumber, with the result that, as the natural and inevitable result of such magnificent plumbing as he now has, there is no more sewer gas in Mr. Fitler's residences.

Of course, the expense will preclude such plumbing for the multitude, but the plumbing of Mayor Fitler's house may be accepted as an ideal to be approached as closely as possible. We would be glad if every one of our readers could see the ideal wash-room on the first floor of Mayor Fitler's residence ; no wood-work,. no paper—*tiles, beautiful tiles* everywhere ; nothing organic to be rotted by the splashing water ; nothing that water can spoil, so that absolutely perfect cleanliness is attainable. The whole house is a dream of refined elegance, but this particular wash-room would especially delight the heart of the sanitarian.

Having now, in a general way, outlined our idea that the efficacies of hygiene are as accessible to the ordinary individual as to this man of unlimited wealth, we feel that to complete our article a brief reference must be made to Mayor Fitler's individuality. We have already given as our reason for selecting His Honor to typify our idea, that, because of his wealth and intelligence he could avail himself of all that there is in hygiene, while, because of his prominence, people would like to read of his doings, and his example would be followed. That Mayor Fitler is a healthy, happy, and contented man, a study of his portrait will demonstrate. As in the case of so many of our great men, domestic felicity has had much to do with Mayor Fitler's success in life. As in all well-regulated households, Mrs. Fitler has been truly a "helpmate" for His Honor, while his family of handsome sons and daughters have been to him a source of justifiable gratification and pride. This is, from a hygienic view, a more important point than will appear at the first glance, for domestic felicity is a mighty hygienic factor.

Mayor Fitler is, as his portrait indicates, a man of great dignity and courtly demeanor, and just here we would give expression to a thought that has been frequently in our mind when we encounter "His Honor" on the street. The late Justice Miller, of the United States Supreme Court, once remarked that he was tired to death of having characterless men in the White House, and that he would like to say good-bye, for a time, to negative Presidents, and to see how the country would get along under a positive one. With Justice Miller, we have often thought it a pity that the Presidents of this great country have been, as a rule, of late years, men not only of but little dignity, but men who for many reasons were not equal to the dignity of this office. We believe that, with Mayor Fitler in the White House, Justice Miller's ideal would be realized. Wealth, health, dignity, culture, a handsome presence, a courtly demeanor, the ability to royally receive and entertain, just such attributes as would best become the ruler of a great nation, these attributes are possessed in a marked degree by Mayor Fitler.

It is with a feeling of great satisfaction that we have learned of Mayor Fitler's great practical interest in hygiene, for it encourages us to believe, as we have always hoped and trusted, that when our glorious science has received the sanction, support, and hearty coöperation of the leaders of men, then it is but a question of time until all humanity will be as a great family of sanita-

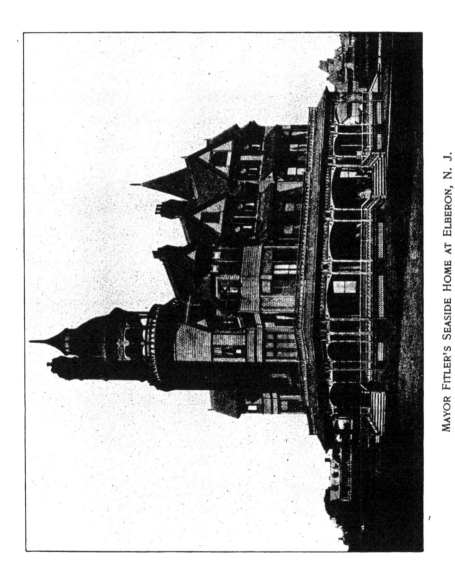

MAYOR FITLER'S SEASIDE HOME AT ELBERON, N. J.

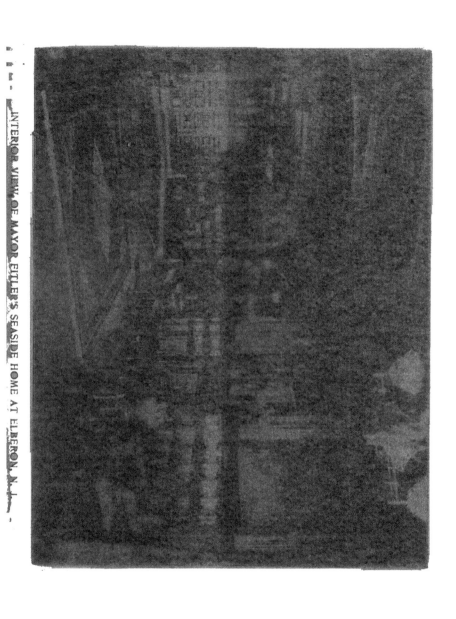

INTERIOR VIEW OF MAYOR FULLER'S SEASIDE HOME AT ELBERON, N. J.

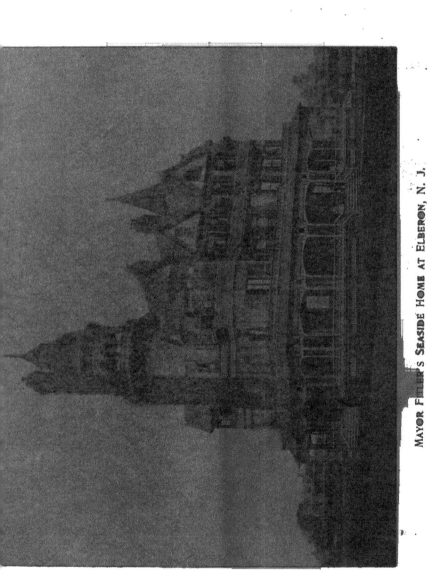

MAYOR FULLER'S SEASIDE HOME AT ELBERON, N. J.

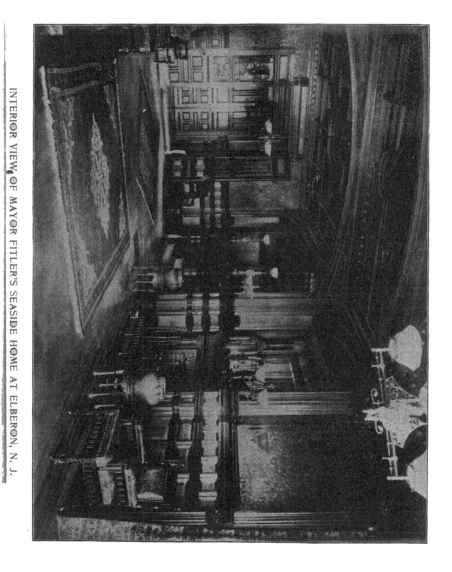

INTERIOR VIEW, OF MAYOR FITLER'S SEASIDE HOME AT ELBERON, N. J.

rians. It is truly a cause for congratulation among those of us who are striving to better the condition of humanity, to ameliorate its woes and to lessen its suffering, to feel that we have in our efforts not only the earnest sympathy but the ardent support of such a strong, loyal, hearty, manly man as the Hon. Edwin H. Fitler, Mayor of the great city of Philadelphia ; truly, it is appropriate that the Chief Executive of the city of "brotherly love" should be a leader in that movement wherein "brotherly love" is best exemplified ; warmly Mr. Mayor, do we welcome you to a leadership in the glorious army of sanitarians.

Observations on Clothing.

BY GEORGE G. GROFF, M.D.,
President State Board of Health of Pennsylvania.

To preserve health, nothing is more important than the proper and sufficient clothing of the body. The object of clothing is to protect delicate parts, to ornament the body, and, principally, to prevent too rapid loss of the body heat. In cold climates, the well clothed need less food than the ill clothed, and should be at all times more vigorous and healthy. The person ill clothed, because unable to resist cold, is weak and debilitated, and a ready victim of any disease which he may contract.

THE ESSENTIALS OF CLOTHING.—1. It should fit loosely ; 2. It should be porous ; 3. It should be light as to weight ; 4. It should be a poor conductor of heat ; 5. It should be of materials easily cleansed ; 6. The color should be adapted to the season ; 7. The material should be durable ; 8. The material should be as good as the wearer can afford, for this looks best and is the cheapest.

THE KINDS OF CLOTHING.—These are *linen, cotton, woolen, silk* and *fur*. The first conducts heat from the body so rapidly that it should never be worn next to the skin. Cotton is good for warm climates, but in cold climates, woolen garments should always be worn next to the skin. Silk is expensive, but is an excellent material for clothing, and furs are very valuable in cold regions.

OBSERVATIONS.—After exercise, always cover the body until it cools. The sedentary need more clothing than the active ; the young and the old more than those in the prime of life. Clothe all parts of the body except the face and the hands. Do not let fashion dictate in matters of dress, for the laws of hygiene are inviolate. Do not attempt to harden children by exposing to the weather their delicate little arms, legs, and chests, but clothe them more warmly than adults. "Clothe thyself neatly, not conspicuously." When the clothing becomes wet, it should be changed as soon as possible, but until it is changed the person should keep in constant motion that he becomes not chilled. Keep the feet dry and warm and the head cool. Woolen socks should be worn at least nine months in the year.   In wet and sloppy weather, good overshoes should always be worn ; thick soles and heavy leather will never keep the feet as dry as they should be.   Always sleep under sufficient bedclothes, and never lie down to sleep without an extra garment thrown over the shoulders.   Change all clothing worn during the day, and allow it to air during the night.   In the morning carefully air the bedclothing for several hours before making the bed. Feather beds are a kind of clothing, and from long use become saturated with the exhalations of the body ; they can be purified by being baked in an oven. The " guest bed" should always be warmed before being used, and the stranger placed between blankets, otherwise the bed may be the gate to the grave. Muffling the throat produces congestions, croup, colds, and other complications. Avoid an excess of clothing over vascular organs, as the lungs, heart, kidneys, etc.   Remove extra clothing on coming into a warm room, and put it on again on going out.   Be always warmly dressed, and have abundant wraps for cases of emergencies.   Do not put on Summer clothing until the presence of Summer in well established.   Clothe warmly when about to take a ride.   Many diseases are promoted by being thinly clad.   Both men and women should carry the clothing from the shoulders and not from the hips.   Women should wear reform-suits.   In cold weather, if possible dress in a warm room. Clothing which has been washed, should be *thoroughly dried* before being again worn. All underclothing should be frequently washed, at least once a week.

The Lesson of Mr. Pulitzer's Life.*

MR. JOSEPH PULITZER, the proprietor and editor of the New York *World*, announced in his paper recently that he retires absolutely from the editorship of that paper.   This announcement has caused universal comment in the community, although it is not a surprise to those who know the condition of Mr. Pulitzer's health.   He has been spending nearly three years now in the hope that he would by care and by competent medical treatment recover the use of his eyes.   He has submitted some of the time to treatment of extraordinary severity.

Once, when in Naples, he was kept in a room absolutely dark for a period of six weeks, and while this treatment benefited the eyes a little, it was altogether harmful in other respects, for Mr. Pulitzer is a man of extraordinary energy and restless mental activity, and the confinement, therefore, produced a sort of nervous prostration and a debilitated state of the system, for which the improvement in his eyesight scarcely compensated.

He subsequently went to Switzerland, where the air seemed to do him good for awhile, but there a severe cold developed asthmatic tendencies.   He went from Switzerland to Paris, and there submitted to rigorous medical treatment, part of which consisted of nourishing him with a diet which some of his friends

*From the Philadelphia *Press.*

here think would have debilitated anybody's system. They fed him on a little oatmeal and he was permitted to eat sparingly of other cereals and gruels, but he could drink nothing, and was practically obliged to fast.

This, with his nervousness and his anxiety, as well as the chafing caused by the attempt to carry on the business of the *World* while laboring under all sorts of annoyances, told seriously upon his general health. When he returned a few days ago he was found by his friends to be very thin, weighing forty pounds less than when he went abroad, and his complexion is of a waxy color, which suggests how debilitated his physical condition is.

In addition to that, Mr. Pulitzer has entirely lost the sight of one eye, and sees but indistinctly with the other. With a magnifying glass of great power he would be able to read, and he can discern objects and faces. But the danger is that he will lose the sight of this eye also, and he therefore is confronted with the appalling possibility of total blindness.

He has recently consulted with Dr. S. Weir Mitchell, of Philadelphia, who, after a careful study of the case, and with the approval of other physicians in consultation, have earnestly advised Mr. Pulitzer absolutely to give up all business and professional work for at least one year.

They tell him to abandon himself entirely to a life of comfort. They urge him to permit of no distraction whatever, and in consideration of no business principle, however simple. They want him to entertain himself with friends, advise him to surround himself with genial company, suggest that he drive in the open air when the weather permits, that he enjoy music whenever possible, and give himself up as completely to a life of ease and comfort as it is possible to do.

Even this regime may not avail, but the physicians are satisfied that only by the adoption of it can Mr. Pulitzer have any hope whatever of entering again into the activities of life.

During all his illness heretofore, Mr. Pulitzer has been in constant consultation with the very capable men whom he associated with him in the management of *The World*. The system which was adopted to keep him informed, both of the business and editorial policy of the paper, as well as of the conduct of journalism generally in this city, was a most comprehensive one. He was kept, while in Europe, as fully in touch with the paper as he would be had he remained at his house on Fifty-first Street.

He has now constituted a Board of Managers who will be wholly responsible for the conduct of *The World*, and who will manage it as though Mr. Pulitzer were not, excepting that they will follow his teachings and be guided by what they believe would be his judgment if he was with them.

Cures for Neuralgia of the Head.

An English physician has recently asserted that headaches and neuralgia could be stopped by blowing a solution of salt up the nose.

Brown's Mills-in-the-Pines.*

BY JOSEPH PARRISH, M. D.,
Burlington, N. J.

FOR nearly one hundred years "The Pines" of New Jersey have been known and visited as a health resort, and also as a place for rest and enjoyment, by the farmers of the county and its neighborhood, after the in gathering of their harvests ; but it is only of late years that the attention of the public has been called to their superior health-giving properties. The pine belt is an extensive forest of pine and cedar trees covering a vast area of the soil of New Jersey, with its base line nearly fifty miles long, crossing the southern part of the State between the bay and Atlantic shore. From this its lateral boundaries rise northward for about a hundred miles, gradually narrowing as they approach its apex or summit in Monmouth County, where it is much narrower than at its base. The New Jersey Southern Railroad traverses it from Eatontown, near Long Branch, to its terminus at Bayside.

In past years the majestic range of native woods was at times visited by forest fires and tornadoes, which, together with the busy woodman's axe, devastated about 25 per cent. of the whole ; though the most serious and most extensive injury was confined to the southern end of the State. There still remains the larger part of close, evergreen forest, with multiplied attractions for those who may seek its shade and healthful breezes.

The soil is sand and gravel. Its chief characteristic is dryness, a most important quality, and much desired for its effect on some forms of disease. This dryness is not occasional, but permanent ; its permanency being due to the absorbing power of the pine woods, which take the humidity from the atmosphere and the excess of moisture from the soil immediately following rain, leaving the air laden with the fragrance of the forest. No remedy is more important in the management of some forms of disease than dry air; and, in view of the effect upon the human system of varieties of temperature, to be assured of uniform degrees and a comparatively even temperature is a boon greatly to be desired and sought for.

An interesting and valuable feature of this locality is the natural beverage known as cedar water, which derives its name from its being always found where the dense cedar forests are within the area of the pine belt.

The variety of the cedar family called the "water tree" grows luxuriantly and of stately proportions in these so-called swamps. The supply of water being exhaustless and always fresh and cool, the source and the cause of so uniform a fact taxes the mind, and allows the imagination freedom to search out the wonderful phenomenon and all its history. The searcher discovers only that it seems to come from some fairy "land of brooks of water—of fountains and depths that spring out of valleys." As it swells up from the depths towards the sunlight, whirling in circling eddies about the polished cedar roots, it takes

* From the Telegraph.

that pale mahogany tint by which it is distinguished. It is possible, as some believe, that it possesses decided sanitary virtues. Be that as it may, all agree that the cedar water is exceptionally pure, refreshing and wholesome.

Iron and sulphur springs, in the pine belt, are unmistakably iron and sulphur, perfectly true to taste and quality. Invalids who require such waters may find them in perfection under the shade of Jersey pines.

The lake is within gunshot of the hotel, and presents a fine picture, with its glassy surface extending for miles among the distant forests and sweeping around the many islands that dot its surface—its coast line turning here and there and forming pleasant coves, retired nooks and little bays or inlets sparkling with lily beds. The miniature ferries, rustic bridges and quiet inlets inviting the visitor to seek for the secret entrance to the jungle, all contribute to make this beautiful lake a most popular resort. Flat-bottom boats are furnished by the proprietors for the use of guests, who may find pleasure in sailing or fishing for the long-snouted pike (*Esoxlucius*), which is the principal inhabitant of these waters.

Brown's Mills-in-the-Pines is not in a patch or group of trees covering a few acres only, but literally in the midst of the great pine wilderness so noted throughout the country, enclosed within the belt, sheltered by the health-promoting foliage, which robs the earth and air of their damp, and gives in return the fragrance and life which the invalid seeks.

The new Forest Springs Hotel is a model building, with every convenience and provision for the comfort of guests. Open wood fires in almost every room, electric lights and steam heating. Large, enclosed verandas, also heated by steam, keeping the temperature about sixty degrees Fahrenheit.

The natural lay of the land, with added appliances, secure almost perfect drainage and ventilation. More than $100,000 have been expended in the new hotel and its surroundings within the last eighteen months, and the fact now to be added will secure confidence and support. The manager is Mr. Peter Addicks, late manager of the Bryn Mawr Hotel. Cleanliness, order, good living and whatever else is needed to make the keeping of the house as perfect as the house itself are added.

The Microscope versus Hygiene.

BY FREDERICK GAERTNER, A.M., MD.,

Of Pittsburgh. Pa., U. S. A.

HE who hates the microscope hates his profession. The man who has made "microscopy" a profession will soon be in demand for his scientific services, not only in making scientific examinations, but especially for making microscopical researches and investigations; *i. e.*, in a hygienic point of view.

The scientist who practices microscopy as a method of investigation and research on the one hand, and for the advancement of every branch of science and art on the other, should receive both great credit and honor as well for his experiments as for the results. But the man who has been called upon to give expert testimony without having a practical knowledge of microscropy and its uses, and without having made a thorough microscopical examination of the subject before him, should be ruled out of the court for want of scientific knowledge. It is impossible for a scientist and hygienist to arrive at a positive and correct conclusion without the assistance of the microscope, together with the accessories, such as the microtome, polariscope, photo-micro-cameras, spectro-polarimeter, etc., etc.

I think that microscopy and its allied branches should be made "compulsory" studies at all the different universities and high schools, and especially at medical colleges. Even at the common schools the fundamental part of microscopy should be taught. In my mind, there is no doubt that the microscope and its application should receive the greatest attention, and that it is certainly of paramount importance not only to the medical man but also to the pharmaceutist (druggist), chemist, botanist, geologist, etc. In Europe, a student attending a university for the purpose of studying a profession, whether it be that of physics, law or divinity, whether his pursuit be mathematics or high grade classics, music or painting, must have completed three semesters in the study of microscopy (compulsory study) before he can be received as a candidate for admission to his final examination. This is necessary whether his career is to be that of a physician, attorney, chemist, botanist, geologist or mathematician, etc., and compulsory even for those who are studying theology or the arts of music and painting.

I think the United States Government (Congress) ought to enact laws making the study of microscopy a compulsory study in all universities and high schools and especially medical colleges. The United States Government, through Congress, should also encourage microscopical researches and investigations for the advancement of every branch of science and the art of hygiene, just as England, Germany, Austria and France have done during the last decade. These foreign nations have gone so far as to encourage the scientist and microscopist by the offer of capital prizes, not only cash prizes, but honorary medals, etc. This is done all in the interest of science, and principally for the protection of humanity. Congress is doing a very noble act in enacting laws for the protection of our home industries and commerce, but the people of our Commonwealth should urge Congress also to enact the most stringent laws for the protection of the people in the maintenance of health. Such protection can be obtained only from the microscope.

There is not the least doubt that the greater number of diseases in this country are due largely to the adulteration and imitations of our food and drink, and especially to the adulterated drinks, including principally our liquors, beers, wines, vinegar, cider and mineral waters on the one hand, and milk, teas, coffees, sugar, flour, etc., on the other.

I think that scientists and microscopists ought to be encouraged by Congress by means of compensations, and that they should prepare statistical reports of all adulterated foods and drinks, and especially as to their comparative adulterated constituents. Such reports ought to be placed before Congress, and Congress should be urged to enact laws to prohibit such adulterations and imitations under penalty of a heavy fine and imprisonment for any violation of. the said laws.

I certainly believe that this would be a "protective tariff" (as good as the McKinley Bill), if our home manufacturers were compelled to produce only pure articles of food and drink and to have everything unadulterated. This would, indeed, be a great protection for this country, and our fellow-citizens would not be compelled to send to Europe for a pure article, as they might be supplied in this country and thus keep their gold. Here, also, what a protection, and all by the aid of the microscope! Would not this be one of the greatest and noblest acts Congress has done since the Declaration of Independence? And if Congress were willing to enact laws prohibiting the adulteration and imitations of our food and drink, how else than by the aid of the microscope could such adulterations and imitations be detected? If the worthy readers of the ANNALS OF HYGIENE were only aware of the unwholesome food and drink they are daily using, how both are adulterated and what are the comparative adulterated constituents, including both quantity and quality, they would rise up in arms and not only boycott our home producers, but would certainly raise an insurrection against such adulterators and imitators. How can these adulterations and imitations be revealed except by the microscope? What a wonderful instrument the microscope is!

The microscope during the last forty years has done "wonders." Just see how Pasteur, the great French chemist, has studied and discovered the process of fermentation, and this, again, was only accomplished by the use of the microscope. Also from a hygienic point of view, had it not been for the microscope, Koch, the greatest bacteriologist that ever lived, would not have discovered the cause of consumption (tuberculosis) and of that deadly and most infectious disease, Asiatic cholera. Just see how Koch ventured to go to India and remain there month after month employing in his labors the highest powered microscopes that were ever invented and manufactured by the shrewdest and finest opticians in the world! With these instruments Koch labored hard and finally succeeded in making the discovery that *Asiatic cholera* is caused by a germ which he called "*comma bacillus.*"

Had it not been for the microscope the great anatomists, and especially the great pathologists, would not have made such wonderful progress and such great discoveries during the past forty years. For instance, they have proved without a doubt the causes of typhoid fever, pneumonia, smallpox, scarlet fever, even of cancer and other grave afflictions. Without the microscope, scientists would never have made the discoveries of the causes, "the etiological conclusions" of all the various diseases. It would still have been neces_sary for the physician to work in the dark, and to treat rather the symptoms of the disease than the disease proper as the scientific physician now does.

' When that greatest of calamities befell the people of Johnstown ; when the great flood had buried beneath its ocean of water nearly 10,000 human beings, was it not a notable and extraordinary fact that the Pennsylvania State Board of Health, and especially the Hon. Benjamin Lee, M.D., of Philadelphia, as soon as the waters of the flood had subsided in the Conemaugh Valley, resorted to the microscope for the protection of the survivors after the *débris* had been removed and disinfectants employed to destroy the germs of disease. Was not the microscope the principal factor in analyzing the food and drink of the survivors after the great calamity ? Just see how the waters of the Conemaugh and Allegheny rivers were examined and analyzed so that it might be positively stated that the waters of both rivers were so polluted and unwholesome as to be unfit for drinking purposes for months after the great catastrophe ! The microscope should be used in every family. Even the grocer, butcher and farmer should make themselves acquainted with the workings and manipulations of a microscope. Of course, a physician simply must have one, otherwise he is considered incompetent.

Just see how the doctors—George E. Fell and Spitzka—jumped upon the microscope when the world-renowned murderer, Kemmler, was executed by electricity—"electrocuted." It was the only reliable apparatus or instrument they could secure in order to determine accurately, first, that the man was dead ; second, what killed him. The cause of death, that is, the result of the electricide, as has been authoritatively stated, and which was revealed by the microscope, was nervous shock. This means simply a destruction and paralysis of the nerve centres of the brain and spinal cord. Scientifically, or rather microscopically, expressed, a disintegration of the protoplasm of the nerves, nerve cells and ganglion of the brain and spinal cord, with a secondary destruction or disintegration of the elements of the blood, producing a hemorrhagic transudation into the ventricles and substance of the brain, coagulation and death. There is not a particle of doubt that Kemmler was dead after the very first shock, even if the papers did call it a "bungled-up job." We know from experimental research the action of electricity upon the living tissue, whether animal or human. When 1000 volts or more are applied to living tissue, whether animal or human, a tremendous lightning-like nervous shock follows, in the first, the destruction of the superficial layers of nerve cells and ganglion of the brain, followed by the destruction of the deeper layers, until the entire brain is destroyed in a similar manner.

I have had the opportunity of experimenting upon the brains of cats and dogs, and these have been my results, all through the aid of that wonderful instrument, the microscope. I think it will require about 1200 to 1500 volts, applied from fifteen to twenty-five seconds, to kill any ordinary human being, especially when applied as near as possible to the nerve centres. Consequently, it is a matter of possibility for a human being to stand 1000 volts, that is, when it has been applied to his extremities, such as his feet or hands, and only for a very short time, say about two or three seconds, and still recover from the shock. Should the poles be applied directly to the head or spine, then it is an impossibility for a human being to recover from the shock, even if applied but for a single second. And if only the very superficial layers of the nerve cells and ganglion are destroyed, he would remain a deformed invalid for life. His hands and feet would be more or less paralyzed, and he would probably die very soon after the shock. Therefore, in Kemmler's execution—electrocution —he was certainly dead after the first shock. The frothing at the mouth, the returning respiration and bleeding from the thumb, were by no means indica- tions that he was still living, or that animation had returned. These symp- toms were nothing else than spasmodic and convulsive contractions of the muscles of the different organs, just as a guillotined head would be dead after it is severed from its body. This, in fact, would be still more certain. I think a human being killed by electricity suffers less pain than a man guillotined or hanged. This fact the microscope has already revealed and demonstrated in a number of cases.

In the year 1884, while I was at the Hospital Generale de Strasbourg, Germany, under the direction of Professor Schwalbe, I was requested to wit- ness a murderer guillotined. The execution took place at Metz. After the operation—" decapitation "—I was directed to hold a post-mortem examina- tion upon the subject. I took particular pains in studying the head, and espe- cially the physiognomy of the subject. Immediately after the head was sev- ered from its body and dropped into the basket, I took charge of it. The following has been my observation and experience, all through the aid of the microscope : His facial expression was that of great agony for many minutes after the decapitation. He would open his eyes, also his mouth in a process of gaping, as if he wanted to speak to me, and I am positive that he could see me for several seconds after the head was severed from the body. There is no doubt that the brain was still active, and this fact the microscope afterward revealed. Just think of the head severed from the body and still in activity ! What agony he must have suffered by the process of guillotining ! His decap- itated body, which had been previously fastened upon a bench, was in continu- ous spasmodic and chronic convulsions, lasting at least from five to six minutes. and indicative of great suffering. I have no doubt that had not his body been previously fastened to the bench, he would have gotten upon his feet and hands. and scrambled all over the " death chamber." That would, indeed, have been a terrible sight. Think of a headless human body performing the gyrations of a chicken just beheaded ! Just as a chicken's body will jump around and spring up into the air from four to six feet, so would that of a man. I have seen chickens actually get upon their feet and run from ten to fifteen feet from the place of decapitation. All this intense suffering would last from five to ten minutes, and still the French nation advocates the use of the guillotine for a death penalty.

Even hanging is a barbarous process. If the neck is not immediately broken, rather dislocated, the sufferer generally lives from ten to twenty minutes, and must certainly endure great agony by the process of strangulation and suffocation. Consequently, electrocution should in every instance be advocated for the infliction of the death penalty. Even the Humane Society ought to compel butchers, and especially killers at abattoirs, to slaughter beef, calves and swine by electricity, which is without doubt a painless death, certainly the quickest, easiest and simplest of deaths. Electrocution is, therefore, to be commended, and this conclusion again is reached through the aid of the microscope.

Pure Air and Sunlight as Preventives and Remedies in Consumption.

BY H. E. BEEBE, M.D.,

Of Sidney, Ohio.

It is with diffidence that I present a subject in which I have no discoveries of my own to ffer, and one that has attracted the attention of so many able workers, the results of whose labors have given us new ideas in the treatment of this formidable disease, and brought hope and encouragement to many who have looked forward, through a long period of suffering, to an untimely grave.

My purpose in this paper is to make an appeal for out-door life on the part of those who have reason to dread the attack of this destroyer, and out-door treatment for those on whom it has already obtained a hold.

Much has been written on the subject, but there seems a strange apathy on the part of the public in adopting as a preventive or remedy what is popularly but erroneously supposed to be the great, if not the principal, cause of the disease. Consumption being found to prevail mostly in regions of cold, late, wet springs, the conclusion has become almost universal that exposure to a climate of this kind is the chief cause ; and in their endeavor to escape the effects of the weather, people have unconsciously, but none the less certainly, intensified the conditions which they were endeavoring to avoid.

The prevalence of the complaint and its nearly uniform fatal termination when once firmly settled, have done much to render the public skeptical concerning almost any proposed means of relief, and constant iteration, with abundant proofs of satisfactoy results, will be necessarry to carry conviction to the minds of sufferers or their friends as to the efficacy of the method of treatment now sought to be adopted, namely, out-door life as far as may be practicable, with an abundant supply of pure air during the hours that must be spent within the walls of a building.

It is only by constant repetition that the general public can be made to heed even the most salutary teachings ; the most strenuous efforts are required to overcome the inertia of popular ignorance and indifference. The necessity for such an attempt, in this connection, is manifest when we consider that consumption is the cause of fully 15 per cent. of all the deaths occurring in the

United States—more than from any other one disease and more than from all other contagious diseases combined. Small-pox, cholera and yellow fever create a panic whenever they appear as an epidemic ; municipalities and States are active in measures of repression and prevention ; national power is summoned to establish quarantine regulations that shall protect the country ; the newspapers daily chronicle the work of the epidemic, and on its near approach to a given locality the inhabitants who are able to do so flee as from an angry demon ; yet these diseases appear only at intervals, and usually may be restricted to certain portions of the territory subject to their ravages, while consumption, more deadly than them all, slays its victims at all seasons, and few places in all our wide domain may be considered exempt from its visitation.

It is a matter of common belief that consumption is largely due to heredity, that its appearance in an individual indicates a similar diathesis in one or both parents, or at least in some ancestor not very remote, while, on the other hand, the child of consumptive parents is very apt, in due time, to follow the same course. Careful statistics, however, show that in not more than 25 per cent. of cases does this hold true ; in the remaining three-fourths, the disease has its inception in the person affected.

Aside from hereditary influence, there are many predisposing causes ; among them we may mention unhealthy occupations ; lack of nutritious food ; dissipation, fashionable or otherwise ; direct contagion ; and, chief of all, the lack of a sufficient amount of pure air. To this last cause, more than to all the others, may the disease be attributed, and while such conditions exist remedial agents will be applied in vain. An impure atmosphere, with an insufficient supply of sunlight, has a very favorable influence on the formation and growth of tubercles, especially in a locality where the soil is of such nature as to retain moisture and thus impede perfect drainage. Fresh air and the direct rays of the sun are the greatest health-giving agencies that exist for mortals, and yet people act as though these life-bearers were their deadliest enemies. A superstitious dread of " night air " causes many persons to keep doors and windows of sleeping-rooms tightly closed in order to shut it out—a proceeding as sensible as an attempt to bottle the sunshine. The fetid odor of such an apartment is sickening to one who may go into it after spending an hour in the bracing air of early morning. It would seem that the instincts of ordinary decency would rebel against such a proceeding, whereas many people labor to accomplish this as if it were something to be desired. We " gag " at the recital of a savage feast, where the host does honor to a visitor by masticating the food until it is in condition for swallowing, and then spitting it into the mouth of the guest ; but wherein is this worse than breathing repeatedly the vitiated air that has time and again been inhaled by another, and each time discharged more heavily laden with the refuse brought by the blood from various internal organs ? How can a diseased lung carry on the recuperative process necessary to bring it to a healthy condition ? How can a sound and healthy lung retain for any great length of time its power for effective secretion under such conditions ? And then in the morning, possibly after a short " airing," the windows and doors must be tightly closed " to keep out the flies " and the blinds drawn " to keep the sun from fading the carpet," so that the room may be practically unventilated for months at a time ; and in such a place consumption finds a congenial home.

Were I restricted to one course of treatment for this malady, it should be abundant exercise in the open air, carried to a degree to make rest feel grateful at night-fall, but never to an extent that would exhaust the patient or induce copious perspiration. In stormy weather he could have the protection of an out-building or a large verandah. Every article of wearing apparel should be made of pure wool, the amount of clothing to be determined by the temperature ; in cold weather, two or even three suits of light undergarments should be worn rather than a single one of heavier material, and by this means we should avoid the stiffness and extra weight of a suit of clothing made of thick, heavy cloth.

At night rest should be sought in a room with windows on at least two sides, and these should be opened wide, that the entire volume of air in the room would be renewed every few minutes, the patient having as many blankets as might be necessary for warmth. The sputum should, of course, be destroyed in some way, preferably by burning, as the bacilli set free by its drying would not only retard, or entirely prevent, healthy lung action, but would imperil those associated with the invalid.

That such a method of procedure would be beneficial is shown by the improved condition of those patients who travel, thus being forced in a measure to breathe more fresh air than when at home, as well as those who spend their time at some resort where the climatic conditions allow a considerable portion of the time to be passed out of doors. The strongest argument in its favor is a recent report from Germany, which informs us that " in the establishment at Falkenstein, at an altitude of 1312 feet, in the midst of woods, the consumptive patients pass their time in the open air at all seasons. The results obtained are very favorable. It is reckoned that there are 25 per cent. of absolute cures and 27 per cent. of relative cures."

By this treatment an increased respiration is gained ; deeper inspirations are taken ; the pulse is quickened and strengthened ; by all which the amount of blood carried to the lungs in a given time is greatly augmented and a larger supply of oxygen brought into contact with it. The skin is stimulated by the friction of the flannel, and a slight perspiration induced by the exercise, thereby relieving the internal organs of a portion of the extra burden imposed upon them by a life of idleness. Finally, the effect upon the mind of the patient is highly important, inasmuch as his attention is called from the contemplation of his condition by the many new and interesting things he sees on every side.

It is not to be inferred that I dispute the benefits to be derived from auxiliary medication ; on the contrary, such a course is of great value. The idea I wish to convey is that, as between a method of treatment which shall include all the appliances of our profession, but at the same time allow the patient to remain in a room practically air tight, and one in which no further change is made in the sanitary or dietetic arrangements of the invalid's every-day life than is necessary in following out the lines above laid down, the latter would be found to yield better results. When we combine this with all that medical skill can furnish we may reasonably hope to convince the people that the present belief in the fatal termination of the disease is without foundation ; and the mental reaction thus brought about will be no small factor in the task of reducing the percentage of mortality to an amount far below that attending diseases of more malignant character, instead of so greatly exceeding them as is the case at present.

Railway Sanitation.

BY G. P. CONN, M. D.,
Of Concord, N. H.,
Third Vice-President of the National Association of Railway Surgeons.

This is an age of immense progress, and the evidences of intelligent and untiring labor are everywhere presented.

During the past quarter of a century preventive medicine has made great strides, and has become so interwoven in the practical work of the surgeon that we must associate it with our everyday labors.

The attention that has been given it by the profession has made itself felt with the public, until a demand is made upon the physicians and surgeons of to-day that was quite unknown until recently.

The progress that has been made, and the proficiency attained in the development of the means to prevent sepsis, is as wonderful as it is commendable.

Modern surgery demands that every known precaution shall be used to prevent septic and putrefactive influences from obtaining a power over the patient.

Sanitary medicine may be far from being an exact science, still the rational application of the principles of hygiene and sanitation have developed such changes in the work of the surgeon and the possibilities of surgery, as to lead the public to expect of the profession results that would not have been dreamed of fifty years ago.

Perhaps no further apology is necessary in placing before this Association a short paper on Railway Sanitation.

It is true that the primary design of this Association was to bring about an interchange of ideas, methods and systems in use by those in the profession having more or less to do with the practical application of surgery to a class of cases where, in consequence of the nature of machinery, weight and momentum of rolling stock, the injuries received are radically different from the incised and lacerating wounds of cutting instruments.

The destruction of tissues and the shock that we find after grave accidents that occur along the line of a road are so much greater than those usually found in gunshot or incised wounds, as to be noticeable even to the non-professional; while the greatest of precautions and the exercise of the soundest judgment are called for, in order to insure good results.

The application of the principles of hygiene underlies and guards the work of the railway surgeon with as much force as it does that of any other department of medicine. Without it we should be powerless to accomplish much that is now known to be perfectly feasible.

To cure disease, to relieve suffering, to bind up wounds, save life and limb after accidental causes have seemingly destroyed all hope of further usefulness of a part of the human body, is indeed a glorious work, and one in which any man may justly take pride.

This may be considered an axiom, yet the knowledge of how to perform such work should lead us to hope to accomplish more.

Dr. Holmes once remarked to his class of medical students that the best time to treat a child was about one hundred years before it was born.

It is scarcely probable, in our limited sphere of action, where our life's work is expressed and represented in deeds rather than words, that we shall ever immortalize our names by devising any plan that will prevent railway accidents; still, we ought to have sufficient influence with the management of our railway systems and with the sanitary authorities of towns and cities along their course, to render it reasonably certain that those coming under our observation and care for the alleviation of their sufferings, whether they be from disease or wounds, shall be free from the influences of contagion or the contamination of preventable disease.

So in railway surgery, if we could throw around the victim of accidental misfortune the mantle of Hygeia, surround his wounds with the dressings of sanitation to that extent that nothing toxic or septic in character should come in contact with the abraded surface, our labors would be very much simplified.

I trust it will not be said of any corporation having representation in this Association that they have neglected to furnish, to employé and patron alike, pure water at every available point, the purest air possible within its cars and tenement houses, and a well-drained and clean soil about its roadways, yards and depot buildings. Anything short of this, at the present time, may be considered culpable neglect and a reason for exemplary damages, and I expect a few years hence any other conditions will be considered derogatory to the management of all first-class roads; for without due attention to sanitation the decay and destruction of material and equipment (owing to dampness, dry rot and want of ventilation) will be second only in importance to their deleterious influence upon the men operating the line.

As an illustration of the fact that the public are becoming critical upon this subject, I will quote from the report of the Railroad Commissioners of the State of Massachusetts for the year 1889. In regard to the ventilation of cars, the Board remarked :

"One of the crying evils of railroad travel at the present time is foul air. The amount of air space in a car is very small, considering the number of people occupying the car, and if no fresh air was admitted, would be used up in a few minutes.

"It is estimated that a human being in an hour would vitiate one hundred cubic feet of air, so that it would be then barely respirable. Supposing that there were sixty persons in a car, they would, therefore, in an hour vitiate six thousand cubic feet of air to such an extent that they would rapidly become asphyxiated. Intsead of having one hundred cubic feet of fresh air per hour, a person ought to have at least five hundred cubic feet, so that sixty persons ought to have thirty thousand cubic feet. As there are only on an average about three thousand cubic feet of air space in a car, all the air in a car containing sixty passengers ought to be changed as often as once in six minutes. The above figures are very conservative. Some of the best authorities claim that each person ought to have as much as three thousand cubic feet per hour. In order to give this supply of fresh air, the air in a car containing sixty people would have to be changed once a minute."

After referring to an examination of the air in railroad cars, made in 1874 by the Massachusetts State Board of Health, and also to a report on ventilation made the same year to the Master Car Builders' Association, the Commissioners say : "The progress of ventilation since that time has not been satisfactory. The problem is undoubtedly a difficult cne. It is claimed that it is more difficult to properly ventilate a car than to properly ventilate a house. Unlike house ventilation, the problem of ventilating cars in the summer is, on account of dust and cinders, as difficult as ventilating in winter.

"In either case there must be a constant supply of fresh, clean air entering the car through apertures, the aggregate area of which shall be sufficient to admit the necessary volume of air, at a low velocity ; and in winter this air must be warmed before entering the main body of the car. Draughts must be avoided. For air thus brought in there must be also good and sufficient means of exit. The problem is by no means so difficult that it cannot be solved, and its solution should go hand in hand with the introduction of the locomotive steam-heating system.

"Death from burning is the most horrible death a man can suffer, and it is on account of the torture connected with it rather than its frequency that we urge so strongly the adoption of locomotive steam-heating systems. It is certain that in railway travel much more of life has been destroyed by poor ventilation of cars than by fire. The destruction is not immediate or obvious, but no person can breathe the air which is sometimes found in cars withont having his life shortened thereby. *On many roads the ventilation of cars is unwarrant-*

ably neglected, to the injury of their business as well as to the injury of the health of the passengers. That road which takes the lead in having conspicuously well-ventilated cars will deserve and will receive public commendation and an increase of patronage."

In speaking of stations, the Commissioners are of opinion that "waiting-rooms in stations are frequently too high studded, and are correspondingly barn-like and cheerless. For the ventilation of stations too much reliance is put on storage of air, while circulation of air is neglected."

I have quoted at length from the report of this commission, because it shows conclusively that men outside the profession, and having to do with the public, are looking for a reform in matters connected with railway sanitation, and as the medical and surgical advisers of the corporations we represent, we should not only comprehend the great work, but we should be the leaders rather than the followers of public opinion.

You can all recall cases of lead poison from water mains ; typhoid fever from want of space and the contaminated atmosphere of crowded offices ; diphtheria, sore throat, tonsillitis and enlarged glands coming from tenement houses situated over pools of filth or standing water in cellars ; erysipelas or septicæmia following minor wounds, apparently of so slight a degree as to require but little or no attention.

These are common occurrences, yet such conditions as might give rise to the development of zymotic diseases should not be allowed to exist on grounds owned and controlled by corporations any more than about the premises of the individual. Every health officer understands and fully comprehends the difficulty of dealing with a corporation, whether it be municipal, commercial, manufacturing or for transportation, for the reason that we scarcely ever find a competent and well-defined department with which to confer; however, grounds, buildings, cars, shops and material under the control of corporate management should present to the public observation evidences of intelligent oversight, rather than the slovenly appearances which characterize those matters over which there is no systematic supervision.

The want of intelligent supervision of buildings and cars, combined with over-work and over-excitement in a vitiated atmosphere, has its sad effects upon individuals composing the board of management as well as upon the individual having constant association with the great army of employés.

Some of our most anxious moments regarding the future of some great corporate management may have been in consequence of the untimely breaking down of some brilliant mind whom nature designed to organize forces and become a leader among strong men.

Such men have extraordinary powers and are able to organize schemes and form business relations that are felt to the very centres of the financial world ; still, many of them have some inherited weakness that only requires a combination of circumstances to develop ill health in the form of nervous exhaustion, neurasthenia, melancholia (even suicide), or such conditions. mentally and physically, as to be a sad ending of an otherwise brilliant career.

Thomas A. Scott, Robert Garrett, —— Clarke and your own Talmage were but examples of the positions men can take at an early period in life, when nature has endowed them with the power of organization, and circumstances combine to develop the latent energies of the brain. Such men devote their entire energies to the work before them, and no class more surely need perfect hygienic surroundings. The hygienic condition of cars, stations and grounds should receive our attention, and while we may not be able to solve the intricate problem of the best form of ventilation for any of these public places, yet we ought to be able to bring about such reform that the means now in use shall be intelligently applied.

At present, trainmen give little or no attention to the atmospheric conditions that obtain in a car, and when one asks a brakeman if he cannot ventilate a car, he opens either all the transoms or the doors, and then goes into another car to get out of the way, or to tell some other trainman of the crank he has in his coach. It will not occur to such a person to go to your assistance when the occupant of the seat in front, clothed in furs sufficient to ride in the open air for miles at a temperature below zero, insists on keeping a window open.

Trainmen should have plain, comprehensive instructions on matters of this kind, and I hope it may not be very long before something of the kind will be published in pamphlet form, after the style of the series of health primers which have been instrumental in developing a vast amount of interest in hygiene and sanitation. Public opinion demands hygienic conditions that were comparatively unknown only a few years since, and nowhere is this more especially true than of stations and cars, about summer watering places and mountain resorts for tourists.

Many a place receives a bad name and is shunned because the station is dark, dismal or so dilapidated as to seem unwholesome, else the trains running to that point are made up of cars that are unkempt, untidy and positively unclean.

Then, again, at some points the boom that is made in making it a place for invalids fills the cars with so many people with such positive evidence of phthisis or syphilis as to cause a great many to avoid such lines unless business renders it imperative to travel on that route. If the catering to invalids is to be indulged, lines running to such resorts should set apart an invalids' car and advertise the same extensively, so that the traveling public may be neither in danger of contagion nor infection, nor subjected to the annoyance and depressing influences of those ill with chronic troubles.

While cars may not always be of the latest type of elegance, still there is no excuse for uncleanliness, as there are always stopping-places where trains remain long enough to allow sweeping and dusting—provided there is some one to see that it is done.

The magic word " Pullman " fades away at once when the passenger realizes that the coach is unclean and unventilated, and a boudoir car having filthy closets destroys the prospective comforts of a journey just as much as though it were a nuisance in any other place. So, too, a stop along a line where ditches are full of offensive water or decaying vegetable or animal matter is as unnecessary as it is to have a shiftless roadmaster or " section boss," and one will naturally follow the other. The progressive spirit of the age in which we live is nowhere better exemplified than in the management of our railways. When we contrast the road-bed with its light iron rail of twenty-five or thirty years ago, with the heavy steel rail and rock ballast of to-day ; the small car with a plain, close top of that period, with the monitor extension vestibule Pullman or Wagner now considered a necessity on almost every line ; the change in the standard weight and speed of the locomotive ; the power brake ; the great system of through trunk line traffic ; the interstate and international lines that practically reduce distance to its lowest conditions of discomfort and time, we are at once confronted with the fact that in our federation of labor the department of railroads has accomplished quite as much as any other.

In some portions of our country great advances have been made in the professional work done by surgeons and in the hospital system that has been developed. In other sections but little as yet has been done towards improvement, and an accident to-day of considerable magnitude, involving injury to several people, would receive at the hands of the corporation substantially the same treatment as was given twenty years since. This is creditable neither to the road, the people along the line, nor the profession, and can only be explained by the fact that the management do not consider it necessary to have a surgical department. To such a management a surgeon is only a necessary evil whose services are required only in an emergency. Too often the results of such labor verify the belief, as he is not prepared for the emergency cases ; and, therefore, a review of his work may not commend itself to the admiration of management, employé or the traveling public.

Fortunately, but few lines continue to operate their roads under a *regime* like the above, and it is evident that the great work of reform that has received substantial shape from the labors of our lamented late ex-president, Dr. Jackson, and his co-laborers, Drs. Outten, King and others, is working its way through every State and Territory of the Union.

Interchange of ideas and the expression of opinions between those whom special training has fitted to be authority upon special subjects, will always command attention from the public and must be fruitful of good professional work. Technically, we have nothing to do with the management of railway lines ; still, in the department of hygiene and sanitation, does not our education particularly fit us to advise ? When men are ill or injured along the line, we are appealed to for advice and assistance, and this is on account of our education.

Parity of reasoning would suggest that every road should have a department of medicine and surgery, the organization of which should take cognizance not only of the sick and wounded, but also of the general interests of the corporation, so far as its hygienic conditions are concerned.

The formulating of rules and regulations for the cleaning, ventilating and inspection of cars and buildings may not attract the attention that would follow the amputation or the saving of a limb after a severe injury, still the great mass of the people who spend so much of their time on trains would be benefited in proportion as the number carried safely over the line exceeds the few that are injured.

It is entirely unnecessary to go into the details of the work of such department before an association like this. You are all conversant with the elements of such work, and a very little reflection would serve to bring about a reform. Car cleansing should be reduced to a scientific basis ; a system of checks should be inaugurated so the responsibility of an unclean car could be traced at once. Every station or other building along the line of a road should have some one who is responsible for its hygienic condition, and also a register of such persons should be kept at the central office, so that in case of complaint it can be at once ascertained who is at fault.

What would be said of a management who left the care and responsibility of the safety of its bridges to the station-agents and section-men ? Yet that is practically what is done in regard to the stations and buildings along the line of roads to-day, and the results are what might be expected ; neither party considers it his business to see that vaults are cleaned or that windows and floors are clean and wholesome. Large stations generally have some sort of a system that partially accomplishes the work, but small stations are usually found to be unwholesome and untidy.

In conclusion, allow me to express my belief that the road having to do with the tourist, that will organize a department of this kind, placing the whole matter under the direction of its chief surgeon, and that will advertise the fact that it has a competent medical officer who will hold the proper person responsible for any neglect of sanitation about its coaches or stations, will find in its increase of patronage an extra dividend upon the investment.

Hotels and boarding-houses have found it necessary to have sanitary inspection and supervision in order to satisfy their guests ; will not railroads have to do the same ? Can they afford to do less ?

Fences for Malaria.

Mr. Stanley endorses the old popular notion that protection against malaria is afforded by trees, tall shrubbery, or even a high wall or close screen, around a house, between it and the wind currents. Emin Pasha told him that he always took a mosquito curtain with him, as he believed that it was an excellent protector against miasmatic exhalations of the night. Stanley suggests a respirator, attached to a veil or face screen of muslin, to assist in mitigating malarious effects, for travellers in open regions. These facts tend to confirm the opinion that malarial affections are caused by microbes, which are unable to pass mechanical obstructions.

THE ANNALS of HYGIENE,

✥ ✥

THE OFFICIAL ORGAN OF THE
State Board of Health of Pennsylvania.

The State Board of Health is not responsible for anything appearing in this Journal except that which bears the official attestation of the Board.

PUBLISHED MONTHLY.

Subscription, two dollars ($2.00 a year, in advance.

Address all communications to

The Hygienic Publishing Company,
224 SOUTH SIXTEENTH STREET,
PHILADELPHIA, PA.

EDITORIAL.

The Lives of Mayor Fitler and Mr. Pulitzer.

IT is not often that one has the opportunity to so strikingly illustrate the efficacy of Hygiene as that which has been offered to us by placing side by side the lives of two distinguished men, the one a success, from a hygienic point, the other a conspicuous and disastrous sanitary failure.

Reading the sketch, which we elsewhere publish, of Mr. Pulitzer, we may well parody Scripture and ask, "What doth it profit a man if he gain the whole WORLD and lose his own health." Because of illy-advised methods of work, because of a disregard of the teachings of hygiene, Mr. Pulitzer is, at 44 years of age, a physical wreck. Because of intuitive wisdom, because of his interest in and observance of the teachings of hygiene, Mr. Fitler, though an older man than Mr. Pulitzer, possesses the health, vigor and keenness of mind that give promise of very many years not only of usefulness to his country but of pleasure and satisfaction to his family and himself.

From a material point of view, Mayor Fitler's life has been certainly even a greater success than has Mr. Pulitzer's. Wealth, position, the establishment of a mammoth commercial enterprise has been accomplished by both in common ; in addition to which, Mayor Fitler has qualified himself as a statesman.

Certainly, the thoughtful man will read a pregnant lesson in the lives of these two great men laid side by side.

Mayor Fitler is a man to be envied ; for with his wealth and position he has yet the health so make these possessions worth having ; but who in this broad land will envy Mr. Pulitzer ; what day laborer, with a keen appetite, a good digestion, vigorous muscles and undisturbed sleep, would accept the New York *World* as a gift if he were compelled to receive along with it the physical bankruptcy of its owner.

Let us earnestly trust that the lessons of these two lives will not be lost. Let us realize that while worldly success is to be aimed at, the preservation of health is never to be lost sight of, and that the truly wise man, like Mayor Fitler, never forgets that wealth without health is a delusion and a snare.

Preservatives.

THIS is certainly an age of artificiality in many things, and it behooves one to be very wide-awake that he may escape the many pit-falls that surround him. Science is a good thing when its revelations are put to good use, but it may, and does, prove a dangerous enemy to mankind when its secrets are utilized for unnatural purposes. We have always maintained that the prolonged preservation, by artificial means, of that which nature intends humanity to consume at an earlier period, is an ·effort to controvert the economy of nature, and can but prove prejudicial to health.

Our attention has been recently called to an article which is being quite extensively advertised as a preserver of various articles of food, especial stress being laid upon the fact that if a certain quantity of this powder is added to milk it will keep for a week, even in warm weather.

We procured a sample of this article and submitted it for analysis to Dr. Charles M. Cresson, who reports that it is composed of equal parts of borax and boric acid.

There may be some who will claim that borax is not, *per se*, a harmful article, but, we would ask, would anyone like to daily consume a certain quantity of these drugs along with their milk?

Yet this is just what a large proportion of the residents of our large cities are doing daily. In our next issue we will give some very interesting information about the milk supply of our own city, which, we are sure, will apply with equal truth to all of the large cities of our country.

The Prevention of Consumption.

It would be premature, as yet, to express an opinion upon the alleged discovery by Dr. Koch, of Berlin, of a species of vaccination or inoculation that will confer immunity from consumption. While we most sincerely trust that the final conclusion will be an affirmative one, we yet fear that the world will never see a material specific against this most fatal of all diseases. We can prevent consumption ;. we know, to-day, how to check its ravages ; but it is not by the agency of any one particular material specific. We would ask our readers not to accept too hastily that which they read in the newspapers about this discovery. We will keep you posted from time to time with reliable information.

Old Plated Ware.

Old plated ware, especially forks and spoons, become, through long use, almost void of silver covering, and many of these goods are made of such metal that the acids of foods act upon it, dissolving it and giving rise to actual poisons, such as salts of copper or lead, in the food—poisons indeed, which are highly injurious to the health, but acting in a most insidious manner.

Silver plating can now be done at so reasonable a price that families would therefore promote their health, in avoiding the risks of poisoning, by having all old plated or " silver " ware replated occasionally, as the best silver plating will, of course, wear off in time.

NOTES AND COMMENTS.

Vinegar

often relieves at once the irritation produced by the bites of mosquitoes and other insects.

Hot Claret

Is said to be an excellent gargle in acute sore throat, being an agreeable astringent, and non-poisonous.—*College and Clinical Record.*

Unhealthy Station Houses.

The Board of Health in Albany, N. Y., has had an inspection made of the police stations in that city, as a result of which many have been found to be in a decidedly unsanitary condition.

Do Quakeresses Have Nasal Catarrh?

Dr. D. Hayes Agnew says that he never saw a case of nasal catarrh among the female members of the community of Friends, and he attributes their immunity to the protection afforded by their peculiar bonnets.

Restrain Enthusiasm.

Enthusiasm is like yeast. Life would be flat enough without it; yet there is such a thing as too much yeast for the dough.'' In other words, business men are apt to go to heaven twenty years before they are wanted often.

Nursing Poison Again.

A case is reported in the *Australian Medical Gazette* of a woman who on taking a dose of chlorodyne for the relief of pain, soon after suckled her twin babies. The children were found the following morning profoundly narcotized, and died before evening.

Bacteria in Drugs.

In a solution of quinine in whiskey which lately produced a severe case of poisoning, there was found a sediment consisting almost entirely of a growth of micro-organisms; evidently of a class with which two of the most deleterious substances in use agree much better than they do with the human organism.

"Deadness Here."

It is very much the custom, especially in the tenement quarters of New York, when a death has occurred, to notify neighbors of the state of things by attaching a mourning badge to the door. A German citizen on the East side accomplished this object economically, by pinning up a bit of paper on which he had inscribed "Deadness Here."

The International Congress of Hygiene.

The Prince of Wales has accepted the post of President of the International Congress of Hygiene, which will be held in London in 1891. He has fixed August 10th as the probable date at which he will open the Congress.

The Death Plant of Java.

The kalimujah, or death plant of Java, has flowers which continually give off a perfume so powerful as to overcome, if inhaled for any length of time, a full-grown man, and which kills all forms of insect life that comes under its influence.

After Sweeping.

It is very necessary, says *Good Health*, after sweeping, to wash out the throat and nostrils with warm water. One would better let the face and hands go without washing in this case than let the nasty dust be absorbed by the delicate lining of these organs.

Law Against Adulteration in Russia.

The Russian Government has recently enacted some very stringent laws against the adulteration of food and drink. Any person guilty of adulterating any article of food will be liable to a fine of $200 or imprisonment for three months for the first offence, double this penalty for the second, and deprivation of all rights as a citizen for the third.

Kerosene Vapor.

Kerosene vapor is a palpable irritant of the throat and air passages, and may well have had something to do with the alleged fact that in a recent epidemic of diphtheria, in Hartford, Conn., the only fatal cases occurred in families who used kerosene lamps, while the families who used gas or candles for light in sick rooms escaped a fatal termination.

Sawing Wood as a "Cure."

Dr. S. Weir Mitchell, of Philadelphia, recently received from a woman patient the singular present of a cord of white oak wood, chopped down and sawed up by her own hands. He had recommended to her an active outdoor life in the woods for nervous invalidism. She had followed his directions, with results of which the cord of sawed wood was one of the evidences.

Willing to Trust Posterity.

A surgeon was called to see a rich but miserly patient, whom he found suffering from advanced cancer of the stomach.

" And what are you going to charge me for treatment, doctor ? "

" Nothing ; not a cent," was the reply.

"Oh, how generous ! How can I thank you ? " said the patient.

" No necessity for thanks, my friend, *your heirs* will see that I am paid."

Is Fair Hair Becoming Extinct?

A recent issue of the *British Medical Journal* prints a long editorial article devoted to this burning question. It concludes as follows: "On various grounds, therefore, it would seem as if the fair hair so much beloved by poets and artists is doomed to be encroached upon, and even replaced by that of darker hue. The rate at which this is taking place is probably very slow, from the fact that nature is most conservative in her changes."

A Universal Panacea.

The acting colonial surgeon of the Victoria Hospital, in Gambia, states that among the inhabitants of that country there is but one recognized treatment of disease. This consists in calling in a man who is supposed to be a "doctor," and who, after looking at the patient, sits down at his bedside and writes in Arabic characters, on a wooden slate, a long rigmarole, generally extracts from the Koran. The slate is then washed, and the dirty infusion drank by the patient.

American Public Health Association.

The next meeting will be held at Charleston, S. C. It will convene December 16th. The sessions will be continued for four days. Among the topics announced are those of sanitary house construction in its various details, the disposal of sewege, isolation of hospitals for infectious and contagious diseases, maritime sanitation at ports of entry, the restriction of tuberculosis, etc. We anticipate the presentation of a valuable series of papers in connection with this meeting.

How to Extinguish Fire.

Take twenty pounds of common salt and ten pounds of sal ammoniac (muriate of ammonia, to be had of any druggist), and dissolve in seven gallons of water. When dissolved it can be bottled, and kept in each room in the house, to be used in an emergency. In case of a fire occurring one or two bottles should be immediately thrown with force into the burning place so as to break them, and the fire will certainly be extinguished, This is an exceedingly simple process and certainly worth a trial.

A Famine Duel.

Jacques, the professional hunger virtuoso of Paris, has sent a challenge to Succi, the famine debauché of Italy, to the following effect: "I, Alexandre Jacques, having been informed that Signor Succi intends attempting a forty-five days' fast in New York, do hereby challenge him once more to fast for endurance under equal conditions. I, the child of France, defy the blatant Italian, Succi. Accept my challenge and starve with me, or be known for evermore as a braggart sailing under false colors.—*Alexandre Jacques.*"

To Abort a Paroxysm of Whooping-Cough.

Dr. Nägeli says that an attack of coughing can be cut short by drawing the lower jaw downward and forward. Patients can readily be taught to make the simple manœuvre, which the author claims is always effective. The regular suppression of the paroxysm affects favorably, he says, the course and duration of the disease, and also prevents many of the complications caused by the violent efforts. The same procedure has been found effectual in restraining spasmodic coughing-fits proceeding from other causes.—*Revue des Sciences Médicales.*

Nightmare in Association with Influenza.

A blonde girl, aged 9 years, of lively disposition and mentally well organized passed through a severe attack of influenza. During the stage of convalescence, she screamed out in sleep, "Father, I grow, I become an animal, I am steadily enlarging, hold me!" Her father did his best to pacify her, and though fully awake and aware of the fact that it was but a delusion, she feared to go asleep again for sometime. An old gentleman who had likewise gone through an attack of "*la grippe,*" said that at the acme of the attack he felt in his sleep as if he was losing the human form and being changed into a plant.

Candy Adulteration.

The National Confectioners' Association will give $100 for evidence that will lead to the conviction of any person adulterating confectionery with poisonous or injurious substances, and the association will assume the cost of prosecuting the offender. The publishers of the *Confectioners' Gazette* will also pay an additional $100 for the same evidence. It is cheering to see the confectioners so much in earnest in their demand for pure goods. When we think of the millions of pounds of candy eaten, and the millions of people who eat it, especially children, it is a matter of national importance that it is made absolutely pure.

The Coffee We Drink.

The United States, is without a doubt, a nation of coffee drinkers. The imports from South America amount to over 525,000,000 pounds annually, of which 69 per cent. comes from Brazil. The second largest shipper to this market is Venezuela, 11 per cent. The first cost in this country averages ten cents and a fraction a pound, aggregating $56,347,600. The first record of production in Brazil begins with 1870, when 180,000,000 pounds were shipped to the United States. Highwater mark was reached in 1885, with 400,000,000 pounds of shipments. One large item of expense in Brazil is to get the coffee to market. Freight charges as high as fourteen cents a ton a mile have been paid, which from a distant plantation to Rio Janeiro means from from $1.75 to $2.50 a sack. The highest charge from Rio to New York is sixty-five cents a bag.

For Tan and Freckles.

Dr. Chevasses' preparation for tan, freckles, pimples, etc. :

℞	Rose water	6 ounces.
	Glycerin,	½ ounce.
	Bitter almond water,	
	Tinct. Benzoin, āā	2½ drachms.
	Borax,	1½ "

Rub the borax with the glycerin, gradually adding the rose and almond-waters; lastly, add the tincture benzoin, agitating constantly. Apply night and morning.—*N. E. Medical Monthly.*

The Incubator Chicken.

Backward, turn backward, O time, in your flight,
Make me an egg again, clean, smooth and white;
I'm homesick and lonely, and life's but a dream,
I'm a chick that was born in a hatching machine;
Compelled in this world sad and lonely to roam—
No mother to shelter, no place to call home.
No mother to teach me to scratch or to cluck;
I, alas! scarcely know if I'm a chicken or duck.
My brothers and sisters have all gone astray;
If a pullet I prove, I will loaf round all day,
And never a bit of an egg will I lay.
So backward, turn backward, yet once more I beg,
Reverse the new process—and make me an egg.

A Physician's Power.

Professor Schwenninger owes his post as the permanent doctor of Prince Bismarck to his extremely frank fidelity. He is a second Abernethy in the brusqueness with which he treats his patients. The great statesman was plagued for years by his incurable nervous excitement and his ever-recurring gout, though it permitted him to eat well, drink well, work prodigiously and smoke amazingly. No doctor could help him until he had the good fortune to get into the hands of the Bavarian professor, the only man, it is said, who has ever had power enough over Bismarck to compel him to obey.

At his first visit, Dr. Schwenninger found the patient in his gloomiest and most hopeless mood. The physician began to catechise the Chancellor about his past life. "That is no matter of yours," said Bismarck; "I want you to deal with my present condition." "If that is the case," said the bold Bavarian, "you had better send for a cattle doctor; he would not be in the habit of putting questions to his patients." He took up his hat and made for the door. But Bismarck, suddenly laughing in the midst of his groanings, laid hold of the independent doctor and said, "I believe, after all, you are my man." He has never lost faith in the doctor from that day till now. He is such a model of docility and compliance toward this one man that there may be some excuse for the notion that Dr. Schwenninger must have hyp-notized him.

Tomatoes as Food.

A somewhat enthusiastic discussion is going on as to the alleged great value of the tomato as food, and its alleged influence on dyspepsia and liver complaints. All this is in a measure apocryphal, but that tomatoes, whether cooked or uncooked, but especially uncooked, form a very wholesome element in diet is unquestionable. No doubt, where it is possible to follow the advice of growing your own tomatoes as well as eating them, the necessary outdoor exercise involved is excellent, and we endorse the advice : Grow your own tomatoes and eat them, if you have a garden.—*British Medical Journal.*

The Chinese now Believe in Vaccination.

The Chinese, who neglect scornfully nearly every application of Western medical science, are, according to the Governor of Hong Kong, firm believers in the advantage gained from vaccination, and submit to the ordeal with a cheerfulness and philosophy which are characteristic of this wily oriental. Protection by vaccination is especially required in Hong Kong, owing, as Sir William Des Vœux points out, to the frequency with which smallpox is introduced by steamers coming from all parts of the world, and to its fatal prevalence when it has once obtained a footing.

Effects of Close Shaving.

A writer in the *Medical Classics* looked through a microscope at a closely-shaved face, and he reports that the skin resembled a piece of raw beef. To make the skin perfectly smooth requires, he says, not only the removal of the hair, but also a portion of the cuticle, and a close shave means the removal of a layer of skin all around. The bloodvessels thus exposed are not visible to the eye, but under the microscope each little quivering mouth, holding a minute blood drop, protests against such treatment. The nerve tips are also uncovered, and the pores are left unprotected, which makes the skin tender and unhealthy. This sudden exposure of the inner layer of the skin renders a person liable to have colds, hoarseness and sore throat.

An Indian View of the Benefits of Civilization.

The impending extinction of the Indian is not viewed with equanimity by all belonging to that race. Here is the speech of an aged warrior, recently reported : " Before the white man came we were strong—we were alive ! We lived in tents, we rode on horseback, we moved constantly from place to place. We ate good meat of buffalo and juicy venison ; we drank pure water. Our young men never coughed, the blood never sprang from their lips ; our girls had not these great swellings on their necks and these pale faces. The white man brought us these things ! He brought us the flesh of diseased cattle, bad bacon, the coffee that takes away our strength. We sit in the white man's houses and eat these things, and we die like the dogs ! There are no old men and old women nowadays ; the very children are dying ! "

Creamery Nuisances.

Many complaints are made to this office of nuisances from creameries, by polluting water supplies, and by producing noxious air. There is perhaps no better way to dispose of the buttermilk than to feed it to hogs, but the troughs and feeding places should be kept clean.

The washings of tubs and of floors may be run off, in underground drain tile to cultivated lands, or run into shallow furrows on cultivated land, and then turned under with a plow. This may be done as frequently as need be, and thus prevent what would otherwise become a bad nuisance.

Amenities of Medical Practice in South Africa.

A native medicine-man of South Africa has just had an experience which should convey a moral to his colleagues. The favorite wife of one of the chiefs in the district was taken very ill, and the medicine-man declared that the only cure was the ingestion of fat from the human heart. The chief on looking around him concluded that the heart of the doctor was most likely to furnish the amount of fat required, and ordered him to be killed, which order was promptly obeyed, and the fat of the heart given to the afflicted chieftainess. The other parts of the body usually eaten by cannibals were, it is said, eaten by the healthy members of the chief's household. The inhuman chief has been placed under arrest by the district magistrate pending a full inquiry by the Government officials.—*Hospital Gazette.*

Women's Feet.

A great and very sensible change has taken place within the last few years with reference to the styles of women's shoes. The high-heeled, short and pointed-toed shoe has given way to the low, broad heel and broad toe. As a result of the former practice it was almost impossible to find a woman with a perfect foot. Bunions, callouses and corns were the common heritage of a woman's foot. In a few years, with the improved styles, her foot will be as neat and perfect as a man's—that is, of a man who is not silly enough to try to crowd a number ten foot into a number eight shoe. High heels greatly contribute to foot deformity, throwing the foot forward and requiring the toes—especially the large toe—to bear the entire weight of the body, especially when walking. As a result the toe is displaced inwardly, either under or over the other toes ; a sharp angle is produced at the point of its joint with the foot, and a painful bunion with deformity—constantly increasing deformity—adds to the trouble.

Such misfortunes befall women much more frequently than men. One of the most encouraging signs of the times is the common sense which prevails in the manufacture and purchase of ladies' shoes. There are still, however, society women and shallow-pated men—generally effeminate young men—who torture their feet to make them look well, but the number is becoming less every year.

Conversation in the Sick Room.

A well-meant desire to avoid disturbing or exciting patients often leads persons to converse in whispers or undertones, perhaps in a remote corner. An exchange wisely suggests that "if patients observe anything at all mysterious, any whispering or conversation intended for others only, excitable and nervous as they are they are almost sure to suspect something which must aggravate their symptoms. The mind has a very marked influence over diseases, and nothing calculated to disturb the nerves should be tolerated in the sick room. "Long faces," and those who are prone to look on the dark side, citing cases "just like this" which proved fatal, should be expelled from the room as certainly as ferocious beasts.—*Sanitary Era.*

Vinegar.

Far too much vinegar is used to be compatible with good health. The general belief is that it is a wholesome and necessary adjunct to our diet, but really it might be dispensed with almost entirely except for pickling purposes. If used it should be used very sparingly. A slice of lemon is far preferable as its substitute, and limes may be used if convenient, or let the vinegar cruet be filled with lime juice. If vinegar must be used, that made from wine is better than that made from cider. One writer says that even "a moderately excessive use of vinegar causes intestinal irregularity, constipation, diarrhœa, flatulency, etc., as well as cough, flushing, and watery eyes." As a rule, therefore, persons having trouble with their digestive organs, should use little or no vinegar.—Dr. W. A. Clarke.

Hygiene Cures at Carlsbad.

What is it that cures at Carlsbad? asks Dr. Guernsey, in the *Hahnemanean.*

To my mind it is : 1. *The living in the open air.* Carlsbad life is entirely open-air life—walking, eating, sitting and resting in the open air.

2. The quiet, restful life one leads here; the early hours he keeps; the entire abnegation of fashion's freaks and follies ; the plain diet.

3. The influence of the place upon the patient's mind. He comes here believing he will get well, and intending to get well. He therefore rigorously leads the hygienic life that best conduces to such an end.

4. The fun of going to the springs in the early morning hours and *watching* the zealous enthusiasts slowly sipping their water, as though their cure really depended upon the imbibing of a given amount of it ; inhaling the pure, sweet and cool air as yet unwarmed by the early sun ; and the delight of listening to the well-trained bands that discourse ravishing music. But does the water itself play no part in the cure? Yes, I think the *heat* of the water is decidedly beneficial. But the chemical or medicinal properties of the waters I do not approve of for general use. Carlsbad water can only prove helpful and curative to those patients whose symptoms correspond to the waters.

Is Man the Highest Type of Animal Life?

When we look about us and observe the instinct, that seems like reason, with which what we are accustomed to call the "lower animals" will be found providing for their coming comfort and necessities, we are constrained to reflect whether, after all, man is so very much above the rest of the animal world in point of intelligence.

Particularly is this thought thrust upon us when we learn, from statistics, that only one man in fifteen in the United States has a life or accident insurance policy of any sort or kind, and only two men out of every thirty-two could leave enough behind them to buy a $25 cemetery lot and pay funeral expenses. Certainly such statistics tend to prove that the general average of men have no care beyond the present, and this conclusion must make us believe that the general average of man is not blessed with much more than average intelligence.

The Values of Vegetables.

All vegetables have an effect on the chemistry of the body, so that we cannot speak too highly of their importance at the table. We will mention a few of these matters first, and dispose of this aspect of the subject, so as not to seem to mix pharmacopœia with the kitchen. Asparagus is a strong diuretic, and forms part of the cure for rheumatic patients at such health resorts as Aix-les Bains. Sorrel is cooling, and forms the staple of that soupe aux herbes which a French lady will order for herself after a long and tiring journey. Carrots, as containing a quantity of sugar, are avoided by some people, while others complain of them as indigestible. With regard to the latter accusation, it may be remarked in passing, that it is the yellow core of the carrot that is difficult of digestion—the outer, a red layer, is tender enough. In Savoy, the peasants have recourse to an infusion of carrots as a specific for jaundice.

The large, sweet onion is very rich in those analine elements which counteract the poison of rheumatic gout. If slowly stewed in weak broth, and eaten with a little Nepaul pepper, it will be found to be an admirable article of diet for patients of studious and sedentary habits. The stalks of cauliflower have the same sort of value, only too often the stalk of a cauliflower is so ill-boiled and unpalatable that few persons would thank you for proposing to them to make part of their meal consist of so uninviting an article. Turnips, in the same way, are often thought to be indigestible, and better suited for cows and sheep than for delicate people ; but here the fault lies with the cook quite as much as with the root. The cook boils the turnip badly, and then pours some butter over it, and the eater of such a dish is sure to be the worse for it. Try a better way. Half-boil your turnip, and cut it in slices like half-crowns. Butter a pie dish, put in the slices, moisten with a little milk and weak broth, dust once with bread-crumbs and pepper and salt, and bake in the oven till it gains a bright, golden brown. This dish, which is the Piedmontese fashion of eating turnips, is quite unsuited to cows and ought to be popular. What shall be said about our lettuces ? The plant has a slight narcotic action, of which a French old woman, like a French doctor, well knows the value, and when properly cooked it is really very easy of digestion. But in our country, though lettuces are duly grown in every garden, you often hear the remark, "I can't eat a salad," and as few cooks know how to use the vegetable which has been refused in its raw state, the lettuces are all wasted, and so is the ground in which they are grown.

Twenty-four Cases of Scarlet Fever from Drinking Milk.

Dr. L. H. Miller thus writes in the *Medical Record*: Late in January last a daughter of one of our dairymen went to the city for a visit. The next day after arriving there she was taken sick, manifesting the symptoms of scarlet fever. It was a mystery to her parents as to where or how the disease had been contracted. Two weeks after her recovery her attending physician stated that it would be safe for her to return home, which she did.

Two weeks later, March 11th, her next younger sister, who slept with her, had her first symptoms of scarlet fever.

The case was reported, the health officer visited the house, quarantined it, and his first and most emphatic injunction was that the dairy business should be conducted entirely away from the house ; that nothing should be taken from the house to the dairy.

All went on well till April 4th, when a number of cases of the fever started in different parts of the village. One adult and two children in each of two different families were taken at about the same time, so that on the 6th twelve cases were reported. The Health Officer at once suspected that the milk had been infected.

A thorough investigation showed that everyone who had the fever had drank the milk, and not one who did not drink it was affected ; that at the quarantine his orders had been scrupulously obeyed ; but that the milkman, however, had washed and wiped his cans with white flannel cloths taken from rags left in the barn by a rag peddler.

After delivering milk on the morning of the 7th, this man was not allowed to sell any more ; and after the 8th no new cases of scarlet fever occurred till the 18th and 19th, when two cases started in the same families where it had been introduced by the milk ; and no other cases have occurred up to the time of writing (April 25th). From April 4th to 8th twenty-four cases developed directly from drinking the milk. The stage of incubation in every one of these cases seemed to have been less than twenty-four hours, and the first symptoms in most of the cases were very severe. Intense pain in stomach and bowels, excessive vomiting, and a profuse diarrhœa. After these symptoms nearly every case has run a mild course, and there has not been a single death.

The facts altogether seem to indicate that the dairyman's children in the first place contracted the fever from the rags, and from the same source the milk became infected.

Von Moltke's View of Life.

When that great old German soldier, Von Moltke, was recently asked whether he believed in the coming of universal peace, he replied that he did not, because, unfortunately, man is a bellicose animal, so that individual life and national life is a struggle for existence. Von Moltke, speaking from the standpoint of a soldier, viewing the grosser aspect of humanity, tells us the same thing that the sanitarian would observe, referring, in his case, to the disease-producing agencies that are ever at work. It is true that the healthy life of man must be dependent upon an unceasing struggle with the causes of disease that are ever about him, but when one comes to rightly comprehend the teachings of hygiene, he will perceive that this struggle, far from being a burden, can be made a real source, not only of profit, but of pleasure as well.

Bacteria in Bottled Beer.

The following story is now "going the rounds" of the daily press:

"Come in and have a smile with me," said a learned young scientist as he took the arm of a reporter and ushered him into a palatial café. Sitting down at one of the tables he tapped the bell and inquired: "What are you going to have?" "Beer," said the newspaper man. The professor ordered something else. A bottle of beer was brought. The beverage shone in the thin drinking glass like liquid gold, and the foam was white as snow. It had so excellent a taste that the scribe was about to pour the remainder into his glass, when the scientific man said: "Wait a moment," and drew from his overcoat pocket a microscope and slide. He placed a few drops of the beer beneath the powerful glass, arranged it so that its magnifying powers were focused on the malt liquor, turned the eye-piece toward his companion and directed him to look.

The reporter started back with astonishment, so huge seemed the multitude of bugs and wriggling, crawling creatures that he gazed upon. "Great Scott! What are these?" "Bacteria," replied his vis-a-vis. "You have already taken a few hundred thousand of them." The reporter grieved that his friend had not made the revelation before. "Oh, never mind," said the professor, lightly. "You drank only one glass, and I don't suppose that will hurt you very much. But did you ever think a bottle of beer was more crowded with living creatures than the most densely populated tenement house?" The reporter confessed that he didn't, and asked if such beer bacteria were harmful. "Of course," was the reply, "I do not mean to condemn and decry all bottled beer, but lots of it is full of such germs as these, invisible to the naked eye, which are the insidious promoters of disease in the system of any one who drinks it. This little lesson of mine," he said "just demonstrates that beer is full of germs, and the question as to whether beer itself is liable to contaminate the drinker and kill him depends on how it is made and bottled. I may tell you plainly that there are bottled beers which it is absolutely unsafe to drink. I have taken samples of various brands of beer, subjected them to analysis, and found them thick with the most harmful sorts of bacteria."

A Living Emetic.

A servant who did not find her way very promptly to the kitchen one morning was visited by her mistress, who found her in bed, suffering from pain and violent sickness. She explained that she had a cold, and had taken some medicine that had been recommended for the children. "How much did you take?" asked her mistress. "Well, mum, I went by the directions on the bottle. It said, '10 drops for an infant, 30 drops for an adult, and a tablespoonful for an emetic.' I knew I wasn't an infant or an adult, so I thought I must be an emetic, and the pesky stuff has pretty nigh turned me inside out."—*Medical Brief.*

The Warning of the "Falling Leaves."

The falling leaves admonish us of the frailty of human life; and that the fashion of this world passeth away. The changing seasons have afforded themes for many a poem—and occasion for much reflection. Some of the saddest reflections of life are associated with the season of leaf-fall. It is a season that is generally trying to the old and to those with chronic affections. Hence, it is a season when great care should be taken. It is not a time to house one's self up—there is no time when that can be done profitably ; but it is a time when clothing and home environments should be so adjusted as to properly meet the changed temperature. "Colds" are taken, fevers are contracted, and intestinal diseases occur, that entail suffering and expense, if not death. The fall of the year should not be regarded as the "melancholy days"—"the saddest of the year." With proper care, they should be the most gladsome of the year, since they bring shorter days, longer evenings, home enjoyments, gathered fruitage, and Winter sports, with hopes of Spring.—*Iowa Monthly Bulletin.*

Anointing with Oil.

A writer in the *Provincial Medical Journal* refers approvingly to the Eastern custom of anointing the body with oil.

We heartily coincide with the author's recommendation of these oleaginous inunctions in the case of infants and weakly adults. Many affections of the skin in infants are chargeable to the use of soap, and the substitution of oil is advantageous. But when the author recommends the oil of mustard for rubbing infants we must enter our protest. Many years ago we gave a prescription for liniment containing a little oil of mustard to an old woman with rheumatism. The result was beyond our expectations. On our next visit we found her so much improved that she was able to get around the room with ease—in fact, it required all the agility of an earlier day to enable us to reach the door slightly ahead of the woman and her broomstick ; while the epithets which she heaped upon the embrocation savored of another, but not a better, world. Oil of mustard, as dispensed in American pharmacies, is a drug of which a very little produces a powerful effect.—*Times and Register.*

Next International Congress of Hygiene.

The Lord Mayor of London issued invitations for a public meeting at the Mansion House on July 3d, on behalf of the International Hygienic Congress, which will be held next year in London. Similar congresses have been held in different continental cities, the last at Vienna, under the presidency of the late Crown Prince of Austria. Already the Universities, the Colleges of Physicians and Surgeons, and the various learned societies have appointed delegates, and a large representative committee is being formed for making the necessary arrangements. The Congress itself will be presided over by the Prince of Wales. We sincerely trust that the Lord Mayor will be well supported, and every effort will be made to give a cordial welcome to the many distinguished foreigners who may attend on the occasion

---

Oatmeal.

"Why is it that oatmeal is frequently found to disagree?" says Dr. O. W. Peck. of Oneonta, New York. It is easily answered. By being used almost exclusively as mush, it is *swallowed so easily that it is not properly mixed with saliva*—the first step in digestion. It is true that mastication and the accompanying admixture of saliva with the food is spoken of by physiologists as the first step in digestion. Yet, as a matter of fact, the saliva has but little, if anything, to do with the digestion of food, its office being almost exclusively, if not wholly, that of a lubricator. Without the saliva or some mucilaginous or slimy substance, it would be almost impossible to swallow many kinds of food. Food that needs no masticating needs no saliva to assist the swallowing process, and yet it will be just as readily digested as masticated food. Milk is a familiar example of such a food. Corn starch and other farinaceous puddings are examples of prepared foods that need no saliva to insure their digestion. Food introduced into the stomach through a tube is thoroughly and easily digested. Food under proper temperature can be digested outside of the body without the aid of saliva. So, then, saliva is not a digester.

Now, as to the digestion of oatmeal. Oats, in common with other grains, are composed, for the most part, of gluten and starch. These two substances, if *sufficiently cooked*, will furnish all the nutriment needed for the growth and maintenance of the body at any period of its existence. (Infants under ten months or a year old cannot, as a rule, digest starch, yet they thrive upon gluten even better than upon milk.) So we say then, don't be afraid of your oat meal, only see to it that it is *thoroughly* cooked and then give no thought to the chewing. If the butter or sugar, or whatever is added, is not well borne, do not blame the oat meal. People who would eat oat meal crackers or a hard baked Scotch loaf need to chew long and thoroughly, not for the purpose of getting it incorporated with saliva for the purpose of digestion, but for the purpose of softening it to facilitate the swallowing and to secure a fine subdivision of the hard mass that the juices of the stomach may the more readily and rapidly digest it.

Silly Mothers and Bandy-Legged Children.

The senseless conduct of many parents in urging their children to walk prematurely is productive of lasting injury. Long before their soft bones ought to have any strain put upon them, you will see these poor infants made to stand and even to walk, and by the time they are fourteen or sixteen months old their little legs have been bent very considerably. Pitiful and permanent deformities produced in this way are seen on every hand. Indeed, a person whose legs have not been bent more or less, either outward or inward, by fond parental ambition, is almost an exception among us. Under a year, let the child creep, but do not let it walk ; seldom indeed stand, and then only for a moment ; and from a year to eighteen or twenty months, do not encourage it to walk much, still less set it up on its feet to make it walk.—*Good Health.*

A Health Code.

An unknown poet has left the following very sensible health code :

> Take the open air,
> The more you take the better ;
> Follow nature's laws
> To the very letter.
> Let the Doctors go
> To the Bay of Biscay   :
> Let alone the gin,
> The brandy and the whiskey.
> Freely exrecise,
> Keep your spirits cheerful.
> Let no dread of sickness
> Make you ever fearful.
> Eat the simplest food,
> Drink the pure, cold water,
> Then you will be well.
> Or at least you *oughter.*

The Deadly Cold Bed.

A writer in *Good Housekeeping* says : "If trustworthy statistics could be had of the number of persons who die every year, or become permanently diseased from sleeping in damp or cold beds, they would probably be astonishing and appalling. It is a peril that constantly besets traveling men, and if they are wise, they will invariably insist on having their beds aired and dried, even at the risk of causing much trouble to their landlords. But the peril resides in the home, and the cold "spare room " has slain its thousands of hapless guests, and will go on with its slaughter till people learn wisdom. Not only the guest but the family often suffer the penalty of sleeping in cold rooms and chilling their bodies at a time when they need all their bodily heat, by getting between cold sheets. Even in warm, Summer weather, a cold, damp bed will get in its deadly work. It is a needless peril, and the neglect to provide dry rooms and beds has in it the elements of murder and suicide."

Swallowing Raw Vermin.

The scrupulous care which we exercise in the selection and preparation of our food contrasts strongly with the indifference which is exhibited with regard to the water we drink. Many of our large cities are supplied with river water which not only represents mere surface drainage, but also the diluted sewage of large communities and the refuse of manufactories. We do not hesitate to consume this in its rawest state, though we have learned to apply heat to most other foods, not only as a preliminary aid to digestion, but also to destroy any deleterious matter which may be attached to or incorporated with them. It has now become generally accepted among authorities in hygiene, that water containing a large number of bacteria should not be used as a beverage unless previously boiled or filtered. The bacteria are evidence that the water represents surface drainage, or filters through a very porous soil more or less impregnated with organic matter and living bacteria. These, it is now known, live in the largest numbers near the surface of the soil.—Dr. Theobald Smith, in *Albany Medical Annals.*

Sewer-Gas and Disease.

Because *all* sewer-gas—that is, because the gas from all sewers and waste pipes which carry sewage is not poisonous, Dr. James N. Campbell, of St. Louis, has undertaken to show by a contribution to *Building Trades Journal* that there is little or no danger from sewer-gas under any circumstances. He ventures to illustrate his proposition, however, |by comparing it with the stagnant air of unventilated sleeping apartments and workshops, but fails to follow his illustration to the practical issue. He should have followed his simile by showing that the air of unventilated sleeping apartments befouled by the putrefaction of organic matter exhaled by the lungs and skin is comparable with that of sewage in process of putrefaction, in consequence of retained sewage by unventilated sewerage works or bad plumbing. He would not then be likely to call in question such testimony as the following—to which more might be added—instead of catering to the popularization of a dangerous doctrine through the trade papers.

At a recent meeting of the Medical Society of the County of Kings, Dr. J. H. Raymond, late Health Commissioner of Brooklyn, stated that, during the prevalence of typhoid-fever in that city in 1885 :

" In almost every instance where a case of typhoid fever was found in a house, I think without exception, there was a condition of plumbing which would account for the entrance of sewer gas, so that if the air of that particular sewer was infected with typhoid fever, we could understand how it might find its way into the house, the sewer air serving as a carrier of the germ."

Dr. Bartley said : " I have seen cases of typhoid fever where the attending physician made no attempt whatever to disinfect the discharges ; and it seems to me, in the light of evidence that Dr. Raymond has brought forward, it is almost criminal to pour those discharges into the sewer and thus infect it.

I had last fall a case from such a source, where the physician who treated the case diagnosed it as what is ordinarily called typho-malarial fever. There were three cases developed in one house below that on the side of a hill, where the plumbing was known to be very bad and afterward taken out and replaced. In one or two houses between where these occurred and where the first occurred, where the plumbing had recently been entirely renovated, no cases occurred, but cases did occur about the same time in the house below. I think that the matter of disinfecting the discharges is so important that it ought to be brought to the attention of physicians, because I do not think they really appreciate it."

Dr.' Hunt, Health Officer of Utica, N. Y., says that unquestionably the cause of nine-tenths of the cases of diphtheria reported' in that city last season was sewer-gas. He founds his opinion upon the fact that in most of the houses inspected where diphtheria existed, the house drainage was so defective as to readily permit the return of gas from the main street sewer into the kitchen.— *The Sanitarian*

Condensed Milk.

A mother in Palatka, Fla., writes to the *Philadelphia Record*, under date of July 16th, as follows :

" I have lately read about babies nursing the bottles, and having to drink impure cows' milk, which causes so many deaths among children. Now, as I have two children, and raised them both with the bottle, I thought my experience may help some mothers.

" I feed my baby on condensed milk. Cow's milk did not agree with either of my children. Under the most favorable circumstances cow's milk is risky, the cows' perhaps eating something that disagrees with them. A good brand of condensed milk is always the same, requires no ice, only clean bottles and nipples. I keep two bottles, three or four nipples, clean them with cooking soda and hot water in the morning, during the day and night. When the baby uses one bottle have the other one full of clean water. Buy new nipples about once a month. Boil about a quart of water morning and evening ; to good half cup of water take two teaspoonfulls of milk, stir it up, and it is ready to use. Directions are on can for age of children. Barley, such as is used for soup, is very strengthening for delicate children, or those having delicate or tender stomachs. I give it to mine, and she is 16 months old and hearty. Take about two tablespoonfulls of barley to a quart of water, put a pinch of salt in it and boil steadily two or three hours. When it boils away add a little water to it so that it is a quart when done, not thick. Use it in place of water with milk. I trust these few hints will do some good. It is in the power of every mother to follow them. Condensed milk is cheaper and easier.to handle than cow's milk, and if properly used will not cause the child to die from impure milk. The main thing is clean bottles, etc. I write these lines simply because I see so much about the mortality among the babies on account of impure food."

The Office Cat.

The office cat has become an historical if not a classic figure in newspaper life. Its use as a " figure" (of speech perhaps) seems, however, if the following be a fact, to have been paralleled at least, in usefulness, by the cat of fact, to one publisher.

Years ago when Henry W. Grady was struggling to bring the Rome *Commercial* into the front ranks, he called one day and asked the Rounsaville Brothers for an advertisement. Mr. J. W. Rounsaville replied : "Why, Grady, nobody reads your paper, it is of no use to advertise in it." A happy thought suggested itself to Mr. Grady. He went to his office and wrote the following advertisement, which appeared next morning in the *Commercial ;* "Wanted : fifty cats ; liberal price for the same. Apply to Rounsaville Brothers."

Well, the picture that presented itself at Rounsaville's corner next morning beggars description. Boys of all ages and sizes, boys of all tints from the fairhaired youth to the sable Ethiopian, bare-foot boys and ragged boys, red-headed boys, freckled-faced boys, town boys and country boys, boys from all parts of Floyd County, blocked up the sidewalk, doorways and streets with bags full of cats—cats of every description, name and order—house cats, yard cats, barn cats, church cats, fat cats, lean cats, honest cats, and thievish cats. Well, to make a long story short, the Rounsavilles told Mr. Grady to reserve a column for their advertisement as long as his paper continued, and that was just what Grady wanted.—*Rome Tribune.*

Bismarck's Regimen.

The details of Prince Bismarck's present dietetic regimen, says the *British Medical Journal*, may be interesting to those interested in the treatment of obesity. He says : "I am only allowed to drink thrice a day—a quarter of an hour after each meal, and each time not more than half a bottle of red sparkling Moselle, of a very light and dry character. Burgundy and beer of both of which I am extremely fond, are strictly forbidden to me ; so are all the strong Rhenish and Spanish wines, and even claret. For some years past I have been a total abstainer from all these generous liquors, much to the advantage of my health and my "condition," in the sporting sense of the word. Formerly I used to weigh over seventeen stone. By observing this regimen I brought myself down to under fourteen, and without any loss of strength—indeed, with gain. My normal weight now is 185 pounds. I am weighed once a day, by my doctor's orders, and any excess of that figure I at once set to work to get rid of, by exercise and special regimen. I ride a good deal as well as walk. Cigar-smoking I have given up altogether ; it is debilitating and bad for the nerves. I am restricted to a long pipe, happily with a deep bowl, one after each meal, and I smoke nothing in it but Dutch knaster tobacco, which is light, mild and soothing. Water makes me fat, so I must not drink it. However, the present arrangements suit me very well."

Two Ways of Living.

The old proverb says that every burden we have to carry offers two handles—the one smooth and easy to grasp, the other rough and hard to hold. One man goes through life taking things by the rough handle, and he has a hard time all the way. He draws a tight harness and it chafes wherever it touches him. He carries a heavy load, and he finds it not worth keeping when he gets it home. He spends more strength upon the fret and wear of work than upon the work itself. He is like a disorganized old mill that makes a great noise over a small grist because it grinds itself more than it grinds the grain. Another man carries the same weight, does the same work, and finds it easy, because he takes everything by the smooth handle. And so it comes to pass that one man sighs and weeps, and another man whistles and sings, on the same road.

Sanitary Administration.

"Sanitary administration, like all other governmental intervention in a free country, can be legitimately exercised alone for the welfare of the community, interfering with the individual only when his actions imperil his neighbor.

"Bearing always in mind the limitations of our present knowledge, our sanitary regulations should be cautiously based upon established truths, and executed with scrupulous discretion.

"The position of health officer should everywhere be a career, not an episode ; and for this he should be specially trained, and his tenure of office should depend solely upon his efficiency.

"For the real advancement of hygiene the people themselves must be trained to coöperate with us for their own good ; every avoidable attempt at coercion arouses opposition and retards the ends we have in view."—*Dr. A. L. Carroll.*

Do You Rizzle ?

Do you rizzle every day ? Do you know how to rizzle ? One of the swell doctors in town says that it is the most wonderful aid to perfect health. " I masticate my food very thoroughly at dinner," he says, "and make sure to have my family or friends entertain me with bright talk and plenty of fun. After dinner it is understood that I am going to rizzle. How do I do it ? I retire to my study, and having darkened the room I light a cigar, sit down, and perform the operation. How to describe it I don't know, but it is a condition as nearly like sleep as sleep is like death. It consists in doing absolutely nothing. I close my eyes, and try to stop all action of the brain. I think of nothing. It only takes a little practice to be able to absolutely stifle the brain. In that delightful condition I remain at least ten minutes, sometimes twenty. That is the condition most healthful to digestion, and it is that which accounts for the habit animals have of sleeping after eating. I would rather miss a fat fee than that ten minutes rizzle every day.—*Chatter.*

Laundry Recipe.

To take oil stains out of linen.—Immerse the goods in a soap bath, which should be kept at nearly a boiling temperature. If the stains are fresh, smear them with tallow or lard, and afterwards rub the goods with soap in cold water. Benzine or turpentine is also sometimes successfully used in removing oil stains. How to remove stains caused by acids, vinegar, etc.—For white cottons and linens : Wash with pure warm water or warm chlorine water. Colored goods or silks : Ammonia diluted according to the fineness of the tissue and delicacy of the color. Coffee and milk stains may be removed from silk, woolen or other fabrics, by painting over with glycerine, and then washing with a linen rag dipped in lukewarm rain water. It is afterwards pressed on the wrong side with a moderately warm iron as long as it seems damp. The most delicate are unaffected by this treatment. For removing grease spots from white linen or cotton goods use soap or weak lyes ; for colored calicoes, warm soapsuds ; for woolens, soapsuds or ammonia ; for silks, benzine, ether, magnesia, chalk, yolk of egg with water.

Sanitary Teaching.

The greatest obstacle to the correct application of sanitary principles is either the ignorance or carelessness of those likely to be benefited. Men of general intelligence will allow their farm yards, their cellars, their ponds and drains to be breeders of disease, which may endanger not only their lives but that of the neighborhood, simply through carelessness, or fear of temporary expense. It is true the health boards have been of inestimable benefit to the community where they are located, but if every physician would constitute himself a health officer in the neighborhood where he resides, pointing out the breeding places of disease, not alone in pond and ditch and swamp, but in the houses and the out-door premises of his patients, he would have a much more satisfactory, if not a lucrative, practice. If the masses of the people possessed that education in sanitary matters which every physician should be prepared to give, the death rate in the rural districts especially would be very much lessened. A striking illustration of the danger to an entire community by the ignorance and obstinacy of a few individuals is seen in the rapid spread of the cholera in Spain ; so great is the opposition of the peasants to any change in those conditions upon which the very existence of the cholera depends that the government physicians will no longer visit them unless protected by a strong military escort. If the lives of those in the immediate district was only endangered through their own obstinacy they might be left to their fate, but the seeds of disease ripening among them are scattered broadcast and spread from nation to nation. Of course, in our own country we seldom meet such ignorance and obstinacy, but every physician will find an abundant use for all his information upon sanitary matters, which information should be volunteered whenever it will be productive of good.—*N. Y. Med. Times.*

Observations on the Movements of Young Children.

M. Alfred Binet has recently published some interesting observations which he has made with regard to the movements of infants. The first question to which he directed his attention was the way in which they learn to walk. He maintains that the attempts to walk are instinctive, and not the result of education (*The Lancet*). Among other grounds he draws attention to the more or less co-ordinated treading movements that even an infant of only three weeks will keep up if the soles of its feet are allowed to touch lightly a suitable surface. He believes that the time at which a child learns to walk depends not merely on bodily conditions, such as firmness of the bones, good muscular power, etc., but also on the mental characteristics of each child. Thus he thinks he has established the fact that a child who can give its attention to placing its steps, and whose attention is not easily distracted, learns to walk at an earlier age and in a shorter time than more restless children. He maintains further, that the boy makes the man, and that such children are characterized in later life by the important faculty of close application to work.

Rest a Little.

Good mother, maker of numerous pies, mender of manifold hose, overseer of a province—rest a little. Have a chair by the stove, and when you peep into the oven, sit while you look, yea, even a moment after. You will work all the faster for the short change of posture. While mending, have your chair in the coziest corner, where good light will come in, if possible, over your left shoulder. Drop your hands occasionally and let your eyes rest, by looking at something interesting out of doors ; thus many a holy thought will enter the chamber of your mind and abide with you. Don't rule all the time. Drop the reins of government for only a little while and be a child with your children. These moments of sympathy with their delights will be remembered gratefully longer than your severe disciplinings, and when commands are necessary, as they often are, they will be the more potential because occasional.

Rest a little, and gather restful things about you, that you may rest. Every woman should have a cot and an easy chair in her working room ; if this is every room in the house, then every room should have these resting appurtenances. I have known houses where there were several unmade dress patterns, folded away in the drawers, bought because they were bargains, regardless of need or fitness. Yet these same houses had not an easy chair to rest the body, a book to entertain the mind, nor a convenience to lighten labor. Nor had the inmates a kindly thought or word for each other, let alone the world outside. Can God bless such homes with children ? He does do it. Yet such surroundings transform the holiest blessings sometimes into what seem curses of unspeakable bitterness. These parents reap but what they have sown. Let home bring rest to each member of the family, and let it be the care of each that mother rests a little.

A Caution for Consumptives.

Dr. Tyrrell, in a late bulletin of the California State Board of Health, quotes Dr. Cornet as "of the opinion that the patient is by indiscriminate expectoration even more dangerous to himself than to his surroundings ; that he can poison himself, and that the inhalation of a few bacilli more, and the consequent starting of fresh foci in his lungs may determine the speedy end of his life." It can be seen how very important it is that the expectoration of all consumptives should be speedily disinfected, especially in hotels, pleasure resorts, and sanitariums which invalids seek for health's sake. Until this is methodically and effectually done, we can hope for no advance in the limitation of a disease which is preventable, and which, Dr. Cornet says, kills one-seventh of the entire population.

Some Primary Conditions for the Promotion of Health.

Another advance that requires notice is the machinery for cheap washing with tepid water. Since its use the death-rate of the German army has been brought down to five per thousand, and it is proved that they have been largely exempted from the recent epidemic ; they have kept down their death-rate to five in a thousand, while the death-date in our home army is about eight in a thousand. The cost of washing one hundred men with tepid water in Germany is about sixpence, but here an advance has been made by Mr. W. Bartholomew, who, with his improved jets, up as well as down, can more effectually wash the same number of men for, probably, not more than fourpence halfpenny. In France they are beginning to try this washing with tepid water on soldiers, and it is shown that it may be done in five minutes of time as against twenty in the bath, and with five gallons of water as against sixty and seventy gallons in the bath. Moreover, it is declared that this is accomplished at the cost of a *centime* per head, soap and towel included.

Rely upon it that I do not over-estimate the importance of recommending to all men, but especially to our public protectors, to pay the utmost attention to the function of the skin.

In the first regulation issued by our Board of Health, we provided for a regular inspection of schools and places of work by the local health officer, who would examine and detect prevailing symptoms of disease. It would follow that this officer would be accompanied by a sanitary inspector who would take charge of the affected workman or child, and carry out the health officer's instruction as to a fitting place for the separate treatment of the patient.

To secure a central authority for this kingdom, a minister who can guide and direct sanitation in all its departments is an object toward which every sanitarian should strive. The fact that a Minister of Agriculture has been appointed, should render us all the more determined to add to the Cabinet a Minister of Health. To you, as sanitary men, in the most practical of practical senses, the appointment is vital. You and your labors will never be understood until you have such an official exponent of what you are and what you do in one of the Houses of Legislature, and I cannot do better than close my present address by urging you to organize and agitate for this much-demanded public department until the thing is done. It must some day be done, and for the Association to take a prominent part in the struggle to get it done will be a lasting honor, and a further surety of continued respect and prosperity.—Sir Edwin Chadwick, in *The Sanitarian* for July, 1890.

Bromine as a Disinfectant.

Bromine as a disinfectant is said to be coming to the front. It is an inexpensive by-product of the manufacture of salt, selling at seventy cents a pound, and in solution containing one part in weight to about eight hundred of water; it may be used freely without affecting anything which it may touch. A few gallons used daily will remove all ammoniacal odors from the stables, or a few quarts will thoroughly deodorize the entire plumbing system of an ordinary house. The undiluted bromine is strongly corrosive, and if it touches the skin causes a painful burn.—*The Pacific Record.*

Some Milk Statistics.

The *American Analyst* says that there are $2,000,500,000 invested in the dairy business in this country. That amount is almost double the money invested in banking and commercial industries. It is estimated that it requires 15,000,000 cows to supply the demand for milk and its products in the United States. To feed these cows 60,000,000 acres of land are under cultivation. The agricultural and dairy machinery and implements are worth $200,-000,000. The men employed in the business number 750,000, and the horses over 1,000,000. There are over 12,000,000 horses all told. The cows and horses consume annually 30,000,000 tons of hay and nearly 90,000,000 bushels of corn meal, about the same amount of oatmeal, 275,000,000 bushels of oats, 2,000,000 bushels of bran, and 30,000,000 bushels of corn, to say nothing of the brewery grains, sprouts, and other questionable feeds of various kinds that are used to a great extent. It cost $450,000,000 to feed these cows and horses. The average price paid to the labor necessary in the dairy business is probably $20 per month, amounting to $180,000,000 a year. The average cow yields about 450 gallons of milk a year, which gives a total product of 6,750,-000,000. Twelve cents a gallon is a fair price to estimate the value of the milk, at a total return to the dairy farmers of $810,000,000, if they sold all their milk as milk. But 50 per cent. of the milk is made into cheese and butter. It takes 27 pounds of milk to make 1 pound of butter, and about 10 pounds to make 1 pound of cheese. There is the same amount of nutritive albuminoids in $8\frac{1}{2}$ pounds of milk that there is in 1 pound of beef. A fat steer furnishes 50 per cent. of boneless beef, but it would require 24,000,000 steers, weighing 1,500 pounds each, to produce the same amount of nutrition as the annual milk product does.

A Few Dollars vs. The Health of a Family.

In February last a physician brought a sample of water to the State Board of Health (says the *Sanitary Volunteer*), and asked to have it analyzed, as he suspected that the water, which was from a family well, was having a bad effect upon the persons using it.   The sample was forwarded to Prof. E. R. Angell, of Derry, N. H., and he made the following report :

" This water is horribly polluted.   If it were not polluted, it contains too much solid matter for domestic purposes."

In a private letter accompanying the above report, Prof. Angell writes : " The sample from ———— contains a wonderfully large amount of solids, and is fearfully polluted.   There can be but little question that the vault has direct communication with the well.   It contains the most nitrous acid of any water I ever met.   After it was diluted with 100 volumes of distilled water it gave a sharp reaction for that acid."

The State Board of Health immediately notified the owner of this well of the result of the analysis, and asked him to fill a blank which the board requires in such cases, giving the location of the well in respect to surrounding dangers of pollution, the effect of the water upon those using it, etc. ; but up to date no information has been received from him.   We have learned, however, through sources believed to be thoroughly reliable, the following facts :   That the owner of the well did not furnish the information asked for, through fear that the same would be published and that he could not then sell his place, which he desires to do, without digging a new well, or providing some other water-supply ; that there has been a large amount of sickness in the family, two members having died from a disease said to be consumption ;   that a son is in a debilitated and poorly nourished state ; that the wife has been ill more or less ; and that the husband has been afflicted with quinsy sores.

This water, which is so horribly polluted, has been used for years for all domestic purposes, and without doubt has been the cause of much sickness in the family.

We give the above facts to illustrate the dangerous degree to which well-water may become polluted without attracting the attention of those using it ; and it further shows the thankless manner in which any attempt to improve or protect the health of a family is sometimes received.   We withhold, for the present, the name of the locality and of the owner of the well, out of consideration for others.

The influence of polluted drinking-water in the causation of disease has been repeatedly proven by the investigations and observations of the State Board of Health, as well as by sanitarians everywhere.   Hundreds of polluted wells have been closed in this State within a few years as a result of such investigations, and this is the first instance that has come to our knowledge in which the owner of a dangerously polluted well has desired to keep the matter secret in order to dispose of the place, with its poisonous water-supply, to some unsuspecting family.

An International Sanitary Commission.

Premier Crispi, of Italy, has just caused to be distributed to the representatives of Italy in foreign countries a circular, in which he proposes the convening of an International Commission with a view to institute a sanitary service for the Red Sea. He suggests that two international sanitary offices be established, one for the medical visitation of ships which enter the Red Sea from the Indian Ocean, and the other for that of ships which pass from the Red Sea to the Mediterranean. Another proposal in his circular is to the effect that in connection with each of the two offices should be instituted an international sanitary station, where the ships must put in for disinfection when found to have cases of infective disease, actual or suspected, on board.

Diphtheria and Manure.

The connection between human diphtheria and cognate maladies of the lower animal creation has now been placed on so firm a basis that it is but a step further to postulate an association between this disease and manurial refuse. Dr. Airy, in a recent report to the Local Government Board, on an outbreak of diphtheria in the Samford Rural Sanitary District of Suffolk, has shown that in a particular village in this district the outbreak was immediately preceded by the passage through it of a cartload of London manure landed from a barge near by. Several children returning home from school complained of the stench from the cart, and sickened soon after. These cases set others going, and the disease was then disseminated by school attendance and the like. Though, as Dr. Airy suggests, the foul effluvia of the manure may have acted by hastening the growth of the diphtheria only, yet he considers some weight should be given to the suggestion that the earlier cases were, in some way or other, due to the introduction of the manure. He states that the traffic in manure has increased greatly in these parts of late, and points to the great increase of diphtheria in London since 1882. Dr. Airy's suspicions as to the ability of manure to convey disease are confirmed by the medical officer of health, Dr. Elliston, who has observed scarlet fever to develop in certain places after the deposit of London manure. Similar experience is also forthcoming from Strood, in Kent. The whole question of this association between infectious disease and manurial refuse deserves the attention of sanitary workers and observers. Whether the association is one of coincidence only, or is truly causative, extended inquiry alone can determine; and if the latter be the case, it will yet have to be said whether the infection is a direct one—that is, whether the poison contained in the manure is derived from a toxic animal's discharge or secretion—or whether the infecting manure acts only as a *nidus*, or multiplying ground for the resting forms of certain specific contagia which may gain access to it. We trust that all who have opportunity of observation will not fail to record any facts bearing on this highly important and interesting problem. —*Medical Press.*

Boiled Water.

If there is the least suspicion that the water supply is polluted, get the small quantity to be used for drinking purposes from some source entirely above suspicion. If this is impracticable, boil all water for drinking, and to remove the insipid taste of boiled water filter it. Even infected water used in cooking, and in making tea or coffee, is undoubtedly entirely safe, providing it has actually been boiled.—*Sanitary Inspector.*

Cremation in Milan.

Two systems of cremation are followed at Milan, by one of which the body is burned in a furnace surrounded by wood and charcoal, while by the other the combustion is brought about through a number of jets of gas which cast their heat upon the furnace from all sides. When wood and charcoal are employed about 600 pounds of wood and one of charcoal are found necessary, and the process lasts two hours. When gas is used, all that is consumable in the body is burned up in less than fifty minutes. The body may, in ordinary cases, be introduced into the furnace with or without the coffin. But if death has been caused by some infectious disease the coffin and body must be burned together. The weight of the remains after cremation, in the form of bones and dust, is about four pounds. They are in color pure white, tinged here and there with a delicate pink; and it is a rule never to touch them with the hand. The bones and vestiges of bones (which are for the most part burned into powder) are taken up with silver tongs, while the ashes are removed from the furnace with a silver shovel, to be placed on a silver dish and then deposited in an urn for retention in the cinerarium. Here the ashes are preserved in separate compartments, each with a suitable inscription beneath it. The cost of cremation is $5 to a member of the Society for Extending Cremation in Italy, or $10 in the case of non-members.

Adulteration of Food.

In his annual address delivered before the Chemical Society of Washington, the retiring president, Mr. Edgar Richards, said that, from want of reliable information in regard to the materials employed in most new food products, there is a general feeling of uncertainty and insecurity on the subject. People, as a rule, imagine that any substance used as an adulterant of, or a substitute for, a food product is to be avoided as of itself being injurious to health ; and when they hear that a certain food is adulterated, or is a food substitute, there is immediately a prejudice excited against the article, which it takes time and familiarity to allay. A moment's reflection ought to show that it would be directly contrary to the food manufacturer's interest to add to, or substitute anything for, a food product which would cause injurious symptoms, as in that case his means of gain would be cut off by the refusal of consumers to buy his product. It is true that the unscrupulous manufacturer or dealer does not hesitate to cheat his customer in the interest of his own pecuniary profit or gain, but he does not want to poison him. Where, through carelessness or ignorance, injurious substances, such as arsenic, copper, aniline, and other metallic and organic poisonous salts sometimes used for artificial colors, are added to foods, their presence is promptly revealed by the dangerous symptoms which they call forth in the consumer. About a year ago some Philadelphia bakers added chromate of lead to color their cakes, and caused the death of several persons, and serious illness in nearly every one who ate any of these products.

The great majority of substances used for food adulterants or substitutes consist of cheap and harmless substances, which are not injurious to health, as the following list of those most commonly met with in the products will show. This list has been compiled from the reports of the State boards of health, the returns of the British Inland Revenue Department, the reports of the British Local Government Board, and those of the Paris Municipal Laboratory.

FOOD PRODUCTS AND THER CHIEF ADULTERANTS.

FOOD PRODUCT.	ADULTERANT.
Milk	Water, removal of cream, addition of oleo-oil or lard to skimmed milk.
Butter	Water, salt, foreign fats, artificial coloring matter.
Cheese	Lard, oleo-oil, cottonseed-oil.
Olive-oil	Cottonseed and other vegetable oils.
Beer	Artificial glucose, malt and hop substitutes, sodium bicarbonate, salt, antiseptics.
Syrup	Artificial glucose.
Honey	Artificial glucose, cane sugar.
Confectionery	Artificial glucose, starch, artificial essences, poisonous pigments, terra alba, gypsum.
Wines, liquors	Water, spirits, artificial coloring matter, fictitious imitations, aromatic ethers, burnt sugar, antiseptics.
Vinegar	Water, other mineral or organic acid.
Flour, bread	Other meals, alum.
Baker's chemicals	Starch, alum.
Spices	Flour, starches of various kinds, turmeric.
Cocoa and chocolate	Sugar, starch, flour.
Coffee	Chicory, peas, beans, rye, corn, wheat, coloring-matter.
Tea	Exhausted tea-leaves, foreign leaves, tannin, indigo, Prussian blue, turmeric, gypsum, soap-stone, sand.
Canned goods	Metallic poisons.
Pickles	Salts of copper.

The use of flours and starches of various kinds—wheat, corn, rye, peas, beans. etc.—as food adulterants cannot be considered injurious to health. However much the people may be cheated in the purchase of such adulterated articles of food, the ground spices, coffee, etc., they are not poisoned by their consumption. It is a question how much the purchaser is himself to blame, in his endeavor to secure a "bargain," when he demands so great a quantity of any given material at less than it can be purchased at wholesale in the market, that he compels the unscrupulous manufacturer to make a compound which has never more and generally less than the proportion of the genuine material represented by the price.

Fatal Results of Lacing Among Savages.

We have been told that the vices introduced by white men are depopulating the South Sea Islands, but now it would appear that white women are also responsible for the rapid depopulation of New Zealand. When female missionaries went among the Maoris, they insisted that the Maori women should wear clothing. The latter could not be induced to overcome their prejudice against skirts, but discovering that the missionary women wore corsets, they decided that the latter was a garment not wholly devoid of merit. The result is that every Maori woman now goes about her daily work neatly clad in a corset laced as tightly as the united efforts of half a dozen stalwart warriors can lace it. Being unaccustomed to tight lacing, the women are dying off with great rapidity, and the repentant female missionaries now regret that they ever asked their dusky sisters to consider the question of clothing.

Catholic Typhus and Jewish.

In Galacia a trial has just taken place which reveals extraordinary ignorance and gross superstition among the peasantry of that province. It was discovered at Rzeszow some time ago, says our Vienna correspondent, that several Jewish graves had been broken open, and that the bodies of two children were missing. The police made inquiries, and found out that in a neighboring village, where typhus fever had broken out, that a so-called "miracle doctor" had prescribed as a cure the burning of the bones of a Jew in the patient's room. When the house of this man was searched human flesh and bones and a child's skull was found. The patient had died, notwithstanding the burning of the bones, and the widow of the deceased described how the "miracle doctor" had set about his cure. He had told her that there were two kinds of typhus. One, the Catholic typhus, could be cured by prayer and exhortation; the other, the Jewish typhus, could only be got rid of by the means described. He brought the bones himself, with water from a well from which no man had ever drunk, and burned the bones on a charcoal fire, nearly smothering them all with its terrible fumes. Then while the room was full of smoke he mumbled some strange words and hunted around the table, pretending to catch the typhus, which he then put into the water bottle, and made all present partake of its contents. The "doctor" was sentenced to five months' imprisonment.

Necessity of National Control in Sanitary Matters.

Before the last meeting of the American Medical Association Dr. E. M. Moore, of Rochester, N. Y. (the president), chose for the subject of his address the necessity of national control in sanitary matters. Hygiene does not receive in this country the attention which it deserves. A certain foreigner once said that Americans cared little for health, and when they lost it they took pills. He was in great measure right, as is shown by the fact that medical men are still therapeutists rather than hygienists. Yet we have no cause to despair, for we are progressing, slowly though it may be, in the right direction. In proof of this assertion the speaker reviewed at considerable length the history of Congressional legislation on sanitary matters since the passage of the first act of that nature in 1796. This act directed the President of the United States to assist the State governments in the execution of the quarantine laws enacted by their respective legislatures. This was followed at infrequent intervals by other similar laws, their execution, however, being entrusted to the Secretary of the Treasury, instead of to the President. This was done because it was this department that was specially affected by the enforcement of quarantine. When State boards of health were first established they met often with great opposition, but when epidemics came the local boards were found in many cases unprepared to cope with them, and then the utility of the State boards was demonstrated. It was through the instrumentality of the latter that local boards were spurred into activity. But the boards in the different States varied much in their powers, and some States even yet have none, hence arises the necessity for central authority in matters of this nature. Epidemics are not confined to single States, and they may be controlled only by an efficient body having authority to force its measures in all the States. The National Board of Health has a glorious record, and it has seldom fallen to the lot of any association to demonstrate in so short a time its utility. The recommendations embodied in the report of this board are still reliable, and are of use in sanitariums.

Dr. Moore then reviewed the evolution of the Marine Hospital service, since its establishment in 1798 to care for sick sailors, into virtually a department of the general Government. He spoke of the excellent sanitary work which it did during the prevalence of yellow fever in Florida, and dwelt upon the vast superiority of such a land quarantine station at Camp Perry over the shot-gun quarantine usually established by individual communities in the absence of any intelligent and authoritative control.

The work of the Department of Agriculture in restraining the spread of pleuro-pneumonia among the cattle throughout the country, and in studying by bacteriological methods the diseases most common among swine, was then referred to. But the control of disease among cattle was not properly the duty of the Secretary of Agriculture any more than disease among men was part of the duty of the Secretary of the Treasury. The minister of finance was not the proper person to protect the health of the community. Disease was like an invading host, and, like such an enemy, was to be opposed by an army. It was customary to speak of the work of sanitary officers as police duty, but it was rather military, and sanitary officers should have military powers. The speaker hoped that the time was not far distant when there would be a bureau of sanitation at the seat of the central government, whose head should be a cabinet officer. The subordinates under his control should have a sure tenure of office, such as is secured by a commission in the army or navy. He did not think it expedient that this secretary of public health should be a physician any more than the Secretary of the Navy need be a sailor, or the Secretary of War an army officer.

The Sanitary Condition of Liverpool.

The position of Liverpool as one of the most frequented ports in the United Kingdom renders it peculiarly liable to the introduction of infectious diseases from abroad, and it suffered severely during the cholera visitations of 1832, 1849 and 1866. It places the system of sanitary inspection of the port in a favorable light, that since the outbreak in 1866, only two cases suspected to be cholera have occurred ; and the experience of the last twenty-four years gives good ground to belieue that cholera in the South of Europe will not spread to that city.

The Hygienic Arrest of Leprosy.

Dr. Sandreczky, of Jerusalem, has described his treatment of a case of leprosy which has been under observation four years, and which he thinks may fairly be said to be "cured." After two years of treatment the progress of the malady appeared to be stayed. There has been no relapse, and all signs of the disease have disappeared excepting the atrophy of the hands, which, of course, is permanent. The case, as given in *Monatshefte für praktische Dermatologie*, was that of a child whose family history was free from leprosy. The treatment was directed principally upon lines of general hygienic management, such as open-air exercise, massage, bathing, iron and quinine. The baths were varied with green soap, sulphur, iron or salt, the water being very hot, and free perspiration being promoted by means of proper coverings over the body after each bath. The tubercles were treated by chrysarobin, green soap or iodine, without any manifest benefit.

Milk and Typhoid Fever.

Dr. Vincent, physician to the Geneva Board of Health, has just published a careful report on the typhoid epidemic which raged in that city last Spring, particularly in the Quartier des Paquis. He succeeded in tracing the outbreak to the milk with which the people in general, and the inhabitants of that quarter especially, were supplied. The most culpably negligent and untidy system of cleansing the milk cans prevailed ; indeed, in one extensive dairy he saw a milkman spitting on his hands in order to lubricate them for the scouring process to which he presently subjected the inside of those receptacles. Another source of the mischief was found in the carelessness with which the watering of the milk was practised—any water, pure or impure, being reckoned suitable. He strenuously urges on all who wish to escape the risk of typhiod to boil their milk, and see it done themselves. Milk sold as already boiled had not, in many cases, according to his experience, been properly boiled at all. The most perfunctory methods of boiling he found in constant practice. The moment the milk began to stir in the boiler and to bubble a little it was regarded as boiling and taken off the fire ! Even had the boiling-point been adequately reached, he insists that the milk should still be kept on the fire for some minutes, if it is to be made perfectly innocuous. On the present system he thinks the microbes it is sought to destroy have every chance of surviving and of propagating their kind to increased activity.—*Lancet.*

Dusters and Disease.

A circular of information has been prepared by Dr. Benjamin Lee, Secretary of the State Board of Health of Pennsylvania, on the precautions to be taken by the patient and others against consumption. In addition to the usual counsel given in such circulars, the feather duster finds prominent mention as follows :.

The duster, and especially that potent distributor of germs, the feather duster, should never be used in the room habitually occupied by a consumptive. The floor, woodwork and furniture should be wiped with a damp cloth. The patient's clothing should be kept by itself, and thoroughly boiled when washed. It need hardly be said that the room should be ventilated as thoroughly as is consistent with the maintenance of a proper temperature.

The feather duster is probably the least sanitary of all the so-called cleansing utensils to be found in our homes. In the sick room it is little better than an abomination.

The Hour of Death.

There is a widespread popular impression that a very large proportion of deaths from disease take place in the early morning hours—between 4 and 6 o'clock. That this is an error is well known to most medical men. From time to time careful observations have been made in hospitals, which have resulted in showing that the act of death takes place with fairly equal frequency during the whole twenty-four hours of the day.

Very recently, as reported in the *Journal de Médecine* of Paris, March 24th, 1889, an investigation has been made, which showed that there was a certain falling off of the number of deaths between 7 and 11 o'clock in the evening, but that, with this exception, the proportion of deaths is about even.

We refer to the matter because some of our readers may be glad to have authority for correcting a misapprehension which is of no very great importance, it is true, but which is held with great tenacity by persons who are hard to convince of error.—*Medical and Surgical Reporter.*

Malarious Africa.

Malarial fever is one sad certainty which every African traveler must face. For months he may escape, but its finger is upon him, and well for him if he has a friend near when it finally overtakes him. It is preceded for weeks or even a month or two, by unaccountable irritability, depression and weariness. This goes on day after day till the crash comes—first cold and pain, then heat and pain, then every kind of pain, and every degree of heat, then delirium, then the life-and-death-struggle. He rises, if he does rise, a shadow, and slowly accumulates strength for the next attack, which he knows too well will not disappoint him. No one has ever yet got to the bottom of African fever. Its geographical distribution is still unmapped, but generally it prevails over the whole east and west coasts within the tropical limit, along all the river courses, on the shores of the inland lakes, and all low-lying and marshy districts. The higher plateaus, presumably, are comparatively free from it, but, in order to reach these, malarious districts of greater or smaller area have to be traversed. There the system becomes saturated with fever, which often develops long after the infected region is left behind. The really appalling mortality of Europeans is a fact with which all who have any idea of casting in their lot with Africa, should seriously reckon. None but those who have been on the spot, or have followed closely the inner history of African exploration and missionary work, can appreciate the gravity of the situation. The malaria spares no man; the strong fall as the weak; no number of precautions can provide against it; no kind of care can do more than make the attacks less frequent; no prediction can be made beforehand as to which regions are haunted by it and which are safe. It is not the least ghastly feature of this invisible plague that the only known scientific test for it at present is a human life. The test has been applied in the Congo region already with a recklessness which the sober judgment can only characterize as criminal. It is a small matter that men should throw away their lives, in hundreds if need be, for a holy cause; but it is not a small matter that man after man, in long and fatal succession, should seek to over-leap what is plainly a barrier of Nature. And science has a duty in pointing out that no devotion or enthusiasm can give any man a charmed life, and that those who work for the highest ends will best attain them in humble obedience to the common laws. Transcendentally, this may be denied; the warning finger may be despised as the hand of the coward and the profane. But the fact remains—the fact of an awful chain of English graves stretching across Africa. —*Drummond.*

State Board of Health and Vital Statistics of the Commonwealth of Pennsylvania.

PRESIDENT,
GEORGE G. GROFF, M.D., of Lewisburg.

SECRETARY,
BENJAMIN LEE, M.D., of Philadelphia.

PEMBERTON DUDLEY, M.D., of Philadelphia.

J. F. EDWARDS, M.D., of Philadelphia.   GEORGE G. GROFF, M.D., of Lewisburg.
J. H. McCLELLAND, M.D., of Pittsburg.   S. T. DAVIS, M.D., of Lancaster.
HOWARD MURPHY, C.E., of Philadelphia.   BENJAMIN LEE, M.D., of Philadelphia.

PLACE OF MEETING,
Supreme Court Room, State Capitol, Harrisburg, unless otherwise ordered.

TIME OF MEETING,
Second Thursday in May, July and November.

THE

ANNALS

OF

HYGIENE

VOLUME V.

Philadelphia, December 1, 1890

NUMBER 12.

COMMUNICATIONS

The Curability of Pulmonary Consumption.

BY FRANK WOODBURY, A.M., M.D.,

Fellow of the College of Physicians of Philadelphia ; Chairman Section of Materia Medica and Pharmacy of
the American Medical Association ; Honorary Professor of Clinical Medicine in the
Medico-Chirurgical College of Philadelphia.

To those who are at all familiar with modern therapeutics, and especially
with the works of Jaccoud, Austin Flint, Sr., and numerous more recent| con-
tributors to the well-tilled field of the pathology and treatment of consumption,
it will not be necessary to prove the curability of pulmonary tuberculosis.   Since
Koch pointed out the existence of a ferment in the lung tissues and in the expectoration, a means of diagnosis has been acquired much more exact than any
previously in the possession of clinical investigators.   In some way the so-called
bacillus tuberculosis has been demonstrated to be associated, in many cases at
least, with what we encounter at the bedside and in the consulting room, and
recognize by other means as consumption of the lungs.   Moreover, the character
of the case is believed by good authorities to be affected by the number of the
bacilli in the sputa, and a favorable conclusion is drawn from their diminution
or total disappearance under treatment.   Just exactly what relation exists
between the bacilli and the occurrence of the disease has not been fully elaborated or determined.   It is important to keep this in mind in all discussions of
treatment, and especially any treatment which aims primarily at destroying or
expelling the tubercle baccilli as the principal means of curing the disease.
Let me affirm positively that those best informed upon the subject, even the
ardent advocates of the infectious character of the bacillus tuberculosis and its
agency in causing pulmonary phthisis, *do not claim it to be the sole cause*, but
acknowledge candidly that there must be a suitable soil for its culture, which in
the human being in health is not found and does not exist.   When this abnormal
condition of the system or of the lungs is found, it is expressed by the word
"vulnerability," or "predisposition," and by some it is regarded as an early
manifestation and is called the "pre-tubercular stage of phthisis."   So much
for the claims of the advocates of the bacillary origin of phthisis.   Now, the

opponents of Koch's theory, among whom stands Prof. Peter, of Paris, affirm that the invasion of the tissues by the tubercle bacillus is merely an incident in the course of the disease, and that its relation to the affection is not of primary importance, and most positively that the relation is not one of cause and effect, but at the most a complication increasing the gravity of the case and hastening its fatal conclusion. This was Niemeyer's teaching, and it has not yet been shown to be untrue or inconsistent with clinical experience.

The great predisposing cause of consumption is admitted by all parties to the controversy, of every shade of medical belief, to be physiological misery or insolvency, where the outcome or expenditure of energy is not equalled by the income. When this occurs the subject begins to lose weight, and the loss of weight is so marked a symptom of the disease that it has given its name to the morbid condition, which is familiarly known as consumption or wasting, the Greek title, phthisis, means the same thing. In common language, a person is said to go into a decline when suffering with this disease.

It has been shown by Koch and others, that the expectoration from phthisical subjects contains a poisonous material, which causes death in animals when introduced into the bloodvessel, sfrom tuberculosis of the lungs, with the symptoms of an acute disease—tubercular pneumonitis in fact, or, if applied locally, introduced into the anterior chamber of the eye, for instance, it will cause local tuberculosis with the growth of colonies of tubercle bacilli. It should be borne in mind here, that the inoculation of animals with cultures of tubercle bacilli does not produce the same clinical group or symptoms that we observe in man, except perhaps in cases of acute phthisis or so-called galloping consumption, when it exhibits all the appearances of an acute infectious disease. In the vast majority of cases of pulmonary tuberculosis in the human subject, the patient presents the symptoms of local disease of a chronic character, bronchitis, pneumonitis, or glandular inflammation. Moreover, Trudeau and Sternberg have showed that if rabbits are allowed to run in the open field and are kept in good condition they do not acquire tuberculosis spontaneously, and if inoculated with tubercle bacilli, they recover ; while other rabbits treated exactly in the same manner, but confined in close hutches, die, as they do in the laboratory of Koch. This agrees with the well-established cases of cure in the human subject by camping out ; indeed, there is nothing better established in medicine than the fact that consumption can be cured by hygienic methods, and especially by change of climate. Upon this is based the reputation of the Adirondacks, of Colorado, of California, and other well-known resorts for consumptives. Thomasville, Aiken, Asheville and Winter Park in the south are known to all as curative in pulmonary phthisis. In addition to the climatic treatment, many remedies have a record for curing phthisis ; among these are cod-liver oil, atropine, arsenic, alcohol, the cyanides, and others, without referring to the important dietetic treatment, of rare beef and hot water, drinking fresh blood, etc., from which well-established cases are constantly being reported.

If consumption, then, is an expression of degeneration or a mode of dying, as usually met with in the human subject, and it is curable by improvement of the physiological status, by change of climate, antiseptic or restorative remedies, and especially by properly selected food, without specific treatment, what can we expect from the recently much-advertised antidote or specific of Koch as a means for relief of suffering patients? Whatever the effect of the lymph may be upon animals inoculated in the laboratory, the question that is of paramount importance is, what effect it will have upon the course of consumption as we encounter it in the hospital and at the bedside? This experiment is now being energetically carried on in Berlin, and it is hoped that, making all allowance for exaggeration, there may be some effect upon the development of the tubercle bacillus, for the benefit of poverty-oppressed patients who are obliged to live in crowded, ill-ventilated rooms amidst filth and infection, who are poorly housed and poorly fed and overworked. It will be a great boon to them, possibly, if the bacilli may be prevented from growing in their lungs, but that they will be much helped physiologically does not appear. To a broken-down, phthisical patient, we cannot inject a few milligrammes of lymph under his skin, and say "Be clothed and fed:" more, much more, must be done to bring him up to a plane on a physiological equality with other men. If *this* is done for him, perhaps, like Trudeau's rabbit, it will be found that he will not need any wonder-working lymph to restore his vital powers and cure his consumption. To those who are wealthy enough to carry out the hygienic method, we would offer the advice not to lose the substantial benefit offered by the climate cure in grasping at the shadow of an illusorp specific for pulmonary consumption.

Working Hours and Working Men.*

BY DR. BENJAMIN WARD RICHARDSON,
Of London, England.

IT is my duty to-night to address working men, and to bring to a close the proceedings of the present Congress of the Sanitary Institute. It is assumed that under existing necessities working men and working women have not the time for attending the daily meetings of the Congress—a fact to be regretted, because so much more service to the great cause of sanitation, or health of the world, is imparted when those who are concerned in that cause—and who is not?—can take personal part in advancing it. It is all very well for me, or for some learned colleague of mine, to give a lecture, but that is a poor substitute for direct personal debate on the matter. In my own case I feel sure I should never have acquired the absorbing interest and the knowledge I have attained on health subjects if I had merely been lectured at and told this is what I must understand and that is what I must do.

When, therefore, the Sanitary Institute, or other organization, holds another

* An address delivered to workingmen at the Congress of the Sanitary Institute of Great Britain, held at Brighton, 1890. Reproduced from *Longman's Magazine*.

health congress, I respectfully suggest that on every evening there should be a meeting for papers and discussions |in which working men and women should take a leading part. It would be good if some of these would write papers for every one to discuss, so that they might lend their knowledge to the professed sanitarians in response to that which has been given to them. It would be well, also, to see one of them occupying the chair and conducting the business of the meeting, because, if they once commenced to take leading parts in this magnificent work, they would continue their efforts. For, indeed, the work is so magnificent and so attractive, and, when understood, so mighty, they who have once become connected with it never cease to carry it forward, notwithstanding the anger of the cynics, a mischievous and bad lot, who, when they cannot confute, abuse.

Perhaps you will say this subject of health is too difficult and scientific for men and women who have to work for their daily bread. Not a bit of it; it is simplicity itself. Not a carpenter who planes a piece of wood by the square, not a bricklayer who lays a wall by the plumbrule, not a plumber who wipes a joint; not a blacksmith who forges a horseshoe; not a watchmaker who cleans a watch; not an engine driver who drives an engine, but does something quite as difficult and quite as scientific as anything done by the cleverest sanitarian. It is all a matter of looking at the question and of facing it. Face it, and it is yours, as much as it is ours or anybody's. Every man could, if he would, soon learn to understand and discuss the sanitary business just as we have done in the past week. Neither need the women be afraid to learn and reason and act in the same manner; for women ought to be the best of the sanitary brood. In classical history a woman was the leader of health. We call her the Goddess of Health to this very day, and we owe that title to the wise old ancients. They had a god who was the founder of the science and art of curing diseases, and this god they called Æsculapius; but Æsculapius had a daughter, as might be expected of so great a personage, and she became the goddess, not of physic, but of health. Æsculapius would say to men and women: "Get ill, and I will cure you." But his daughter, who was named Hygeia, Goddess of Health, would say: "My children, my father is a clever old fellow enough, and I am proud of him; but he, belonging to the male side, and always wanting to be master, lets you go wrong in order that he may be called in to show his power and his skill in putting you right. I, however, belonging to the female side, wish to tell you something better. I would advise you never to require his assistance at any time. Live well and keep well. Then those diseases he is so proud of naming and curing will never get into your homes at all. The women can keep the homes in such a healthy state that a home which contains a sick person, with a doctor flitting in and out, will be like a churchyard at midnight, with the usual ghost, a spot to be marked out and shut up." Then, also, the women, coming to a meeting like the present, instead of listening to what is to be taught here, might tell us so much, as goddesses of health, that the Sanitary Institute of Great Britain itself would soon have to go into a position where it could enjoy its dignity at its leisure. And be sure of it, discussions on health by working people will come, although at this moment the fates are against us. We must, therefore, have an address, and now what shall be the topic?

Health is fertile and offers a thousand topics. But many are worn out or require rest; others are deep and require preparatory study; others are pleasant, but theoretical. I propose one that is practical, one that we all know something about if we are worth our salt, which isn't much, though we talk so much about it. I propose that we consider *work* and *working* hours, or hours of work in relation to working men. You needn't start, or begin to get up steam as if a political engine were about to be brought out to run on a line which may have rails, but which certainly is not smooth. Have no fear! To-night let us throw politics, as if they were physic, to the dogs. We are sanitarians looking down on politics and politicians with all the pity that should be felt by the followers of the Goddess of Health. We will study work only as a measure of health. How does work run with health, and how far does health sustain work to the benefit and the happiness of the worker? Let that be our text.

WORK EVERY MAN'S PORTION.

We may start on this inquiry by the assurance that work, manual work—and that, too, of rather a resolute kind—is absolutely necessary for every man. The old saying that man shall live by the sweat of his brow is as true to-day as on the day when it first went forth. The work of man has been compared to that of a gardener, and the similitude is good; for the world at large is a garden, nothing more, nothing less. The true destiny of man is to make the garden a paradise, and until this is done there will be no peace, no garden of peace, no paradise. Every one of us here, probably, has been working all the day for and toward the completion of this greatest work, though we have not been thinking of this object of our labors. Every man, everywhere, who deserves to be called a man, has worked for this unrecognized object. I press this point because it leads us on to understand what is the best idea of work. The idea cannot be too hopeful. We often meet with a good workman who, having completed some really excellent task—shaping a stone, carving a panel of wood, building a wall, painting a wall, decorating a ceiling, or what not—having finished his job, turns from it, glad to get rid of it, and caring not what shall become of it. This is because he does not realize the importance of his labor; does not grasp the fact that nothing done is lost, and that everything well done, if the true worth of it be properly realized, is an addition to the garden of the world, the future Paradise. But when he does realize it, let the following story, true in every word, and resting on my own observation, illustrate how good it is for him.

On the eastern coast of Scotland there is a beautiful old city called St. Andrews. The city claims as its own the oldest of the great universities of

Scotland. In the beautiful lecture hall of the university there is now and then held a kind of gala day, when the learned professors invite an outsider to give a lecture to the students and to those inhabitants of the city, besides the students, who choose to come and listen. On a bright day in the early part of a year not long gone by I was invited to give one of these extra lectures in the morning, and to listen to a lecture in the evening by another outside teacher. I did not know my colleague, who delivered the evening lecture, personally, but I heard that he filled an important judicial office in Scotland, and was considered to be one of the most powerful, able, learned, and, withal, wittiest men in Scotland. He chose for the subject of his lecture ''Self-culture,'' and for an hour he held us in a perfect dream of pleasure. I could not, for my part, realize that the hour had fled, and had difficulty in preventing myself committing the very improper act, for such an occasion, of calling out ,, encore '' with all my might. You may depend upon it that we cheered the lecturer vigorously, and we one and all said: '' What a wonderful lecture ! What a treat, to be sure !'' The lecture ended at 7 o'clock, and at 8 I found myself seated at dinner by the side of the lecturer, at the house of Professor Bell Pettigrew, whose great researches on flight some of you may have heard of, and who is the most genial of men. In the course of the dinner I made some reference to the hall in which the lecture had taken place—how good it was for sound, and what a fine structure to look upon.

'' And did you like the way in which the stones were laid inside ? '' was a question from my new friend to whose lecture I had listened.

'' Immensely,'' I replied. '' The man who laid those stones was an artist who must have thought that his work would live through the ages.''

'' Well, that is pleasant to hear,'' he said ; '' for the walls are my ain doing.'' He had the Scotch accent when he was in earnest.

'' Fortunate man,'' I replied, ''to have the means to build so fine a place ;'' for I thought, naturally enough, that, being a rich man, he had built the hall at his own expense, and had presented it to the university.

'' Fortunate, truly,'' he answered, ''but not in that sense. What I mean is, that I laid every one of those stones with my ain hand. When that place was being built, I was a working mason, under the father of our friend, the professor opposite us, a builder in St. Andrews, who had the contract, and he gave me the contract of laying the inside stonework, and I never had any job in my life that gave me so much pride and so much pleasure.''

My audience, that workman still lives, and is one of the heads of the university. While he was working with his hands he was working also with his brain. He took his degree, he went to the bar, he signalized himself there, and now he is what he is—one of the honored of honored names of his country. But I refer to him here only as the mason at his work, adorning the garden of the world, and proud of his labor. That man had the idea of the paradise. It sweetened his work ; it made it great ; and whatever else he had done, or may do, that was one of his best works, one of which he may be most proud in his own soul. We applauded his brilliant lecture ; but those silent, beautiful stones before him, which echoed our applause, must, I think, have been to him one cheer more, and a big one, too.

The illustration is valuable because it meets an objection which some too refined and overwise people make as to the sentiment which must, as they imagine, always prevail among those who work for their living with their limbs. "What is the use," they ask, "what is the use for you to hold out to working men that they ought to consider the value of their work ? Why, they will laugh you in your face. They live to toil; and the toil is such that they can't be expected to look upon it, or have it referred to with pleasure. It is something they they know they must get through each day, and there it ends." But my new friend gave a direct contradiction to this vulgar prejudice; and I am hopeful that among the ten million workers of these islands there is a large percentage possessed of the same spirit, who take a pride in their work, and who like it best when it is best done. These are the happiest of all their class, and they are the healthiest, which is the point most affecting us at this moment. Under this sentiment the work hours are both shortened and lightened, in so far as strength and health are concerned, since nothing saves the body and keeps it in good order like the tranquil mind which feels the value as well as the dignity and necessity of labor. I am quite sure, for my own part, that I should have given up the supplementary hours of work each day of my own life many years ago but for the feeling that the labor might be of some value in the "garden of the world"—might be helping to make the Paradise which is to be; helping in some very small degree, of course, and in a degree up to my level best.

WILL FOR WORK.

Working hours are sweetened, shortened, and lightened by the idea of the value of the work ; they are directed, in the same manner, by what may be called *will for work.* When will goes with work, half the work is done ; when will does not go with work, the work is doubled, trebled, quadrupled. I like tricycling ; but if I were a man working for a master, who said to me in London : "Now, then, it's 6 o'clock in the morning; get on that tricycle and deliver this letter at Bath before 6 to-night," I should, I fear, be rather inclined to tell him to go to Bath himself, and might even, in my disgust, give him a bit of insane advice as to what he ought to do in connection with the journey. Or, if I took the task by necessity, how I should fume and wear and tear as I went along! Yet, very likely, I should find a man, mounted like me, doing, for his own pleasure, the same task as jollily as Mr. Mark Tapley himself, feeling no fatigue, and determined to add a second hundred miles to his day's work after he has left me at my destination with my master's note. Herein is the difference produced by will:

Against the will no work will run,
But willing work is working fun.

I am convinced that many employers, many employed, fail to understand the importance of this fact. "Employers are practical men, sir," I heard one say. "They care nothing about likes or dislikes, will or no will. The work has to be got through, and if a man don't like it he can chuck it up." "I make it a "point," I heard another employer say, "to study, as far as I can, the tastes of my people, because I find that they do twice the work that comes to them with a will, to what they do when it goes across the grain, and I often regret that my establishment is limited in its resources for variety of work, since I am sure with sufficient variety I could make our work half a holiday, and could get double the amount of work as well or better, carried out."

The cynics, not remembering the low vulgarity of the word, would call this last employer a "faddist;" I call him the real practical man, who in the results he obtained was by far the more successful of the two.

LIMITATION OF WORKING HOURS.

And now I light upon the vexed question: Is it right that hours of work should be limited ; and, if so, how many hours should be allotted to work?

The old saying on this point runs :

> Eight hours' work, eight hours' play,
> With eight hours' sleep makes one good day.

So it does, and there is an immense amount of sound common sense in these two lines. Supposing that meal-times are included in the eight hours' play, the sanitary teacher has little to add, little to take away from the rule in its general application. In the garden of the world no one need be obliged to do more work than can be done in eight hours if the work were carrried out on a scientific and proper system. Unfortunately it is not, and is not likely to be, for an age or two, so that we have to meet a big difficulty in the face and to do the best we can to help to lessen it.

As a matter of health the rule is good. Whose fault is it that it is not generally applied? One says tyranny is the faulty cause; another says necessity. We may admit, in some instances, necessity; but I should say that the fault, pretty universal in its nature, is based on ignorance or thoughtlessness rather than on any systematic oppression or absolute necessity.

I spot one illustration here. Why should shopkeepers be forced by all classes, rich, middle, and poor alike, to keep their places of business open for more than eight hours a day? Who is benefited by the notion which every tradesman seems to have that it is his duty to beat every other tradesman of his sort in the plan of keeping his shop open to the public to the last possible moment, and beginning again at the first possible moment? The man does not like it. Those employed by him do not like tt. It is the outside public who demand it and will have it. The draper, as one of the outside public, will have it of the grocer; the grocer of the baker, the baker of the butcher, and every sort of the liquor seller. Was there ever such an absurdity? There are a few who never can shut up. But how few! Name the policeman, the fireman, the sick nurse, and that most taxed of all living men, the family doctor, and how many more need be employed beyond eight hours out of the twenty-four in constant daily work?

What a grand thing it would be to lessen pressure of business to this extent! In some instances it would cause the rate of mortality to go down as certainly as the barometer goes down when the pressure of air is taken off the mercury. And what a grand example it would be, affecting for the best all sorts and conditions of men! What healthy habits it would produce; what economy! Think of buying all provisions under the light of the sun instead of the flare of gas, paraffin, or naphtha! Look at a purchase made in the light of the morning by the side of one made in the light of the night! Why, I tell you, working men and women, that there are persons who keep what they could not sell in the daytime in order that it may be sold at night, for the simple reason that customers cannot see so well then what they are buying; and I am sure you must all have observed that well-to-do-people never go out at night to buy if they can help it; that their great stores close early, and that the transaction is followed by better health in buyer and seller alike. The old curfew bell that made everybody shut up at one fixed hour was a good bell for many reasons, no reason more than that it carried with it the sound of health. We want a new and still earlier health bell in these times; not one rung by legal order, but by good feeling, good sense, and common humanity; a bell that should not sound to the ear, but should ring in every heart.

It is of no use blaming employers or employed until the public lends its mind to the resolution that it will do no business in unreasonable hours. There is an inconsistency about this subject which is appalling. A philanthropic lady may come to me to ask, will I not do something, will I not say something, will I not write a few lines to the *Times* to help to cure this great an crying evil? Yet a few days afterwards this philanthropist may take away her custom rom her neighboring draper for no other reason than that his shop is closed when at the last moment she requires a piece of ribbon for an evening party to which she is about to go.

EIGHT HOURS A FAIR TIME.

Taking it all in all, we may keep our minds on eight hours as a fair time for work. We may consider justly that a person who works hard and conscientiously for eight hours has little to be ashamed of, and that for health's sake he has done what is near to the right thing; if he takes an hour to get to and from work, two hours for meals, three hours for reading or recreation, and one hour for rising and going to bed, including in this the daily bath which is so essential to health, he is in good form for good health. It matters little then what his occupation may be, since this laying out of time is well laid out for mind and body.

I am quite aware that in the present state of things this rule cannot be made absolute, and that eight hours is rather to be taken as a standard than as a rule. It may be accepted as not positively necessary in some classes of work, and as positively necessary in other classes.

We will, if you please, follow this out a little on the health and life side of the question, and on that alone.

THE BODILY POWERS AND HOURS OF WORK.

The human organization is so far after the manner of a mechanism or engine that it is destined always to perform a certain fixed measure of work. Be it ever so idle, it must do a certain measure of work. We brought nothing into this world, and it is certain we can carry nothing out; but all along the line, from coming in to carrying out, we are all at work. The richest man who thinks he never has occasion to work at all, has within him a working pump called his heart, and a working bellows called his lungs, and a working-vat called his stomach, and a working condenser called his brain, and a working evaporator called his skin, with other parts, all of which must be at work, whether he will or not. He may not know it, but the heart of the laziest lout you can imagine is expending over his body, day by day, one hundred and twenty-two foot-tons weight of work. This is work he can't escape, and he carries it on a longer or shorter time, according as he is constituted to do it. He is born to lift so many millions of tons in so many years, and as each piece of work is done it is finished for good, not a stroke of it ever recalled. If he meets with no accident, the time will come when the last stroke in his capacity will be played out, and then he will die.

A rule of a similar kind applies to all other parts and organs, and that person lives longest who so lives and works that all parts wear out together. There are very few such persons; the larger number break down from one point, the rest of the body being good for long to come. You know the rule in machinery, that the strength of a chain lies in each link; let one link give way, and where is the chain? It is the same with the chain of life.

(This article will be concluded in our issue for January, 1891.)

The Control of Typhoid Fever.

BY CHARLES N. HEWITT, M.D.,

Secretary State Board of Health of Minnesota.

THE better sanitary control of typhoid fever is possible, if we are guided by the following facts, which may be assumed as proven.

1st. Typhoid fever is infectious by the discharges of the sick—from the bowels, certainly—and not unlikely by the urine. The specific poison can live some time in water, in dust, and in soil. It grows, under favorable conditions, in those things, and they (water particularly), are carriers of the poison. That poison is a living plant of the lowest type. It is a matter of experiment that it grows best in a feebly alkaline medium ; but that a strong alkali is speedily and surely fatal to it.

2d. The clothing, bedding and other material of the kind may be soiled by the discharges, as may the floor, walls or furniture. From all these, dried and infectious matter may become dust, which in this way is easily made a carrier of the poison. But the discharges themselves are the sources from which all the rest are infected, and so in proportion to the promptness and thoroughness of their disinfection will be the proportion of all other danger.

3. Disinfection of the discharges is best done in this way : Put into the vessel before use (keep in it all the time it is waiting for use in the room of the patient, and under his bed), a coffeecupful of the limewater described below. It will then be impossible to use the vessel without instant disinfection, which is the essential thing. After use let the mixture stand, covered half an hour, and then bury it, or after adding another cup of the limewater and stirring the mixture, pour it into the water closet.

4th. All soiled clothing, bedding, towels and the like, to be put immediately into as hot water as possible and boiled for twenty minutes. That disinfects positively, and the things can then be treated as any other '' wash.''

5th. Cloths used in bathing the sick, and the water used for each bathing, should be disinfected after use, by boiling the cloths in the water, and so both are disinfected.

6th. Do your dusting with a moist cloth and sweep with moist sawdust, tea leaves, or with a broom covered with a damp cloth. Put the cloths after use in the hot water, and the dust in the stove.

7th. The same rules apply to the disinfecting of the room and furniture, after the disease has ended, as to them while in use, only now be more thorough, and after cleaning, use also abundant sunlight and pure air.

8th. The limewater, as everyone knows, loses its strength by exposure to the air. That is the only drawback to this use of it, but it is easily overcome in this way : Take the best quicklime in lumps and pour on it in a pail, or other suitable vessel, water in the proportion of about one-third water to two-thirds lime, by weight. Cover closely and let it slack till it is in fine powder or a creamy fluid. One part of this to three of water will give a saturated solution, and they should be mixed in the fruit-jar or bottle, in which it is kept for use. A little kerosene or oil poured on the surface will exclude the air, which a common cork will not always do. It is always well to keep a quantity of this limewater on hand for disinfecting sinks, cesspools and the like, when removing their contents.* The bottles, or jars, should be kept plainly labeled '' limewater,'' to prevent accident, and kept in a cool, dark place. Chloride of lime, sold in pound packages in the shops, is more costly, less easy to get and more odoriferous, but no better for the end in view, to kill the poison of typhoid fever.

9th. *Isolation for the Control of Typhoid Fever.*—From what has gone before, it is evident that isolation in the sense of the word as applied to scarla-

---

*For bedroom use, take the clear solution ; to disinfect walls or ceilings, mix residue and clear solution into whitewash, and apply with a brush or broom. Pour it into vaults and drains. Always prepare it fresh when dealing with typhoid fever.

tina, diphtheria or smallpox, is needless. If disinfection has been used constantly, as directed, the danger to others having the direct care of the sick is almost nothing, nor need others be excluded from the house.

10th. Now it will be evident why prompt notification of this fever must be insisted on from physicians and householders. It is to enable boards of health to know where to guard against danger from this poison which is so dangerous in water that the discharges of a single patient might start an epidemic and destroy many lives.

Diphtheria from Cats.*

BY P. C. COLEMAN, M.D.,
Of Colorado, Texas.

IN a recent editorial in the *Medical Record* it is said : '' There seems to be quite strong evidence that there is a natural malady in cats which, when conveyed to man, is diphtheria ; also, that there is a disease occurring in cows which gives rise to this peculiar cat diphtheria when the milk of the infected cow is drank by cats.''

After a residence of five years in western Texas I saw the first case of diphtheria in December, 1888, the case occurring in a child 4 years old, and living thirty miles in the country, and in a region so sparsely settled that the nearest neighbor lived six miles away. The child had not been in contact with other children for months, and yet developed a violent case of diphtheria, which came very near being fatal, and which was followed by paralysis six weeks after recovery. The other members of the family contracted the disease from the child.

I was puzzled to account for the origin of this case for a long time. The child lived at an elevation of two thousand feet above the sea, in a dry atmosphere, was almost continuously isolated, far from any source of contagion, and rarely ever saw other children. The father of the child asked me, some time afterward, if children ever contracted diphtheria from cats, and stated that two kittens died from some disease which he believed to be similar to the disease the child suffered from, and that he believed the kittens communicated the disease, as the child nursed them almost constantly, and had often been noticed kissing them. I am confident this case was communicated by the cats. I reported it in full at the time, but could not account for its origin, as the father had not then spoken of the cats being affected.

Women's National Health Association.

The Women's National Health Association of America was organized in Philadelphia, July 23d, with Caroline Dodson, M.D, as president. Its object is to bring the laity and the medical profession into closer relations by the discussion of health topics.

* From the *Medical Record.*

THE ANNALS of HYGIENE,

THE OFFICIAL ORGAN OF THE

State Board of Health of Pennsylvania.

The State Board of Health is not responsible for anything appearing in this Journal except that which bears the official attestation of the Board.

PUBLISHED MONTHLY.

Subscription, two do lars 2.00 a year, in advance.

Address all communications to

The Hygienic Publishing Company,

224 SOUTH SIXTEENTH STREET,

PHILADELPHIA, PA.

EDITORIAL.

Koch's Consumption Cure.

WE do not like the title of this editorial, and we believe that Professor Koch himself would object to it. From a scientific point of view (and it would be from this view that Koch would consider it), it is misleading, but it expresses the popular idea that is now agitating the civilized world, and it is from this standpoint that we wish to discuss it.

The general public believe (and they so believe greatly because they so *want* to believe), that this great German Professor has discovered some easy way to cure consumption, a disease so frightfully prevalent that its proposed cure excites universal interest. That Professor Koch has discovered a matter, a particular, specific material, that when injected into the body of a consump-tive, will cure|the disease, or that any other man will ever make such a discovery, we do not believe. We make this assertion not hastily, thoughtlessly, pas-sionately, or through any prejudice, but calmly, dispassionately, reflectively, thoughtfully and as the results of well-grounded convictions in reference to the real cause, the real cure and the real prevention of consumption. We are not bacteriologists, we do not work in laboratories, isolating, cultivating and seek-ing the means of destruction of the various bacilli ; but we read the writings of those who do, and we peruse the arguments of those who oppose the bacteri-ologists' claims, and we think and reflect and discuss and reach a conclusion. It is not the lawyer for the plaintiff, nor yet the counsel for the defendant, who formulates the decision in the court of justice, but the judge who has listened to the arguments of both. So, in these debated questions of medicine, it is not the man who, because of his leaning toward, because of his love for, any particular line of argument, should formulate a decision ; it should be, rather, the province of one who, impartial because of his not being specially inter-ested in any particular line of research, is able to view all produced evidence with an impartial eye.

In the first place, to accept the idea that Koch has found a means of curing consumption by injecting a something that will destroy the bacillus tuberculosis, is to assume that this bacillus is the cause of consumption. This assumption has been made by Professor Koch, but it has not been accepted by the profession as a fact ; the assumption is disputed by many of the leaders of our profession. Many good men believe, with the late distinguished Professor Austin Flint, of New York, that while this bacillus is always present in consumption, it is not necessarily the cause thereof ; it may be the result or it may be coincident therewith. Let it be clearly understood that we are not saying that Koch's bacillus is not the cause of consumption, but we are alleging that it has not yet been conclusively proven that it is the cause.

We have, as yet, had no official communications from Berlin, but as we read the published statements we do not understand that Professor Koch himself claims that his procedure will cure consumption as the disease is understood by the laity ; the claim made by Koch is, we believe, that his inoculations will abort the disease in its very earliest stages. This means a stage of the disease when it is not perceptible to the general public, and when, generally, it can be recognized only by the most expert of diagnosticians. When the disease is fairly established, thsee inoculations will have no retarding effect upon it.

Let it be clearly understood that we do not mean to belittle either Dr. Koch or the value of his very great contributions to preventive science. We merely wish to check the mad enthusiasm which the popular announcement of his discovery has occasioned ; we feel that the flocking of medical men to Berlin, many of them sent out as official representatives of learned institutions, will cause the public to feel that there must be something in this discovery, and they will consequently have their hopes raised high only, we fear, to be doomed to disappointment. *Let us clearly, plainly, definitely, dogmatically and unequivocally understand that consumption is a preventable, and, in its early stages, a curable disease.* But let us once for all equally forcibly realize that this prevention and this cure are not to be brought about by the injection of any material specific. Any well-informed physician can tell anyone predisposed to the disease how to avoid it, or anyone who is in the very early stages how to cure it, and the advice so given will be much more potent than will any inoculation or medication. There is no royal, easy road to this prevention or this cure ; it can be realized only by persistent methods of life ; the hygienic prevention and cure of consumption is the only means of prevention and cure from which we can ever hope to realize any real benefit.

Though we know that our publication will not create any such intense interest as has that of Koch, yet in our issue for February next we will publish an illustrated article on "THE PREVENTION AND CURE OF CONSUMPTION IN ITS EARLY STAGES." We name our February issue for this publication, because we feel that by that time the feverish excitement caused by Koch's announcement will have been succeeded by the chill of disappointment at its failure to do that which the public expect of it, and that therefore, the people will be ready to listen to and act upon the only suggestions that are sure to give relief from this great "*white plague.*"

NOTES AND COMMENTS.

The "Schweninger Cure."

Dr. Schweninger, who has become world-famous because he is Bismarck's physician, has a sanitarium, the course of treatment in which is thus detailed by one of his patients :

"Rising, 6.30 A. M.: Cold bath and free towel friction over the whole body. 7 A. M.: Staff and dumb-bell exercise for an hour, with frequent rests. 8 A. M.: Rest and gentle exercise. 8.30 A. M.: First breakfast (meat, eggs or milk). 9 A. M.: Work at the Zug apparatus. 9.30 A. M.: Rest and gentle exercise. 10 A. M.: A walk. 10.30 A. M.: Second breakfast (meat or fish and a glass of white wine). 11 A. M.: Work at the ergostat (a kind of crank) for half an hour. At noon a walk, and at 1 P. M. dinner (meat, vegetables and fruit *compote*). During the afternoon some additional gymnastic work is done, and at 7 P. M. supper of one dish of meat and fruit *compote* or salad, with a glass of white wine, or in some cases beer. Meals, as a rule, are taken without drinking, fluids being only used some time afterward, though in my own instance this rule was not insisted on. In many cases at 4.30 P. M. a slight additional meal is recommended, thus making four meals a day, which in my own case I found impracticable. Weight, strength and chest girth are tested weekly. Coffee, tea, soup, shell-fruit (*Hülsenfrüchte*), potatoes, rice and red wine are, as a rule, prohibited."

Physiology in the Schools.

The following question and answer record what actually happened in a "deestrict school" in this State within a few months, in a junior class in physiology :

Teacher.—What teeth come last?

Pupil.—False teeth.

Ventilation of School Houses.

The German Minister of Education sent out instructions early in the summer in regard to the airing of school houses. He advises, where it can be done with safety, that the school-room windows shall be left open nights, and when this will not do, that the windows shall be opened at 4 o'clock mornings, and left open after school until dusk.

Are Children Happy?

People have a great deal to say about the happiness of childhood, but they are grown up before they say it. For, after all, children have a harder life of it than their elders do. To begin with, there is the constant discipline life gives them in such Scripture measure—the things they want and are forbidden to have ; the things they do in ignorance, to be punished for without clearly understanding the offence ; the imaginative terrors of darkness and evil spirits and unknown powers, to say nothing of an offended Deity, who is angry when they eat too much bread and jam. And then there is the school, with its hard discipline of having to study Chapter XX in the big book of learning, which is the Long Division, when their legs are aching to be at Chapter XLI, which is playing "tag" on the village green. And there is their wondering misapprehension of their elders, and the vague but awful sense of suffering they have at hearing impending calamities spoken of, which they can apprehend as sharply as their elders, but which they see no earthly means of escaping—the possible death of a dear one, a coming scourge of disease, the loss of money, or the end of the world. And there is—oftener, perhaps, than all else—the sharp grief of being misunderstood ; of having their thoughtlessness and ignorance taken for wilful disobedience ; of feeling their natural, healthy fearlessness taken for pertness and forwardness ; of having even their very love thrust aside because it is manifested at an inconvenient moment—of finding themselves, in short, in a great big world, where everything is to be learned, and where the only persons who can teach them are most given to bejuggling and bewildering them.

Dangers of Medical Practice in Spain.

A doctor's life is not a happy one in Spain just now, an ignorant and superstitious population having testified to their dislike for sanitary precautions by assassinating three medical officers in the discharge of their duties. Apart from these regrettable and disgraceful occurrences, it has been found necessary to send soldiers along with the medical officers on their errand of mercy, though even this precaution does not seem to have secured them against personal violence in many instances.—*Hospital Gazette.*

Responsibility of the State for Infectious Fevers.

A citizen will bring suit against the city of Salem to recover damages for a case of typhoid fever alleged to have been caused by the offensive contents of a barn cellar on the adjoining estate. The plaintiff's wife was taken with the fever, and is now seriously ill. The attention of the Board of Health has been repeatedly called to this cellar, but the nuisance was not permanently abated until after the outbreak of the disease, when, by order of the Board of Health, the cellar was filled up.—*Boston Medical and Surgical Journal.*

The Park Acreage of Pittsburgh.

Mr. James B. Scott, of Pittsburgh, thus writes us : "In the October number of ANNALS OF HYGIENE, Dr. J. M. Andres has an article on the "Ventilation of Cities," in which he paid his respects to Pittsburgh, and stated that ' there is scarcely a representative city, *excepting Pittsburgh of course*, which *is not bestowing some attention* to park improvements, etc.,' and that ' it is a disgrace to Pittsburgh, etc., etc.'

" I do not for a moment suppose that the gentlemen wrote his article with "malice prepense' towards the city, but I submit that he should have more carefully inquired of the proper authorities on the subject before advertising Pittsburgh in the way he did.

" Pittsburgh has not only large areas of open spaces in various sections (in addition to others, such as Arsenal Park, belonging at present to the government), but it is in municipal possession of

Schenley Park, }	. . . . 415 acres
" " now under negotiation, }	. . . . 19 "
Highland "	. . . . 162 "
Herron Hill Park,	 13

609 acres

with a considerable additional acreage under contemplation.

" This condition of things you will admit to be different from that to which the Doctor assigns us, and which, I suggest, merits a correcting notice."

SPECIAL REPORT.

Precautions to be Adopted by Funeral Directors to Prevent the Spread of Contagious and Infectious Diseases.

The State Board of Health has recently considered it expedient to issue a circular addressed to ministers of religion, requesting them to use their influence to prevent the holding of public funerals in the case of persons who have died of contagious diseases. If it can succeed in putting an end to this fertile source of epidemics, it will have accomplished much. There is, however, a period between the death and the obsequies, after the ministrations of the physician have ceased, and before those of the clergyman have begun, which is fraught with danger to the community. During this interval the sick room now becomes the chamber of death; the body of the deceased, the contents of the room, and, to some extent, the arrangements of the house, come under the care and supervision of the undertaker or funeral director. In such cases as we have been considering, when the room itself, its furniture and the corpse are all centres of infection, his position becomes one of the gravest responsibility. Whether the infection shall be stamped out then and there, or whether it shall make this room a fresh starting-point for invading other homes and desolating other firesides, depends on his knowledge, energy and firmness. It follows from this that it is of the utmost importance that the members of this craft should be men of sufficient intelligence to be able to appreciate the exigencies of the occasion, of such technical education as will enable them to take the proper scientific steps to overcome the danger, and of such respectability that their recommendations will carry weight with their patrons, and that they need not hesitate to assert their authority. This desirable end can only be accomplished by a State system of registration and examination. That this will ultimately be obtained through the efforts of the many intelligent members of the calling who are urging its adoption, there can be little doubt. In the meantime the board desires to assist them to an understanding of the requirements of what the Hon. Josiah Pearce, of this State, President of the Funeral Directors' Association, has aptly denominated "Sanitary Undertaking." .

PRECAUTIONS IN REGARD TO THE FUNERAL.

In the first place, then, the undertaker can and should use his influence to induce the family of the deceased to dispense with a public funeral in the case of any person who has died of scarlet fever (scarlatina), diphtheria, membranous croup, diphtheritic sore throat, smallpox, varioloid, typhus fever, yellow fever or measles. As his advice will be purely disinterested—in fact, opposed to his own interests pecuniarily—it will be the more likely to be heeded ; and as the minister may be relied upon to second his suggestion, their agreement in the matter will have great weight. The members of the Funeral Directors' Association might very properly agree to refuse their ministrations in public in such cases.

In the second place, he can and should use his influence to prevent friends, neighbors and even relatives from coming to view the remains while they are awaiting sepulture. What terrible results may follow carelessness and the indulgence of idle curiosity in this respect is well illustrated by the following statement which occurred in the course of an address upon "The Dangers Arising from Public Funerals in the Case of Contagious Diseases," delivered by the Rev. S. Bridenbaugh, before the State Sanitary Convention, held at Norristown in May last, and which forms a part of the circular addressed to the clerical profession on this subject :

"About twelve years ago, while pastor in a town of Western Pennsylvania, malignant diphtheria became epidemic. A child died of this disease in a house opposite the public school building. Burial did not take place until the third day after the occurrence of death. During a considerable portion of that time the remains were exposed to public gaze. More than a hundred pupils of the school availed themselves of the opportunity to linger around the corpse and take a last look at the remains of their departed schoolmate. The disease spread. In the town and surrounding country at least one hundred and fifty persons were infected with it. About forty died. This will not be surprising when I assure you that all the funerals were public. Whether held in the house or in the church, in most instances crowds thronged to view the remains and aid in spreading the disease. There was no board of health, and a majority of the people were, doubtless, unaware of the danger to the living in their efforts to show respect for the dead."

In the third place, he can and should avoid taking chairs, palls or other articles of furniture or decoration, which are liable to be used on other like occasions, to houses in which a death from one of the above-mentioned diseases had taken place. And this because so subtle are the germs of contagion that every room in an infected house may contain them.

Among the articles to come under this restriction is the ice-box. *An ice-box should never be used for a body dead of an infectious disease.* Cases of shocking recklessness have been reported to the board in which the ice used to preserve such bodies has been emptied out on the public street.

Fourthly, he can and should urge that the private burial of the deceased take place at the earliest possible moment after death—within twenty-four hours, unless the local board of health fixes a limit of its own.

Fifthly, he can and should refuse to carry, or cause or allow to be carried, in a carriage the corpse of a child dead of an infectious disease.

Sixthly, he can and should insist on the disinfection of every carriage, in which the occupants of the house in which such death took place have ridden in attending the funeral.

Seventhly, he can and should take pains not himself to be the means of spreading the contagion. It would be well for him to have a separate suit of clothes to wear in such cases, and to keep the same well aired and disinfected. He should also take the precaution to take a bath after preparing every such body for burial, and to sponge his entire body with a disinfectant solution. Should he be called upon to attend several of this nature in one day, as may often be the case during epidemics, he should take these consecutively and then take the personal precautions mentioned, before going to others.

PRECAUTIONS IN REGARD TO THE CORPSE.

The corpse should be handled as little as possible. No more washing should be done than is demanded by the slightest requirements of decency. The water for this purpose should contain a disinfectant. If the implements are at hand—and the educated and skilful undertaker will never be without them—the cavities of the chest and abdomen should be injected with a strong solution of chloride of lime or other antiseptic fluid of full strength unless the body is to be kept for a length of time or transported, arterial embalmment is unnec-essary and adds to the risk incurred by the operator. The body should then be at once wrapped in a sheet saturated with a strong disinfectant solution, of which corrosive subli-mate should be the principal ingredient, and this sheet should be moistened with the same at frequent intervals.

EMBALMMENT.

The act of embalming, which is practiced more generally and more successfully in this country than anywhere in the world, must be looked upon as a decided advance over the plan of preservation by the use of ice, from a sanitary point of view. The fluids which are used for the purpose are all antiseptic to a greater or less extent. A careful arterial injection with a powerful antiseptic or germicidal solution, must certainly go a great way towards de-stroying all specific germs of disease in a body. Instead of the paraphernalia required for the application of cold, all that is needed are a few surgical instruments, and there is no pol-luted water to be disposed of. To offer suggestions as to the manner of performing the opera-tion as the places of selection would be entirely beyond the province of this Board. They may be found in full in that valuable compendium, The National Funeral Directors' Official Text Book, which should be studied by every one who aspires to prepare the dead for sepul-ture and conduct their obsequies. Still less is it the duty of the Board to recommend any par-ticular embalming fluid. But it is right that it should state that many substances which will act as preservatives have little or no value as disinfectants. Such are the arsenical prepara-tions and hydrate of chloral. The great germicides are chloride of lime, hypochlorite of soda, corrosive sublimate, and carbolic acid. Chloride of lime, in the proportion of 5 per cent. is also an agent of considerable value. Hence the embalming fluid to be used in inject-ing a body dead of an infectious disease should contain at least one of the first-mentioned articles.

Every undertaker is aware of the fact that embalming has been objected to on the ground that the fact of death from poison may thus be concealed. The objection is a valid one and will probably lead to legislative enactment on the subject. A written certificate of the cause of death should therefore always be procured from the attendant physician before performing the operation. It should never be attempted in the face of suspicious circumstances.

PRECAUTIONS IN REGARD TO DISINFECTION OF ROOM, FURNITURE AND CLOTHING.

Unless in cities where the Board of Health undertakes the work of disinfection in pri-vate houses, the undertaker should feel that he has a moral responsibility in regard to this important matter. The occupants of the house will usually accept his suggestions, espe-cially if he can show them that they are strictly in accordance with the instructions of the State Board of Health.

The following are

STANDARD DISINFECTING SOLUTIONS RECOMMENDED BY THE BOARD.

1. *Standard Solution, No. 1.*—Dissolve chloride of lime or bleaching powder of the best quality (containing at least 25 per cent. of available chlorine) in soft water in the propor-tion of six ounces to the gallon.

2. *Standard Solution, No. 2.*—Dissolve corrosive sublimate and permanganate of potash in soft water in the proportion of two drachms of each salt to the gallon.

(NOTE.—1. This solution is highly poisonous. 2. It requires a contact of one hour to be efficient. 3. It destroys lead pipes. 4. It is without odor.)

3. *Standard Solution, No.* 3—To one part of Labaraque's solution of hypochlorite of soda (*liquor sodæ chloratæ*,—U. S. P.,) add five parts of soft water.

4. *Standard Solution, No. 4*—Dissolve corrosive sublimate in water in the proportion of four ounces to the gallon, and add one drachm of permanganate of potash to give color to the solution as a precaution against poisoning. One fluid ounce of this solution to the gallon of water is sufficiently strong. Articles should be left in it for two hours.

(NOTE.—Corrosive sublimate solutions should be kept in wooden or crockery vessels.)

TO DISINFECT DISCHARGES FROM THE BODY.

Use standard solutions Nos. 1, 2, or 3, keeping a pint of the solution used constantly in a vessel ready for any emergency. Let the discharges be emptied directly into the solution, and then let a pint more of it be added, and allow the whole to stand for some time before being thrown into the sewer, or being buried.

TO DISINFECT CLOTHING, TOWELS, NAPKINS, BEDDING AND SUCH TEXTILE FABRICS AS CAN BE WASHED.

Use standard solution No. 4, *one ounce to the gallon of water*, or use one gallon of solution No. 1, in nine gallons of water. Let the goods soak in the solution for at least two hours—better four hours—before they leave the room. Stir them up so that the solution gets all through them. After disinfection, boil the goods thoroughly.

FOR THE DISINFECTION OF WATER-CLOSETS, URINALS, SINKS AND CESS-POOLS.

5. *Carbolic Acid Solution.*—Mix one pint of carbolic acid with two and a half gallons of water.

Standard solution, No. 4, diluted with three parts of water, may also be used in the proportion of one gallon (of the solution) to every four (estimated) of the contents of the vault. Standard solution, No. 1, would require to be used gallon for gallon of the material to be disinfected. Dry chloride of lime may be sprinkled over the contents of a privy, or standard solution, No. 2, may be made up by the barrel, and four or five gallons be applied daily during an epidemic.

TO DISINFECT THE SICK ROOM AFTER IT IS VACATED.

If it is possible, let the room be thrown wide open for several days, for a thorough airing. If papered, let the paper be all removed with care, and burned. Then let all the walls, the doors and the woodwork of the room, as well as the furniture, be washed with standard solution, No. 4, one pint to four gallons of water, or, of solution, No. 1, a quarter of a pint to a gallon of water. Let this work be done most carefully, getting the solution into all the crevices. If any dust be present in the corners and crevices, wipe it out with a rag wet in the disinfecting fluid. *Don't stir it up with a brush or broom.* Last of all, whitewash the walls and the ceiling.

SULPHUR FUMIGATION

Is believed in by many as very efficacious, but should not be allowed to take the place of the scraping and scrubbing. It is performed in the following manner : Open wide all the drawers and closet doors. Hang on lines, opened up as much as possible, all the woolen articles which have been in the room during the sickness and which have not been disinfected and washed, then burn two pounds of sulphur for every thousand cubic feet of air space in the room. Every opening in the room—flues, doors, windows, cracks and crevices—must be closed, except the door by which the disinfector is to escape. The sulphur is to be burned in an iron kettle or other vessel set in a tub, containing a little water to guard against fire. A little alcohol or kerosene must be poured upon the sulphur by means of which it may be ignited. Leave the room quickly, for the fumes are highly poisonous when breathed, and close the door tightly. Let the room remain closed twenty-four hours or more. Then air thoroughly for several days.

BEDS WHICH HAVE BEEN SATURATED WITH THE DISCHARGES OF THE PATIENT.

Children's playthings, used during sickness, paper books, articles of fur and wool such as strips of carpet and pieces of badly-infected woolen clothing should be burned ; never given away. If there is an open fireplace or a stove in the room many small articles may at once be burned on the spot. In a city, this is best done by making them into a compact bundle in the sick room, thoroughly dampening the outside of the bundle with a solution of chloride of lime or corrosive sublimate in water, and then carrying it to the glowing furnace under a large boiler in some industrial establishment. If in the country, these things should be carried into a field or a woods far from any human habitation, and there made to burn thoroughly and quickly, to do which the bundle should be opened and saturated with petroleum. Under no circumstances should these things be thrown into an open space or into running water.

PRECAUTIONS TO BE OBSERVED IN REGARD TO THE DISINTERMENT AND TRANSPORTATION OF DEAD BODIES.

Too scrupulous care cannot be observed in the transportation of the bodies of those who have died of infectious diseases to a distance from the place of death. The following extract from the last quarterly report of the State Board of Health of Maryland furnishes only one of a hundred instances which might be adduced in proof of this statement :

"About the middle of June last, a child died of diphtheria in a city in a neighboring State and upon a certificate furnished by a physician of that city that the child died of pneumonia the corpse was transported into this State by the Philadelphia, Wilmington and Baltimore Railroad Company in an ordinary casket without metal lining or any antiseptic precautions. On the arrival of the body at Conowingo Station, it was immediately removed to the residence of the grandfather, at Prospect, where the coffin was opened and the remains viewed by the family. In a few days thereafter there was an outbreak of diphtheria in the house, and in less than a month six or seven members of the family were attacked, and five died of the disease in a malignant form. It then spread to other families in the neighborhood."

The Board therefore earnestly calls the attention of all Funeral Directors throughout the Commonwealth to the following Regulations. No railroad can be compelled to take a body unless they have been complied with.

Regulations of the State Board of Health of Pennsylvania.

DISINTERMENT OF BODIES.

RULE 1.—The removal of any body from its place of original interment is declared to be a nuisance dangerous to the public health, and is prohibited, unless the same be done under the direction and by permission of the State or Local Board of Health or Borough Council.

RULE 2.—The above rule applies as well to the removal of a body from one grave or vault to another, in the same cemetery, as to its removal to another burial ground or place.

RULE 3.—The removal of dead bodies from any burial ground situated within the built up portions of any city or borough is forbidden between April 1st and October 15th.

RULE 4.—The disinterment of the body of any person who died of any contagious or infectious disease is strictly prohibited unless by special authority, and upon such conditions as the State or Local Board of Health or Borough Council may impose.

TRANSPORTATION OF BODIES.

RULE 1.—The transportation of bodies of persons dead of small-pox, varioloid, Asiatic cholera, leprosy, typhus fever or yellow fever is strictly forbidden.

RULE 2.—The bodies of persons dead of diphtheria, membranous croup, anthrax scarlet fever, puerperal fever, typhoid fever, erysipelas, measles, whooping-cough or dysentery must be wrapped in a sheet thoroughly saturated with a strong solution of bichloride of mercury in the proportion of one ounce of bichloride of mercury to a gallon of water, and encased in an air-tight zinc, tin, copper or lead-lined coffin ; or in an air-tight iron casket, hermetically sealed, and all enclosed in a strong, tight, wooden box ; or the body must be prepared for shipment by being wrapped in a sheet disinfected by a solution of bichloride of mercury as above, and placed in a strong coffin or casket, and said coffin or casket encased in a hermetically sealed (soldered) zinc, copper, or tin case, and all enclosed in a strong, outside, wooden box of material not less than one inch and a half thick.

RULE 3.—In the case of contagious, infectious, or communicable diseases the body must not be accompanied by persons who, or articles which have been exposed to the infection of the disease. And, in addition to the permit from the Board of Health or proper health authority, agents will require an affidavit from the shipping undertaker, stating how the body has been prepared and the kind of coffin or casket used, which must be in conformity with Rule 2.

RULE 4.—The bodies of persons dead of diseases that are not contagious, infectious, or communicable, may be received for transportation to local points in this State when encased in a sound coffin or metallic case, and enclosed in a strong wooden box, securely fastened so that it may be safely handled. But when it is proposed to transport them out of the State (unless the time required for transportation from the initial point to destination does not exceed eighteen hours) they must be encased in an air-tight, zinc, tin, copper, or lead-lined coffin, or an air-tight iron casket, or a strong coffin or casket encased in a hermetically sealed (soldered) zinc, copper, or tin case, and all enclosed in a strong outside wooden box of material not le s than one inch thick. In all cases the outside box should be provided with four iron chest handles.

RULE 5.—Every dead body must be accompanied by a person in charge, who must be provided with a transit permit from the Board of Health, or proper health authority, giving permission for the removal, and showing name of deceased, age, place of death, cause of death (and if of a contagious or infectious nature), the point to which it is to be shipped, and the names of medical attendant and undertaker.

RULE 6.—The transit permits must be made with a stub and two coupons ; the stub to be retained by the person issuing it ; the first coupon to be detached by agent at initial point and sent to the general baggage agent, and the second coupon by the last train baggage-man, while the permit itself must accompany the body to its place of destination. The stub, permit and coupons must be numbered so that one will refer to the other, and on the back of the permit there must be a space for the undertaker's affidavit to be used in case of contagious or infectious diseases, as required by Rules 2 and 3.

RULE 7.—The box containing corpse must be plainly marked with a paster, showing name of deceased, place of death, cause of death, point to which it is to be shipped, number of transit permit issued in connection, and name of person in charge of the remains. There must also be blank spaces at the bottom of the paster for the station agent at the initial point to fill in the form and number of the passage ticket, where from, where to, and route to destination of such ticket.

RULE 8.—It is intended that no dead body shall be moved which may be the means of spreading disease ; therefore, all *disinterred* bodies, dead from any disease or cause, will be treated as infectious and dangerous to public health, and must not be accepted for transportation unless said removal has been approved by the State or Local Board of Health, and the consent of the health authority of the locality to which the corpse is consigned has first been obtained ; and the disinterred remains have been enclosed in a hermetically sealed (soldered) zinc, tin, or copper-lined coffin or box, or a box encased in a hermetically sealed (soldered) zinc, tin, or copper case.

FORM OF PASTER.

CERTIFICATE OF UNDERTAKER.

.... Date, ... 18....

Name of deceased ....

Place of death, ...

Cause of death, ...

For interment at..

Name of person in charge..

Number of transit permit..

Signed............................... Undertaker.

.... P. O. Address.

The above to be filled out by undertaker and attached to box containing corpse.

From.................. to.................. State...................

Number of ticket,... .... Form No. of ticket,..............

From........................ To ....

Via.......................... R. R......................... Junction

Via.......................... R. R......................... Junction

Via.......................... R. R......................... Junction

Via.......................... R. R......................... Junction

Signed,.......................... Station Agent.

The above to be filled out by Agent or Baggageman at the initial point, showing description of ticket, exact route, and via what junction points the ticket reads which is held by passenger in charge of corpse.

(INSTRUCTIONS TO PRINTER.—This paster to be printed on stout yellow paper. Size, 7¼ x7¼ inches.)

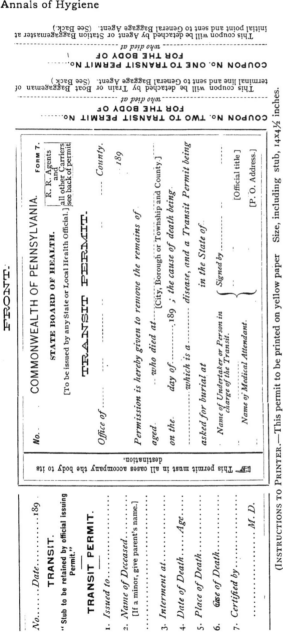

FRONT.

This coupon will be detached by Agent or Station Baggagemaster at initial point and sent to General Baggage Agent. (See Back.)

.... who died at ....

COUPON No. ONE TO TRANSIT PERMIT No. ....
FOR THE BODY OF ....

This coupon will be detached by Train or Boat Baggageman of terminal line and sent to General Baggage Agent. (See Back.)

.... who died at ....

COUPON No. TWO TO TRANSIT PERMIT No. ....
FOR THE BODY OF ....

No. .... COMMONWEALTH OF PENNSYLVANIA. FORM 7.

STATE BOARD OF HEALTH.

[To be issued by any State or Local Health Official.]

R. R. Agents and all other Carriers see back of permit

TRANSIT PERMIT.

Office of .... County.

.........189

Permission is hereby given to remove the remains of ....

aged .... who died at .... [City, Borough or Township and County.]

on the .... day of .... 189 ; the cause of death being ....

.... which is a .... disease, and a Transit Permit being

asked for burial at .... in the State of ....

Name of Undertaker or Person in charge of the Transit. } Signed by ....

Name of Medical Attendant. .... [Official title]

.... [P. O. Address.]

☞ This permit must in all cases accompany the body to its destination.

No. .... Date 189

TRANSIT.

" Stub to be retained by official issuing Permit."

TRANSIT PERMIT.

1. Issued to ....

2. Name of Deceased ....
[If a minor, give parent's name.]
....

3. Interment at ....

4. Date of Death ..... Age ....

5. Place of Death ....

6. Cause of Death ....

7. Certified by .... M. D.
....

(INSTRUCTIONS TO PRINTER.—This permit to be printed on yellow paper Size, including stub, 14x4½ inches.

FIRST COUPON. } *Taken at*...........................

By ....

SECOND COUPON. } *Taken at*...........................

By ....

Undertaker's Affidavit—In case of Infectious or Contagious disease.

BACK.

State of Pennsylvania,.....................189

I Hereby Certify, That the body of.................*named in this transit permit has been prepared by me for transportation by being*......................

....

(*Signed*)....................*Undertaker.*

State of....................

County of....................} *On this*........*day of*........*A. D.* 189 *before me, a*........(*Notary Public, Justice of the Peace*) *in and for the County and State aforesaid, personally appeared*........*to me known, and made oath and says that all of the statements contained in the foregoing are true.*

Sworn and subscribed to before me this........*day of*........*A. D.* 189

....

[SEAL]

It is expected that Local Boards of Health and Borough Councils will have blanks printed in conformity with these models. Until this has been done, however, the State Board will furnish copies to any undertaker on application to

BENJAMIN LEE, M. D., *Secretary*,

1532 Pine Street, Philadelphia.

Sixth Annual Report of the Secretary of the State Board of Health of Pennsylvania.*

PROF. GEORGE G. GROFF, M. D., LL. D.,
> *President of the State Board of Health and Vital Statistics of the Commonwealth of Pennsylvania.*

SIR:—During the year which has elapsed since your Secretary, in obedience to Article V, of the By-Laws, made "full report of his official acts," the Board has been steadily prosecuting its important work of educating the public mind in the elementary principles of sanitary reform, and, at the same time, rendering aid to citizens in all parts of the State in their efforts to cope with individual outbreaks of communicable and preventable diseases.

Three regular and three special meetings have been held. The former took place on November 13th, 1889, May 8th, 1890, and July 10th, 1890 ; and the latter on February 22d, May 28th, and August 30th, 1890.

There has been no change in the composition of the Board. Prof. George G. Groff, who, on the withdrawal of Dr. David Engelman from the Board, had been called to fill the vacancy in the presidency *pro tempore*, was, at the regular meeting in July, elected President. It is with pride and gratification that the Secretary is able to testify that the cordial relations which have existed between himself and the other members of the Board since its formation continue unimpaired, and that the readiness of each member to co-operate with him in the practical work of the Board, often at the expense of serious loss of time and personal inconvenience, have contributed greatly to its usefulness. He believes that it will not be deemed invidious if he calls attention in this connection to the valuable services rendered by the President and by the Chairman of the Committee on Water Supply, Sewerage, Drainage, Topography, and Mines, in making special inspections. The Chairman of the Committee on Public Institutions and School Hygiene, who went abroad the previous year with credentials from the Board to health authorities in Europe, was cordially received by them, and was afforded opportunities for inspecting sanitary works of various kinds. On his return he presented an interesting report of an inspection of the system of water purification in use in the City of Antwerp.

DECLARATION OF ABATEMENT OF NUISANCE IN THE SUSQUEHANNA AND JUNIATA VALLEYS.

In accordance with the instructions of the Board, the Secretary, soon after the last annual meeting, addressed a communication to his Excellency, the Governor of the Commonwealth, stating officially that the conditions in the valleys of the West Branch of the Susquehanna, the Juniata, and the Susquehanna Rivers and their tributaries had so improved, that there was no longer any ground for State aid, and declaring the nuisance abated.

RESOLUTION OF REGRET AT DR. ENGELMAN'S WITHDRAWAL.

The following resolution, passed at the same meeting, was forwarded to Dr. Engelman :
"*Resolved*, That the State Board of Health of Pennsylvania desires to place on record its high appreciation of the value of the services rendered by the Hon. David Engelman,

---

* Presented to the Board at its meeting in Harrisburg, November 13th, 1890.

M. D., its late President, both as a member of the Board, and as its presiding officer for more than two years.

"Not only his sagacious counsel, but his urbane demeanor and agreeable companionship made his presence welcome at its deliberations. The Board trusts that the severance of his official connection, which it regards with sincere regret, will not lessen the interest of their late colleague in the progress of sanitary reform in the State, or deprive the Board of his valuable aid in its prosecution."

POLLUTION OF STREAMS.

The question which has given your Secretary the most uneasiness during the past year, and to which he has felt it necessary to call the attention of the Board on several occasions, is that of the pollution of streams by drainage and sewerage. With the rapidly increasing density of population which distinguishes this Commonwealth, the question of the disposal of sewage in rural districts and small towns becomes every year more serious.

The whole theory of the modern gospel of sanitation is founded on the belief that man is his brother's keeper ; and the whole theory of American freedom is based on the idea that the inherent rights of one man or community to the enjoyment of "life, liberty, and the pursuit of happiness," are to be so exercised that they shall interfere with the enjoyment of the same inalienable rights by no other man or community. It needs no argument to prove that the wholesale poisoning of a stream in a populous region does so interfere with the enjoyment of those rights by all who live on its banks, or through whose property it passes below the point of contamination. Hence, the pollution of streams has become one of the most urgent problems with which the sanitarian has to deal. In Great Britain it has led to the establishment of the "Rivers' Pollution Commission," which has now been in existence for many years, and has spent thousands of pounds in its investigations. It must be remembered that what are there called rivers, would by us often be called runs, brooks, or creeks. There are, it is true, few general statutes in this Commonwealth bearing on the subject ; but it must be borne in mind that, in the language of Judge Thayer, of Philadelphia, in the case of the Commonwealth vs. Soulas, et al., November 25th, 1884, "it is a very old and well-settled law, that to pollute a public stream is to maintain a common nuisance. It is not only a public injury, but it is a crime, a crime for which those who perpetrate it are answerable in a tribunal of criminal jurisdiction."

The length of time during which such material has been deposited in any one locality, so far from constituting an excuse, only adds to the gravity of the question. The longer the pollution of the soil or of the banks and bed of a water course has been going on, the more complete will be their saturation with organic filth, and the greater the danger. "No length of time (says Judge Thayer in the opinion above alluded to) can justify a public nuisance. . . . Public rights are not destroyed by private encroachments, no matter how long they have endured. Nor is it any defense that the river is also polluted from other sources. . . . No man can excuse himself for violating the law upon the ground that others violate it. . . . It is no defense to say that the premises are in the same condition, and the drainage conducted in the same manner as when the defendants obtained possession and began their occupancy. The law is perfectly well settled that no man can prescribe for a public nuisance, or defend himself by showing that others have violated the law before him."

The decision given eo die (that is, without taking much time to advise or consult, showing that the case was a perfectly clear one to the court) in the case of Albertson vs. The City of Philadelphia et al., in the Court of Common Pleas, July 15th, 1882, established a precedent which no judge will be likely to set aside. In this instance the City of Philadelphia and William Baldwin, Commissioner of Highways, had contracted to build (under alleged authority of an ordinance of March 7th, 1882), and were building a sewer, which was intended to drain into a small stream running through Albertson's lot, and finally emptying into the Schuylkill River. Previously to this time, only pure water had passed through the stream.

The proposed sewer would discharge into it fecal and other filthy material from many dwelling houses, the stables of a railroad company, a hospital and an institution of learning. The city was enjoined from using or permitting the said sewer to be used for any purpose other than surface drainage.

It is evident that, if a city which possesses the right of eminent domain and is, by the terms of its charter, especially authorized to construct sewers, can be enjoined from discharging its filth into a small stream running through private property, so much the more can private individuals, hotels, schools, hospitals or jails.

This matter is forcing itself upon the attention of borough authorities, hotel proprietors, mill owners and other employers of large bodies of operators throughout the entire Commonwealth. Numerous plans have been suggested for rendering sewage inoffensive and innocuous. These include irrigation both on and under the surface, filtration, precipitation, oxidation and disinfection. One system will be better suited for one location, quite a different one for another.

Your Secretary feels that it is not the province of this Board to indicate, save in the most general way, what means should be adopted in any particular instance to attain the desired end. Competent and thoroughly educated sanitary engineers are now to be found in every large city, whose advice should be sought. It would be well, however, to submit any proposed plans to the Board before they are finally adopted.

Among the complaints of this nature which have reached the Board during the year, several have been due to the disposal of the sewage of public buildings. Recognizing the fact that all State establishments, such as asylums, hospitals, colleges and schools, and all county institutions, such as jails and almshouses, which derive a portion, if not all, of their support from the public funds, are generally looked upon as models by the communities in the midst of which they are placed, the Board felt it to be a matter of importance that such institutions should set the example to municipalities and private individuals of making proper provision for the purification of their sewage before it is permitted to enter any stream. Such establishments often contain within their walls a population twice as large as that of an ordinary village. But instead of disposing of their filth in small deposits over a large area, they are enabled by the modern appliances of plumbing to pour it in a concentrated form into the nearest stream. So far as the health of their own inmates is concerned this is often (not always, as recent investigations of this Board have shown) the best plan. But so far as the health of those who live farther down the streams, and of the domestic animals which pasture along their borders is concerned, it is the very worst plan, and one which civilized communities will not much longer tolerate.

In view of these facts the Board deemed it expedient to instruct the Secretary to prepare a circular, addressed to the trustees or other responsible heads of all such institutions throughout the State, representing the gravity of this growing evil, and earnestly urging that no time be lost in remedying any offensive or dangerous conditions found to exist in connection with the edifices over which they have control.

Such a circular has accordingly been prepared and issued, constituting Circular No. 30.

PURIFICATION OF SEWAGE.

Closely allied with this subject is that of the possibility of the purification of sewage.

In response to an admonition of the Board that the sewage and drainage of their building was a source of serious pollution to a stream, the proprietors of a large summer hotel have introduced, at a very considerable expense, an apparatus known as the Rimmer Oxidizer, with the laudable desire of abating the nuisance. On the invitation of the sanitary engineer of the hotel, the Board accompanied the Secretary in making a personal inspection of the working of this system. While it was evidently accomplishing something toward remedying the offensive character of the outflow, it was still of too recent construction to be able to judge fairly of its merits. The proprietors of, the hotel however, are deserving of commendation for the promptness with which they have responded to the notice of the Secretary, and their evident desire to spare no expense to free their establishment from the stigma of being a source of annoyance to their neighbors or of injury to the public health.

PURIFICATION OF DRINKING WATER.

So long as water continues to be used as a beverage, so long will the pollution of streams which are the natural and most reliable sources of drinking water for towns and cities render the subject of the purification of water supplies one of intense interest to the sanitarian.

Even supposing the millennium to have arrived, when proper laws for the prevention of the contamination of public waters shall be enacted and strictly obeyed by a regenerated community, with consciences alive to the wickedness of filth, there will still be a certain amount of unavoidable pollution, which will make it advisable to purify a water before drinking it. Allusion has already been made to the report of a member of the Board on a system which has been in successful use for four or five years for purifying the exclusively filthy water with which the citizens of Antwerp are supplied. This is known as the Anderson System. It consists briefly in passing the water through a shower of small pieces of metallic iron and then through a filter. On the invitation of the agent for the company in this country, the Board, together with the Boards of Health and of Trade of Philadelphia, made a visit of inspection to Lardner's Point on the Delaware, where a plant had been erected for purposes of demonstration, in order to satisfy themselves as to its efficiency. While not in any sense endorsing it, the Secretary feels justified in saying that the members were favorably impressed with what they could see of its working in their limited time of observation.

PHILADELPHIA THE ONLY CITY WHOSE WATER SUPPLY IS PROTECTED BY LEGISLATIVE ENACTMENT.

Before leaving this subject, it is the duty of the Secretary to call attention to the singular fact that the water supply of the city of Philadelphia is the only one in the entire State, so far as he has been able to discover by a diligent examination of the statutes, which the Legislature has thought it worth while to protect.

Why the life of a Philadelphian is of so much more value than that of a citizen of Reading or Pottsville, or any other town in the State, in the eyes of our legislators it is difficult to understand.

In a judicious spirit of compromise, however, while extending the ægis of their protection over the milk supply of all smaller cities, they turn a deaf ear to the repeated importunities of the health authorities of the great city, to aid them in checking the slaughter of the innocents within her borders, by causing the provisions of this salutary enactment to apply also to cities of the first class. This subject might properly be referred to the consideration of the Committee on Sanitary Legislation.

Very valuable contributions to the question of the purity of water supplies will be found in the appendices to the Reports of the Board for the year 1889 and the present year; in the Reports of the State Sanitary Conventions held at Pittsburgh and Norristown. Among them may be mentioned one by Col. Thomas T. Roberts, Chief Engineer of the Monongahela Navigation Company, on the "Future of our Rivers as Sources of Water Supply," and one by Dr. C. W. Chandler, Secretary of the State Board of Health of Maryland, on "The Purification of Water Supplies." The State Board of Health of Massachusetts, with the aid of a liberal appropriation from the legislature, is engaged upon a series of elaborate and comprehensive experiments on the purifaction of sewage and of potable waters which will undoubtedly produce very valuable practical results. One of the facts at which the committee appears to have arrived may be stated for the benefit of those whose faith in the benefits of filtration has been shaken by the statements of amateur microscopists. It is this: That the presence of a certain quantity or number of harmless, or, as they may even be termed, benevolent, bacteria in a filter-bed, so far from rendering a water injurious to the health, positively adds to its purity.

EPIDEMICS.

The only wide-spread epidemic which has visited the State has been that of influenza, which, in itself, will render the year a memorable one. Reaching our shores from Europe about December 10th, the first cases were reported in the city of Philadelphia on the 20th of that month. The disease began to appear as a factor in the mortality tables of the city on the fourth day of January, when one death is recorded from the disease. An increase in the number of deaths from inflammation of the lungs, however, from thirty-three in the week previous to seventy-one in the first week in January, sufficiently indicates that the epidemic had become fairly seated. It spread with a rapidity which is scarcely conceivable, and gained in intensity as the numbers of its victims increased. By the 23d of December it was estimated that there were 2000 cases in the city. On the 9th of January 6000 of the pupils of the public schools were reported as prostrated with the disease. The number of deaths increased the first week in January from 404, in the week previous, to 492. In two weeks it reached the startling figure of 770, more than twice as great as the mortality of the corres‑ponding week of the year of 1889. The over-worked physicians were prostrated both by fatigue and by the disease itself, and many succumbed finally.

Business was now almost at a standstill. In several instances places of business or manufacture were compelled to close for want of hands. Whole families were confined to the bed at once, so that neighbors were obliged to provide them with food and nursing care. This week, ending January 18th, marked the high tide of pestilence so far as mortality was concerned, the city death rate having fallen to its normal by the end of February. In the meantime the epidemic influence had spread like wild-fire, literally "on the wings of the wind" throughout the entire State. On the 27th of December the disease was rife in Lancaster, and genuine cases had appeared in Pittsburg on the extreme western border and Wilkes-Barre on the northern border of the State.

It is probable that not a single individual entirely escaped its pernicious effects. Its manifestations were so various, affecting in one the bronchial tubes, in another the nervous system, now the brain and now the bowels, here peritonitis and there pneumonia, that it was a long time, comparatively, before physicians even recognized it in its protean forms. It is scarcely conceivable that a disease which spreads with such astonishing rapidity, goes through the process of re-development in each person infected and is only communicated from person to person by infected articles. And yet this theory has been maintained by a few authorities who claim that it is always more prevalent along lines of travel and that it did not progress more rapidly than modern means of communication would enable it to do.

Whatever theory we may adopt of its means of propagation, it was felt by your Sec. retary that an affection so fatal in its results and so widespread in its domain, possessed an importance which entitled it to especial study. He therefore prepared the following circular, cyclostyle copies of which, to the number of 7000, were distributed to the members of the medical profession throughout the State :

Dear Doctor :—

I am desirous to obtain reliable statistics in regard to the recent pan-demic of influenza as observed in this State ; will you, therefore, kindly furnish the information called for below, by filling up the blanks from the data in your visiting list or note book and returning the sheet to me as early as practicable ? Yours very respectfully,

(Signed) BENJAMIN LEE, M. D.,
Superintendent of Vital Statistics.

Residence.................................County....................................
Date of first case..
Number of cases.....................Adults...................Children...................
Predominant type (nervous)...
(Catarrhal) ....
(Inflammatory)...

Number of deaths (directly caused)..

(indirectly caused)..

Immediate cause of death :

Bronchitis.....................Adults....................Children....................

Pneumonia...................... " .... " ....

Phthisis........................ " .... " ....

Nervous affections................ " .... " ....

Up to the first of May 4500 of these letters had been sent out.

The following is an analysis of the results obtained at that date :

Number of physicians reporting..................................... 265

Number of cases... 37,275

Adults 26,302

Children 10,973

Number of cases, nervous.. 6,913

"   "   catarrhal... 16,434

"   "   inflammatory..................................... 5,829

Number of deaths directly caused..................................... 56

"   "   indirectly caused 205

Immediate cause of death, bronchitis... 8

"   "   "   pneumonia............................... 217

"   "   "   phthisis................................. 42

"   "   "   nervous................................. 21

Supposing, which there is no reason to doubt, that the 265 physicians who replied represent a fair average of the practitioners of the State, this would give us 88,416 persons as having been sufficiently ill with this disease to demand medical aid. We know that there were many who suffered mild attacks who never sought advice, and many more whom physicians, in their excessive haste, never entered on their visiting lists, although they may have prescribed for them.   •

The Board has aided the local authorities in their attempts to suppress local epidemics of typhoid fever in fourteen instances, and of diphtheria in twelve instances.

TYPHOID FEVER.

Those of typhoid fever could, in every instance, be traced directly to the use of polluted water, generally from wells. In that of Lock Haven a connection seemed to be traceable between the floods of the previous summer as affecting the reservoir and the supply pipes and the existence of the disease.

DIPHTHERIA.

Diphtheria has invariably been found in the midst of conditions of the greatest filth' and has been distinctly propagated by gross disregard of sanitary regulations, and especially in the matter of public funerals.

PUBLIC FUNERALS IN CONTAGIOUS DISEASES.

So strongly has this last fact impressed the Board, that the Secretary was authorized to issue two circulars, one addressed to the clerical profession throughout the State, earnestly requesting its members to discourage the practice of holding public or church funerals in the case of persons who have died of contagious or infectious diseases, more particularly of diphtheria, scarlet fever, and measles ; and another to undertakers and funeral directors, warning them of this danger, and also urging the adoption by them of certain precautions in the preparation of such bodies for burial, the conduct of the funeral, and subsequent disinfection of vehicles and apartments.

The former of these has been printed and already widely circulated. The latter has been prepared, and is now submitted to the Board for its consideration, as it involves points of considerable importance. (See page 629.)

The epidemic of diphtheria in Delaware County is so widespread and persistent, and the conditions so unusually detrimental to health, that the Secretary has deemed it necessary to issue the following proclamation in the name of the Board :

COMMONWEALTH OF PENNSYLVANIA, STATE BOARD OF HEALTH.

EXECUTIVE OFFICE, 1532 Pine Street,

PHILADELPHIA, *November 4th, 1890,*

PROCLAMATION.

In consequence of an inspection, made on the twenty-seventh day of October, 1890, by the Medical Inspector of the Delaware District, the State Board of Health hereby declares diphtheria to be epidemic in the township of Middletown, Delaware County, including the villages of Glen Riddle, Lima, Parkmount, and Lenni ; and in the township of Ashton, Delaware County, including the villages of Crozerville, Rockdale, and Village Green.

In the absence of any local health authorities in these townships, the Board establishes the following

REGULATIONS.

First.—There shall be no public or church funeral of any person who has died of diphtheria, or of any person who has died of any other disease in a house in which diphtheria was present at the time of such death.

Second.—The body of any person who has died of diphtheria shall not be exposed to view. Such body shall be immediately after death wrapped in a sheet which has been soaked in a solution of corrosive sublimate, in the proportion of two drachms to the gallon of water, and privately buried within twenty-four hours.

Third.—No person shall unnecessarily visit any house in which diphtheria is known to exist, or has existed within a period of six weeks.

Fourth.—No member of a family in whose house diphtheria exists should attend school, Sunday-school, church, theatre, or any other public assembly.

Fifth.—Every school, among members of which there have been cases of diphtheria, should be closed ; and no child should be received into a non-infected school who has been attending one, among the pupils of which the infection is known to have existed.

Sixth.—No person recently recovered from an attack of diphtheria, or in whose family diphtheria exists, shall go to work in any factory or mill in which their work requires them to be in close contact with their fellow workmen in confined rooms, without a certificate from their attending physician stating that in his opinion they run no risk of conveying the contagion.

Seventh.—The period during which a person who has had diphtheria is in danger of conveying the contagion is from four to six weeks.

Eighth.—All rooms and houses in which diphtheria has occurred, and all clothing, bed clothing, and articles of furniture which have been exposed to infection should be disinfected in accordance with the subjoined instructions.

Ninth.—No dead animal, garbage, or filth of any kind shall be thrown into any stream, race, dam, pond, or other water, or upon any public road or place. All such material should be either burned or buried.

Tenth.—All cellars should be thoroughly cleaned and whitewashed, and all house yards and privies disinfected with copperas, and kept clean.

NOTE.—The State Board of Health has "power and authority to order the cause of any special disease or mortality to be abated and removed." Any person who shall fail to obey or shall violate such order becomes liable to a fine of $100 for each such act of neglect or violation.

The circulars of the Board (No. 19, Precautions against Diphtheria, and No. 29, on The Dangers Arising from Public Funerals, of those who have died from contagious and infectious diseases), can be obtained of the minister of the Calvary Church at Lenni, of Dr. Morton P. Dickinson, of Glen Riddle, or by addressing Benjamin Lee, M. D., Secretary of the State Board of Health, 1532 Pine Street, Philadelphia.

To this proclamation were appended careful instructions, taken from the circulars of the Board, as to disinfectants and the mode of using them.

SMALLPOX.

Smallpox has appeared only in three places, namely, Pittsburg, Canonsburg, Washington Co., and Glen Lyon, Luzerne Co., and by the prompt action of the State or local authorities has, in each instance, been at once crushed out.

LEPROSY.

Leprosy has occurred in two cities, Philadelphia and Chester. Both cases were promptly isolated by the local health boards, and are under strict surveillance. The Secretary has addressed a communication to the Surgeon-General of the United States Marine Hospital Service, suggesting that in accordance with the new regulations of that service, inasmuch as the patient is not a naturalized citizen of the United States, he is extradited to his native country, Sweden, where he could be comfortably cared for, in a leper colony, where he could enjoy the society of his fellows, instead of enduring the torture of solitary confinement.

In view of the rapid spread of this disease both in the East and West Indies during the last decade, it will undoubtedly become necessary, at no distant period, either for the United States to found leper colonies, or for each large city to establish its leper house. The former plan is evidently the more practical and rational. At the National Conference of State Boards of Health which met in Nashville in the month of May, your Secretary suggested that the United States should, either by purchase or cession, obtain possession of three tracts of land, one in the northwest, one in Louisiana, and one in California, already to some extent occupied by lepers, and establish thereon as many colonies, to the nearest of which every leper discovered should be removed, and on which he should be detained with every provision for his comfort until death should come to his relief. At the meeting of the American Public Health Association in the City of Brooklyn in October, 1889, which your Secretary and Dr. Edwards attended as delegates, the former presented a resolution at the close of a paper, detailing the results of his observation of leprosy in the island of Cuba, which read as follows :

"*Resolved*, That this Association, recognizing the admirable precautions taken by the United States Marine Hospital Service and by the State Board of Health of Florida to prevent the introduction of yellow fever in this country, respectfully request Supervising Surgeon-General Hamilton, of the United States Marine Hospital Service, the Honorable the State Board of Health of Florida, and all quarantine commissioners of ports having intercourse with Cuban ports, to exercise the same vigilance with regard to leprosy that is already observed in the case of yellow fever during what is known as the quarantine season.

"*Resolved*, That the Secretary be instructed to transmit copies of the above resolution to the several officials therein indicated."

The resolution was adopted and forwarded as directed. In compliance with this request, the following circular was issued by the Treasury Department of the United States :

CIRCULAR.

REGULATION TO PREVENT THE INTRODUCTION OF LEPROSY.
1889.
Department No. 130.

TREASURY DEPARTMENT.

OFFICES SUPERVISING SURGEON-GENERAL, MARINE HOSPITAL SERVICE, }
WASHINGTON, D. C., December 23d, 1889. }

To Medical Officers of the Marine Hospital Service, Collectors of Customs, and others Concerned:

The National quarantine act, approved April 29th, 1878, entitled, "An act to prevent the introduction of contagious or infectious diseases," provides that no vessel or vehicle coming from any foreign port or country where any contagious or infectious disease exists, or any vessel or vehicle conveying persons or animals affected with any contagious disease, shall enter any port of the United States, or cross the boundary line between the United States and any foreign country, except in such manner as may be prescribed.

Attention is now directed to the increased prevalence of the contagious disease known as leprosy in several foreign countries, and the danger of its increase in the United States, through the immigration of persons affected with leprosy, and by direction of the Secretary of the Treasury, the following regulation is framed under authority of the foregoing act, subject to the approval of the President, to protect the people of the United States from the introduction of leprosy :

1. Until further orders, no vessel shall be permitted to entry by any officer of the customs until the master, owner or authorized agent of the vessel shall produce a certificate from the health officer or quarantine officer at the port of entry, or nearest quarantine United States officer, that no person affected with leprosy was on board the said vessel when admitted to free pratique, or in case a leper was found on board such vessel, that he or she with his baggage has been removed from the vessel and detained at the quarantine station.

2. Medical officers in command of United States quarantines are hereby instructed to detain any person affected with leprosy found on board any vessel, but such officer will permit the departure on outgoing vessels of persons detained at quarantine in pursuance of this regulation, provided such vessel shall be bound to the foreign country from which the said leper shall have last sailed.

JOHN B. HAMILTON,
Supervising Surgeon-General Marine Hospital Service.

Approved :
WILLIAM WINDOM, *Secretary.*
Approved :
BENJ. HARRISON.

The anxiety which is felt upon this subject in California, which is in intimate communication with leprosy-breeding centres, is sufficiently indicated by the following resolution, adopted by the State Board of Health of that State, which was forwarded to the Secretary in the early part of this year :

DEAR SIR : At a regular meeting of the State Board of Health of the State of California, held January 11th, 1890, it was

" *Resolved*, That the California State Board of Health recommend that the Congress of the United States do enact a statute,

" First, That no person affected with leprosy should be permitted to enter the United States.

" Second, That every person immigrating to the United States from any place where leprosy prevails shall procure a certificate from a competent physician, properly attested by some United States consul or health officer, certifying that he or she is not affected with leprosy, is not a descendant from a leprous family, and has no relations in the co-lateral line who are lepers.

" Third, That every immigrant coming to the United States who has sojourned or resided where leprosy prevails shall be reported to the Board of Health of the State of his destination, so that he may, during his residence in the United States, be inspected not less than twice a year by some competent physician or person appointed by the health authorities of the place wherein he resides for a period of ten years.

" That the penalty for the violation of the first two sections of this statute shall be the immediate return of such person to the place from whence he or she came.

"*Resolved*, That the California Representatives in Congress be and they are hereby earnestly requested to vote for the enactment of such a statute, and that the Secretary of this board be instructed to furnish said Congressmen a copy of these resolutions, duly signed by the President and attested by the Secretary.

" HENRY S. ORME, M.D., *President*.

' G. G. TYRRELL, M.D., *Secretary*,"

CHOLERA ON THE MEDITERRANEAN—AND SPANISH RAGS.

At the regular meeting of the board in July the Secretary reported as follows in reference to the prospects of the arrival of cholera from Spain :

The appearance of Asiatic cholera almost simultaneously at six different points in Spain, covering a distance of 250 miles in a straight line and probably 400 by rail, indicates a very considerable survival of germs of that disease from last Summer along the shores of the Mediterranean. Their wide dissemination and early maturity make a grave epidemic in that region, and it may be in Southern Europe generally, probable. We in this country have little to fear, however. Our quarantine stations, National, State and municipal, were never before so well equipped. That of the port of New York, which is our most vulnerable point, is fully twice as well prepared as it was when it so successfully checked the invasion of the disease at the threshold three years ago. Philadelphia, the next most likely point of attack, has a double line of intrenchments, the Lazaretto, or Municipal Quarantine Station, twelve miles down the Delaware River, and the United States Quarantine Station, eighty miles below, at Cape Henlopen. The latter is provided with a fumigating steamer, just finished, which is capable of disinfecting the largest vessel in a few hours.

The Baltimore Station is well equipped and under intelligent management, and suspected vessels at that port, as well as for Norfolk, are also detained at Cape Charles by the United States Marine Hospital Service. The efficiency of the New Orleans quarantine has been frequently demonstrated. Its plant is the most complete and the most scientifically constructed of any in the country. Should the disease pass these barriers, however, its mode of propagation is now so thoroughly understood that it will be a reproach to local health authorities if it is not at once stamped out.

It is their duty immediately to put their cities and towns into such a condition of cleanliness that the germs will find no congenial soil. The Secretary has in preparation a new circular on this subject, which will shortly be issued.

Since making the above report, the disease has extended somewhat, and still exists in Valencia and neighboring provinces. The conservative " Local Government Board of Great Britain " has considered the condition of sufficient gravity to lead it to modify its somewhat lax regulations in regard to quarantine—an order to that effect having been issued August 30th.

This was followed up on the 4th of September by the issue of regulations forbidding the importation of rags from Spain until the 31st day of December, 1890. The period of danger from this source in our own country is not until an epidemic abroad has existed for many months. It may be said to be just now beginning. The Secretary, therefore, suggests the passage of a resolution calling upon the Board of Health of the City of Philadelphia to prohibit the importation of rags from any Spanish port, or of rags which there is reason to suppose have been gathered in Spain, from the 1st day of December, 1890, to the 1st day of December, 1891. The Secretary has already had a personal conference with the health officer of Philadelphia upon the subject, calling his attention to the action of the English authorities.

NOTIFICATION OF TYPHUS FEVER IN THE PORT OF NEW YORK.

On the 6th of January the following letter was received from the Secretary of the New York State Board of Health :

STATE BOARD OF HEALTH OF NEW YORK,
ALBANY, *January 6th, 1890.*

SIR : Six cases of typhus fever occurring among immigrants who arrived in New York the 5th of November last in the steamship "Westernland," are reported from New York city. I send you a list of the steerage passengers of the "Westernland," who have scattered in various directions. The places to which they were booked could not be obtained. In case of typhus fever breaking out in your jurisdiction, it was thought the list might be an aid. .Very respectfully,

Your obedient servant,
LEWIS BALCH,
Secretary.

To BENJAMIN F. LEE, *Secretary State Board of Health of Pennsylvania.*

The list referred to contained 284 names. Copies of the same were made and sent to the boards of health of all the large cities in the State, with the request that all newly-arrived immigrants be closely watched for indications of the disease.

PROPOSED WATER SUPPLIES OF TOWNS.

In compliance with the instructions of the Board, a communication has been addressed to the authorities of the Borough of Muncy, advising them to be cautious about accepting a new water supply, which a member of the Board had found, upon personal inspection, to have its sources in an agricultural water-shed, and to be in danger of serious pollution.

At the request of prominent citizens of Berwick, Columbia County, an inspection was made by Dr. Leiser, Medical Inspector of the Northumberland District, of a proposed new source of water supply. The report showed certain objectionable features, which, however, might be removed by proper precautions. A copy of the report was forwarded to the petitioners.

OLD CANAL·BEDS.

Frequent complaints reach the board of nuisances created in small towns by collections of stagnant water in the beds of old canals, which have fallen into a "desuetude" the reverse of "innocuous." This is especially true of the old State Canal and of portions of the Schuylkill Navigation Company's canal. The right of the State to leave such a source of disease unremedied may well be questioned. Some general system of drainage should be adopted which would either dry up these malaria-breeding ditches or keep streams of clean water running through them.

DOES THE HABIT OF TOBACCO SMOKING RETARD OR PREVENT THE DEVELOPMENT OF PULMONARY CONSUMPTION?

At the request of the board, the following circular has been widely distributed among physicians :

STATE BOARD OF HEALTH OF PENNSYLVANIA,
EXECUTIVE OFFICE, 1532 Pine St.,
PHILADELPHIA, *March 10th, 1890.*

DEAR DOCTOR: The State Board of Health is desirous of obtaining authentic information as regards the effect of tobacco smoking, either in promoting or retarding the development of pulmonary tuberculosis or consumption. It has been stated that inveterate smokers are, to a great extent, exempt from the disease. If this is true, the fact ought to be made widely known. If it has no foundation, it ought to be authoritatively contradicted. The board has, therefore, instructed me to address you this communication, asking if you will kindly forward, at as early a date as convenient, the results of your own observation and experience in regard to this subject.   Yours very truly,

(Signed)   BENJAMIN LEE,
Secretary.

The entire indifference with which this circular was received may safely be regarded as an indication that such a theory has no hold upon the minds of the profession in general. Only about two hundred replies were received. Of those fifty-six were affirmative of the belief that inveterate tobacco smoking does sometimes act as a preventive. One hundred and nine scouted the idea, and thirty-five were non-committal. On the face of the returns, therefore, the "nays have it." The decision is, however, stronger than the mere numerical showing, as many of those who considered tobacco smoke a prophylactic, acknowledged a strong personal bias in favor of the habit; and there was also much more positiveness in the tone of those who believed in its efficacy. So far, therefore, as the investigation has had a value, it has tended to prove that there is no real scientific foundation for the theory.

THE CONEMAUGH DISTRICT.

A new inspection district has been formed comprising the counties of Cambria, Westmoreland, Indiana and Armstrong. These counties previously formed a portion of the Central and the Western Slope Districts, which were both very large and in parts difficult ot access. Dr. W. E. Matthews, of Johnstown, who so faithfully and acceptably discharged the duties of Chief Deputy Medical Inspector, in charge of the Sanitary Corps of the State Board of Health at Johnstown, during the operations for the renovation of the site of that ruined city, has been appointed medical inspector to the new district.

SPECIAL INSPECTOR ON THE PENNSYLVANIA RAILROAD.

At the request of the Pennsylvania Railroad Company, Dr. R. C. Town, a company surgeon, has been appointed special inspector to the Board, with authority to burn bundles of clothing, rags, etc., suspected of danger of conveying infection, left upon the premises or in the stations of the company, reporting such action to the Board.

SANITARY CONVENTIONS AND CONFERENCES.

The Secretary has attended as delegate from this Board the following meetings, viz.: those of the Tri-Sanitary Convention at Wheeling, West Virginia; of the National Conference of State Boards of Health of Nashville, Tenn., and of the Section on State Medicine of the American Medical Association.

TRI-SANITARY CONVENTION.

On the 28th day of February the Secretary represented the Board at the meetings of the Tri-State Sanitary Convention at Wheeling, West Virginia, occupying the chair in the absence of the President, Dr. Harvey Reed, who was detained at home by illness. The special object of this convention was to consider the problems presented to sanitarians by devastating floods. Many interesting papers were presented, several of them founded on the experience of the writers in the Johnstown disaster. The progress of the convention and papers read as published in the ANNALS OF HYGIENE are herewith submitted.   •

NATIONAL CONFERENCE OF STATE BOARDS OF HEALTH.

This body is composed entirely of executive officers of Boards of Health of States and provinces in the United States and the Dominion of Canada. It possesses, therefore, an official character which gives its deliberations great importance and its action an executive weight. Sanitary regulations thus become to a considerable extent uniform throughout the continent, and the different boards aid one another in their enforcement. As chairman of a committee, your representative read a report on the subject of the "Spread of Leprosy in its Relation to the United States;" showing that during the past ten years this loathsome disease has been making rapid progress and that it behooves the sanitary authorities of the country to be on the alert to prevent its gaining a foothold here. The following resolution offered by him was passed :

Resolved, That it is the sense of this Conference that all State and Local Boards of Health should keep all cases of leprosy existing in their respective districts under surveillance, and should require physicians to report all cases of the disease which may come to their notice.

The following resolution offered by your Secretary was also passed :

Resolved, That this Conference respectfully urges upon the sub-committee on Forestry of the Committee on Public Domains of the Congress of the United States to pass such laws as shall check the reckless destruction of trees on public lands.

A full report of the proceedings of the Conference are herewith submitted.

SECTION ON STATE MEDICINE.

The section on State Medicine of the American Medical Association was presided over by Supervising-Surgeon General Hamilton, of the U. S. Marine Hospital Service. This officer has charge of the entire quarantine establishment of the country, and his selection as presiding officer was therefore a very fitting one.

One of the most interesting papers read before this Section was by Dr. Henry B. Baker, Secretary of the State Board of Health of Michigan, on the "History and Causation of the Influenza Epidemic."

It is a significant fact that the President of the Association chose for his theme, not some practical subject connected with medicine or surgery, but "The Relation of Hygiene to the Government." In this connection the attention of the Board is called to the following important

CIRCULAR.

INTER-STATE QUARANTINE ACT.

1890.
Department No. 18.

TREASURY DEPARTMENT.

OFFICE OF THE SUPERVISING SURGEON-GENERAL,
U. S. MARINE HOSPITAL SERVICE,
WASHINGTON, D. C., *March 29th, 1890.*

To Medical Officers, Marine Hospital Service, Officers State Boards of Health, and others concerned :

The following Act of Congress, approved March 28th, 1890, is hereby published for the information of the persons to whom it is addressed.

JOHN B. HAMILTON,
Supervising Surgeon-General.

Approved :
WILLIAM WINDOM,
Secretary.

AN ACT to prevent the introduction of contagious diseases from one State to another, and for the punishment of certain offenses.

Be it enacted by the Senate and House of Representatives of the United States of America in Congress Assembled, That whenever it shall be made to appear to the satisfaction of the President that cholera, yellow fever, smallpox, or plague exists in any State or Territory, or in the District of Columbia, and that there is danger of the spread of such disease into other States, Territories, or the District of Columbia, he is hereby authorized to cause the Secretary of the Treasury to promulgate such rules and regulations as in his judgment may be necessary to prevent the spread of such disease from one State or Territory into another, or from any State or Territory into the District of Columbia, or from the District of Columbia into any State or Territory, and to employ such inspectors and other persons as may be necessary to execute such regulations to prevent the spread of such disease. The said rules and regulations shall be prepared by the Supervising Surgeon-General of the Marine Hospital Service, under the direction of the Secretary of the Treasury. And any person who shall wilfully violate any rule or regulation so made and promulgated shall be deemed guilty of a misdemeanor, and upon conviction shall be punished by a fine of not more than five hundred dollars, or imprisonment for not more than two years, both at the discretion of the court.

SEC. 2. That any officer, or person acting as an officer or agent of the United States at any quarantine station, or other person employed to aid in preventing the spread of such disease, who shall wilfully violate any of the quarantine laws of the United States, or any of the rules and regulations made and promulgated by the Secretary of the Treasury as provided for in Section 1 of this act, or any lawful order of his superior officer or officers, shall be deemed guilty of a misdemeanor, and upon conviction, shall be punished by a fine of $300 or imprisonment for not more than one year, or both, in the discretion of the court.

SEC. 3. That when any common carrier or officer, agent, or employé of any common carrier shall wilfully violate any of the quarantine laws of the United States, or the rules and regulations made and promulgated as provided for in Section 1 of this act, such common carrier, officer, agent, or employé shall be deemed guilty of a misdemeanor, and shall, on conviction, be punished by a fine of not more than $500, or imprisonment for more than two years or both, in the discretion of the court.

Approved March 28th, 1890.

The Fourth State Sanitary Convention was held at Norristown, May 9th and 10th, and was presided over by the Hon. Thomas J. Stewart, Secretary of Internal Affairs, assisted by their honors, Judges Weand and Schwartz. The attendance was large, the speakers able, and the papers of great interest. The annual address was delivered by Mr. A. Arnold Clarke, of Lansing, Michigan, and was a lucid and forcible exposition of the germ theory of disease. The learned professions of Norristown all contributed representative men to the discussions. The proceedings will form a volume of no little value to the sanitarian.

REGISTER OF PHYSICIANS.

As Superintendent of Vital Statistics, the Secretary has issued the first official "Register of Physicians in Pennsylvania by Counties," a volume of 425 pages, giving the date of registration, full name, sex, place of birth, residence, medical degrees, institution and dates, other degrees, institutions and dates, place or places of continuous practice since 1871, of those having no diploma, and removals and deaths as nearly as can be ascertained, of every physician in the State. In the work of revision and proof reading of this immense list the Secretary has availed himself of the services of Prof. William B. Atkinson, Medical Director to the Board for the Delaware district, whose long familiarity with the profession throughout the State in the capacity of Secretary of the State Medical Society has peculiarly fitted him for the task.

The Secretary desires it to be understood that, in publishing this list of the practitioners of medicine and surgery, he does not in any way endorse the character of those whose names appear. He simply reports the fact that these persons have registered. There has been considerably laxity on the part of the registration officers. The law has not always been fully understood, and in some instances, even where it has, its requirements have been slighted.

There are many names recorded of persons holding diplomas from those infamous *bogus* faculties which disgraced Philadelphia some years since. In many instances the prothonotary had no choice but to admit these pretenders to registration, the charters of the colleges (so called) not having been revoked at the time the diplomas were purchased. In each instance, however, the name of the college from which the physician was graduated is given, or, in case he possesses no diploma, the length of time during which he has been in continuous practice at the time of the passage of the act of 1881. To this the Secretary has thought it well to add a list of the colleges from which the physicians of the State have received their credentials, noting each case in which there has been a taint of fraudulence· This will enable the public to be somewhat on their guard.

It will be noted that the number reported in the tables of comparison is less than that given in the general list. This is owing to the fact that these tables were prepared by the Secretary of Internal Affairs, whose report was published much in advance of our own, and that a considerable number of delinquents have since reported. Many corrections also require to be made for deaths and removals. The value of this register is therefore mainly that it formed a broad, and in the main, corrèct basis for future work which will result in the completion, at no distant date, of one which shall be complete and accurate. Any one who is in the habit of making deductions from tables, figures and statistics, knows how voluminous the manuscript of such work becomes, and how much easier these records are to manipulate when reduced to print.

In the following list it is to be understood that all colleges not annotated have an actual and legal existence so far as the Board has been able to ascertain.

NAMES OF COLLEGES AND NUMBER OF GRADUATES FROM EACH COLLEGE.

Jefferson Medical College of Philadelphia,	2,000
University of Pennsylvania,	1,945
Hahnemian Medical Colege of Philadelphia,	470
Woman's Medical College of Pennsylvania, Philadelphia,	140
Bellevue Hospital Medical Collège of New York,	203
Western Reserve Medical College of Ohio,	176
College of Physicians and Surgeons of Baltimore, Md.,	198
University of Michigan,	112
University of New York,	117
Pennsylvania Medical College (extinct),	122
Cincinnati Medical College (Medical College of Ohio),	101
University of Maryland,	101
Homœopathic Medical College of Philadelphia,	95
Medico-Chirurgical College of Philadelphia,	64
University of New York City,	69
Eclectic Medical College (became fraudulent, extinct),	91
Homœopathic Hospital College of Cleveland, Ohio,	65
American University of Pennsylvania, Philadelphia (fraudulent, extinct),	63
Cleveland Medical College (Western Reserve),	53
Philadelphia Medical College (extinct)	48
Medical College of Worcester, Mass.·(extinct),	44
University of Medicine and Surgery of Philadelphia (fraudulent, extinct),	59
College of Physicians and Surgeons of New York,	29
Baltimore Medical College,	49
Long Island College Hospital,	38
Eclectic Medical College of New York City,	49
University of Vermont,	25
Ohio Medical College,	38
University of Kentucky,	19
Berkshire Medical College of Massachusetts (extinct 1867),	13
College of Physicians and Surgeons of Maryland,	12
Royal College of Physicians and Surgeons, Canada,	16

Homœopathic Medical College of New York, ... 15
Homœopathic Medical College of Chicago, ... 17
Physico-Medical Institute, Cincinnati (extinct 1880), ... 14
Eclectic College of Medicine and Surgery of Ohio (Eclectic Medical Institute), ... 16
Dartmouth Medical College of Vermont, ... 11
Pulte Medical College of Cincinnati, Ohio, ... 17
Columbia, of District of Columbia, ... 12
Howard University of District of Columbia, ... 12
Starling Medical College of Ohio, ... 17
Albany Medical College, New York, ... 24
University of Buffalo, New York, ... 67
Miami Medical College of Ohio, ... 48
Castleton Medical College of Vermont (extinct 1854), ... 10
Rush Medical College, Illinois, ... 22
Geneva Medical College (Syracuse University, New York), ... 17
American Medical College of St. Louis (Eclectic), ... 15
Washington University of Baltimore (College of Physicians and Surgeons), ... 10
Queen's University of Ireland, ... 11
University of Heidelberg, Germany, ... 6
Royal College of Surgeons of England, ... 3
Medical Department University of Georgetown, D. C., ... 9
University of Nashville. 4
University of Geissen, Germany, ... 7
College of Physicians and Surgeons of Iowa, ... 7
College of Physicians and Surgeons of Missouri, ... 5
University of Georgia (Medical Department), ... 7
Willoughby University of Ohio, ... 7
Boston University (fraudulent, extinct), ... 4
Hygeo-Therapeutic College of New Jersey (extinct), ... 8
University of Hudson, ... 8
United States Medical College, New York (eclectic, illegal, extinct), ... 8
College of Medicine and Surgery of Baltimore, ... 9
Detroit Medical College, ... 8
Medical College of Columbus, Ohio, ... 6
National, D. C. (Medical Department of Columbian University). 4
Harvard Medical College, ... 7
College of Physicians and Surgeons of Chicago, ... 7
Medical Department of Yale College, Connecticut, ... 9
New York Medical College (merged into Bellevue Hospital Medical College), ... 7
Charity Hospital Medical College, Ohio, ... 6
Bowdoin Medical College, Maine, ... 6
University of Glasgow, Scotland, ... 8
Royal College of Medicine of Edinburgh, Scotland, ... 9
University of Wurtzburg, Germany, ... 9
University of Berlin, ... 7
University of Vienna 7
University of Jenna, Germany, ... 6
Woman's Medical College of Germany, ... 7
Albert Medical College of Canada, ... 4
University of Koenigsberg, Germany, ... 4
McGill University of Montreal, Canada, ... 4
Columbian Medical College of Michigan, ... 4
Columbia of New York (College of Physicians and Surgeons), ... 6

Homœopathic Medical School of Massachusetts (Boston University),	4
Metropolitan, of New York (extinct),	4
Homœopathic Medical College of Missouri,	4
Franklin Medical College,	3
Medical Department of Victoria College, Canada (extinct),	3
Bolomidico Generale, Nicaragua,	3
University of Keoskenell, Russia,	3
Evansville Medical College of Indiana (suspended),	3
University of Marburg,	2
University of Amsterdam,	2
Hoscomic Insular Longo,	2
Germania Medical College of Austria,	2
State University of Iowa,	2
Chicago Medical College,	2
University of Erlingen, Germany,	2
University of Padua, Italy,	2
University of Coburg, Canada,	2
University of Stuttgart, Germany,	2
University of Indiana (fraudulent, extinct),	4
Bennett College of Eclectic Medicine and Surgery, Illinois,	2
Virginia University,	2
Syracuse Eclectic Medical College of New York (extinct),,,	2
New York Ophthalmic Hospital,	2
College of Medicine and Surgery of Keokuk, Iowa,	2
Julio Hospital College,	2
Royal College of Physicians and Surgeons of Ontario, Canada,	2
Fairfield Medical College of New York (extinct, 1840),	1
Eclectic Medical College of Atlanta, Georgia,	1
Pacific Medical College,	1
University of Tennessee,	1
Eclectic of New Jersey,	1
University of Louisiana,	1
Medical College of South Carolina,	1
University of Gratz, Austria,	1
University of Breslau, Prussia,	1
University of Munich, Bavaria,	1
Ac. Maximilian,	1
University of Basel, Switzerland,	1
Medical College of Virginia,	1
Toledo Medical College,	1
New York Medical College for Women,	1
Reformed Medical College of New York (Eclectic, extinct),	1
Manchester Medical College, New Hampshire (fraudulent, extinct),	1
Savannah Medical College (extinct, 1880),	1
Indiana Medical College,	1
Academica Indovicenia,	1
University of Freyburg, Switzerland,	1
College of Augsburg,	1
University of Naples,	1
University of Herford, Prussia,	1
Institute of Midwifery,	6

Total, ... 7,315

NATIONALITY OF PHYSICIANS OF FOREIGN BIRTH IN PENNSYLVANIA.

The returns fail to show the place of birth of many of the Physicians. Of the 8,248 reported, 642 are of foreign birth. The following table gives the number of foreign born, and shows the number of each nationality :

Germany,	131	Saxony,	3
England,	153	Austria,	5
Ireland,	100	South America,	2
Canada,	58	Baden,	2
Scotland,	32	New Brunswick,	2
Prussia,	27	Bavaria,	2
Wales,	24	Mexico,	1
France,	19	Roumania,	1
Switzerland,	14	Turkey,	1
Nova Scotia,	7	Island of Malta,	1
Russia,	7	Isle of Man,	1
Cuba,	7	Brazil,	1
Sweden,	6	Prince Edward's Island,	1
West Indies,	4	Bermuda,	1
Italy,	5	Australia,	1
Poland,	4	Jerusalem,	1
Hungary,	4	Geneva,	1
Nicaragua,	3	Bohemia,	1
India,	3	Belgium,	1
Holland,	3	Iceland,	1
	611		31—642

It will be seen from this table that of the 642 foreign-born physicians, Great Britain is the birthplace of 152 and Germany of 131. The registration indicates that 7,316 are graduates of medical colleges, 2,009 being among the alumni of Jefferson Medical College, and 1,945 among the alumni of the University of Pennsylvania. The returns further show that there are 932 physicians without diplomas, who are now practicing under the provisions of the fifth section of the act of 1881, which allowed those who had been in constant practice for ten years to continue without certificates of graduation. Of 8,248 reported, 7,932 are males and 316 females. In the counties of Allegheny and Erie about nine per centum of the physicians are females.

DISTRIBUTION OF PHYSICIANS BY COUNTIES.

The following table shows (in each county) the number of persons to each physician, the number of male and female physicians, the number practicing without diplomas, the number who are foreign born and the total number registered :

	Number of persons to each physician in each county.	The number of male physicians.	The number of female physicians.	The number practicing without a diploma.	The number who are foreign born.	The total number registered.
Allegheny	677	431	44	100	135	525
Armstrong	554	35	1	5	5	86
Beaver	404·	97	1	20	6	98
Bedford	17,464	2	....	....	2	2
Berks	371	320	10	53	22	330
Blair	398	129	3	4	7	132
Bradford	321	175	7	43	1	182
Butler	530	98	1	14	2	99
Cameron	322	16	....	2	1	16
Centre	499	76	....	....	....	76
Chester	488	164	7	25	13	171
Clearfield	353	122	1	24	1	123
Columbia	459	71	1	1	1	72
Crawford	406	160	9	38	8	169
Cumberland	370	123	1	15	4	124
Dauphin	382	194	5	21	8	199
Delaware	637	84	4	3	7	88
Elk	1422	9	....	....	1	9
Erie	410	167	15	39	16	182
Fayette	467	125	1	24	6	126
Forest	208	20	1	3	1	21
Franklin	402	122	2	10	1	124
Huntingdon	506	67	....	7	2	67
Indiana	698	58	....	9	1	58
Jefferson	417	67	....	6	....	67
Juniata	623	29	....	....	....	29
Lackawanna	384	219	13	36	8	232
Lancaster	425	320	8	39	1	328
Lawrence	362	90	2	11	4	92
Lebanon	323	116	3	16	2	119
Lehigh	5497	12	....	1	....	12
Luzerne	375	349	5	57	44	354
Lycoming	479	116	4	6	2	120
Mercer	390	143	1	16	9	144
Mifflin	343	56	1	2	2	57
Monroe	448	44	1	7	4	45
Montgomery	548	170	6	4	4	176
Montour	515	30	....	1	1	30
Northampton	385	182	3	13	8	185
Northumberland	563	92	2	16	5	94
Perry	423	64	1	4	2	65
Philadelphia	405	1952	138	95	265	2090
Pike	878	11	....	....	2	11
Potter	1724	7	1	3	1	8
Schuylkill	797	163	3	22	....	166
Sullivan	323	24	1	8	3	25
Susquehanna	463	85	2	17	3	87
Union	318	52	1	1	2	53
Venango	580	77	....	13	1	77
Warren	325	82	2	6	....	86
Washington	401	138	....	27	6	138
Wayne	515	63	2	12	6	65
York	410	212	2	23	5	214

UNITED STATES FUMIGATING STEAMER.

An act of great importance on the part of the National Government, acting through the U. S. Marine Hospital Service, is the placing of a substantial boarding and fumigating steamer, "The Pasteur," at the quarantine station at the mouth of Delaware Bay. The Secretary took occasion to inspect this vessel on different occasions while it was building, and believed it to be well adapted to this peculiar service. This acquisition will add much to the value of the station.

NOMENCLATURE OF DISEASES.

An effort is now making to secure greater uniformity in the return of diseases and deaths by registration officers throughout the entire State. A scheme of nomenclature prepared by the Secretary, in conjunction with other physicians, is submitted for your consideration and criticism. It is founded mainly on that adopted by the Royal College of Physicians of England.

SANITARY LEGISLATION.

It is made the duty of the Secretary in his annual report to suggest amendments to the Sanitary Code of the Commonwealth. The preceding report of the work of the office for the last year should in itself be sufficiently suggestive. The two crying needs of the State for legislation which shall aid in the preservation of the public health and check the unnecessary mortality which is carrying thousands to premature graves, are, first, an act to prevent the pollution of streams and protect the purity of water supplies ; and, secondly, an act to provide for the sanitary organization of the State. It is unnecessary to remind the board how seriously it is crippled in its efforts to carry out the beneficent designs of the law establishing it, by want of funds. This, however, is a minor evil. It can go on accomplishing much good by dint of practicing a severe economy, as it has done for the past five years, but the two former necessities are absolute and will brook no delay.

INSPECTIONS.

The following is a list of places at which inspections have been made either by members of the board or its medical inspectors :

Natrona,	Allegheny Co.
Mansfield,	Tioga County.
Devon Inn,	Montgomery Co.
Berwick,	Columbia Co.
McKees' Rocks,	Allegheny Co.
Greensburg,	Westmoreland Co.
Norristown,	Montgomery Co.
Uniontown,	Fayette Co.
Millersville,	Lancaster Co.
Bridgeport,	Montgomery Co.
State College,	Centre Co.
Sunbury,	Northumberland Co.
Horatio,	Jefferson Co.
Punxsutawney,	"
Beaver River,	Beaver Co.
Harrisburg,	Dauphin Co.
Bulger,	Allegheny Co.
Loyalhanna River,	"
Pottstown,	Montgomery Co.
Altoona,	Blair Co.
Edge Hill,	Montgomery Co.
Sharon Hill,	Delaware Co.
Norwood,	"
Eddington,	Bucks Co.
Blairsville,	Indiana Co.
Chambersburg,	Franklin Co.
Farrandsville,	Clinton Co.
Wallingford,	Delaware Co.
Anderson Water Purification System,	Lardner's Point.
Bethlehem,	Northampton Co.
Newville,	Cumberland Co.
State Line,	Bedford Co.
Brownsville,	Fayette Co.
Bethlehem Township,	Northampton Co.
Lenni,	Delaware Co.
Chester,	Delaware Co.
Patterson,	Juniata Co.

Making, in all, thirty-seven, of which thirty were made by medical inspectors, five by the entire board, and two by individual members of the board.

REGISTER OF PHARMACISTS.

At the request of Mr. Alonzo Robbins, Secretary of the State Pharmaceutical Examining Board, and on the suggestion of His Excellency the Governor, the first annual report of the

Board has been incorporated, as an appendix, with the report of our own Board, and a limited number of copies of the same, with a "list of registered pharmacists and qualified assistants," has been issued for distribution by their officers.

CENSUS OF THE PHYSICALLY DEFECTIVE CLASSES.

The effort of the officer in charge of department of vital statistics of the United States Census Bureau, Dr. John S. Billings, appeared to your Secretary to offer an opportunity of obtaining information of great value to the Bureau of Vital Statistics in this Commonwealth. Finding that many physicians hesitated to reply to the interrogatives propounded with regard to the defective classes, from motives of professional delicacy, he addressed a communication to the department at Washington, asking for a guarantee of absolute secresy. This was cheerfully and explicitly given. A circular was then addressed to the profession throughout the State, informing them of this guarantee, and requesting their co-operation. The following letter indicates the appreciation of this effort on the part of the Superintendent of Census:

ELEVENTH CENSUS OF THE UNITED STATES. C. S. C.

DEPARTMENT OF THE INTERIOR.

CENSUS OFFICE, WASHINGTON, *June 11th, 1890.*

SIR: I beg to acknowledge the receipt of your kind favor of the 7th inst., and to thank you for the manner in which you have encouraged the physicians of Pennsylvania to make returns to this office regarding the defective classes of your State. I have read your circular to the "Physicians of Pennsylvania" with great care, and appreciate the spirit that prompted you to so forcibly urge upon the medical fraternity the advantage of making prompt and accurate returns.

Again expressing my thanks, I remain,

(Signed) ROBERT P. PORTER, *Superintendent of Census.*

BENJAMIN LEE, M.D.,
  Supt. Vital Statistics of Pa., Philadelphia, Pa.

The following is a list of the places where disease has prevailed epidemically, or contagious diseases have occurred and been reported to the board:

TYPHOID FEVER.

1. Lock Haven, ... Clinton Co.
2. Johnstown, ... Cambria Co.
3. Lancaster, ... Lancaster Co.
4. Manor, ... Westmoreland Co.
5. State College, ... Cambria Co.
6. Beaumont, ... Wyoming Co.
7. Farrandsville, ... Clinton Co.
8. East Reading, ... Berks Co.
9. Auburn, ... Schuylkill Co.
10. Dallas, ... Luzerne Co.
11. Wallingford, ... Delaware Co.
12. Bethlehem, ... Northampton Co.
13. Dauphin, ... Dauphin Co.
14. Shade Valley, ... Huntingdon Co.

DIPHTHERIA.

1. Weatherly, ... Carbon Co.
2. Lehman, ... Luzerne Co.
3. East Stroudsburg, ... Monroe Co.
4. Oxford, ... Chester Co.
5. Lincoln University, ... Chester Co.
6. Langhorne, ... Bucks Co.
7. Monroeton, ... Bradford Co.
8. Middletown, ... Dauphin Co.
9. Waterville, ... Lycoming Co.
10. Pen Argyle, ... Northampton Co.
11. Lenni, ... Delaware Co.

SMALLPOX.

Cannonsburg, ... Washington Co.
Glen Lyon, ... Luzerne Co.
Pittsburg, ... Allegheny Co.

LEPROSY.

Philadelphia, ... Philadelphia Co.
Chester, ... Delaware Co.

The following is a list of circulars which have been issued during the year :

4. Regulations in Regard to the Disinterment and Transportation of Dead Bodies (revised).

Circular No. 28. Precautions against Consumption.

Circular No. 29. The Dangers Arising from Public Funerals of Those who have Died from Contagious or Infectious Diseases. Addressed to the Clerical Profession.

Circular No. 30. The Disposal of the Sewage of Public Edifices. Addressed to the Trustees and Managers of Public Institutions.

Circular No. 31. Precautions to be Observed by Undertakers in Case of Infectious Diseases.

Circular No. 7 (revised). Precautions against Cholera, Cholera Infantum, Cholera Morbus, Summer Diarrhœa, and Dysentery.

Invitations to Fourth State Sanitary Convention, held at Norristown, May, 1890.

Programmes for Fourth State Sanitary Convention, held at Norristown, May, 1890.

The total number of written communications received during the year has been 1,960, and the total number sent 1,835.

The total number of books received by exchange with other boards and scientific bodies during the year has been 44, and the total number of pamphlets during the same period 181·

The total number of books purchased during the year has been 13.

Permits for the disinterment and transportation of bodies have]been issued in the following cases :

George L. Bowan, cause of death diphtheria, from North East, Erie Co., to Savanna, Illinois. Permission of health officer of Savanna obtained.

Dr. H. Schill, cause of death phthisis, from California to Pennsylvania.

Twenty-nine bodies of persons identified, and a general permit for the bodies of the unidentified at Johnstown, cause of death drowning, to be transported from other cemeteries to Grand View Cemetery, Johnstown.

Theresa E. Mahratta, cause of death non-infectious, from Rochester, Beaver Co., to Minneapolis, Minn. Permission of health officer of Minneapolis obtained.

Kate O. Obley, cause of death drowning, from Johnstown to Lower Yoder.

Young woman buried in Grand View Cemetery, Johnstown, grave marked 715–N–47, name not given, cause of death drowning, record of destination not preserved.

Adam Ferg, cause of death blood poisoning, from Bremen, Germany, to Pennsylvania·

Milton Acker, cause of death croup.

Jane Acker, cause of death convulsions.

Charles W. Acker, cause of death croup, all from one grave to another in Rich Valley Cemetery, Tylersport.

Harry Seipel, cause of death intestinal catarrh, from Gum Tree, Chester Co., to Frankford, Philadelphia.

Two children of Henry Riddle, of Media, from one grave to another in churchyard at Middletown, Dauphin Co.

The following is a list of the circulars distributed during the past year :

No. 7. Cholera, etc., revised edition. 287
8. Smallpox. 387
18. Typhoid Fever 1,129
19. Diphtheria 1,901

And 508 box envelopes, containing each Circulars Nos. 18, 19, 20, 21, 24, 26, 28, a total of 22,028.

INTER-STATE NOTIFICATION OF COMMUNICABLE DISEASES.

During the year, notification of the existence of contagious or infectious diseases has been received from the secretaries of the boards of the following States and Provinces :

SMALLPOX.

Minnesota, on two occasions, covering three outbreaks.
Ohio, on three occasions, covering three outbreaks.
Michigan, on five occasions, covering five outbreaks.
Ontario, on one occasion, covering one outbreak.
Connecticut, on five occasions, covering five outbreaks.
Illinois, on one occasion, covering two outbreaks.
Massachusetts, on two occasions, covering two outbreaks.
Kansas, on one occasion, covering one outbreak.
Maine, on two occasions, covering one outbreak.

TYPHUS.

New York, on one occasion, covering one outbreak.

Similar notification of the occurrence of communicable diseases in Pennsylvania has been sent to the secretaries of all the State and Provincial boards. .

Smallpox, on three occasions, covering three outbreaks.

Leprosy, on two occasions, covering two outbreaks.

Respectfully submitted,

(Signed)   BENJAMIN LEE, M.D.,

Secretary and Executive Officer.

State Board of Health and Vital Statistics of the Commonwealth of Pennsylvania.

PRESIDENT,
GEORGE G. GROFF, M.D., of Lewisburg.

SECRETARY,
BENJAMIN LEE, M.D., of Philadelphia.

PEMBERTON DUDLEY, M.D., of Philadelphia.

J. F. EDWARDS, M.D., of Philadelphia.   GEORGE G. GROFF, M.D., of Lewisburg
J. H. McCLELLAND, M.D., of Pittsburg.   S. T. DAVIS, M.D., of Lancaster.
HOWARD MURPHY, C.E., of Philadelphia.   BENJAMIN LEE, M.D., of Philadelphia.

PLACE OF MEETING,
Supreme Court Room, State Capitol, Harrisburg, unless otherwise ordered.

TIME OF MEETING,
Second Thursday in May, July and November.

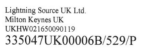

Lightning Source UK Ltd.
Milton Keynes UK
UKHW021650090119
335047UK00006B/529/P

9 780483 112315